Women's Health Across the Lifespan

A Comprehensive Perspective

Karen Moses Allen, PhD, RN
*Associate Professor, Department of Psychiatry,
Community Health and Adult Primary Care
University of Maryland at Baltimore School of Nursing
Baltimore, Maryland*

Janice Mitchell Phillips, PhD, RN
*Assistant Professor, Department of Acute and Long Term Care
American Cancer Society Professor of Oncology Nursing
University of Maryland at Baltimore School of Nursing
Baltimore, Maryland*

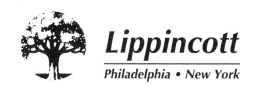

Lippincott
Philadelphia • New York

Acquisitions Editor: *Jennifer E. Brogan*
Coordinating Editorial Assistant: *Danielle J. DiPalma*
Project Editor: *Erika Kors*
Production Manager: *Helen Ewan*
Production Coordinator: *Nannette Winski*
Design Coordinator: *Melissa Olson*
Indexer: *Katherine Pitcoff*

Library of Congress Cataloging-in-Publication Data

Allen, Karen M. (Karen Moses)
    Women's health across the lifespan: a comprehensive perspective/
Karen Moses Allen, Janice Mitchell Phillips
        p. cm.
    Includes bibliographical references and index.
    ISBN 0-397-55216-5 (alk. paper)
    1. Women – Health and hygiene – Sociological aspects. 2. Women – Diseases.
3. Health education of women. I. Phillips, Janice Mitchell. II. Title.
RA564.85.A46 1997   96-22832
613'.04244—dc20   CIP

Care has been taken to confirm the accuracy of the information presented and to describe generally accepted practices. However, the authors, editors, and publisher are not responsible for errors or omissions or for any consequences from application of the information in this book and make no warranty, express or implied, with respect to the contents of the publication.

The authors, editors and publisher have exerted every effort to ensure that drug selection and dosage set forth in this text are in accordance with current recommendations and practice at the time of publication. However, in view of ongoing research, changes in government regulations, and the constant flow of information relating to drug therapy and drug reactions, the reader is urged to check the package insert for each drug for any change in indications and dosage and for added warnings and precautions. This is particularly important when the recommended agent is a new or infrequently employed drug.

Some drugs and medical devices presented in this publication have Food and Drug Administration (FDA) clearance for limited use in restricted research settings. It is the responsibility of the health care provider to ascertain the FDA status of each drug or device planned for use in their clinical practice.

9 8 7 6 5 4 3 2 1

Women's Health
Across the Lifespan

A Comprehensive Perspective

*I dedicate this book to my parents, George and Claudia Moses.
Because of their health beliefs, which led to incorporating a
healthy lifestyle, my five sisters and I are wholesome.
And we exemplify healthy women across the lifespan.
Thanks Mamma and Daddy!*

KMA

*This book is dedicated to all the many women who have touched my life
with their love, inspiration, and wisdom,
most notably to my mother Ernestine Mitchell;
my life-supporting friends Irma Johnson and Rev. Kathy Reeves;
and to all the women of St. John Baptist Church,
who continue to enrich my spiritual journey.
I love you.*

JMP

Contributors

Karen Allen, PhD, RN
Associate Professor
Department of Psychiatry,
Community Health and Adult Primary,
Care
University of Maryland at Baltimore
School of Nursing
Baltimore, MD
Chapter 13: Alcohol and Other Drug Use,
Abuse, and Dependence

Deborah Antai-Otong, MS, RN, CS
Certified Psychiatric Clinical
Specialist
Director, Employee Assistance
Program
Department of Veteran's Affairs
Medical Center
Dallas, TX
Chapter 16: Mental Disorders

Consuelo M. Beck-Sague, MD
Associate Director
Minority and Women's Health
National Center for Infectious Diseases
Centers for Disease Control and
Prevention
Atlanta, GA
Chapter 12: Infectious Diseases

Ami B. Becker, PhD
Research Psychologist
National Research Council Fellow
National Institute for Occupational
Safety and Health
Cincinnati, OH
Chapter 25: Women's Health
in the Workplace

Janine A. Blackman, MS
Doctoral Candidate
MD/PhD Program
Department of Epidemiology
University of Maryland, School
of Medicine
Baltimore, MD
Chapter 2: Demographic Overview of
Women Across the Lifespan

Linda Burnes Bolton,
DrPH, RN, FAAN
Immediate Past President, National Black
Nurses Association
Director, Nursing Research and
Development
Cedars-Sinai Medical Center and
Research Institute
Assistant Professor
UCLA School of Nursing
Los Angeles, CA
Chapter 24: Poverty

Linda Burhansstipanov,
MSPH, DrPH, CHES
Director, Native American Cancer Research
Program
AMC Cancer Research Center
Denver, CO
Chapter 20: American Indian Women

Vivian T. Chen, ScD, MSW
Associate Director of Policy
Division of Quality Assurance
Bureau of Health Professions
U.S. Public Health Service
Rockville, MD
Chapter 18: Asian and Pacific Island
Women

Jenny H. Conviser, PsyD
Assistant Professor
Department of Psychiatry and
Behavioral Sciences
Northwestern University Medical
School
Chicago, IL
Chapter 14: Eating Disorders

Karin Coyne, RN, MPH
Clinical Research Coordinator
The Cardiovascular Research Institute
George Washington University
Washington, DC
Chapter 9: Vascular Disease

Cynthia Dailard, JD
Staff Counsel
National Women's Law Center
Berkely Law Foundation Fellow
Washington, DC
Chapter 23: Incarceration

Lucille Davis, PhD, RN, FAAN
Dean and Professor
College of Nursing and Allied Health
Chicago State University
Chicago, IL
Chapter 6: Health Promotion:
The Mature Years (64 and Older)

Connie Dresser, RDPH, LN
Public Health Nutritionist/Analyst
National Cancer Institute
Bethesda, MD
Chapter 20: American Indian Women

Elaine Feeney, MS, RN, C
Doctoral Student
Community Addictions Nursing
University of Maryland, School of
Nursing
Baltimore, MD
Chapter 13: Alcohol and Other Drug Use,
Abuse, and Dependence

Carol Fennelly
Activist
Washington, DC
Former Director
The Community for Creative
Nonviolence and Medical Services
for the Homeless
Political Commentator
WAMU Radio and NPR Affiliates
Meltin, DE
Chapter 22: Homelessness

Marian L. Fitzgibbon, PhD
Associate Professor
Department of Psychiatry and Behavioral
Health Sciences
Director,
Eating Disorders Program
Northwestern University Medical
School
Chicago, IL
Chapter 14: Eating Disorders

Kelly Garry, RN, MBA
Special Assistant to the Director
Bureau of Primary Health Care
Health Resources and Services
Administration
United States Public Health Service
Bethesda, MD
Chapter 17: African American and
Caribbean Island Women

Marilyn H. Gaston, MD
Assistant Surgeon General
Director, Bureau of Primary
Health Care
Health Resources and Services
Administration
United States Public Health
Service
Bethesda, MD
Chapter 17: African American and
Caribbean Island Women

Aida L. Giachello, PhD
Associate Professor and Director
Midwest Latino Health Research,
Training and Policy Center
University of Illinois at Chicago, Jane Addams College of Social Work
Chicago, IL
Chapter 19: Latino/Hispanic Women

Karyn Holm, PhD, RN, FAAN
Professor and Chair
Department of Medical-Surgical Nursing
Marcella Niehoff School of Nursing
Loyola University Chicago
Maywood, IL
Chapter 8: Coronary Heart Disease

Judith Hsia, MD
Associate Professor of Medicine
Division of Cardiology
George Washington University
Washington, DC
Chapter 9: Vascular Disease

Nancy E. Isaac, ScD
Instructor and Research Associate
Harvard Injury Control Center
Harvard School of Public Health
Boston, MA
Chapter 21: Violence

Abby C. King, PhD
Assistant Professor of Health Research and Policy, and Medicine
Stanford Center for Research in Disease Prevention
Stanford University School of Medicine
Stanford, CA
Chapter 7: Preventive Health Issues: The Mature Years (64 and Older)

Bernardine Lacey, EdD, RN, FAAN
Director and Associate Professor
School of Nursing
Western Michigan University
Kalamazoo, MI
Chapter 22: Homelessness

Judith H. LaRosa, PhD, RN, FAAN
Former Deputy Director
Office of Research on Women's Health
National Institutes of Health
Professor and Chair
Department of Applied Health Sciences
Tulane University School of Public Health and Tropical Medicine
New Orleans, LA
Chapter 1: Women's Health Policy and Research

Trent MacKay, MD, MPH
Medical Epidemiologist
Division of STD Prevention
National Center for HIV/AIDS, STD and TB Prevention
Centers for Disease Control and Prevention
Atlanta, GA
Chapter 12: Infectious Diseases

Mary Maryland, PhD, RN, C
Staff Nurse, Independent Consultant
Bethany Hospital Advocate Healthcare
Chicago, IL
Chapter 6: Health Promotion: The Mature Years (64 and Older)

Judith McDevitt, MS, RN, CS
Doctoral Candidate
College of Nursing
University of Illinois at Chicago
Chicago, IL
Chapter 4: Health Promotion: The Perimenopausal to Mature Years (45-64)

Beverly McElmurry, EdD, RN
Associate Dean
Professor, Public Health Nursing
University of Illinois at Chicago
College of Nursing
Chicago, IL
Chapter 3: Health Promotion and Preventive Health Issues: Young Adulthood to the Perimenopausal Years (15-45)

Arlene Michaels Miller, PhD, RN, CS
Associate Professor
Department of Public Health, Mental Health
and Administrative Studies in Nursing
College of Nursing
University of Illinois at Chicago
Chicago, IL
Chapter 4: Health Promotion:
The Perimenopausal to
Mature Years (45-64)

Ellen Sullivan Mitchell, ARNP, PhD
Associate Professor, Family and Child
Nursing
University of Washington
School of Nursing
Seattle, WA
Chapter 6: Health Promotion: The Mature
Years (64 and Older)

Janice Mitchell Phillips, PhD, RN
Assistant Professor
Department of Acute and Long Term Care
American Cancer Society Professor of
Oncology Nursing
University of Maryland at Baltimore
School of Nursing
Baltimore, MD
Chapter 2: Demographic Overview of
Women Across the Lifespan

Deborah Prothrow-Stith, MD
Assistant Dean,
Government and Community Programs
Professor of the Practice of Public Health
Department of Health Policy and
Management
Harvard School of Public Health
Boston, MA
Chapter 21: Violence

Janet Scherubel, PhD, RN
Professor
Loewenberg School of Nursing
Memphis State University
Memphis, TN
Chapter 8: Coronary Heart Disease

Mary Sexton, PhD, MPH
Professor of Epidemiology
Director of Graduate Programs
Department of Epidemiology
University of Maryland, School of
Medicine
Baltimore, MD
Chapter 2: Demographic Overview of
Women Across the Lifespan

Phyllis W. Sharps, PhD, RN
Assistant Professor
Department of Maternal/Child Health
University of Maryland at Baltimore
School of Nursing
Baltimore, MD
Chapter 10: Reproductive, Gynecologic,
and Urinary Tract Conditions
and Disorders

Brenda V. Smith, JD
Senior Counsel
Director, Women in Prison Project
National Women's Law Center
Washington, DC
Chapter 22: Incarceration

Naomi G. Swanson, PhD
Chief, Motivation and
Stress Research Section
National Institute for
Occupational Safety and Health
Cincinnati, OH
Chapter 25: Women's Health
in the Workplace

Junko Tashiro, MS, RN
Doctoral Candidate, Nursing Science
College of Nursing
University of Illinois at Chicago
Chicago, IL
Chapter 3: Health Promotion and
Preventive Health Issues:
Young Adulthood to the
Perimenopausal Years (15-45)

Martha J. Tenney, MPH
Public Health Educator
Native American Cancer Research Program
AMC Cancer Research Center
Denver, CO
Chapter 20: American Indian Women

Suzanne D. Vernon, PhD
Microbiologist
Division of Viral and Rickettsial Diseases
National Center for Infectious Diseases
**Centers for Disease Control and
    Prevention**
Atlanta, GA
Chapter 12: Infectious Diseases

JoEllen Wilbur, PhD, RN, CS
Associate Professor
*Department of Public Health, Mental
    Health and Administrative Nursing*
College of Nursing
University of Illinois at Chicago
Chicago, IL
**Chapter 4: Health Promotion:
    The Perimenopausal to
    Mature Years (45-64)**

**Jacqueline A. Walcott-McQuigg,
    PhD, RN**
Assistant Professor
*Department of Public Health, Mental Health,
    and Administrative Studies in Nursing*
**University of Illinois at Chicago
    College of Nursing**
Chicago, IL
Chapter 15: Obesity

Roma D. Williams, PhD, CRNP
Assistant Professor, School of Nursing
**University of Alabama
    at Birmingham College of Nursing**
Birmingham, AL
Chapter 11: Cancer

**Nancy Fugate Woods,
    PhD, RN, FAAN**
*Director, Center for Women's Health
    Research*
Professor, Family and Child Nursing
**University of Washington
    School of Nursing**
Seattle, WA
**Chapter 5: Preventive Health Issues:
    The Perimenopausal to Mature Years
    (45-64)**

Deborah Rohm Young, PhD
Assistant Professor
*The Johns Hopkins Center for Health
    Promotion*
Division of Internal Medicine
The Johns Hopkins School of Medicine
Baltimore, MD
Former Research Fellow
Geriatric Medicine Program
John A. Burns School of Medicine
University of Hawaii at Manoa
**Chapter 7: Preventive Health Issues:
    The Mature Years (64 and Older)**

Foreword

Susan J. Blumenthal, M.D., M.P.A.
Deputy Assistant Secretary for Health (Women's Health)
Assistant Surgeon General
U.S. Department of Health and Human Services

The last several decades mark a period of tremendous change and increased opportunity in the lives of American women. Women are living longer. Since the turn of the century, women's lifetimes have been extended by 30 years, from 49 years of age in 1900 to an average of 79 years today. Women today represent more than half of the American population, and, as we age, the proportion of women to men rises dramatically. On average, women live seven years longer than men. For those lucky enough to reach 100 years of age, there will be five women alive for every two men.

The extension of women's lives comes at a price, however. For many women, the bonus years of life may not be better years. Chronic diseases and illnesses never dreamed about at the turn of the century have taken the place of acute illnesses and childbirth as the leading causes of death. Women today face a broad constellation of diseases and disabilities associated with aging, including osteoporosis, depression, heart disease, cancer, and Alzheimer's disease. Diseases like heart disease, lung cancer, and stroke—once thought to be the province of men alone—today are among the leading killers of women. Today, women are the fastest growing group with HIV/AIDS; violence against women has become a public health epidemic in our country today.

Just as women have had to play catch-up in the workplace and in the ivory towers of academia, so, too have they had to play catch-up in securing their health. The effort began only in this last decade of the 20th century.

A landmark report by the U.S. General Accounting Office in 1990 shook the health care system to the core by disclosing the significant gaps in research on women's health issues. It exposed the historical inequities in research, health care services, and public and health professional education that have placed the lives of American women at risk.

Until that turning point year, little notice was paid to the fact that, despite well-documented differences in the bodies and experiences of women and men, most research studies were conducted only in male populations, with the findings generalized to women. Clinical interventions (including the development of new medical devices and medications) and medical school education focused on the male model as if man were the "generic" human. In research, health care service delivery and education, findings about men were simply extrapolated to guide the diagnosis, treatment, and prevention of disease in women. Further, there was a minimum of public and health professional education on women's health issues and a shocking dearth of senior women scientists and health care professionals in our nation's public and private sector health care organizations and research institutions.

However, since 1990, there has been the greatest focus on women's health in the history of our country. The new national focus on women's health has mobilized all agencies of the Federal government through the work of the U.S. Public Health Service's Office on Women's Health to collaborate with other public and private sector organizations to improve the health of American women. Our nation's health policy and programs increasingly are addressing women's health issues in the structure and content of health care research and services, in the recruitment, promotion, and retention of women in leadership positions in academic and research careers, and in public and health care professional education and training.

Because of new attention and increased investments in women's health research, new discoveries are being harvested to improve women's health. For example, researchers working at the cutting edge of science have discovered genes responsible for inherited breast cancers. Improved methods to detect breast cancer, ranging from safer mammography to the use of high-speed precise stereotactic biopsy mechanisms, are making possible more accurate and earlier diagnosis of breast cancer, when there is the best chance for effective treatment. New medications to reduce the risk of osteoporosis—dangerous bone thinning found predominantly in older women—have been introduced. The largest longitudinal research study ever undertaken in women or men—the Women's Health Initiative, supported by the National Institutes of Health—is examining major causes of death, the disability, and frailty in postmenopausal women, such as heart disease, breast and colon cancer, and osteoporosis, to examine how dietary patterns, calcium and Vitamin D supplements, and hormone replacement therapy may help prevent or reduce the risk of these disorders.

Those in the field of women's health are working to translate research findings into improved clinical care for women, ending the days when treatment decisions for women are simply extrapolations from standardized treatments based on a male model. At the same time, women are being better educated to the role their own behavior and lifestyle play in safeguarding or damaging their current and future health. After all, behavioral and lifestyle factors—years of smoking, alcohol, substance abuse, poor diet, lack of exercise—now contribute to over 50% of the causes behind the ten leading killers of women in America, including heart disease, cancer, chronic lung disease, stroke, and diabetes. By changing behaviors and their lifestyles, women can help write a healthier future for themselves.

These efforts also target the powerful social, economic, and environmental factors that influence women's health: poverty, illiteracy, violence, teen pregnancy, substance abuse, unemployment, environmental and occupational hazards, and cultural and financial barriers to health care. As we educate health care professionals and women themselves about their physical and mental health, we must also educate about the social context on which our health depends.

This volume does just that. It places women's health into an environmental context, focusing not only on specific illnesses, but also on disease prevention and the social and economic factors that affect women's health. It makes an important contribution to the new prescription being written today to improve women's health in this decade and beyond into the 21st century. I commend it as an important volume that will inform a broad range of health care professionals for whom it has been so ably written.

Preface

According to the National Institutes of Health, at the end of the 1980s irrefutable national data and statistics pointed to a crisis in women's health. As the statistics on death and disease specific to women were interpreted, individuals became acutely aware that health problems specific to women were worsening and that the following issues are now glaringly undeniable truths:

- Women will constitute the larger population and will be most susceptible to disease in the future.
- Although women outlive men by approximately seven years, women have worse health than men.
- Certain health problems are more prevalent in women than in men.
- A greater percentage of women than men report chronic conditions and restricted activity.
- Certain problems are unique to women or affect women differently than they do men.

These and other factors have led to increased interest, momentum, and activity surrounding the issue of the women's health movement, which began in the mid 1970s with the establishment of self-help groups and political action organizations. As a result, great strides have been made in identifying, researching, and addressing women's health issues. This is evidenced by the establishment of the Office for Research on Women's Health in 1990, within the National Institutes of Health. This office was charged with the responsibility of promoting women's health and increasing the related knowledge base through research.

In addition, in 1991 the U.S. Department of Health and Human Services created the Office of Women's Health to stimulate, coordinate, and implement a comprehensive women's health agenda on research, service delivery, and education across the agencies of public health service. The content and special features of this book reflect the increased interest, momentum, and activity that has been started, and offer a substantial contribution to the area of women's health.

Section I: Introduction presents an overview of women's health policy and research, as well as a demographic overview of women's health across the lifespan.

Section II: Health Promotion and Preventive Health Issues, a unique feature of this text, presents a discussion on health promotion and disease prevention among women aged 15-64 and older. Age-specific recommendations for promoting health and preventing disease are highlighted. In addition, this section provides definitions for health promotion and disease prevention and strategies for maintaining health and preventing disease across the lifespan.

Section III: Systems and Other Health-Related Concerns provides in-depth information on the major illnesses and health concerns of women across the lifespan, based on the leading causes of morbidity and mortality outlined by the Report of the National Institutes of Health on "Opportunities for Research on Women's Health." The following topics are discussed in this section: coronary heart disease, vascular disease, gynecologic and urinary tract conditions, cancer, infectious diseases, problems related to alcohol and other drugs, eating disorders, and obesity. Under these topics, the following areas are addressed, as they specifically relate to women: etiology; antecedents and risk factors; epidemiology; symptoms, disease patterns and responses to disease; relevance across the lifespan; clinical, therapeutic, and behavioral interventions; and implications for policy, practice, and research.

Section IV: Cultural Diverseness and Women's Health presents a well-researched overview of the status of women's health among African-American, American Indian, Asian American/Pacific Island, and Hispanic/Latino cultures. Disparities in health status; impact of economics and culture; health beliefs, values, and practices; cultural strengths; and implications for policy, practice, and research are emphasized.

Section V: Issues Impacting Women's Health provides insight into significant social and economic factors that influence women's health. The chapters on violence, homelessness, incarceration, poverty, and women's health in the workplace discuss the magnitude of the problem, contributing factors, health-related concerns, societal and political responses and strategies for intervening.

Written by women's health experts from multiple disciplines, *Women's Health Across the Lifespan: A Comprehensive Perspective* is sure to meet the needs of educators, students, practitioners, policymakers, and researchers from various backgrounds and specialty areas. We strongly believe that everyone from novice to expert on the topic of women's health will be intellectually as well as emotionally enhanced by reading this text.

Karen Moses Allen
Janice Mitchell Phillips

Acknowledgments

First, I thank God—the greatest contributor overall—for the success of this book. Then, I would like to acknowledge that a book of this caliber is a result of the commitment of expert contributors. In addition, I would like to acknowledge those grassroots organizations, lobbyists, policymakers, researchers, educators, and practitioners who have provided me with the idea, the impetus, and the information to make this valued resource a reality.

KMA

My deepest thanks to:

My Father who art in Heaven from whom all blessings flow, including the production of this book.

Valerie Williams, for providing the opportunity to publish this text; the staff at Lippincott, but especially Jennifer Brogan, Danielle DiPalma, and Erika Kors, our editors, for their ongoing support and insightful comments; and our many contributing authors, who took time out of their busy schedules to write chapters for this first edition.

My dearest of friends, Dorothy Booker, Dorthea Daley, Yvonne Holmes, Lennette Meredith, Judy Smith, Jacqueline Waggonner, and Sandra Webb for their love, encouragement, and support.

Annie Mae Earles, Dr. Eva Smith, Dr. Sandra Underwood and Dr. Anne Belcher, my mentors, who continue to encourage me to strive for excellence in all my endeavors.

Rev. Dr. Robert Turner, my pastor, whose inspirational messages affirm that all things are possible through Jesus Christ.

Robert Phillips, who always believed in me.

JMP

Contents

UNIT 1

Introduction

CHAPTER 1

Women's Health Policy and Research

Judith H. LaRosa

Introduction

Women's health research has inched forward unevenly during the past several centuries. The last quarter of the 20th century, however, has seen an explosion of focused action and has extended scientific inquiries from those limited largely to women's reproductive organs to encompass all organ systems and behaviors, as well as the interactions between them (LaRosa & Pinn, 1993; Mastroianni, Faden, & Federman, 1994). In the past 20 years, directed efforts in women's health research have been written into law and specific areas of research have been targeted for action (Food and Drug Administration [FDA], 1993; National Institutes of Health Revitalization Act, 1993). Furthermore, women who had often been ignored in past investigations, most notably women of color, are now mandated for appropriate inclusion in such basic and applied research. The purpose of this enhanced effort is to provide biomedical[1] data to achieve two major objectives: the appropriate prevention, identification, treatment, and control of the diseases, disorders, and conditions that affect women of all racial and ethnic groups across the lifespan and a more complete understanding of normal biologic, behavioral, developmental, and aging processes.

Historical Perspective

In 1986, the Public Health Service (PHS) of the U.S. Department of Health and Human Services (USDHHS) convened a task force on women's health issues. The charge was to examine women's health issues and to recommend a course of action to address gaps in knowledge. The task force subsequently published those recommendations (USDHHS, 1987). One of the recommendations was to advance gender equity in biomedical research. In response, the National Institutes of Health (NIH) established guidelines for the inclusion of women into clinical studies supported by the NIH.[2]

---

1. Biomedical includes both physiologic and psychological/behavioral data.
2. The NIH is the preeminent Federal biomedical research institution in the United States.

Several years later, however, an inquiry by the General Accounting Office, at the request of the Congressional Caucus for Women's Issues, revealed that the 1986 NIH guidelines had not been implemented uniformly across the NIH. Particular areas of research had not appropriately included women—for example, heart disease, aging, and human immunodeficiency virus/acquired immunodeficiency syndrome (HIV/AIDS) (Nadel, 1990). In 1990, the NIH implemented strengthened guidelines and established the Office of Research on Women's Health (ORWH) within the Office of the Director, NIH. In April 1991, Bernadine Healy, MD, was appointed the first woman director of the NIH. Spurred on by these events, women's health research surged forward across the spectrum of women's diseases, disorders, and conditions.

Today, women's health research is firmly ensconced at NIH and in the PHS agencies,[3] with resources allocated to ensure that such investigations move forward vigorously. Furthermore, the ORWH was mandated by law in 1993 along with more focused guidelines on the inclusion of women and minorities into clinical studies supported by NIH (U.S. Congress, June, 1993).

Mortality and Morbidity in Women

Mortality

Overall, the trend in the health of both women and men has been positive since the beginning of the 20th century. Recent data (Table 1–1) indicate that, at birth, children in the United States can generally expect to live well into their sixties or seventies, depending on gender and race (Kochanek & Hudson, 1995).

Furthermore, death rates for 10-year age groups have declined for both genders with the important exception of ages 35 to 44, wherein the death rates have increased primarily because of HIV/AIDS (Kochanek & Hudson, 1995). The ratio was 7:1 men/women for HIV infection. The smallest gender differential was for diabetes mellitus, where the ratio was 1:1 (Kochanek & Hudson, 1995).

Although the trend in health is positive, more remains to be accomplished if individuals are to maximize health and live as fully as possible until they die. Overall, the leading causes of death for women, as for men, remain heart disease, cancer, and cerebrovascular disease. They are followed less dramatically by chronic obstructive pulmonary disease (COPD), diabetes mellitus, pneumonia and influenza, and a host of other diseases and conditions. Examination of the data by age and racial/ethnic groupings provides even more refined information. Table 1–2 indicates the rank order of the leading causes of death among women by racial group.

Clearly, important differences exist between the racial groups concerning causes of death. The rates also differ by age. The leading causes of death among girls and younger women (aged 1–24 years) are accidents, homicide, suicide, HIV/AIDS, and complications of pregnancy. For women aged 25 to 64, the leading

3. Such agencies include the Food and Drug Administration, Agency for Health Care Policy and Research, Health Resources and Services Administration, PHS Office of Women's Health, Indian Health Service, and Centers for Disease Control and Prevention.

Table 1-1. Life Expectancy at Birth, 1992

White females	79.8 yrs	White males	73.2 yrs
Black females	73.9 yrs	Black males	65.0 yrs

causes of death are malignant neoplasms, HIV/AIDS, heart disease, and COPD. The leading causes of death in women over age 65 are heart disease, cancer, cerebrovascular disease, and pneumonia and influenza (Kochanek & Hudson, 1995). These diseases and conditions do not generally appear suddenly and mysteriously. In addition to genetic predisposition and family history, they are often caused by lifestyle, environmental, and social factors, which are often first manifested as chronic risk factors, such as alcohol and drug use and abuse, unprotected sex, cigarette smoking, hypertension, elevated blood cholesterol level, obesity, lack of exercise, and the myriad environmental threats posed by toxins, poverty, and physical and mental abuse.

Morbidity

Younger women, overall, tend to be affected by different chronic conditions than are older women (Verbrugge & Patrick, 1995). For example, the leading chronic conditions in younger women are chronic sinusitis and hay fever followed by or-

Table 1-2. Rank Order of Causes of Death Among U.S. Women by Racial Group, 1991

	Racial Group Rank			
Cause of Death	W	B	NA	A/PI
Heart disease	1	1	1	1
Malignant neoplasms	2	2	2	2
Cerebrovascular disease	3	3	5	3
Unintentional injury	4	4	3	4
Pneumonia and influenza	5	7	7	7
Diabetes mellitus	6	5	6	5
Atherosclerosis	7			
Chronic obstructive pulmonary disease	8			
Chronic liver disease/cirrhosis	9	9	4	
Conditions of perinatal period	10	6	8	6
Nephritis, nephrotic syndrome, etc.		10	9	
Homicide/legal intervention		8	10	10
Congenital anomalies				8
Suicide				9

W, White; B, Black; NA, Native American; A/PI, Asian/Pacific Islander.
Adapted from National Center for Health Statistics (1994). *Health United States, 1993.* Washington, DC: Public Health Service.

thopedic problems such as scoliosis and arthritis. For middle-aged women, arthritis is the leading cause of chronic disease followed by hypertension. During these middle years, COPD is beginning to manifest itself as a leading cause of impairment. For women over age 65, arthritis and hypertension remain the leading chronic conditions but are now followed by afflictions of older age: hearing and vision impairment. COPD and arteriosclerosis now become seriously limiting and life-threatening diseases (Verbrugge & Patrick, 1995).

Prevention

The presumed goal of most individuals is to live a healthy, disease-free, and fulfilling life for as long as possible. Certain risk factors are uncontrollable: genetic predisposition, family history, and accidents. However, where free will is possible and desirable, the individual requires education, an interest in controlling her own health, and the ability to achieve a healthy lifestyle. Unfortunately, not all women can or do exert their will. A 1993 survey conducted by Louis Harris for the Commonwealth Fund indicated that the health of many women in the United States remains in jeopardy (Commonwealth Fund, 1993). Key features of the report follow.

- Many women do not receive needed health care because of lack of adequate health insurance and vulnerable economic status.
- More than one third of women are at risk for undetected treatable conditions.
- Women are at serious risk of heart disease, lung cancer, and osteoporosis, and they lack sufficient knowledge about how to protect themselves.
- Depression and low self-esteem are pervasive problems for American women.
- Three in 10 women—nearly 30 million—report having suffered some type of abuse as a child; the effects can be lasting.
- Women of color are more likely to be poor and uninsured and to lack needed medical care than are Caucasian women.
- Chronic, disabling conditions limit the quality of life for millions of women, particularly the elderly.

This glance at selected data underscores the magnitude of the problem. Furthermore, it heightens not only the tremendous need to direct studies toward the many diseases, disorders, and conditions that affect women, but toward the myriad factors that prevent and influence them. Finally, the data demonstrate that racial and ethnic groupings, as well as genetic and environmental origins, are important in women's health and must be considered in studies.

Constant vigilance is required to determine where gaps in knowledge still exist, especially among different groups of women. Scientists, clinicians, and policymakers cannot remain static in the face of changing issues and times. Thus, the national, state, and local databases must be sufficiently comprehensive and inclusive to provide data for targeted action. Not only is health the responsibility of the individual, but it is the responsibility of the highest levels of state and federal government.

The Office of Research on Women's Health— Research Issues

Women's health research had been historically focused on diseases and conditions affecting reproductive organs. The initial challenge for ORWH and its partners has been to discern where gaps in knowledge exist and then to implement targeted efforts in women's health research across the biomedical research spectrum.

An identification of such gaps in 1991 emerged initially from two sources: a public hearing and a scientific workshop. At the public hearing, more than 90 local and national organizations[4] provided testimony on future research directions. The scientific workshop produced substantive guidance on how such research action might be achieved in basic and applied studies. The underlying guidance was, of course, scientific and relied on the latest epidemiologic, morbidity, and mortality data. One concept was stressed throughout—women's health research had to expand from the traditional focus on reproductive organs to include all organ systems and behavioral factors. The recommendations from the workshop are presented in the *Report of the National Institutes of Health: Opportunities for Research on Women's Health* (ORWH, 1992a).

From these recommendations, ORWH implemented a plan of action, in cooperation with its NIH partners, the 23 NIH institutes and centers. ORWH focused attention on two large-scale efforts: providing funds to add women to ongoing NIH studies and to target four focused areas of research.

Adding women, especially women of color, to ongoing studies has proved particularly fruitful. Since its inception, ORWH has provided funds to include women in more than 350 studies examining such issues as the identification and treatment of sexually transmitted diseases (STDs); risk factors for disease among women of different racial and ethnic groups; factors associated with mental and physical health among women suffering physical and emotional abuse; lung cancer; and cardiovascular and peripheral disease (ORWH, 1995). An increasing percentage of the principal investigators on these studies have been women.

Myriad studies surrounding women's health are now supported by NIH. A perspective on the changes in focus and funding in the last several years can be found in documents demonstrating the tremendous diversity of women's health research. These documents, produced originally by the NIH Advisory Committee on Women's Health Issues,[5] reflect the continuing NIH commitment to women's health.[6] The most recent and comprehensive of these documents (NIH, 1994b) chronicles the many studies currently underway. Selected examples follow to illustrate the comprehensive nature of women's health research supported by NIH.

- The National Center for Nursing Research supports a specialized center that examines the health needs and societal demands of middle-aged women.

---

4. For example, the American Heart Association, the American Cancer Society, the National Organization for Women, and others.
5. This committee was the immediate precursor to the Office of Research on Women's Health and was comprised of representatives from each of the NIH institutes, centers, and divisions. It was disbanded in 1992.

- The National Eye Institute has supported the Optic Neuritis Treatment Trial investigating the acute inflammation of the optic nerve, which occurs primarily in women aged 18 to 45.
- The National Heart, Lung, and Blood Institute currently supports the Women's Health Study, a randomized, placebo-controlled trial of aspirin use to prevent heart disease.
- The National Cancer Institute currently maintains the Prostate, Lung, Colorectal, and Ovarian Clinical Trial, which considers the impact of early detection and screening on these diseases. Biologic markers are an important facet of this trial.
- The National Institute of Dental Research supports ongoing studies investigating Sjoegren's syndrome, a chronic, systemic, autoimmune disease that presents as dryness of mucosal membranes. The etiology is presently unknown. Over 90% of those with Sjoegren's syndrome are women.
- The National Institute of Environmental Health Sciences supports research on environmental hazards such as the effects of cigarette smoke on the fetus and the ability of women to store fat-soluble toxins.
- The National Institute of Arthritis, Musculoskeletal, and Skin Diseases supports both basic and applied studies aimed at osteoporosis, a disease that affects four times as many women as men. Research into autoimmune diseases, especially systemic lupus erythematosus, which occurs nine times more frequently in women compared with men, has focused on a variety of approaches. Most recent work focuses on the immunogenetic component.
- The National Institute of Child Health and Human Development has a comprehensive program aimed at women's health. Some selected examples of support to scientists include a focus on STDs and the efforts to improve barrier contraception. A better understanding of endometriosis and uterine leiomyomata is underway through basic research studies.

The reports (NIH, 1994b; ORWH, 1992a), coupled with recommendations from NIH and external scientists, led ORWH to select four areas for special research attention: autoimmune diseases, reproductive health from menarche through menopause, urologic diseases and conditions, and occupational and environmental effects on women's health. Although research had clearly been accomplished in these areas, ORWH believed that a more focused approach was required to advance the state of the science.

The process has generally been one in which scientists, clinicians, and advocates in a workshop or conference setting delineate issues and make specific recommendations. Then ORWH and specific NIH institutes and centers determine where and how to implement research action. Throughout the process, ORWH has underscored the need to consider all aspects of the questions being posed—from the basic mechanisms through the clinical interventions.

Reproductive Health

The ORWH has initiated a trans-NIH coordination effort among nine NIH institutes and centers to guide future research initiatives. As part of this process, ORWH col-

6. These documents can be obtained from the Office of Research on Women's Health, National Institutes of Health, Building 1, Room 201, Bethesda, MD 20892.

laborates with the National Cancer Institute, the National Institute for Environmental Health Sciences, and the National Institute for Child Health and Human Development to support studies that survey and monitor the continuing effects of diethylstilbestrol (DES) on affected mothers and their offspring. DES-related educational materials are being developed to educate the public and physicians concerning the need for continued attention to this important issue, especially in affected offspring and even in their children.

Substantial information deficits exist concerning the effects of menopause on physiology and psychology during the aging process. ORWH cosponsored, with the National Institute on Aging (NIA) and the National Institute for Nursing Research (NINR), a conference on menopause and its effects. Using guidance from this conference, the three groups are cofunding a six-center natural history study of menopause. In addition, ORWH and NINR are cofunding a study of the decision-making process between a woman and her health care providers surrounding whether or not to perform a hysterectomy.

The STDs, not including HIV, number more than 13 million cases annually and cause enormous and often long-lasting health problems: pelvic inflammatory disease, ectopic pregnancies, low-birthweight babies, and congenital defects (Centers for Disease Control and Prevention, 1993). In seeking to understand the basic mechanisms of action, ORWH cooperated with the National Institute on Allergy and Infectious Disease on two conferences: an examination of the use and effectiveness of topical microbicides as a spermicide and viricide and an examination of the basic mechanisms of human papillomavirus and subsequent pathology in women. Both conferences have led to additional investigations.

Perhaps the most notable effort in this arena is the Women's Health Initiative (NIH, 1994d). This prospective clinical trial, probably the largest clinical trial ever mounted, considers prevention for the three leading causes of death and disability among postmenopausal women: heart disease, cancer, and osteoporosis. The two-part trial consists of the observational study of over 160,000 women and the clinical trial of over 60,000 women. The clinical trial examines three primary interventions: a low-fat diet, hormone replacement therapy, and vitamin and calcium supplements. When the 10- to 15-year trial ends, scientists and health care practitioners will have a wealth of information regarding primary intervention in postmenopausal women of different racial and ethnic groups.

Urologic Health

Why do urinary tract infections plague some women more than others? What factors contribute to urinary incontinence and how can they be averted? What is the pathobiology of bladder disorders? Seeking answers to this largely overlooked area of women's health, ORWH cooperated with the National Institute on Diabetes, Digestive, and Kidney Disorders (NIDDK) to cosponsor a conference on basic bladder pathophysiology and to direct research funds in related studies. ORWH and NIDDK are cosponsoring an investigation on normal and abnormal functioning of the urinary bladder in women. This basic study should elucidate more clearly some of the basic mechanisms and provide data for further studies on the appropriate identification of risk factors and intervention. In addition to the ongoing studies,

NIDDK recognized that this area of women's health required considerably more attention and established the Women's Urological Health Branch.

Autoimmune Diseases

Graves and Hashimoto's diseases have a 15:1 ratio of women to men; rheumatoid arthritis has a ratio of 3:1; systemic lupus erythematosus affects nine times more women than men and is especially prevalent among African American women (ORWH, 1992b). These autoimmune diseases cost billions in disability and tremendous suffering by those affected and their families. Yet, scientists do not fully understand the underlying pathobiology nor the reasons behind the striking gender differences. The immune response requires considerably more investigation at the cellular level and the nexus of the communication between the endocrine and immune systems. Therefore, ORWH, the National Institute on Allergy and Infectious Disease, the National Institute of Arthritis, Musculoskeletal, and Skin Diseases, and the National Institute for Child Health and Human Development have joined together to support the study of the sex steroid regulation of autoimmunity. Such efforts promise long-overdue information on a puzzling and complex problem for women. Understanding the etiology in women should also provide important guidance on understanding the diseases in men as well.

Occupational Health

Although women have been in the workplace for hundreds of years, information on the effects of hazards and toxins on their health has been limited. In 1993, ORWH joined the National Cancer Institute and the National Institute on Environmental Health Sciences to sponsor the NIH Occupational Cancer and Women Conference, which underscored the need for directed action in occupationally related diseases and disabilities and proffered important recommendations (Zahm & Pottern, 1995). One of the most pressing and immediate needs noted by conference participants is to establish more complete and comprehensive databases (cancer registries, death registries, exposure data, and other disease databases) and combine them with accurate sociodemographic information. It is only from these more complete data that pertinent exposure information can be applied to disease consequences. Based on these and other recommendations, ORWH has joined with these institutes to consider further efforts.

Miscellaneous Initiatives

In addition to the strengthened and targeted action in women's health, ORWH and its partners have turned their attention to the health needs of often ignored groups of women: lesbians and the disabled. Although it has been noted on many occasions that an individual with disabilities has many challenges to meet, the actual depiction of those challenges and mechanisms to meet them has been sparse. In 1994, ORWH joined with the National Institute of Child Health and Human Development to cosponsor a conference directed toward the health problems of women with disabilities. The participants outlined many of the physical and psychological issues that disabled women face in their daily lives and the diseases and conditions that impair their well-being and self-esteem. Several initiatives have been implemented at NIH as a result of this conference and heightened attention to this issue. The book, *Women with Physical Disabilities: Achieving and Maintaining Health and Well-being* will be released in spring 1996. The National Institute of Child Health and Human Development has delineated two areas for women with disabilities: reproductive health (OB/GYN and contraceptive) and the ramifications of stressors, including abuse, on health. In addition, they are seeking opportunities to further educate professionals and patients and are issuing requests for grant applications on health promotion for women with disabilities. (Personal communication with Dr. Danuta Krotoski, National Institute of Child Health and Human Development, March 20, 1996.)

Lesbians have often found the simple acknowledgment of their sexuality to be troublesome for some health care providers. Lesbians often report feeling that their health concerns are not always dealt with fully and with knowledge specific to their concerns and needs. In addition to providing funds to study specific issues, such as breast cancer in lesbians, ORWH has joined with the National Cancer Institute to explore further target efforts in lesbian health.

Research, to be effective, must remain dynamic. Emerging research answers some questions, but raises others that must be addressed if data are to be realized and women's health continually advanced based on reliable information. Thus, the cycle perpetuates itself, looping back with new information and new puzzles. Figure 1–1 illustrates this process.

The Office of Research on Women's Health— Inclusion Issues

In the past, some scientists and clinicians have assumed that the findings from studies on men might apply reasonably well to women. After all, biologic homogeneity exists. Yet, notable differences exist. Women and men differ in the amount of steroidal sex hormone concentrations they have, and in the effect of these hormones on fetal and cellular development, organ systems, and disease. These differences are only now being appreciated. It is poor science to assume that what applies to a woman in her childbearing years, with the continuous rise and fall of her sex hormones, would also apply to a man of the same age. Similarly, it is illogical to assume that older men and postmenopausal women will respond equally to medication and devices designed for one particular gender. These gender differences must be understood and appreciated for appropriate medical practice and good health.

These and other issues have been at the root of the recent legislation to include women in clinical studies. The NIH Revitalization Act (1993) states that:

> In conducting or supporting clinical research for the purposes of this title, the Director of NIH shall . . . ensure that
> A. women are included as subjects in each project of such research.

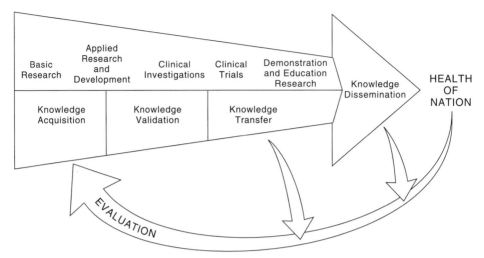

Figure 1-1. Biomedical research spectrum (Source: National Heart, Lung, and Blood Institute.)

Furthermore, the statute continues:

> In the case of any clinical trial in which women or members of minority groups will be included as subjects, the Director of NIH shall ensure that the trial is designed and carried out in a manner sufficient to provide for valid analysis of whether the variables being studied in the trial affect women or members of minority groups, as the case may be, differently than other subjects in the trial.

On this basis, the NIH has implemented guidelines on the inclusion of women and minorities into clinical studies supported by the NIH. The guidelines state:

> It is the policy of NIH that women and members of minority groups and their subpopulations must be included in all NIH-supported biomedical and behavioral research projects involving human subjects, unless a clear and compelling rationale and justification establishes to the satisfaction of the relevant Institute/Center Director that inclusion is inappropriate with respect to the health of the subjects or the purpose of the research. Exclusion under other circumstances may be made by the Director, NIH, upon the recommendation of an Institute/Center Director based on a compelling rationale and justification. Cost is not an acceptable reason for exclusion except when the study would duplicate data from other sources. Women of childbearing potential should not be routinely excluded from participation in clinical research. All NIH-supported biomedical and behavioral research involving human subjects is defined as clinical research. This policy applies to research subjects of all ages (NIH, 1994a).

In short, women and minorities must be included in studies of diseases, disorders, or conditions that apply to them, unless compelling rationale is provided. If not, the study cannot be funded.

This legislation is powerful and assures that now women will not only be included, but that in Phase III clinical trials[7] they will be included in sufficient numbers to detect gender differences in the intervention effect. For example, if the study seeks to understand the effect of beta-blockers on hypertension, enough women and men must be included to discern whether the medication affects either gender differently. Furthermore, minority women must be included to understand different racial or ethnic effects.

Because of the impact these guidelines would have on the scientific community, the National Institutes of Health Revitalization Act (1993) further directed that:

> The Director of NIH, in consultation with the Director of the Office of Research on Women's Health and the Director of the Office of Research on Minority Health, shall conduct or support outreach programs for the recruitment of women and members of minority groups as subjects in the projects of clinical research.

Such efforts are important in the full and ethical implementation of these guidelines. Indeed, the legislation, and the ensuing guidelines, underscore that women of childbearing age are eligible for inclusion. This issue alone demands careful attention surrounding informed consent, contraception, and embryo/fetal safety. Such issues must be considered even more thoughtfully in women who may not be native English speakers or who may have difficulty understanding the language of the study requirements. Yet these factors alone do not preclude their participation. Older women, rural women, women with children, and disabled women may also have barriers that require attention for their appropriate inclusion into studies. Scientists and study designers must be sensitive to special considerations and incorporate them into planning efforts.

The NIH is intent on continuing and enhancing its partnership with the scientific community surrounding this important endeavor. To that end, NIH staff prepared a notebook, a primer, on recruitment and retention of women and minorities into such research studies (NIH, 1994c). The notebook is intended to stimulate appropriate study design among scientific teams as they consider the research question and the individuals it will require to supply the answers. Key issues in recruiting and retaining individuals and the communities in which they reside as well as ethical concerns are considered throughout the process.

Research Efforts of Other Federal Agencies

The NIH is not alone in its timely and vigorous response to research needs to promote and protect women's health. The FDA has established an Office of Women's Health with a director and resources to address issues relevant to the FDA mandate. Furthermore, the FDA has also altered its guidelines on the inclusion of women in

---

7. For the purpose of the guidelines, a "clinical trial" is a broadly based prospective Phase III clinical investigation, usually involving human subjects, for the purpose of evaluating an experimental intervention in comparison with a standard or control intervention or comparing two or more existing treatments. Often the aim of such investigation is to provide evidence leading to a scientific basis for consideration of a change in health policy or standard of care. The definition includes pharmacologic, nonpharmacologic, and behavioral interventions given for disease prevention, prophylaxis, diagnosis, or therapy. Community trials and other population-based intervention trials are also included.

studies (FDA, 1993). The 1977 FDA guidelines excluded "women of childbearing potential from participation in early studies of drugs" (FDA, 1993). The new guidelines state that:

> . . . [E]xclusion of women from early trials is not medically necessary because the risk of exposure can be minimized by patient behavior and laboratory testing, and initial determinations about whether that risk is adequately addressed are properly left to patients, physicians, local IRBs, and sponsors with appropriate review and guidance by FDA, as are all other aspects of the safety of proposed investigations (FDA, 1993).

The Agency for Health Care Policy and Research has established an Office of Women's Health with appropriate resources for action. Part of the efforts within this agency have been to develop guidelines on the appropriate screening and intervention for diseases and disorders. One excellent example is the set of guidelines for clinicians and radiologists on screening and diagnostic mammography. These exhaustive guidelines provide a comprehensive overview along with specific recommendations for action (USDHHS, 1994).

The Health Resources and Services Administration has established an Office of Women's Health. One of the major efforts of this agency, in addition to its research portfolio, has been the work of the Bureau of Health Professions. This group, in cooperation with the ORWH, has created a focused effort to direct appropriate and gender-specific education in medical schools and subsequently in all health professions schools. Until recently, gender differences have not been fully appreciated in most health professional education with the result that health professionals, especially physicians, do not always appreciate the need for such refinement in patient diagnosis and treatment. This educational effort has had strong support from the Congressional Caucus for Women's Issues.

Other agencies have developed similar initiatives. As a result of this wellspring of activity, the Federal agencies have come together in a unified effort coordinated by the PHS Office of Women's Health. This coordination is critically important in disseminating information and enhancing mutually beneficial activities across the agencies and those they serve.

Women's Health Research Across the Nation

Research action is not confined to the Federal agencies. Colleges, universities, and medical centers profit from this expanded support. Not only is scientific endeavor enhanced, but many of these institutions have developed or are developing women's health centers. Although these centers vary widely in their intent and purpose, many have research activities within their core. Unfortunately, to date, no known effort has been made to catalogue and annotate all these activities.

State and local health departments are similarly involved. Because funding differs in amount and administration within each agency, no one unified effort in women's health research has been identified throughout the public health service regions or states. Some states, however, have directed efforts in delineating the status of women's health within their state or region. One interesting example is the work of NC Equity, an organization within North Carolina. This group has produced a document (North Carolina Equity, 1993) that is being used by the state to guide women's health intervention.

Many pharmaceutical corporations have increased their attention and efforts in women's health research. The Pharmaceutical Research and Manufacturers Association (PhRMA) surveys their membership annually and documents the action in women's health drug development in key disease areas. Their 1994 survey (PhRMA, 1994) shows that most major companies do include women in testing and in drug development and do assess gender differences. These latest data indicate a change from earlier surveys that showed gaps in drug development across major areas of women's health, for example, cardiovascular disease. Now, not only are drugs in development, many are well into Phase III or are being reviewed by the FDA.

Summary

The need for biomedical research studies directed toward women is unquestionably important. Furthermore, the need for studies that delineate and test the differences not only between women and men but among racial and ethnic groups is also critical. The recent attention to women's health and research underscored by the congressional mandate demonstrates that such efforts are becoming an integral part of the scientific and clinical infrastructure of this country. Yet, considerable effort must be expended to assure full integration. Many are working toward a time when the issue of whether women should be included in studies or whether studies directed toward women's health issues are necessary is an historical footnote.

References

Centers for Disease Control and Prevention, Division of STD/HIV Prevention. (1993). Sexually transmitted disease surveillance, 1992. Atlanta, GA: Author.

Commonwealth Fund. (1993). *The Commonwealth Fund Survey of Women's Health.* New York: Author.

Food and Drug Administration. (1993, July 22). Guidelines for the study and evaluation of gender differences in clinical evaluation of drugs. *Federal Register, 58* (139), 39406-39414.1.

Kochanek, K. D., & Hudson, B. L. (1995). Advance report of final mortality statistics, 1992. *Monthly Vital Statistics Report Suppl., 43*(6), 1. Hyattsville, MD: National Center for Health Statistics.

LaRosa, J. H., & Pinn, V. W. (1993). Gender bias in biomedical research. *Journal of the American Medical Women's Association, 48*(5), 145-151.

Mastroianni, A., Faden, R., & Federman, D. (1994). *Women and health research: Ethical and legal issues of including women in clinical studies, 1.* Washington, DC: National Academy Press.

Nadel, M. V. (1990, June 18). *National Institutes of Health: Problems in implementing policy on women in study populations.* United States General Accounting Office. Statement before the Subcommittee on Health and the Environment, Committee on Energy and Commerce, House of Representatives.

National Center for Health Statistics. (1994). *Health United States, 1993.* Washington, DC: U.S. Public Health Service.

National Institutes of Health Revitalization Act of 1993, Pub. L. No. 103-43, 107 Stat. 22 (1993).

National Institutes of Health. (1994a, March 29). The NIH guidelines on the inclusion of women and minorities as subjects in clinical studies. *Federal Register 59,* 14508-14513.

National Institutes of Health. (1994b). *NIH support for research on women's and men's health is-sues* (NIH Publication No. 94-3717). Bethesda, MD: Author.

National Institutes of Health. (1994c). *Outreach notebook on the inclusion of women and minori-ties as subjects in clinical research.* (Available through the National Institutes of Health of NIH GOPHER on Internet.)

National Institutes of Health. (1994d). *Women's health initiative* [patient recruitment brochure]. Bethesda, MD: Author.

Office of Research on Women's Health. (1992a). Executive summary. *Report of the National Institutes of Health: Opportunities for research on women's health* (NIH Publication No. 92-3457, pp. 19-34). Bethesda, MD: Author.

Office of Research on Women's Health. (1992b). Immune function and infectious diseases, T. C. Quinn & P. H. White (cochairs). *Report of the National Institutes of Health: Opportunities for research on women's health* (NIH Publication No. 92-3457, p. 195). Bethesda, MD: Author

Office of Research on Women's Health. (1995). *Research initiatives.* Bethesda, MD: Author.

North Carolina Equity. (1993). *The status of women's health in North Carolina.* Raleigh: Author.

Pharmaceutical Research and Manufacturers of America. (1994). *New medicines in development for women, 1994 survey.* Washington, DC: Author.

U.S. Department of Health and Human Services. (1987). *Women's health: Report of the Public Health Service Task Force on Women's Health Issues, Vol. II.* (DHHS Publication No. PHS 88-50206). Washington, DC: Author.

U.S. Department of Health and Human Services, Agency for Health Care Policy and Research. (1994). *Quality determinants of mammography. Clinical practice guide* (AHCPR Publication No. 95-0632). Washington, DC: Author.

Verbrugge L., & Patrick, D. L. (1995). Seven chronic conditions. The impact on U.S. adults' activ-ity level and use of medical services. *American Journal of Public Health, 85*(2), 173-182.

Zahm, S. H., & Pottern, L. M. (1995). Future directions for research on occupational cancer among women: Summary of conference panel discussions. *Journal of Employment Medicine, 37* (3), 363-365.

CHAPTER 2

Demographic Overview of Women Across the Lifespan

Janice Mitchell Phillips
Mary Sexton
Janine A. Blackman

Introduction

Today, in the mid-1990s, the average American woman is 34 years of age and is more likely to be college educated when compared with the average American man. Although women and men differ by cause of death overall, American women outlive their male counterparts by approximately 7 years. Despite these advantages, American women are disproportionately represented among the poor, single heads of households, and the chronically ill and disabled. This chapter presents a demographic profile of women living in the United States and briefly discusses gender differences in mortality and morbidity.

Characteristics of American Women

Today's average American woman is 34 years old. By the middle of the next century, however, the average American woman could be about 45 years old. However, this average age hides much of the diversity and disparity among American women. Among 100 women today, 84 are Caucasian, 13 are African American, 3 are of other races, and 8 are of Hispanic origin (may be of any race). By the middle of the next century, projections indicate that among 100 women, 75 will be Caucasian, 16 will be African American, 9 will be other races, and 17 will be of Hispanic origin. Hence, the racial and ethnic diversity is expected to increase among women over the next several decades (Table 2–1). Early in the next century, when the baby-boom generation (born 1946–1964) begins to reach age 65, the female elderly population will grow rapidly. After 2030, baby boomers will begin to reach age 85 and care of our oldest old, most of whom will be women, could become one of the most significant issues during this period (Taeuber, 1991).

Proportion and Longevity

The secondary sex ratio, the sex ratio of human fetuses that reach viability, has consistently been 105 males to 100 females for the past two decades (U.S. Bureau of the Census, 1993). On the one hand, since the primary sex ratio, or the ratio at the

Table 2-1. Percent Distribution for Females by Age and Race:1988 and 2030

Age	1988			2030*		
	Caucasian	African American	Other	Caucasian	African American	Other
	84.1%	12.6%	3.3%	77.9%	15.1%	7.0%
<15	80.2	15.6	4.2	75.2	17.3	7.5
15–24	81.4	15.1	3.5	74.8	17.4	7.8
25–34	83.0	13.4	3.6	75.1	16.6	8.3
35–44	84.7	11.6	3.7	77.1	15.5	7.4
45–54	85.4	11.4	3.2	77.4	13.1	9.5
55–64	87.2	10.1	2.6	79.0	14.4	6.6
65–74	89.1	8.9	2.0	81.3	13.5	5.2
75–84	90.8	7.6	1.6	83.5	7.6	8.9
85+	91.3	7.5	1.2	85.2	9.6	5.2

*Middle series projections
The 1988 data are from Table A1-1 of Taeuber, C. M. (1991). *The statistical handbook on women in America.* The 2030 projection data are from Table A1-9 of Taeuber, C. M. (1991). *The statistical handbook on women in America.*

time of fertilization, should theoretically be one, the secondary sex ratio of 105:100 suggests that more female than male fetuses are lost during the early months of pregnancy. On the other hand, females have an expected life that averages 7 years longer than males. This difference has been fairly constant over the last 25 years and is projected to be about the same for the next 25 years (U.S. Bureau of the Census, 1993). Males, overall, have higher age-adjusted mortality rates than females, an observation that is seen throughout the 1900s (1.4 in 1900 and 1.8 in 1980). Despite a small decrease in the differential, it is not likely that the ratio will approach one in the foreseeable future. Because males are more likely to die at every given age, the proportion of females to males increases over the lifespan. For example, at age 65 to 70, there are about 10% more women than men (55% versus 45%) and for those 85 and older, there are about 44% more women than men (72% versus 28%) (U.S. Bureau of the Census, 1993).

Educational Status

Education is positively associated with health status regardless of gender. From 1970 to 1993, there has been a steady increase in the proportion of women who have completed college. The number of college graduates doubled from 8.1% to 19.3% (Table 2–2). For African American women, the proportion has more than doubled, increasing from 4.6% in 1970 to 12.4% in 1993. For women of Hispanic origin, the proportion of women college graduates has also increased from 4.3% to 8.5% during the same interval. However, of all racial groups in 1980, Asian women were the most likely to be college educated, as shown in Figure 2–1. An increasing percent-

Table 2-2. Percent of Persons 25 Years and Over Who Have Completed College, by Race, Hispanic Origin, and Sex: 1970 to 1993

	Caucasian		African American		Hispanic Origin*	
	Male	Female	Male	Female	Male	Female
1993	25.7	19.7	11.9	12.4	9.5	8.5
1990	25.3	19.0	11.9	10.8	9.8	8.7
1985	24.0	16.3	11.2	11.0	9.7	7.3
1980	21.3	13.3	8.4	8.3	9.4	6.0
1975	18.4	11.0	6.7	6.2	8.3	4.6
1970	14.4	8.4	4.2	4.6	7.8	4.3

*Persons of Hispanic origin may be of any race.
Adapted from Table No. 233, U.S. Bureau of the Census. (1994). *Statistical abstract of the United States: 1994* (114th edition).

age of advanced degrees have been awarded to women. Although women represent the majority of all college students, including graduate students, men are still more likely than women to have completed college (Fig. 2–2) (Taeuber, 1991).

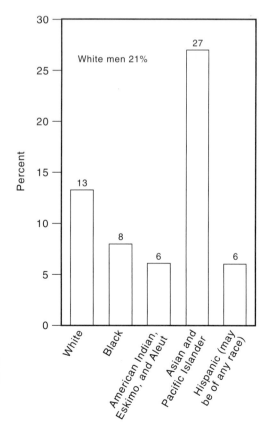

Figure 2-1. Percentage of women 25 years and over with four or more years of college: 1980.(Taeuber, C.M., Statistical Handbook on Women in America, P. 311, 1991)

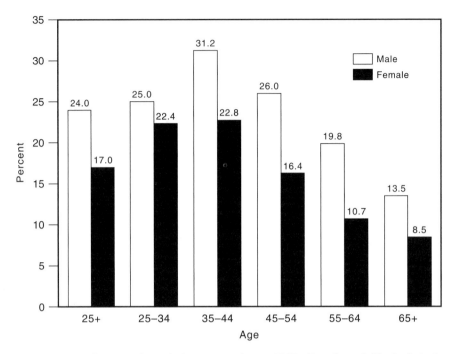

Figure 2-2. College graduated, by age and sex: 1988. (Taeuber, C. M., Statistical Handbook on Women in America, *P. 312, 1991)*

Employment

Educational status is related to earning power and being in the workplace. More men than women are in the labor force at any given time of their life. In 1970, for example, 80.0% of Caucasian men were in the labor force versus 42.6% of Caucasian women. In 1992, these participation rates were 76.4% and 57.8%, respectively. The employment rate for men has perhaps declined slightly, but for women it continues to increase with about three of four women in their thirties now working. More women are working at younger ages. For example, about 70% of women who were 30 to 34 years of age in 1987 worked when they were 25 to 29; however, only about 35% of women who were 50 to 54 years of age in 1987 worked when they were 25 to 29 (Taeuber, 1991).

There are significant differences in the labor participation rates between African American and Caucasian women. The proportion of African American teenagers (ages 16–19) who work is considerably lower than that for Caucasian teenagers and for women over age 20 of both races. For example, in 1987, only 39.6% of African American teenagers were in the labor force compared with 56.5% of Caucasian female teenagers, with 55.6% of adult (age 20 and over) Caucasian women, and with 60% of adult African American women (Taeuber, 1991). From the 1950s through the early 1980s, Caucasian women were traditionally more likely to be in the labor force when they were teenagers than when they were older, but since the late 1980s, about the same proportion of teenagers and the same proportion of older

Caucasian women are working. For African American women, however, the proportion of adults working has remained much larger than that of teenagers from the 1950s to the present.

Earnings

Whether African American, Caucasian, or Hispanic, women earn less than men. In 1986, women aged 35 to 44 earned a median annual wage of $18,179, which is 65% of the $27,991 median annual wage earned by men in the same age group (Table 2–3). Further, a higher level of education does not overcome the deficit in wages for women. In 1986, women who were college graduates and who were aged 25 to 34 years earned a median salary of $21,900; comparable men earned $27,700 (see Table 2–3). Also, the more education a worker has, the less likely he or she is to experience poverty. For example, in 1986, the median income for a woman with 4 years or more of college was $23,300 compared with $10,100 for a woman with 8 years or less of school (see Table 2–3). Nevertheless, the rate of poverty is consistently higher among women than among men. In 1987, 13.4% of all women, compared with 9.1% of all men, were below the poverty level. Even among adults with 1 year or more of college education, 5.5% of women were below the poverty level compared with 4.2% of men (Taeuber, 1991).

Marital Status

From 1970 to 1993, smaller proportions of women married (Table 2–4). In 1993, about three in five women in their early twenties had never married compared with only one in three in 1970. Even among those aged 25 to 29, 30% of the women had never married compared with only 11% in 1970 (Taeuber, 1991). Also, both men and women are delaying marriage. The median age at first marriage for women in 1988 was 23.6 compared with a low of 20.1 in the late 1950s. For men, the comparable median ages were 25.9 and 22.5. It is interesting to note that these more recent ages at first marriage are similar to those in the late nineteenth century of 22.0 for women and 26.1 for men (Taeuber, 1991).

Characteristics Related to Childbearing

Historically, the trend in births is a more important element in the growth of the national population and its distribution by age and race than either of the other components of population change—mortality and net migration.

Fertility and Birth Rates

Overall, fertility rates during the 1980s were stable and averaged 70 births per 1000 women aged 18 to 44. Among Hispanic women, the 1988 rate was 94 compared with 87 for African American women and 66 for Caucasian women (Taeuber, 1991). The biggest difference between Caucasian and African American women was the fertility rate for young women: African American rates were higher for women under age 25; after age 35, there is much less difference between the two races (Taeuber, 1991).

Table 2-3. Median Annual Earnings of Full-Time, Year-Round Wage and Salary Workers, by Sex and Years of School Completed: 1986

Sex and Age	Total	8 Years or Less of School	1–3 Years of High School	4 Years of High School	1–3 Years of College	4 or More Years of College
Women						
Total, 16 and over	$16,323	$10,088	$11,815	$14,698	$16,724	$23,276
25–34	16,813	10,269	11,710	14,424	16,946	21,883
35–44	18,179	10,358	11,679	15,761	18,936	25,326
45–54	17,450	10,314	12,637	16,206	18,750	25,861
55–64	16,066	10,616	12,464	16,085	16,989	24,211
65+	13,217	8,239	9,860	13,601	12,300	21,403
Men						
Total, 16 and over	25,400	15,503	17,829	22,670	25,852	32,288
25–34	22,607	12,101	15,905	20,540	23,469	27,693
35–44	27,991	15,714	19,959	25,633	28,070	34,189
45–54	28,955	18,989	23,930	26,969	29,636	39,932
55–64	27,326	17,881	21,725	26,957	28,143	39,366
65+	23,922	15,843	17,568	24,488	26,724	38,976

Adapted from Table B2-6 of Taeuber, C. M. (1991). *The statistical handbook on women in America.*

Table 2-4. Marital Status of Women, by Race:1970, 1980, 1990, and 1993*

Marital Status	African American				Caucasian			
	1970	1980	1990	1993	1970	1980	1990	1993
Total, 14 years and over	7.1	9.2	11.2	11.7	62.2	72.8	80.6	82.1
Percent total	100.0	100.0	100.0	100.0	100.0	100.0	100.0	100.0
Never married	17.4	27.4	32.5	34.9	13.2	15.7	16.9	16.8
Married	61.7	48.7	43.0	41.1	69.3	64.7	61.9	61.6
Widowed	15.8	14.3	12.4	12.0	13.8	12.8	12.2	11.6
Divorced	5.0	9.5	12.0	12.0	3.8	6.8	9.0	10.0

*Numbers in millions, except percent. Excludes members of the Armed Forces except those living off post or with their families on post.
Adapted from Table No. 59, U.S. Bureau of the Census. (1994). *Statistical abstract of the United States: 1994* (114th edition).

Baby boomers are nearing their forties and fifties, and most will reach the end of their childbearing years in the 1990s. The numbers of total births and Caucasian births are expected to drop sharply during the 1990s. Total births would drop about 9% and Caucasian births about 14% because of the decline in the number of women of childbearing age as baby boomers continue to age. The annual number of African American births is projected to remain close to 600,000 (slightly below the current level) for at least the next half century. The "other races" group is the only one whose future number of births is projected to be even 5% above the current level (Taeuber, 1991).

Out-of-Wedlock Births

Childbearing for women over age 30 has increased since the mid-1970s, whereas the birth rate for teenagers has declined since 1960. This decline is projected to continue through 2050 and beyond. In 1960, the birth rate for women aged 16 to 19 was 91.0 (the number of live births per 1,000 women in that age group), whereas in 1985, the birth rate was 51.9. By 2050 and beyond, the birth rate for women aged 16 to 19 is projected to drop to 40.0 (Taeuber, 1991). However, the relatively large number of out-of-wedlock births is new in the United States. In 1940, there were about 90,000 out-of-wedlock births reported. In 1987, there were more than 10 times that number. Of all births to African American women in 1988, 56% were to unmarried women compared with 15% and 26% for Caucasian and Hispanic women, respectively (Taeuber, 1991). The increase in premarital childbearing among teenagers is a matter of concern because these mothers and their children tend to face economic hardship. In the period from 1970 to 1974, just under half the women under age 25 with a premaritally conceived first birth married before the baby was born; that proportion dropped to about one fourth by 1985 to 1988 (Taeuber, 1991).

Employed Mothers

Over 50% of women with an infant were in the labor force in 1988, which is up from 35.3% in 1978 (Taeuber, 1991). As indicated in Table 2–5, the percentage of new mothers who work tends to increase both with age and with education. Sixty-one percent of women with 1 to 3 years of college who had a birth in the previous year were in the labor force in 1988 compared to 49% of these women who have only a high school education. Also, 68% of new (first birth) mothers aged 30 to 44 years were in the labor force compared to 50% of new mothers aged 18 to 24.

Head of Household

The mix of households has changed dramatically in the last two decades, with one of the biggest changes being the proportion of family households maintained by women alone. As listed in Table 2–6, the term "family household" refers to a group of two or more persons related by birth, marriage, or adoption and residing together in a household. From 1970 to 1993 the proportion of Caucasian family households headed by a woman increased from 9% to 14%. For African American family households, the percentage increased from 28% to 47%, and for Hispanic households, the percentage increased from 15% to 23%. The large difference in the proportion of Caucasian and African American households headed by a women is primarily a result of the fact that African American women are much more likely than Caucasian women to be divorced, separated, have their husband absent, or to have never married over the last two decades (see Table 2–4).

Health Status

Several indicators are essential to assessing the health status of any population. More specifically, a review of life expectancy, morbidity, and mortality figures both past and present provides a general perspective on the nation's health.

Life Expectancy

Life expectancy has been defined as the "average (mean) number of years for which a group of individuals of the same age are expected to live" (Harper & Lambert, 1994). Life expectancies are summary measures of mortality and thus are calculated from the age-specific death rate of the population at a particular time (Harper & Lambert, 1994).

Life expectancies have consistently increased since the turn of the century. Although overall life expectancies have increased for both males and females, Caucasian females have experienced the greatest gain when compared with Caucasian males or non-Caucasian males and females. In 1990, the life expectancy for Caucasian females at birth is 79.4 years followed by African American females (73.6

Table 2-5. Women Who Gave Birth and Their Percentage in the Labor Force, by Selected Characteristics:1988 and 1976 (Numbers in Thousands)

Characteristic	July 1987 to June 1988		July 1975 to June 1976	
	Number of Women Who Gave Birth	Percent in Labor Force	Number of Women Who Gave Birth	Percent in Labor Force
Total	3,667	50.9	2,797	31.0
Years of school completed				
Less than high school	656	33.7	783	26.0
High school, 4 y	1,583	49.1	1,273	31.6
College, 1–3 y	778	61.6	413	32.1
College, 4 y or more	649	59.8	328	39.0
Age:				
18–24 y	1,146	46.3	1,291	30.9
25–29 y	1,238	52.3	929	33.1
30–44 y	1,283	53.6	577	27.6
Birth order and age of woman at birth:				
First birth	1,282	57.7	1,082	39.0
18–24 y	628	50.3	694	35.7
25–29 y	382	62.2	306	45.0
30–44 y	273	68.4	82	44.4
Second or higher order birth	2,385	47.2	1,715	25.9
18–24 y	518	41.3	597	25.3
25–29 y	857	47.8	623	27.2
30–44 y	1,010	49.7	495	24.9
Race and Hispanic origin*:				
Caucasian	2,894	49.4	2,328	28.6
African American	595	58.6	407	43.2
Hispanic	406	36.6	N/A	N/A
Not Hispanic	3,261	52.6	N/A	N/A
Marital status:				
Married, husband present	2,700	51.6	2,331	30.4
Widowed, divorced, or separated†	361	50.3	225	32.3
Never married	606	47.9	241	34.8

NA, not available.
*Persons of Hispanic origin may be of any race.
†Includes married, husband absent.
Adapted from Table A2-14 of Taeuber, C. M. (1991). *The statistical handbook on women in America.*

years), Caucasian males (72.7 years), and African American males (64.5 years) (National Center for Health Statistics [NCHS], 1993). Overall, women live longer than men by about 7 years (Mastroianni, Faden, & Federman, 1994).

Table 2–7 depicts life expectancies at birth by sex and racial group for six different years (NCHS, 1993). Life expectancy has increased for both sexes and racial groups; however, Caucasian females have experienced the greatest gain. Between 1900 and 1990, life expectancy increased 30.7 years for Caucasian females and 40.1

Table 2-6. Family Households by Race, Hispanic Origin, and Type: 1970–1993

Race, Hispanic Origin	Number (1,000)					Percent Distribution				
	1970	1980	1985	1990	1993	1970	1980	1985	1990	1993
Caucasian, total	46,166	52,243	54,400	56,590	57,858	100%	100%	100%	100%	100%
Married couple	41,029	44,751	45,643	46,981	47,601	89	86	84	83	82
Male householder*	1,038	1,441	1,816	2,303	2,409	2	3	3	4	4
Female householder*	4,099	6,052	6,941	7,306	7,848	9	12	13	13	14
African American, total	4,856	6,184	6,778	7,470	7,888	100	100	100	100	100
Married couple	3,317	3,433	3,469	3,750	3,748	68	56	51	50	48
Male householder*	181	256	344	466	460	4	4	5	6	6
Female householder*	1,358	2,495	2,964	3,275	3,680	28	40	44	44	47
Asian or Pacific Islander, total†	NA	818	NA	1,531	1,662	NA	100	NA	100	100
Married couple	NA	691	NA	1,256	1,335	NA	84	NA	82	80
Male householder*	NA	39	NA	86	95	NA	5	NA	6	6
Female householder*	NA	88	NA	188	232	NA	11	NA	12	14
Hispanic, total‡	2,004	3,029	3,939	4,840	5,318	100	100	100	100	100
Married couple	1,615	2,282	2,824	3,395	3,674	81	75	72	70	69
Male householder*	82	138	210	329	407	4	5	5	7	8
Female householder*	307	610	905	1,116	1,238	15	20	23	23	23

NA, not available.

*No spouse present.

†1980 data as of April and are from 1980 Census of Population.

‡Hispanic persons may be of any race. 1970 data as of April.

Adapted from Table 71 of the U.S. Bureau of the Census. (1994). *Statistical abstract of the United States: 1994* (114th edition).

Table 2-7. Life Expectancy at Birth by Sex and Racial Group: 1900, 1950, 1960, 1970, 1980, 1990

Year of Birth	1900	1950	1960	1970	1980	1990
Caucasian						
Male	46.6	66.5	67.4	68.0	70.7	72.7
Female	48.7	72.2	74.1	75.6	78.1	79.4
African American						
Male	32.5	58.9	60.7	60.0	63.8	64.5
Female	33.5	62.7	65.9	68.3	72.5	73.6

Adapted from National Center for Health Statistics. (1993). *Healthy People 2000 Review: Health, United States, 1992.*

years for African American females. In contrast, between 1900 and 1990, Caucasian and African American males experienced an increase in life expectancy of 26.1 years and 32 years, respectively (NCHS, 1993).

Improvements in life expectancies for females reflect the identification, treatment, elimination, and control of various diseases, particularly infectious, parasitic, and cardiovascular diseases. Additional factors responsible for improving the life expectancy for females include better prenatal and antenatal care and improved protection from environmental and worksite hazards (Alexander & LaRosa, 1994). Furthermore, the increase in life expectancy is primarily due to the reductions of deaths from both cardiovascular disease and cancer, reductions that have been more pronounced for women than for men (Overfield, 1995).

In a review of the literature, Waldron (1994) found that sex roles, genetics, environmental factors, and gender differences in risk taking and preventive behavior influence gender differences in mortality. For example, because men are employed in jobs that tend to be more hazardous than women's jobs, men are exposed to a greater number of carcinogens in the workplace, contributing to an increased incidence of lung and bladder cancer when compared to women. Men experience a higher influence of job-related injuries than women, indicating a link between gender differences in mortality (Waldron, 1994). In addition, when compared with women, men often engage in more risk-taking behaviors, namely, behaviors that involve physical daring, use of psychoactive substances, and illegal actions. Evidence suggesting that women are more likely to engage in preventive behaviors to preserve and enhance their health varied across studies (Waldron, 1994).

Projections indicate that life expectancies will continue to increase for both sexes and racial groups. By the year 2010, Caucasian women will continue to experience the greatest life expectancy (81.5 years), followed by African American women (77.0 years), Caucasian men (75.1 years), and African American men (67.3 years) (U.S. Bureau of the Census, 1993).

Mortality

Mortality rates—the total number of deaths for an identified disease over a specified period of time—are another indicator of the nation's health. Crude, specific, and adjusted death rates are used to identify the frequency of deaths occurring in a specific population. Category-specific and adjusted rates are more beneficial in identifying and comparing the causes of death among subgroups of the population.

Table 2–8 illustrates the 10 leading causes of death for men and women in the United States for 1992 and the ratio of age-adjusted death rates according to sex and race (Centers for Disease Control and Prevention [CDC], 1994b). As shown, heart disease was the leading cause of death for both men and women in the United States. Deaths from heart disease have continued to decline since the 1950s; men have experienced the greatest decline in cardiovascular deaths (American Heart Association, [AHA], 1993b).

As shown in Table 2–8, mortality patterns revealed that the ratio of age-adjusted death rates differed according to both sex and race. According to these patterns, death rates from infection with immunodeficiency virus (HIV), suicide, homicide, and unintentional injuries were higher for men than for women (CDC, 1994b). When compared with Caucasians, African Americans had a higher ratio of age- adjusted deaths rates for most of the leading causes of death. Only deaths from suicide and chronic pulmonary obstructive disorders and allied conditions were more prevalent among Caucasians than African Americans (CDC, 1994b).

Table 2-8. Ten Leading Causes of Death and the Ratio of Age-Adjusted Death Rates According to Sex and Race: United States, 1991

Rank	Cause of Death (ICD-9)	Male/ Female	African American/ Caucasian
1	Heart disease (390–398, 402, 4404–429)	1.9	1.5
2	Malignant neoplasms, including neoplasms of lymphatic and hematopoietic tissues (140–208)	1.5	1.4
3	Cerebrovascular diseases (430–438)	1.2	1.9
4	Chronic obstructive pulmonary diseases and allied conditions (490–496)	1.7	0.8
5	Accidents and adverse effects (E800–E949)	2.6	1.3
	Motor vehicle accidents (E810–E825)	2.3	1.0
	All other accidents and adverse effects (E800–E807, E826–E949)	3.0	1.6
6	Pneumonia and influenza (480–487)	1.7	1.4
7	Diabetes mellitus (250)	1.1	2.4
8	Human immunodeficiency virus infection (042–044)	7.0	3.7
9	Suicide (E950–E959)	4.3	0.6
10	Homicide and legal intervention (E960–E978)	4.0	6.5

Per 100,000 population, age adjusted to the 1940 U.S. population. Centers for Disease Control. 1994. Mortality patterns: United States, 1992. *Morbidity and Mortality Weekly Report,* 43(49), 916–920.

Consistent with previous rates, in 1992, the age-adjusted death rates for men were higher when compared with women. However, a comparison of 1991 and 1992 age-adjusted death rates revealed that both sexes experienced a decline in age-adjusted death rates. For men there was a decline from 669.9 to 656.0, respectively, and for women a decline from 386.5 to 380.3, respectively (CDC, 1994b).

A further review of mortality patterns indicated a variation in the leading causes of death for men and women across the various age groups. Table 2–9 shows the leading causes of death for men and women according to age group in 1991. As shown, accidents were the leading cause of death for women aged 15 to 24. Malignant neoplasms accounted for the greatest number of deaths for women aged 25 to 44 and 45 to 64, and heart disease was the leading cause of death for women aged 65 and over (U.S. Bureau of the Census, 1994). In contrast, accidents were the leading cause of death for men aged 15 to 24 and 25 to 44, and heart disease accounted for the greatest number of deaths for men aged 45 to 64 and 65 and over (U.S. Bureau of the Census, 1994).

The leading causes of deaths for women differ not only according to age group but also by age group and racial group combined. A more detailed delineation of these differences is needed to develop appropriate health-related interventions and health policies that will improve the health status of all women. Although a more detailed discussion of these differences is beyond the scope of this chapter, subsequent chapters examine variations in health status among women of various minority groups. Table 2–10 illustrates the leading causes of death according to racial group (NCHS, 1993). Although not depicted, the five leading causes of death among Hispanic women include cardiovascular disease, followed by cancer, accidents, diabetes, pneumonia/influenza, and HIV infection (AHA, 1993b).

Cardiovascular Disease

Cardiovascular disease and cerebrovascular disease are leading killers of women in the United States today, ranking first and third, respectively. These diseases claim more women's lives than do cancer, accidents, and diabetes combined (AHA, 1993b). Annually, about 236,000 women die of a heart attack and another 87,000 die of a stroke. In 1991, 478,179 women died of cardiovascular disease, about 51.6% of all female deaths. In that same year, 447,900 men died of cardiovascular disease, about 48.4% of all male deaths (AHA, 1993b). A review of cardiovascular mortality trends revealed that from 1979 to 1990, men experienced the greatest decline in cardiovascular deaths.

In contrast, in 1990, death rates from cardiovascular disease were 244.2/100,000 for Caucasian men and 353.1 for African American men (45% higher). The age-adjusted death rate for cardiovascular disease is six times higher for African American women and four times higher for Caucasian women (AHA, 1993a). In 1990, the death rate from heart disease was higher in African American women than in Caucasian women (225.5 versus 134.8/100,000 population—67% higher) (AHA, 1993b).

Epidemiologists indicated that one of nine women aged 45 to 64 has some type of cardiovascular disease and that after age 65 the ratio increases to one in three

Table 2-9.   The Leading Causes of Death According to Sex and Age Group: 1991

	Death Rate Per 100,000 Population		
	Total	Male	Female
15–24 y			
All Causes	**100.1**	**148.0**	**50.0**
Leading causes of death			
Accidents	42.0	62.0	21.0
Motor vehicle	32.0	45.5	18.0
Homicide and legal intervention	22.4	37.2	6.9
Suicide	13.1	21.9	3.8
Malignant neoplasms (cancer)	5.0	5.8	4.1
Heart disease	2.7	3.4	2.0
HIV infection	1.7	2.4	0.9
25–44 y			
All Causes	**179.9**	**255.2**	**105.3**
Leading causes of death			
Accidents	32.3	50.3	14.4
Motor vehicle	18.4	27.3	9.5
Malignant neoplasms (cancer)	27.1	24.9	29.2
HIV infection	26.5	47.1	6.0
Heart disease	19.3	28.1	10.5
Homicide and legal intervention	15.1	23.9	6.3
Suicide	14.9	24.1	5.9
45–64 y			
All Causes	**788.9**	**1,011.2**	**582.6**
Leading causes of death			
Malignant neoplasms (cancer)	286.9	320.9	255.4
Heart disease	253.4	330.1	128.3
Cerebrovascular (stroke)	30.9	34.6	27.5
Accidents	29.3	43.3	16.3
Chronic obstructive pulmonary disease	27.3	30.6	24.3
Chronic liver disease and cirrhosis	22.5	32.5	13.2
Diabetes	21.5	22.8	20.3
65 years and over			
All Causes	**4,924.0**	**5,719.9**	**4,387.0**
Leading causes of death			
Heart disease	1,881.0	2,131.3	1,712.0
Malignant neoplasms (cancer)	1,117.3	1,469.3	879.7
Cerebrovascular (stroke)	394.1	366.6	412.7
Chronic obstructive pulmonary disease	240.4	334.7	177.2
Pneumonia and influenza	217.2	240.1	201.7
Diabetes	115.0	114.1	115.7
Accidents	83.3	102.9	70.0
Motor vehicle	22.2	30.9	16.3

Source: U.S. Bureau of the Census. (1994). *Statistical abstract of the United States:* 1994 (114th ed.).

(AHA, 1993a). For all ages under age 75, death rates from cardiovascular disease are higher for African American women than for Caucasian women (Douglas, 1993).

Cancer

Cancer is the second leading cause of death for both men and women living in the United States (American Cancer Society [ACS], 1995). Although both races and sexes have experienced a decrease in cancer mortality over the last 30 years, in general, cancer incidence and mortality rates are higher among African Americans than among Caucasians. Recent findings indicate that in 1991, overall cancer incidence rates were 439/100,000 for African American and 406/100,000 for Caucasians. In 1991, the mortality rates were 228/100,000 for African Americans and 170/100,000 for Caucasians (Wingo, Tong & Nalden, 1995).

Lung cancer followed by breast cancer are the two leading causes of cancer death among women living in the United States. In 1991, approximately 51,000 women died of lung cancer compared with 44,500 deaths from breast cancer (CDC, 1993). It is interesting that in 1986, lung cancer surpassed breast cancer as the leading cause of cancer death among Caucasian women (27.5 versus 27.3 per 100,000, respectively) and among African American women in 1990 (32.0 versus 31.7 per 100,000, respectively; CDC, 1993). Recent epidemiologic data indicate that changes in smoking habits are primarily responsible for the recent decline in lung cancer incidence among American men; however, increases in lung cancer incidence and

Table 2-10. Rank Order of Selected Causes of Death in Women According to Race: United States, 1990

	Caucasian	African American	Native American	Asian Pacific Islander
Heart disease	1	1	1	1
Malignant neoplasms	2	2	2	2
Cerebrovascular disease	3	3	4	3
Chronic obstructive pulmonary disease	5	10	8	7
Pneumonia and influenza	4	6	7	5
Chronic liver disease and cirrhosis	11	13	6	13
Diabetes mellitus	7	4	5	6
Nephritis, nephrotic syndrome, and nephrosis	10	9	10	12
Septicemia	9	11	13	14
Atherosclerosis	8	16	15	16
Human immunodeficiency virus infection	23	12	29	22
Unintentional injuries	6	5	3	4
Suicide	12	20	13	10
Homicide and legal intervention	18	8	11	11

Adapted from National Center for Health Statistics. (1993). *Healthy People 2000 Review: Health United States, 1992.*

mortality are consistent with increased smoking patterns noted among both African American and Caucasian women.

Projections indicate that there will be 182,000 new invasive cases of breast cancer in the United States in 1995 and 46,240 deaths attributable to breast cancer (46,000 women, 240 men) (ACS, 1995). Breast cancer incidence rates for women have increased about 2% annually since 1980; however, mortality rates have remained constant for the last 50 years (ACS, 1995). Epidemiologic data suggest that the rise in breast cancer incidence is primarily due to increases in earlier detection and mammography use. Other factors thought to play a role include the changing prevalence of certain reproductive factors (delayed childbirth), diet, alcohol consumption, and long-term use of menopausal estrogens (Kelsey & Gammon, 1991; Miller, Feuer, & Hankey, 1993). The overall incidence of breast cancer is higher among Caucasian women and lower among African American women; however, African American women who develop breast cancer have a 5-year survival rate of 63% compared with 76% for Caucasian women (ACS, 1994).

Cerebrovascular Disease

Cerebrovascular disease is the third leading cause of death in the United States and the leading cause of disability for both men and women. Since 1972, stroke mortality has declined by more than 50%, much of which can be attributed to advances in hypertension control (AHA, 1993b). In 1990, 87,391 women died of cerebrovascular disease, about 60.7% of all female deaths. In the same year, 56,697 men died of cerebrovascular disease, about 39.3% of all male deaths (AHA, 1993b). In all stages of life, women in the United States experienced a higher mortality from cerebrovascular disease than men (Douglas, 1993).

The age-adjusted death rate for cerebrovascular disease is higher for African American women than for Caucasian women. In 1990, the death rate from cerebrovascular disease for African American women was 42.8/100,000 population compared with 23.8/100,000 population for Caucasian women (AHA, 1993b).

Chronic Conditions and Restricted Activities

Because women live longer than men, a greater percentage of the chronically sick elderly are women. Despite the gains in life expectancy, women appear to have greater morbidity than men (Rodin & Ickovics, 1990). Morbidity, defined as generalized poor health or the total number of illnesses, can be identified through self-reported occurrence, that is, number of physician visits or hospitalizations, restricted activity, or actual health screening (Rodin & Ickovics, 1990). Consistent with higher morbidity prevalence rates, more women than men report higher rates of chronic conditions. More specifically, for every 1 man, 6.5 women seek care for thyroid disorders, 1.6 for arthritis, 2.0 for chronic bronchitis, 3.5 for constipation, and 1.6 for gallstones (Office of Research on Women's Health [ORWH], 1992). Interestingly, a greater percentage of African American women reported poor health when compared with Caucasian women (NCHS, 1993).

In addition to cardiovascular disease, cerebrovascular disease, and cancer, women also suffer disproportionately from a variety of chronic illnesses including, but not limited to, arthritis, auditory, visual, and orthopedic impairments, and digestive disorders (Taeuber, 1991). For example, although arthritis is a major chronic condition affecting both sexes, data from the National Health Interview Survey 1989–1991 showed higher rates of arthritis among women than men (17.1% versus 12.5%). Women also reported higher rates of activity limitation due to arthritis. Estimated prevalence rates were similar for both African Americans and Caucasians; however, African Americans reported higher rates of activity limitation (CDC, 1994a).

Other chronic conditions occurring more frequently in women than men include osteoporosis, autoimmune disorders, and diabetes mellitus. According to the ORWH, the incidence for osteoporosis increases dramatically with age—from 17.9% for women aged 40 to 49 to 89% for women aged 75 (ORWH, 1992). Fifty percent of all women over age 45 and 90% of women over age 75 will develop osteoporosis, which results in at least 1.3 million fractures in the United States each year (ORWH, 1992). A greater percentage of Caucasian than African American women are affected by osteoporosis primarily because of differences in bone mass and density (Horton, 1995). When compared to men, women suffer disproportionately from a variety of autoimmune disorders. For example the female/male ratio for rheumatoid arthritis is about 3:1, systemic lupus erythematosus about 9:1, and multiple sclerosis about 4:1 (ORWH, 1992).

Diabetes represents the seventh leading cause of death in the United States, affecting more than 8 million people (Kahn & Weir, 1994). In general, the prevalence increases with age and is higher in women than men except in the age group 65 through 74 (Kahn & Weir, 1994). In 1990, the age-adjusted death rate from diabetes for African American women (25.4/100,00) was more than double that for Caucasian women (9.5/100,000) (NCHS, 1993).

Finally, research showed that in 1987, African American women had the highest age-adjusted rate of hospitalizations related to diabetes; 36% higher than the rate for African American men, 95% higher than the rate for Caucasian women, and 109% higher than the rate for Caucasian men (Kahn & Weir, 1994).

Consistent with the higher morbidity prevalence rates, when compared with men in 1990, women reported higher rates of restricted activity, disability, and physician visits (Table 2–11). In contrast, men have longer hospital stays (6.9 versus 6.1 average hospital days) (U.S. Bureau of Census, 1993). Although women reported higher rates of disability and restricted activity, data showed no difference in the total work-loss days between men and women (U.S. Bureau of the Census, 1993). Women reported having made more visits to physicians than men, yet research shows that women received fewer interventions than men when confronted with the same diagnosis. (Horton, 1995). This is particularly true with medical interventions related to coronary heart disease, lung cancer, and kidney dialysis.

Summary

This chapter only begins to highlight some of the multiple and complex factors and issues influencing the health and well-being of women. Despite the gains and longevity for women, when compared with their male counterparts, women con-

Table 2-11. Morbidity Indices by Sex and Sex Ratios in the United States, 1990

Morbidity Indices	Women	Men	Sex Ratio Women/Men
Restricted activity days total days of disability (millions)	2,135	1,558	1.37
Days/person	16.7	13.1	1.27
Bed disability days total days of disability (millions)	896	625	1.43
Days/person	7.1	5.2	1.36
Work loss days total (millions)	319	303	1.0
Days/person	5.9	4.7	1.25
Hospitalization utilization rates patients discharged per 1000 persons	144	102	1.41
Days of care per 1000 persons	875	704	1.24
Average stay (days)	6.1	6.9	0.88
Physician visits total (millions)	806	558	1.44
Visits/person	6.4	4.7	1.36

Adapted from U.S. Bureau of the Census. (1993). *Statistical abstract of the United States: 1993* (113th ed.).

tinue to suffer disproportionately from a variety of chronic conditions and disabilities. Although current research indicates that biologic, behavioral, sociocultural, and environmental factors contribute to this disparity, still much is not known about these factors and the full extent of their contribution to the differences in mortality and longevity noted between the sexes. Further investigation of these and other factors and issues is essential to the development of interventions, women's health initiatives, and policies directed toward improving the health and well-being of women.

Given the heterogeneity among women, future research endeavors must use samples of women representative of the various cultural, ethnic, and socioeconomic backgrounds. Particular attention should be paid to lifespan issues, health promotion, disease prevention, women's social roles, and health care service delivery and utilization. Finally, an ongoing analysis of the gender differences in morbidity and mortality and responses to illness and disability is central to protecting and promoting the health of all women.

References

Alexander, L. L., & LaRosa, J. H. (1994). *New dimensions in women's health.* Boston: Jones & Bartlett.

American Cancer Society. (1994). *Cancer facts and figures—1994.* Atlanta, GA: Author.

American Cancer Society. (1995). *Cancer facts and figures—1995.* Atlanta, GA: Author.

American Heart Association. (1993a). *Cardiovascular disease in women.* Dallas, TX: Author.

American Heart Association. (1993b). *Heart and stroke facts: 1994 statistical supplement.* Dallas, TX: Author.

Centers for Disease Control and Prevention. (1993). *Priorities for women's health.* Atlanta, GA: Author.

Centers for Disease Control and Prevention. (1994a). Arthritis prevalence and activity limitations–United States, 1990. *Morbidity and Mortality Weekly Report, 43*(24), 433-437.

Centers for Disease Control and Prevention. (1994b). Mortality patterns: United States, 1992. *Morbidity and Mortality Weekly Report, 43*(49), 916-920.

Douglas, P. S. (1993). *Cardiovascular health & disease in women.* Philadelphia: Saunders.

Harper, A. C., & Lambert, L. J. (1994). *The health of populations: An introduction* (2nd ed.). New York: Springer.

Horton, J. A. (1995). *The women's health data book.* Washington, DC: The Jacobs Institute of Women's Health.

Kahn, C. R. & Weir, G. (1994). *Joslin's diabetes mellitus* (13th ed.). Philadelphia: Lea & Febiger.

Kelsey, J. L., & Gammon, M. D. (1991). The epidemiology of breast cancer. *CA: A Cancer Journal for Clinicians, 41*(3), 146-165.

Mastroianni, A. C., Fader, R. L., & Federman, D. (1994). *Women and health research: Ethical and legal issues of including women in clinical studies, 1.* Washington, DC: National Academy Press.

Miller, B. A., Feuer, E. J., & Hankey, B. F. (1993). Recent incidence trends for breast cancer in women and the relevance of early detection: An update. *CA: A Cancer Journal for Clinicians, 43*(1), 27-41.

National Center for Health Statistics. (1993). *Healthy people 2000 review: Health United States, 1992.* Hyattsville, MD: Public Health Service.

Office of Research on Women's Health. (1992). *Report of the National Institutes of Health: Opportunities for research on women's health* (NIH Publication No. 92-3457). Washington, DC: U.S. Government Printing Office.

Overfield, F. (1995). *Biologic variations in health and illness: Race, age, and sex differences* (2nd ed.). Boca Raton, FL: CRC Press.

Rodin, J., & Ickovics, J. R. (1990, September). Women's health: Review and research agenda as we approach the 21st century. *American Psychologist,* 1018-1034.

Taeuber, C. (1991). *Statistical handbook on women in America.* Phoenix, AZ: Oryx Press.

U.S. Bureau of the Census. (1993). *Statistical abstract of the United States: 1993* (113th ed.). Washington, DC: Author.

U.S. Bureau of the Census. (1994). *Statistical abstract of the United States: 1994* (114th ed.). Washington, DC: Author.

Waldron, I. (1994). What do we know about causes of sex differences in mortality? A review of the literature. In P. Conrad & R. Kern (Eds.), *The sociology of health and illness: Critical perspectives* (pp. 42-53). New York: St. Martin's Press.

Wingo, P. A., Tong, T., Balden, S. (1995). Cancer Statistics 1995. *CA: A Cancer Journal for Clinicians, 45* (1), 8-30.

UNIT 2

Health Promotion and Preventive Health Issues

Health Promotion and Preventive Health Issues: Young Adulthood to the Perimenopausal Years (15–45)

Beverly J. McElmurry
Junko Tashiro

Introduction

Insufficient attention has been given to the study of programs for promoting the health of women from young adulthood to their middle years. This chapter presents concepts of health promotion, outlines the disease prevention issues that women in this age group encounter, and describes what is known about their response to these issues— especially health-promoting behaviors. These ideas are discussed within the context of a developmental perspective on women. Overall, the conclusions we reached about promoting the health of women are based on a review of study findings on health behaviors and programs for women.

In discussing the promotion of women's health, we use a broad or general understanding of health such as that found in the World Health Organization's (WHO) definition of health as "a state of complete psychological, mental, and social well-being" (WHO, 1948). Whether or not any of us has ever experienced such a state of complete well-being, it can serve as a goal, albeit a moving target over the lifespan, toward which we can aspire. By focusing on the middle 30 years (15–45) in the lifespan of women we are able to look closely at developmental concerns women face during this period.

Goals for Health Promotion and Disease Prevention

In recent years, health promotion has become a major goal in many countries of the world. If this aim is to be achieved, encouraging a lifestyle based on health-promoting behaviors must be an essential aspect of health promotion programs. Breslow (1990) emphasized two factors that have contributed to the health promotion movement: 1) the remarkable improvement in health in terms of mortality; and 2) the increasing recognition that illness care plays a limited role in health. Globally, as mortality rates have decreased and the average life expectancies at birth have increased in many countries, it is becoming possible to envision the attainment of WHO's goal of "absence of disease." As people live longer, "a state of complete physical, mental, and social well-being" has become a realistic health goal. It has been recognized that individual health behaviors affect health status. Since the early 1970s, studies (Belloc, 1973; Belloc & Breslow, 1972; Breslow & Enstrom, 1980) have provided evidence that an individual's good health practices are positively associated with health status and mortality. In response we have focused on individual health behaviors to improve health status and prevent disease.

In the 1990s (the decade for the Fourth World Conference of Women in Beijing), the global community is urged to improve the health of women in four fundamental areas (United Nations Children's Fund, 1994):

- the educational attainment of women
- the provision of family planning services
- attention to the specific health and nutrition needs of women
- improvement in the technology that women use to perform their work

Conceptual Issues in Health Promotion and Disease Prevention

Definitions of Health Promotion

In 1986, more than 200 participants from 38 countries attended the first International Conference on Health Promotion, which was held in Ottawa, Canada. The conference adopted the Ottawa Charter, which refers to health as "a resource for everyday life" and "a positive concept emphasizing social and personal resources, as well as physical capacities." Health promotion was defined as "the process of enabling people to increase control over, and to improve, their health" (International Conference on Health Promotion, 1986).

The term "health promotion" has various definitions. Display 3–1 highlights some of the definitions and goals of health promotion efforts. In synthesizing these differing definitions, health promotion can be defined as a process, action, program, or endeavor to obtain the goal of "complete physical, mental, and social well-being" (WHO, 1947), which includes the empowerment of people, encouragement of health-promoting behaviors (self-care), and the facilitation of advocacy for health. One of the essential elements of health promotion programs is to promote community health while recognizing the contribution of individual members of that community. In a broader sense, promoting healthy behavior includes preventive, protective, and promotive behaviors. In a narrower sense, the promotion of healthy behaviors can be carried out by any basically healthy individual, group, or community where the goal is a higher level of health, well-being, or self-actualization.

Conceptual Issues in Disease Prevention

In clarifying the notion of disease prevention, two terms, "health protection" and "primary prevention" are found in the literature and both concepts include

DISPLAY 3-1
Definitions and Goals of Health Promotion

- "efforts to enhance positive health, and prevent ill-health, through the overlapping bases of health education, prevention, and health protection" (Downie, Fyfe, & Tannahill, 1990, p. 64)

- behaviors "initiated by basically healthy people who seek the development of community and individual measures which can help them develop lifestyles that maintain and enhance the state of well-being" (U.S. Department of Health, Education, and Welfare, 1979, p.119)

- "the combination of education and environmental supports for actions and conditions of living conducive to health" (Green & Kreuter, 1991, p. 4)

- any program that "targets healthy individuals to maintain or enhance their state of well-being by using community and individual approaches for healthy lifestyle development" (Elder, Geller, Hovell, & Mayer, 1994, p. 15)

- to "help the person to maintain [his/her] stability, to foster ongoing development" (Murray & Zenter, 1985, p. 20)

- to increase "the level of well-being, and self-actualization, of a given individual or group" (Pender, 1987, p. 57)

- to "facilitate the development of young people who are healthy, happy, and prepared to assume their place as adults in society" (Crockett & Petersen, 1993, p. 13)

prevention of disease and health promotion. Both terms are based in behavioral perspectives.

In this chapter, health and disease are viewed as distinct entities. This position differs from the view of health as a continuum from absence to presence of disease. It is a curious phenomenon that interest in defining health is a more recent development than the emphasis on understanding diseases.

An early definition of "health-protective behavior" was "any behavior" carried out to "protect, promote, or maintain...health, whether or not such behavior is objectively effective toward that end" (Harris & Guten, 1979, p. 18). Since then, the term "health-protective behavior" has been used frequently in health behavioral science, although the above definition is different from the U.S. Surgeon General's (1992) emphasis on reduction of community and environmental threats to health. Duffy (1986) used the term "primary prevention behaviors," as an adaptation of the "primary prevention" concept of Leavell and Clark (1965), to refer to "those health practices to promote health or prevent illness" (p. 116) that were identified by individuals. Shamansky and Clausen (1980) referred to primary prevention as "generalized health promotion as well as specific protection against disease" (p. 106). Conversely, Pender (1987) conceptually differentiated the term "health-protecting [preventive] behavior" from the term "health-promoting behavior" because of "motivational mechanisms" (p. 38), and referred to "health promotion and prevention" as "complementary processes" (p. 5). "Health-protecting [preventive] behaviors" are motivated by the need to guard or defend an individual or group against illness or injury, whereas "health-promoting behavior" is motivated toward the goal of positive health.

In short, there is a lack of consensus on how the terms "health promotion" and "disease prevention" are used in the literature. However, each concept emphasizes self-care as essential to promote the health and wellness of people.

Women's Health Promotion and Disease Prevention Issues

Like women in many other countries, American women are living longer than men. However, the health status of women is not ideal (Verbrugge & Wingard, 1987). Life expectancy at birth for American women in 1995 was 79, compared with age 73 for men (United Nations, 1995). The leading causes of death for women included injuries (unintentional, suicide, and homicides), heart disease, cancer, acquired immunodeficiency syndrome (AIDS), and liver disease (Kochanek & Hudson, 1994). These conditions are affected by behavioral factors, namely lifestyle or health behaviors such as smoking, alcohol and drug abuse, poor diet, physical inactivity, unsafe driving, unsafe sex, and inappropriate stress management.

In contrast to mortality data, the census data commonly indicate that women have greater morbidity than men; consequently, women are consuming more health services. Rodin and Ickovics (1990) have noted that gender differences in morbidity emerge from various sources, some of which are psychological (women's perceptions of their health status and health-related behavior), whereas others originate in socioeconomic factors.

Gender differences in perceptions of and attitudes toward health can be observed in childhood; Cohen, Brownell, and Felix (1990) and Radius, Dillman, Becker, Rosenstock, and Horvath (1980) reported that girls perceived themselves as less healthy than boys. Duchen Smith, Turner, and Jacobsen (1987) noted that 61% of boys reported their overall health as "very good," whereas 68% of girls stated their health as "average." However, women are more engaged in health-promoting behaviors than their male counterparts throughout their lifespan (Lonnguist, Weiss, & Larsen, 1992; Mechanic & Cleary, 1980; Oleckno & Blacconiere, 1990; Pender, Walker, Sechrist, & Frank-Stromberg, 1990; Perry, Griffin, & Murray, 1985; Volden, Langemo, Adamson, & Oechsle, 1990; Waller, Crow, Sands, & Becker, 1988). Perry et al. (1985) found that girls reported making significantly more healthful food choices than boys at all age groups, whereas boys reported significantly more exercise outside of school than girls. Such findings are consistent with other studies as well as other age groups (Cohen et al., 1990; Kadota, 1991; Lonnguist et al., 1992; Nishida, 1992; Teuful, 1992; Vinal et al., 1986). Perry et al. (1985) stated that health behavior patterns are "learned early in life, are seen to consolidate in adolescence, and then persist into adulthood" (p. 379). However, little is known about the process of developing health-promoting behaviors in women.

Health promotion must become a major goal in enhancing the health of American women. Nancy Woods's (1988) review of women's health research from

1980 to 1985 urged a research agenda for the 1990s that places greater emphasis on adolescence and midlife. Furthermore, she urged that the agenda incorporate theoretical models for understanding the dynamic interplay of biologic, psychological, social, and environmental conditions for women that are so crucial to understanding their health at different developmental points. Although Woods found such a dynamic focus in women's health research underdeveloped, she noted that there was even less attention paid to clinical trials of health promotion interventions for women.

Given the above situation, several challenges become obvious in constructing a chapter on health promotion and disease prevention for women from adolescence through midlife. For the most part, the research available has dealt with conceptualizations of health (Newman, 1991), health promotion (Pender, 1984), women's health (Woods, 1988) and human development (Stevenson, 1992) as separate entities. We do not find research integrating the above areas in studies of women, particularly examining women by age categories.

Developmental Perspectives in Health-Promoting Behaviors of Women

This chapter focuses on developmental perspectives; therefore, it is important to emphasize that the majority of women aged 15 to 45 are experiencing the most productive years of their lives. Their contribution and importance to personal, family, and community activities has been recognized in literature on women's health and in the economic development of entire countries (National Institutes of Health, 1991). During these years, women are expected to develop their physical, psychological, and social health, as well as the capacity to care for themselves (including their sexuality, reproductive functions, and other health issues). Health promotion programs enable women to "increase control over, and to improve, their health" (International Conference on Health Promotion, 1986). However, the number of studies on health-promoting behaviors of adolescents and women is still limited compared to the total number of studies on health problems (Elliot, 1993).

Given the above recognition of an insufficient examination of health promotion for women, there are a number of studies that provide information concerning the antecedents of health-promoting behaviors for various adult samples (men and women). Demographic variables including age, gender, marital status, education, and income are associated with many health-promoting behaviors (Eaton, Nafziger, Strogatz, & Pearson, 1994; Gottlieb & Green, 1984). Gillis (1993) reviewed the studies of these antecedents and reported that self-efficacy was a powerful predictor of health-promoting behaviors, whereas the demographic considerations cited above were viewed as mediating factors.

An understanding of the antecedents of health-promoting behaviors in women must begin with an examination of the positive health behaviors of young women, and the socially dominant expectations of girls during the teenage years. It is essential to assess the current body of knowledge about young women's health. Thus, we begin our discussion with a focus on adolescence.

Adolescence

Values and health concerns are important motivating factors or antecedents for health-promoting behaviors of female adolescents. Prokhorov, Perry, Kelder, and Klepp (1993) studied changes in values and the importance of adolescent behaviors (6th to 12th graders). They found that "relations with family members," "school performance," and "physical appearance" were valued by 6th graders, and (although the importance of physical appearance increased for 7th graders) these values persisted through the 12th grade. Duchen Smith, et al. (1987) reported two areas of health concerns for 9th grade adolescents: social personal (future, emotions and feelings, and relationships with family members) and physical appearance (body weight, muscles, skin, and hair). Girls listed more health concerns than boys and ranked "body weight" as their number one concern.

Although boys reported fewer health worries, they ranked "future" as their number one concern. Cohen et al. (1990) noted that older girls (7th to 12th graders) reported greater internality (self-direction) than boys their age. They also found that older girls reported more smoking habits than boys. The same study noted that although girls reported healthier food habits than boys, the percentage of girls who reported feeling overweight increased. Further, more girls than boys perceived their families as spending time thinking about health.

Perceived health or health status is considered an incentive to motivating behaviors. A number of studies have examined the mechanism of health-promoting behaviors. Mechanic and Hansell (1987) affirmed that perceived health was an antecedent of health-promoting behaviors, especially for physical exercise or participation in sports. When the authors examined the relationships among self-assessed physical health (perceived health), competence of school achievement, sports and exercise, and social activities with peers, they found three variables with the following recursive relationships:

- Perceived health was related to adolescent competence.
- Competence was positively associated with psychological well-being.
- Psychological well-being was also associated with perceived health.

Terre, Ghiselli, Taloney, & DeSouza (1992) assessed the relationships among health behaviors, demographic data (including age, gender, and socioeconomic status), as well as affection, anxiety, depression, and hostility. They found low socioeconomic status was associated with unhealthful eating habits and tobacco use.

The influence of parents and peers, and the relationships between them that influence health behaviors, have been studied by a few investigators. Nutbeam, Aar, and Catford (1989) reported several characteristic health behaviors of adolescents (aged 11–16) in Norway and Wales. When the data for Norwegian adolescents were examined, two groups of health behaviors were observed: 1) a health-negative group of behaviors (health-compromising behaviors) consisting of monthly alcohol consumption, weekly smoking, daily coffee consumption, and unhealthy food consumption; and 2) a health-positive group of behaviors (health-promoting behaviors) consisting of healthy food consumption, good oral hygiene, use of vitamins, and regular physical activity. Health-promoting behaviors were associated with three predictors: 1) positive attitude toward school and education; 2) parents' occupational status; and, 3) relationship with parents. By contrast, health-promoting be-haviors were negatively related to the health-compromising behaviors of drinking alcohol, smoking, eating unhealthy food, and having irregular meals. Relationships with peers were associated with both health-promoting and health-compromising behaviors.

Donovan, Jessor, and Costa (1991) have defined a "conventionality-unconven-tionality" orientation as "a dimension underlying and summarizing an orientation toward, commitment to, and involvement in the prevailing values, standards of be-havior, and established institutions of the larger American society" (p. 52). Furthermore, most measures of conventionality-unconventionality were related to the index of involvement of adolescents in health behavior (7th to 12th graders). The dimensions of conventionality-unconventionality consisted of personality, so-cial environment, and behaviors classified as problem behaviors (Jessor, 1987). The five variables related to greater involvement in health-promoting behavior were: value placed on health; self-descriptions affirming health and fitness; greater inter-nal locus of control; lower external locus of control; and belief that exercise serves a variety of positive personal functions.

In summary, the studies cited above indicated interrelationships among health-promoting behaviors. Various studies have found the antecedents of health-pro-moting behaviors of school children and adolescents to be:

- the value placed on health or health concerns
- self-concept
- self-competence
- health locus of control
- the influence of parents and peers
- environmental or situational factors

These antecedents can be considered mechanisms for influencing health behav-iors. Parents are assumed to be key players or influences on the cognitive/perceptual behavior of female adolescents; however, few studies have been conducted in this area. Further study is critical to a better understanding of the antecedents and expla-nations of health behaviors of female adolescents. In fact, following a three-year as-sessment of adolescent health and health services, the United States Congress' Office of Technology Assessment (OTA) suggested that "a definition of adolescent health should include health-related behavior, positive components of health such as social competence, health and well-being from the perspective of adolescents themselves, and consideration of the impact of social and physical influences on health" rather than "the absence of physical and mental disorders" (Dougherty et al., 1992, p. 167).

Young Adulthood

The dominant social concern for late adolescence or young adulthood is further preparation for gainful employment and the establishment of relationships that fre-quently involve reproduction and parenting activity. Thus, in the following section we will examine health promotion as described for female college students and employed or parenting women.

Female College Students

The health concerns, needs, and behaviors of female college students are unique. Vinal et al. (1986) surveyed female college freshmen and described their expressed health concerns or needs as:

- management of stress (58%)
- handling anxiety (67%)
- increasing social skills (42%)
- preventing rape (57%)
- preventing minor illness (54%)
- increasing control over their sexuality (66%)

They also found that 58% of the students they studied perceived themselves to be overweight, and 74% practiced some kind of dieting measures to reduce weight. Also, a number of health-damaging coping styles were used by students, including over- or undereating (48%), frequent alcohol or drug use (12%), and frequent cigarette smoking (8%). Lonnguist et al. (1992) reported that predictors of positive health behaviors of female students were peer practices and the value placed on health, with female students participating in more positive health behaviors than male students. Furthermore, female students participated in more positive behaviors as they matured. Lonnguist et al. (1992) also noted that a primary motivator of female students was the desire to improve their physical appearance.

The characteristic health perceptions and behaviors of female students raise questions. What are additional antecedents of women's health perceptions and behaviors? Schank and Lawrence (1993) suggested that the career orientation of female students might be an antecedent of differences in health behaviors and locus of control. For example, compared to nonnursing female students, nursing students participated in more positive health behaviors and indicated more internality of locus of control. Schank and Lawrence (1993) discussed the influence of health information and training as well as self-identity as predictors of positive health behaviors. In comparing females with male students, Oleckno and Blacconiere (1990) found that female students' scores were higher on health-related attitudes and behaviors than those of males. They also found an inverse relationship between health-related attitudes and behaviors and smoking.

In summary, the studies indicated that young women in college engaged in more health-promoting behaviors than men, and developed healthy behaviors, although a number of female college students engaged in health-damaging stress-coping behaviors. The possible antecedents of health-promoting behaviors of female college students include:

- health information and training
- value placed on health
- sense of responsibility for health
- internal locus of control
- self-identity or concept, which relates to career choice or gender roles

Employed or Parenting Women

The economic (employed or unemployed, supported or unsupported) and social roles (daughter, sibling, mother, wife) of women are factors that influence their health-promoting behaviors. Duffy (1986) emphasized that situational or environmental factors such as time and money, social resources, parental and marital status affect the health of women and their family members. For example, Duffy reported that female-headed, single parent families engaged in two types of health behaviors: health care system related behaviors and behaviors routinely learned during childhood (ie, attention to the basic food groups, hygiene, rest, and proper clothing). However, they participated less in other positive health behaviors (eating a low salt or low fat diet, examining the breasts, using seat belts, checking the home for safety) because of barriers such as lack of motivation, time, money, and lack of support from others. Duffy discussed the social support system as an antecedent of health-promoting behavior. Teufel (1992) reported that overall, full-time employed women were within the recommended range for body weight, whereas men were marginally overweight. The explanations for these differences were that women were more active outside of the workplace and engaged in domestic activities more than men. For Duffy (1989), the 33% of variance in the health status of employed women aged 21 to 65 was explained by "diagnosed health problem," "internal locus of control," "self-actualization," "low chance health locus of control," "health responsibility," and "exercise." Furthermore, Duffy (1988) reported that 25% of the variance in health promotion behaviors for employed women (aged 35–65) was explained by the following variables: "Low chance health locus of control," "self-esteem," "current health," "health concern," "education," and "internal locus of control." Duffy (1988) concluded that the findings of the study supported previous research findings on health status and health-promoting behaviors.

Hibbard and Pope (1987) affirmed women's roles as essential antecedents of health-promoting behaviors. They indicated, for example, that the women's "family health officer" role was a predictor of health interests and concerns, and proposed a model to explain health-promoting behaviors of young women. In this model, the authors explained three types of women's roles (parental, marital, and employee) were related to health interest and health concerns. Level of interest in and concerns about health were also significantly related to health behaviors.

Walker and Best (1991) also emphasized the influence of situational factors on health behaviors and found that more homemakers engaged in health-promoting behaviors than employed mothers. Walker and Best noted several reasons why employed mothers experienced more stress:

- conflicts or problems about going back to work
- lack of time, fatigue, and sleep disturbance
- work overload
- illness of a child

Midlife

In general, health-promoting behaviors of women throughout their adulthood often depend on their roles (eg, socioeconomic or cultural) or situations (eg, access to social resources), which in turn influence their cognitive and perceptual understanding, management of health, and disease prevention. However, when considering economic and social roles as factors influencing women's health-promoting behaviors, it is important to understand the dynamic nature of these roles. The period of midlife is complex, multidimensional, and marked with many developmental changes. This is a time when career development and transitions occur, physical appearance changes, social roles shift, the care of aging parents becomes a concern, losses are experienced, and (in general) multiple demands are placed on women with too little discretionary time, energy, and disposable resources (Woods, 1993). During the last decade there has been increasing attention drawn to the need for studies of women in midlife (Woods, 1993).

By focusing this chapter on women up to the age of 45, we have omitted discussion of menopause. This decision was based on the fact that the majority of women experience menopause in their fifties, but it is also useful in drawing attention to the point made by Woods (1993) that there is more to midlife than concern about menopause. Chapters 4 and 5 provide a full discussion of menopause, the care of menopausal women, and hormonal therapy replacement.

Empowerment and Self-Care for Women

There are many theories about ways to promote women's health, prevent disease, and improve the social situations that most gravely affect women's health. Some of these ideas are cited in a report published by the United Nations Development Program (1995, p. 23). The report comments on:

- the relationships between human development and economic growth
- the importance of external environments on human and economic growth
- the need to restructure allocation of resources to meet human priorities
- the need for political will to achieve change
- the participation of people in the decisions that affect their lives
- the assurance of human security in homes, work settings, and communities

If these situations were to improve, women would be empowered and more capable of participating in health-promoting and disease- preventing behaviors.

An important activity for those wishing to promote the health of women is to search for ongoing innovative programs and learn more about what is being studied in these programs. Large urban cities face enormous challenges in trying to understand how to provide inner city women (who often have very diverse cultural, economic, and personal situations) with the health information and education they need to implement self-care and access the health care system. A variety of innovations are merited, including those that seem to work at the grassroots level and incorporate the use of peers prepared as community workers and health promoters (McElmurry, Swider, & Norr, 1991). Regardless of where we work (urban or rural) it is important to read and discuss what others are attempting and ascertain if it might work in our own settings.

Where to locate health promotion activities and practice is another area for health professionals to consider. The move to greater use of community-based settings for health care delivery offers an opportunity to examine possible changes in our practice. For example, although there has been an emerging body of literature on school-based clinics for high school students, we are now beginning to see some multidisciplinary innovations in school-based and school-linked services for K-12 students and their families (Behrman & Richard, 1992). In Chicago there have been a variety of primary health care projects that have been very useful in enlarging our understanding of how to ensure community residents' participation in the identification, implementation, and evaluation of health and health care concerns. There are some ideas that hold true across communities, such as the importance of:

- designing services that the public can afford to continue over time
- ensuring the appropriate use of health technology
- attending to the literacy levels of the people with whom you work
- avoiding the professional arrogance embedded in the assumption that "you know best what people need"
- creating dialogue around the essentials or basics in health care that should be available to all people

However, the design of services that will work must in the end be tailored to the specific community in which they will be implemented. The report of the National Institute of Nursing Research (NINR) Priority Expert Panel on Health Promotion (1993) provides numerous examples of health promotion research questions for youth that can be investigated in traditional and nontraditional settings. A caution here is that regardless of which settings we use, we need to approach those settings with fresh views and a willingness to try innovations.

Research and Policy Issues in Health Care for Women

Although the social situation is ripe for change, the systematic study of factors that promote health and prevent disease in women has not been realized as a research base for clinical practice with women. What to do when there is insufficient research to guide the practice of health care for women is a concern, and is further emphasized in the following review of some of the reports that can be found in the literature.

Young Adulthood

It is important for health professionals to act as advocates for changes in health care delivery and policies. Generally, the health care provider can help the public become more aware of the need for attention to adolescent health. This can be done through collective action and support of advocacy groups in the development of a constituency that speaks on behalf of needed changes. One example is the project of the Illinois Caucus for Adolescent Health, a state-wide membership group that has been developing networks of increased services, including: creation of a healthy school model; advocacy on minors' access to reproductive health services; integration of pregnancy prevention, family planning education, and service with STD and HIV/AIDS prevention programs; projects for young parents, and counseling to help teenage mothers speak on their own behalf (Illinois Caucus for Adolescent Health, 1993, 1995).

Midlife

Recognizing the lack of information on health promotion and disease prevention issues for women in midlife, Woods (1993) encouraged the use of DeLorey's (1984) recommendations on what to do until the knowledge base for practice is established. These recommendations can be applied to all age groups (Woods, 1993, pp. 174–175):

1. Establish priorities of health care reflecting women's experiences as well as the findings from social, behavioral, and medical sciences.
2. Establish an information base considering precursors of health.
3. Redefine research priorities to include nonclinical populations and prospective studies about women's experiences.
4. Present a more realistic view of women in midlife to health professionals in their training.
5. Support environments in which women can develop realistic expectations about the health issues of midlife.

The area of disease prevention has been addressed in recent years through the process of establishing national health goals (United Nations Development Program, 1995). Often, the practitioner is faced with decisions about how to distinguish between women who are well informed about self-care and management, those who require some assistance or information about their health, and those who require more intensive health relevant interventions. In evaluating women's requirements for care to prevent disease, the United States Department of Health and Human Services, Public Health Service (USDHHS, PHS, 1994), has formulated a useful handbook that combines reports of scientific investigations, policy statements and documents, educational reports, and consultation with experts to arrive at age-appropriate timelines for health tests, examinations, immunizations, and health guidance. Although this does not recognize a comprehensive definition of women's health, it is a start.

The Perry & Jessor model for health promotion (1985), although published over a decade ago, can serve to illustrate the complexity of studying health promotion. Their model illustrates a multidimensional concept of health that identifies strategies to change behaviors and provides an analysis of interventions from three levels of focus. This model helps make the logical connections between definitions of health and intervention strategies. Thus, a definition of health that includes a social component might appropriately focus on a community mobilization program (such as the preparation of community workers or indigenous leaders). The intervention studies that might accomplish tests of a comprehensive health promotion model, especially at community or social levels of intervention, will most likely be large scale, costly, multidisciplinary, and complex. Eventually these studies will be done, and there is every reason to believe that women health professionals will provide leadership in such investigations. Until then, we must continue to work on smaller scale interventions and encourage attention to environmental, social, and political interventions as well as individually focused actions.

Conclusion

Overall, when thinking about the future of health promotion and disease prevention for women aged 15 to 45, consider the inadequacies of past approaches and strive to improve on them. First, we have reported a general confusion of terms and concepts about health and its promotion. Fortunately, nursing has generally favored a broad notion of health that encompasses physical, emotional, social, political, and environmental components. Other disciplines are now beginning to embrace a holistic perspective regarding health care.

Second, we have noted a persistent lack of information about successful health promotion interventions for women. Few studies on the health-promoting and disease-preventing behaviors of women have been conducted and further study is needed to determine the antecedents of health-promoting behaviors, the relationships among those antecedents, health behavior, and health status. Yet, even though comprehensive and systematic studies of women are still to be realized, the number of professional and lay books on women's health has grown rapidly. The emerging literature presents several challenges to scholars:

- Reexamine your views of women's health. (Dan, 1994)
- Look for the themes that characterize unique yet universal experiences such as motherhood or the loss of a child or caring relationships. (Munhill, 1994, 1995)
- Study vulnerable populations such as immigrants or minorities (Aday, 1993) with a personally constructed perspective on women's health (Maher & Thompson-Tetreault, 1994).
- Integrate in-depth reviews of knowledge about specific health topics such as sexually transmitted diseases. (McElmurry & Parker, 1993, 1995)

Finally, there is a need for a more comprehensive focus for interventions to promote health. The literature reports more studies that focus on individuals rather than on environmental, social, or community contexts for intervention. Becker (1993) called the failure to look beyond individual determinants one of the dark sides of the health promotion developments of the past few decades.

...[T]o turn our attention beyond the individual—to recognize the social and economic determinants of disease, health and wellness—is complex and threatening. Doing something about poverty, racism, unemployment, inequitable access to education and other issues involves notions of planned social and economic change...(p. 4)

To move forward with studies of health promotion practice in women's health, we encourage the use of perspectives that incorporate or synthesize age and developmental attributes of women with clarity about concepts of health and its promotion that are relevant to the diverse situations of women.

References

Aday, L. (1993). *At risk in America: The health and health care needs of vulnerable populations in the United States.* San Francisco: Jossey-Bass Publications.

Becker, M. H. (1993). A medical sociologist looks at health promotion. *Journal of Health and Social Behavior, 34*(3), 1-6.

Behrman, & Richard E. (Eds.). (1992). *The future of children: School linked services.* 2(1): David and Lucille Packard Foundation.

Belloc, N. B. (1973). Relationship of health practices and mortality. *Preventive Medicine, 2,* 67-81.

Belloc, N. B., & Breslow, L. (1972). Relationship of physical health status and health practices. *Preventive Medicine, 1,* 409-421.

Breslow, L. (1990). A health promotion primer for the 1990's. *Health Affairs, 9,* 6-21.

Breslow, L., & Enstrom, J. E. (1980). Persistence of health habits and their relationship to mortality. *Preventive Medicine, 9,* 469-483.

Cohen, R. Y., Brownell, K. D., & Felix, M. R. (1990). Age and sex differences in health habits and beliefs of schoolchildren. *Health Psychology, 9*(2), 208-224.

Crockett, L. J., & Petersen, A. C. (1993). Adolescent development: Health risks and opportunities. In S. G. Millstein, A. C. Petersen, & E. O. Nightingale (Eds.), *Promoting the health of adolescents: New directions for the twenty-first century.* New York: Oxford University Press.

Dan, A. (Ed.). (1994). *Reframing women's health: Multidisciplinary research and prevention.* Thousand Oaks, CA: Sage.

DeLorey, C. (1984). Health care and midlife women. In G. Baruch & J. Brooks-Gunn (Eds.), *Women in midlife* (pp. 277-301). New York: Plenum.

Donovan, J. E., Jessor, R., & Costa, F. M. (1991). Adolescent health behavior and conventionality-unconventionality: An extension of problem-behavior theory. *Health Psychology, 10* (1), 52-61.

Dougherty, D., Eden, J., Kemp, K. B., Metcalf, K., Rowe, K., Ruby, G., Stobel, P., & Solarz, A. (1992). Adolescent health: A report to the U.S. Congress. *Journal of School Health, 62* (5), 167-174.

Downie, R. S., Fyfe C., & Tannahill, A. (1990). *Health promotion: Models and values.* New York: Oxford University Press.

Duchen Smith, K. L., Turner, J. G., & Jacobsen, R. B. (1987). Health concerns of adolescents. *Pediatric Nursing, 13*(5), 311-315.

Duffy, M. E. (1986). Primary prevention behaviors: The female-headed, one-parent family. *Research in Nursing & Health, 9,* 115-122.

Duffy, M. E. (1988). Determinants of health promotion in mid-life women. *Nursing Research, 37*(6), 358-362.

Duffy, M. E. (1989). Determinants of health status in employed women. *Health Value, 13* (2), 50-57.

Eaton, C. B., Nafziger, A. N., Strogatz, D. S., & Pearson, T. A. (1994). Self-reported physical activity in a rural county: A New York county health census. *American Journal of Public Health, 84*(1), 29-32.

Elder, J. P., Geller, E. S., Hovell, M. F., & Mayer, J. A. (1994). *Motivating health behavior.* Albany, NY: Delmar.

Elliott, D. S. (1993). Health-enhancing and health-compromising lifestyles. In S. G. Millstein, A. C. Petersen, & E. O. Nightingale (Eds.), *Promoting the health of adolescents: New directions for the twenty-first century.* New York: Oxford University Press.

Gillis, A. J. (1993). Determinants of a health-promoting lifestyle: An integrative review. *Journal of Advanced Nursing, 18,* 345-353.

Gottlieb, N. H., & Green, L. W. (1984). Life events, social network and health: An analysis of the 1979 National Survey of Personal Health. *Health Education Quarterly, 11*(1), 91-105.

Green L. W., & Kreuter, M. W. (1991). *Health promoting: An educational and environmental approach* (2nd ed.). Mountain View, CA: Mayfield Publishing.

Harris, D. M. & Guten, S. (1979). Health-protective behavior: An exploratory study. *Journal of Health and Social Behavior, 20,* 17-29.

Hibbard, J. H., & Pope, C. R. (1987). Women's roles, interest in health and health behavior. *Women & Health, 12*(2), 67-84.

Illinois Caucus for Adolescent Health. (1993). *Improving the health of adolescent women in Chicago: A policy report*. Chicago: Author.

Illinois Caucus for Adolescent Health (1994). *A state-wide action plan for improving the health of adolescents in Illinois*. Chicago: Author.

Illinois Caucus for Adolescent Health (1995). *Teenage mothers talking for themselves: A public policy report*. Chicago: Author.

International Conference on Health Promotion. (1986). *Ottawa charter for health promotion*. Ottawa, Canada: Author.

Jessor, R. (1987). Problem-behavior theory, psychological development, and adolescent problem drinking. *British Journal of Addiction, 82,* 435-446.

Kadota, S. (1991). Kyoikubakubu gakusei no kenko to syokuseikatsu yoin tono kanren ni tuite [The relationship between the health status and eating habits of college students majoring in education]. *Okayama Daigaku Kyoiku Kenkyu Syuroku, 86,* 1-8.

Kochanek, K. D., & Hudson, B. L. (1995). Advance report of final mortality statistics, 1992. *Mortality Vital Statistics Report Suppl., 43*(6). Hyattsville, MD: National Center for Health Statistics.

Leavell, H. R., & Clark, E. G. (1965). *Preventive medicine for the doctor in his community: An epidemiologic approach* (3rd ed.). New York: McGraw-Hill.

Lonnquist, L. E., Weiss, G. L., & Larsen, D. L. (1992). Health value and gender in predicting health protective behavior. *Women, & Health 19* (2/3), 69-85.

Maher, F. A. & Thompson-Tetreault, M. K. (1994). *The feminist classroom*. New York: Basic Book.

McElmurry, B. J., & Parker, R. S. (Eds.). (1993). *Annual review of women's health, Vol I*. New York: National League for Nursing.

McElmurry, B. J., & Parker, R. S. (Eds.). (1995). *Annual review of women's health, Vol II*. New York: National League for Nursing.

McElmurry, B. J., Swider, S. M., & Norr, K. (1991). A community-based primary health care program for integration of research, practice and education. In *NLN curriculum revolution: Community building and activism* (pp. 77-90). (NLN Publication N15-2398). New York: National League for Nursing

Mechanic, D., & Cleary, P. D. (1980). Factors associated with the maintenance of positive health behavior. *Preventive Medicine, 9,* 805-814.

Mechanic, D., & Hansell, S. (1987). Adolescent competence, psychological well-being, and self-assessed physical health. *Journal of Health and Social Behavior, 28,* 364-374.

Munhill, P. L. (1994). *In women's experience, Vol I*. New York: National League for Nursing.

Munhill, P. L. (1995) *In women's experience, Vol II*. New York: National League for Nursing.

Murray, R. B., & Zentner, J. P. (1985). *Nursing concepts for health promotion* (3rd ed.). Englewood Cliffs, NJ: Prentice-Hall.

National Institute for Nursing Research. *Health promotion for older children and adolescents: A report of the NINR Priority Expert Panel on Health Promotion*. National Nursing Research Agenda, Developing Knowledge for Practice: Challenges and Opportunities. (NIH Publication No. 93-2420). Bethesda, MD: Author.

National Institutes of Health. (1991). *Report of the National Institutes of Health: Opportunities for research on women's health*. Bethesda, MD: Author.

Newman, M. (1991). Health promotion and illness prevention. In H. H. Werley & J. J. Fitzpatrik (Eds.), *Annual review of nursing research* (Vol. 2, pp. 83-105). New York: Springer.

Nishida, T. (1992). Raifusutairu kara mita shintai katsudouryo ni kansuru kenkyu. [The amount of physical activities and life style of college students]. *Shukutoku Tankidaigaku Kenkyu Kiyo, 31,* 215-221.

Nutbeam, D., Aar, L., & Catford, J. (1989). Understanding children's health behavior: The implications for health promotion for young people. *Social Science and Medicine, 29* (3), 317-325.

Oleckno, W. A., & Blacconiere, M. J. (1990). A multiple discriminant analysis of smoking status and health-related attitudes and behaviors. *American Journal of Preventive Medicine, 6*(6), 323-329.

Pender, N. J. (1984). Health promotion and illness prevention. In H. H. Werley & J. J. Fitzpatrick (Eds.), *Annual review of nursing research* (Vol. 2, pp. 83-105). New York: Springer.

Pender, N. J. (1987). *Health promotion in nursing practice* (2nd ed.). Norwalk, CT: Appleton & Lange.

Pender, N. J., Walker, S. N., Sechrist, K. R. & Frank-Stromberg, M. (1990). Predicting health-promoting lifestyles in the workplace. *Nursing Research 39* (6), 326–332.

Perry, C. L., Griffin, G., & Murray, D. M. (1985). Assessing needs for youth health promotion. *Preventive Medicine, 14,* 379-393.

Perry, C. L., & Jessor, R. (1985). The concept of health promotion and the prevention of adolescent drug abuse. *Health Education Quarterly, 12*(2), 169-184.

Prokhorov, A. V., Perry, C. L., Kelder, S. H., & Klepp, K. (1993). Lifestyle values of adolescents: Results from Minnesota heart health youth program. *Adolescence, 28* (111), 637-647.

Radius, S. M., Dillman, T. E. Becker, M. H., Rosenstock, I. M., & Horvath, W. (1980). Adolescent perspectives on health and illness. *Adolescence, 15* (58), 375-384.

Rodin, J., & Ickovics, J. R. (1990). Review and research agenda as we approach the 21st century. *American Psychologist, 45* (9), 1018-1034.

Schank, M. J. & Lawrence D. M. (1993). Young adult women: Lifestyle and health locus of control. *Journal of Advanced Nursing, 18,* 1235-1241.

Shamansky, S. L., & Clausen, C. (1980). Levels of prevention: Examination of the concept. *Nursing Outlook,* February, 104-108.

Stevenson, J. S. (1992). Review of the first decade of the Annual Review of Nursing Research. In J. Fitzpatrick, R. L. Taunton, & A. K. Jacox (Eds.), *Annual Review of Nursing Research 10,* 1-22. New York: Springer.

Terr, L., Ghiselli, W., Taloney, L., & DeSouza, E. (1992). Demographics, affect, and adolescents' health behaviors. *Adolescence, 27* (105), 13-24.

Teufel, N. I. (1992). Diet and activity patterns of male and female co-workers: Should work site health promotion programs assume homogeneity? *Women and Health, 19* (4), 31-54.

United Nation Children's Fund. (1994). Gertrude Mangella. Commentary: Change for the last and the least (pp. 30-31). *The progress of nations.* New York: UNICEF.

United Nations Development Program. (1995) *Human development report.* New York: Oxford.

United Nations. (1995). *The world's women, 1995: Trends and statistics.* New York: Author.

U.S. Department of Health, Education, and Welfare. (1979). *Healthy people: The Surgeon General's report on health promotion and disease prevention.* Washington DC: Superintendent of Documents (#017-001-00416-2).

U.S. Department of Health and Human Services (1994). *Clinician's handbook of preventive services.* Washington, DC: U.S. Government Printing Office.

Verbugge, L. M., Wingard, D. L. (1987). Sex differentials in health and mortality. *Women & Health, 12* (2), 103-145.

Vinal, D., Wellman, C., Tyser, K., Stites, I., Leaf, J., Larson, & Graves, J. (1986). A determination of the health-protective behaviors of female adolescents: A pilot study. *Adolescence, 21*(81), 87-105.

Volden, C., Langemo, D., Adamson, M., & Oechsle, L. (1990). The relationship of age, gender, and exercise practices to measures of health, life-style, and self-esteem. *Applied Nursing Research, 3*(1), 20-26.

Waller, P. R., Crow, C., Sands, D., & Becker, H. (1988). Health related attitudes and health promoting behaviors: Differences between health fair attenders and a community comparison group. *American Journal of Health Promotion, 3* (1), 17-24.

Walker, L. O., & Best, M. A. (1991). Well-being of mothers with infant children: A preliminary comparison of employed women and homemakers. *Women and Health, 17* (1), 71-89.

Woods, N. F. (1988). Women's health. In J. J. Fitzpatrick, R. L. Taunton, & J. Q. Benoliel (Eds.), *Annual Review of Nursing Research, 10,* 209-237. New York: Springer.

Woods, N. F. (1993). Midlife women's health: There's more to it than menopause. In B. J. McElmurry & R. S. Parker (Eds.), *Annual review of women's health* (pp. 161-196). New York: National League for Nursing.

CHAPTER 4

Health Promotion: The Perimenopausal to Mature Years (45–64)

Arlene Michaels Miller
JoEllen Wilbur
Judith McDevitt

Definition

Health Promotion in a Developmental Context

The years from approximately 45 to 64 are considered midlife, the period of mature adulthood during which significant physical and psychosocial changes and challenges occur. Women who are now in midlife were born between 1930 and 1950 and became young adults during the post-World War II and Vietnam War eras of U.S. history. These historical contexts define their experiences and affect their perspectives, expectations, and interpretations of life cycle events.

The onset of menopause is one commonly used indicator for the transition to midlife. Menopause is usually defined as the final menstrual period experienced by a woman and is identified retrospectively as being a year without menstruation. The mean age of menopause for women in North America is 51.3 years (McKinlay, Brambilla, & Posner, 1992); by age 58, 99% of women are postmenopausal.

Although the menopause is a singularly important physiologic change in women's lives, the transition to midlife is much broader, involving significant psychosocial changes as well. In terms of the family life cycle, midlife is defined as the time children leave home. Other role-related indicators of midlife include a change in emphasis on a woman's primary role as mother to that of worker or wife (Fogel & Woods, 1995). In addition to these shared markers used to delineate midlife, women often have their own perceptions about whether they are middle-aged (Murray & Zentner, 1993).

The onset of significant changes in roles and physical abilities or appearance during midlife creates a new awareness of personal mortality and a revised perception of the future as "time left to live" (Neugarten, 1968, p. 97). This is accompanied by a new preoccupation with taking stock and finding personal meaning in life. Generativity (Erikson, 1982), which may be expressed by women as caring for family members or mentoring younger colleagues at work, assumes important meanings during midlife (McAdams, de St. Aubin, & Logan, 1993). Developing satisfying leisure time, including a range of enjoyable community, social, physical, and solitary activities, supports healthy development during midlife and helps prepare for retirement and successful aging.

Age-Related Changes and Symptoms During Midlife

Symptoms common during midlife include those related to normal physiologic aging as well as to menopause. Vulnerability to adverse symptoms is multidetermined, a combination of predispositional and situational factors. Physical, nutritional, environmental, and genetic factors contribute to the formation of symptoms, whereas cultural background, social support, coping strategies, and other psychological resources affect their appraisal and interpretation. Symptom inventories are useful in assessing complaints of midlife (Kaufert, Gilbert, & Hassard, 1988).

The symptoms of aging experienced most frequently by women in midlife include joint pains, backaches, fatigue, and sleep disorders (Wilbur, Holm, & Dan, 1992). Visual changes leading to an inability to accommodate as easily to close items are common in women after age 40, whereas the hearing loss that occurs with aging generally does not begin until after age 50 (Youngkin & Davis, 1994). Cognitively, memory changes begin to occur as well and are manifested most commonly as mild forgetfulness and decreased word retrieval (Hoyer & Rybash, 1994). Qualitative changes in sleep during midlife include a decrease in rapid eye movement sleep and waking more easily during the night. These changes are sometimes attributed to the co-occurrence of hot flashes or night sweats.

Although psychological symptoms may increase during the premenopausal period while women are still menstruating (Wilbur et al., 1992), recent research has not demonstrated an increase in depressive symptoms in women experiencing a natural menopause (Busch, Zonderman & Costa, 1994; Matthews et al., 1990). Disturbances of mood appear to be more common among women who seek care for other menopausal symptoms, and the development of depressive symptoms may be greater in women experiencing surgical menopause (Sherwin, 1994). A negative attitude toward menopause appears to be related to increased reporting of physical and psychological symptoms (Avis & McKinlay, 1991; Wilbur, Miller, & Montgomery, 1995). Nevertheless, women's attitudes toward menopause are generally positive (Avis & McKinlay, 1991). The factors most consistently associated with women's attitudes toward menopause are age and menopausal status, with older, postmenopausal women having the most favorable attitude (Avis & McKinlay, 1991; Wilbur et al., 1995).

The most common symptom of menopause is hot flashes, which are indicators of the vasomotor instability that occurs in approximately 50% of women at some time during the menopausal years (U.S. Congress, Office of Technology Assessment [OTA], 1992). There appears to be no association between hot flashes and age at menarche, age at menopause, height, or medical problems (Sherman, Wallace, Bean, Chang, & Schlabaugh, 1981). In relation to weight, Erlik, Meldrum, and Judd (1982) found that women with a lower body mass index (BMI) reported more hot flashes than women with a higher body mass, but heavier women aged 35 to 65 had more vasomotor symptoms in our recent study (Wilbur, Miller, & Montgomery, 1995, June). After the menopause, from 10% to 30% of women experience vaginal and other genitourinary changes, including urinary frequency, urgency, and stress incontinence as well as vaginal dryness and dyspareunia (Wilbur et al., 1992).

Physical Health Risks During Midlife

The most significant health risks facing women in midlife are those related to cardio-vascular disease and osteoporosis. The risk of heart disease in women begins to rise around the age of 45 (American Heart Association, 1991). The Framingham study reported that the risk of coronary heart disease for women triples after menopause and that premature menopause increases this risk (Gordon, Kannel, Hjortland, & McNamara, 1978). Elevated levels of serum cholesterol and phospholipids increase the risk of cardiovascular disease and are believed to be associated with decreased ovarian function (Engeland et al., 1990; Stampfer, Colditz, & Willett, 1990).

Loss of bone mineral density begins in women around the age of 30. Women lose bone at a rate of 0.3% to 0.5% per year after age 40, and this rate escalates after menopause (Riggs & Melton, 1986). According to Avioli (1991), 5 to 10 million women in the United States will be diagnosed as osteoporotic by the year 2000 and thus will be subject to fractures of all types. There is an abrupt rise in hip fractures in women as early as ages 40 to 44 (Avioli, 1991). In addition to age and menopausal status, bone loss is influenced by heredity (Dequeker, Nijs, Verstraeten, Guesens, & Gevers, 1987), race, and body weight. African Americans have significantly denser bones than Caucasians (Silverman & Madison, 1988), whereas low body weight is a risk factor for hip fracture in both African American and Caucasian women (Pruzansky, Turano, Luckey, & Senie, 1987). Modifiable lifestyle factors related to cardiovascular disease and bone mineral density include physical activity (Dalsky et al., 1988; Haskell et al., 1992), high-fat diet (U.S. Department of Health and Human Services, 1991), dietary intake of calcium (Smith et al., 1989), alcohol consumption (Wardlaw, 1988), and smoking (American Heart Association, 1991; Hopper & Seeman, 1994).

Health Promotion Activities

Exercise and Physical Activity

Studies that have quantified occupational and leisure activity indicate that more active or physically fit people tend to develop less coronary heart disease and that physical fitness is associated with a decrease in mortality from all causes (Blair et al., 1989). When active people do develop coronary heart disease, it occurs at a later age and tends to be less severe (Haskell et al., 1992). The benefits of physical activity in relationship to bone health are not as clearly defined; however, Wilbur, Dan, Montgomery, and Holm (1994) found a significant correlation between spinal bone mineral density and aerobic fitness, suggesting that fitness protects against loss of bone mineral density.

Exercise is also associated with improved psychological health symptoms; however, the major psychological benefit of exercise for healthy individuals may be prevention of depression and anxiety (Raglin, 1990). Choi, Van Horn, Picker, and Roberts (1993) found that women exercising at both low and high intensities experienced increased positive affect and decreased negative affect immediately after an aerobics exercise class. Few studies have looked at exercise in relation to vasomotor symptoms. Hammar, Berg, and Lindgren (1990) found that hot flashes and sweating were only half as common in physically active than in inactive postmenopausal women. Dennerstein et al. (1993) found less dysphoria (nervous tension, feeling sad, difficulty concentrating, lack of energy, and trouble sleeping) and fewer digestive and cardiopulmonary symptoms in women who exercised at least once a week.

The exercise patterns of women in midlife are notably poor. The majority of women are sedentary (Centers for Disease Control and Prevention, 1993), and their leisure activity decreases in midlife (Dan, Wilbur, Hedricks, O'Connor, & Holm, 1990); thus, increasing physical activity is a primary objective for health promotion (U.S. Department of Health and Human Services [USDHHS], 1991). Physical activity is any bodily movement produced by skeletal muscles that results in energy expenditure, whereas physical fitness relates to the ability to perform physical activity. The components of physical fitness include aerobic fitness, body composition, muscular strength and endurance, and flexibility (Baranowski et al., 1992). Exercise is physical activity undertaken to maintain one or more components of physical fitness. Studies indicate that women in midlife can improve their aerobic fitness by following an exercise program of moderately intense activity (King, Haskell, Taylor, Kraemer, & DeBusk, 1991; Notelovitz, 1990).

An exercise prescription for midlife includes intensity, duration, frequency, and mode. The optimal intensity levels most often recommended to develop and maintain aerobic fitness are those sufficient to attain 60% to 90% of the maximum heart rate, estimated by subtracting the age of the individual from 220 (Pollock & Wilmore, 1990). Moderate-intensity effort at 50% to 74% of maximum is recommended for the average person, however, not only to account for the probable lower threshold of previously sedentary individuals, but also to avoid increased musculoskeletal injuries and cardiovascular symptoms and events associated with high-intensity effort. Additionally, women are more likely to adopt and maintain moderate activities, and moderately intense activity can be tolerated comfortably by most persons for 20 to 30 minutes, the recommended duration (Pate et al., 1995). A schedule of three to four times per week is frequent enough to improve aerobic fitness and body composition (Pollock & Wilmore, 1990). Alternatively, moderately intense activity totaling 30 minutes a day can be accumulated in short sessions (Pate et al., 1995).

Women's leisure time may be fragmented and depend on the priorities of others, so that finding time for exercise is often a problem. Finding a mode of activity suitable for women's lifestyles is important for successfully establishing an ongoing exercise program. Women often choose activities that can be done in and around the home, using time as it becomes available. Walking, exercising with a stationary bike or video, and dancing are examples of home-based activities of moderate intensity that women enjoy (Wilbur, Holm, & Dan, 1993).

Nutrition

Nutritional needs for women during midlife are determined by the changes that characterize this period of life, including menopausal status, changes in body composition, and a decrease in the amount of physical activity, as well as by the health risks that become salient during this time. Menopause equalizes the risk for cardiovascular disease between women and men. This makes limiting fat intake even more important during midlife than it may have been during earlier life stages. The most important change in body composition during midlife is a decrease in lean body mass; the daily calorie requirement for energy also decreases (Rosenberg, 1991). If physical activity does not increase, maintaining the same caloric intake with a reduction in basal metabolic rate leads to weight gain. Upper body or abdominal pattern obesity appears to be a risk factor for non–insulin-dependent diabetes mellitus, whose onset is mainly in postmenopausal women aged 45 to 60. Obesity and high-fat diets have also been implicated in the development of breast cancer (Heber, McCarthy, Ashley, & Byerly, 1989).

An appropriate guide throughout the lifespan is now believed to include a daily dietary intake of 15% protein, 55% carbohydrates, and no more than 30% fat. The Food Guide Pyramid provides a graphic representation of current dietary principles and recommendations (Gizis, 1992). There are several changes in recommended daily allowances (RDAs) of calories and selected minerals and vitamins after age 50 (U.S. Departments of Agriculture and Health and Human Services, 1990). First, after age 50, the RDA for women is 80% to 85% of the 2200 calories of younger adults (RDA Subcommittee, 1989). Second, an increase in calcium and phosphorus is essential for maintaining or slowing the decline in bone mineral density. The usual dietary recommendation for calcium, 800 mg/d, is sufficient for active women aged 25 to 50; after menopause the intake should be increased to 1200 to 1500 mg/d and up to 2000 mg/d for postmenopausal women who are not on hormone replacement therapy (HRT) (Murray & Zentner, 1993). Third, the need for iron decreases from 15 to 10 mg/d for postmenopausal women, who no longer experience monthly iron losses associated with menstruation. Thiamine, riboflavin, and niacin requirements are also somewhat smaller due to decreased energy metabolism. Other vitamin and mineral recommendations remain the same for adults over age 18. Finally, a diet high in complex carbohydrates may reduce the incidence of colon cancer, and fiber is important to avoid the constipation that may become more common during midlife.

Recent research suggests that antioxidant nutrients, including beta-carotene, vitamin C, and vitamin E, help the body maintain its network of defenses against free radicals, which are highly reactive molecules causing oxidative stress or damage when they unite with body cells. These micronutrients may protect against the development of some forms of cancer, cataracts, and cardiovascular disease (Monti et al., 1992), but current RDAs do not yet reflect this research.

Desirable body weight during midlife is the subject of continued controversy. Height and weight tables such as those developed by the Metropolitan Life Insurance Company are often used as guides but must be interpreted carefully because they may underestimate weights that are truly related to health and longevity. Another simple measure is the BMI, the weight in kilograms divided by the height in centimeters squared. This measure is a somewhat better estimate of overweight than the tables (USDHHS, 1994). Women should be advised not to decrease their weight too quickly and to avoid the cycle of repeated weight loss and gain. Each round of weight loss and gain increases the proportion of regained adipose tissue. The best long-term strategy for controlling weight is to reduce dietary fat intake to an average of 30% of calories and to maintain a program of regular physical activity and exercise (USDHHS, 1991). In midlife, the challenge for women is to modify food choices to reflect the increased need for calcium while reducing saturated fat within lower requirements for overall caloric intake.

Stress Management

Among environmental factors influencing health at midlife, participation in multiple roles is an important consideration. Women are increasingly entering, reentering, or continuing jobs; in 1991, 75% of women in this country were in the labor force at midlife (Women's Bureau, 1992). Approximately 75% of these employed women were married and about half had children under age 18 years. Although the independent and cumulative effects of being a worker, daughter, mother, and wife were once thought to be linked to psychological distress and physical illness, multiple roles may in fact ease distress and enhance health (Barnett, Marshall, & Singer, 1992). The number of roles appears to be less critical than their subjective quality (Waldron & Jacobs, 1989). For employed women who are also parents and partners, the quality of family roles seems to be more important to psychological well-being than job roles (Barnett, Marshall, & Singer, 1992; Miller, Wilbur, & Montgomery, 1995).

It is useful to consider stress as a reaction to life events in which intervention can occur at several points and using several modalities. Adequate rest and sleep, exercise, and nutrition should not be disregarded because each of these has an important impact on maximizing resources available to deal with stress (Manderino & Brown, 1992). Using medications, cigarettes, and alcohol should be discouraged as means of responding to stressful life events.

Healthy coping methods can forestall some of the mental and physical reactions to stress that lead to illness. Before initiating a stress management program, however, the nature and sources of stress should be assessed. Stress assessment instruments include the Social Readjustment Scale (Holmes & Rahe, 1967), although some consider this measure less useful than those that measure daily annoyances (Kanner, Coyne, Schaefer, & Lazarus, 1981), the common daily stressors that may add up over a period of time. The Ways of Coping Questionnaire (Folkman & Lazarus, 1988) may also be helpful for identifying usual methods or styles of coping with stressful events (Rich, 1991).

Stress management programs should include cognitive and behavioral skills such as problem solving, time management, and assertiveness training as well as relaxation techniques (Manderino & Brown, 1992). Learning time management is important for women in midlife, for whom setting priorities within multiple role responsibilities is essential. Assertiveness training may also be useful, particularly for women who are entering or reentering employment or school after participating in roles that did not require assertive behavior. Otherwise, stress management techniques need not be different for this age group than for other adults. Relaxation methods include progressive muscle relaxation, a series of isometric contraction and relaxation of large muscle groups, which increases awareness of the difference between tense and relaxed states; guided imagery, in which women can picture themselves in a relaxed, comforting place; and abdominal deep breathing (Rich, 1991).

A useful program of stress management has been developed by the Center for Nursing Research and Clinical Practice at Pace University. It includes assessment, education, and management strategies that can be easily adapted to the needs of women in midlife (Rich, 1991).

Sexuality and Contraception

Sexual function in women as well as men is affected by both biologic and psychosocial factors. The exact role of hormones remains unclear. Lower estrogen levels associated with menopause alter the integrity of the vaginal tissues and blood flow to the pelvic organs, which may affect sexual functioning (Sherwin, 1994). Some women experience changes in their sexual function just before and after the menopause, expressed as a decline in sexual interest, responsiveness, and sexual satisfaction.

Despite the lower levels of hormones in midlife and beyond, sexual desire and activity remain. Women and their partners need information about the physiologic changes of midlife that affect sexual performance. Sexual behaviors may need to be modified, such as allowing adequate time for stimulation, using alternative positions during coitus, using water-soluble lubricants, and identifying alternative forms of sexual behavior. In some instances estrogen or estrogen and androgen therapy may be warranted. One of the effects of estrogen replacement therapy is the return of vaginal circulation to premenopausal levels. Sexually active women, regardless of hormone levels, have less vaginal atrophy and report fewer vaginal symptoms than women who are not sexually active (Bachmann, 1993). Most importantly, couples need to share their problems and desires to successfully deal with the sexual changes that occur with aging.

During the perimenopausal years fertility declines, with a sharp decrease starting at age 40. Evidence suggests, however, that as long as women are having menstrual periods they are potentially fertile. Among women who do become pregnant in midlife, the incidence of miscarriages is higher than for women in their twenties and thirties. Estimates available for U.S. women between 40 and 44 years of age suggest that 71% are at risk of pregnancy, but of these, 46.9% have had tubal ligation and 21.4% have partners who have had a vasectomy (Trussell & Vaughan, 1991).

Many women who delay marriage or remarry do not wish to close the opportunity for childbearing, and so there is a continued need for reversible contraceptive methods for pre- and perimenopausal women. The general recommendation is for women to continue to use contraception for a year after the last menstrual period. Among hormonal methods, recent recommendations are that birth control pills with low doses of estrogen may be used for women in midlife who do not smoke, are not diabetic or hypertensive, or do not have an elevated cholesterol level (Hatcher et al., 1994). Progestin-only methods include the minipill, Depo-Provera injections, and Norplant implants. Depo-Provera produces amenorrhea in the majority of women, so it may be good for perimenopausal women with irregular bleeding and cyclic symptoms (Thorneycroft, 1993). The main drawback with progestin-only methods is that they may cause irregular bleeding, at least initially. If persistent, such bleeding will require further evaluation (Hatcher et al., 1994).

The intrauterine device may be particularly suitable for women over 40 who are parous, do not have dysfunctional bleeding, and are in a mutually monogamous relationship (Thorneycroft, 1993). Barrier methods, including condoms, foam, and diaphragms, remain safe contraceptive options. Condoms are the most frequently used reversible contraceptive method in women aged 40 to 44 (Hatcher et al., 1994). The condom may not be as acceptable to a male partner for whom it takes longer to obtain an erection (Jarrett & Lethbridge, 1990), but for unmarried and divorced women in midlife who are in new relationships and who may be at increased risk for sexually transmitted diseases, the condom affords the same protection as with younger women. The diaphragm has the advantage of offering additional lubrication in women who have less natural lubrication with decreasing estrogen levels. This method may not be suitable, however, for women experiencing pelvic relaxation (Jarrett & Lethbridge, 1990). Natural family planning methods may no longer provide reliable contraception as menstrual cycles become less regular and more cycles are anovulatory.

Strategies for the Maintenance of Health Promotion Behaviors

What motivates individuals to modify their lifestyles to better promote personal health and how individuals maintain these changes is only beginning to be understood. The research to date has been largely empirical and suffers from limited internal or external validity due to design and measurement problems; additionally, there has been little analysis of age or gender differences and few studies have specifically targeted women aged 45 to 64. Because of these problems, it is not yet possible to identify any strategies for health promotion maintenance that are unique for women in midlife. Considering the issues of women's health at midlife in a developmental context, however, offers some important insights for guiding age-appropriate health promotion strategies.

Health Promotion Models

Health Behavior Models

Two models originally developed to assist in changing addictive behaviors have useful applications for health promotion behaviors such as physical activity (Dishman, 1991; King et al., 1992) and weight management (Rimer, 1990). In their Transtheoretical Model, Prochaska and DiClemente (1985) have proposed that behavior change occurs in stages, including contemplation (thinking about change), determination (deciding to change), action (undertaking change), and maintenance. The processes of change differ by the stage of change and include consciousness raising, self-evaluation, self-liberation, contingency management, helping relationships, and stimulus control. In general, verbal processes prepare individuals for action, whereas behavioral strategies are more important in the action and maintenance stages (Rimer, 1990). The stages of change are similar across behaviors and occur regardless of whether change is professionally or self-guided; also, individuals may enter, exit, and reenter at any stage (Rimer, 1990). The Relapse Prevention Theory (Marlatt & Gordon, 1985) complements and supports the Transtheoretical Model. This theory recognizes that relapse is possible at any stage of behavior change, and because different processes operate at each stage, different strategies for preventing and managing relapse are necessary for each stage (Rimer, 1990). Identifying high-risk situations for relapse; planning how to cope with or avoid such situations; expecting and planning for relapses; and techniques for blocking self-talk rationalizing relapse are examples of strategies that support the maintenance of desired changes. Both of these health behavior models emphasize the importance of assessment in identifying the individual's stage of change and of providing a range of options and strategies in managing and maintaining processes of change.

Nursing Models

Pender's Health Promotion Model (HPM) is a complex model proposing that cognitive-perceptual factors of benefits and barriers; definitions, importance, and control of health; and self-efficacy predict the likelihood of engaging in health-promoting behaviors. These cognitive-perceptual factors may be modified by demographic and biologic characteristics, interpersonal influences, and situational and behavioral factors (Pender, 1987). The HPM has had limited application to women in midlife. Gillis and Perry (1991) found that, for women in midlife, the situational factors of homogeneity of age and fitness level, flexible time offerings, and program accessibility as well as the interpersonal influences of family and professional support promoted adherence to a dance exercise program. Duffy (1988) used the HPM to describe the health behaviors of 262 women in midlife. Control of health, self-esteem, health concerns, and education explained 25% of the variance in engaging in health-promoting lifestyle activities, but the issues of maintenance were not explored.

The Interactional Model of Client Health Behavior (IMCHB) (Cox, 1982) relates elements of client singularity (eg, demographic characteristics, intrinsic motivation, cognitive appraisal, and affective response) to health outcomes (eg, adherence to care recommendations). Outcomes result from the interaction between the client and health care provider, in which the professional provides affective support and health information tailored to the client's singularity while supporting the client's decisional control. The IMCHB is unique among the models discussed here because it specifically proposes tailoring health care interventions to the individual as a strategy for maintaining health promotion behaviors. A long-standing problem in women's health care has been that providers have not been sensitive to contextual factors affecting women's lives or supported their decisional control (Dan & Wilbur, 1990). Unfortunately, the tailoring element of the IMCHB has not yet been tested nor have women in midlife been studied using the full model.

Orem's Theory of Self-Care (Orem, 1991) proposes that self-care requisites, or the purposes for which individuals care for themselves, are of three types: universal, performed by all people at all ages (eg, food, activity, rest); developmental, associated with various stages of the life cycle; and health deviation, associated with "human structural and functional deviations" (Orem, 1991, p. 125). Hartweg (1993) used Orem's classification to explore self-care actions related to physical, social, and psychological developmental changes affecting well-being during midlife. The self-care actions used to promote well-being addressed physical, personal, emotional, psychological, vasomotor, and relationship changes the women experienced during middle age, including positive changes such as the increased sense of freedom and a reworking of relationships for greater personal satisfaction first reported by Neugarten (1968). In a more specific analysis of self-care actions of women in midlife, McElmurry and Huddleston (1991) critically reviewed the research regarding how women care for their menopausal symptoms. These two studies are important because they address the lived experiences of women during the developmental changes of midlife and describe how women promote their own health during this time by caring for themselves.

Strategies for Maintaining Specific Behaviors

Exercise and Physical Activity

Enhancing self-regulatory skills through behavioral modification and cognitive-behavioral approaches supports activity maintenance (Dishman, 1991; King et al., 1992). These skills include contracting, preparing a decision balance sheet summarizing the expected benefits and costs of activity, effective goal setting, self-monitoring of progress, self-reinforcement for progress, contingency management, and managing relapses, all of which have been associated with a 10% to 25% increase in activity frequency (Dishman, 1991).

Although individuals may begin a program of physical activity because they know about and believe in the health benefits of exercise, they are most likely to maintain such activity if they enjoy it and do not encounter significant barriers to continuing it (Dishman, 1991; Fogel & Woods, 1995). Women in midlife cite walking for pleasure, walking to a social event, aerobic exercise, using a stationary bike, dancing, swimming, and yoga as their most frequently performed leisure-time physical activities (Wilbur et al., 1993). All of these activities can be performed at a moderate level of intensity, which has been associated with lower dropout rates (Dishman, 1991) and is more likely to allow the participant to feel refreshed and relaxed rather than exhausted (Fogel & Woods, 1995). Convenience, low cost, and flexibility are program factors that support maintenance, with home-based programs providing one model for how these factors can be optimized and barriers minimized (King et al., 1992). Social support from family, friends, and program staff enhances maintenance, with long-term adherence in home-based programs supported through occasional staff phone calls and ongoing reinforcement of self-regulatory skills (King et al., 1992). The overall goal is the flexible integration of moderate physical activity into daily life, either intermittently through several routine activities such as walking or stair climbing or in a single planned exercise session (Pate et al., 1995). Health care providers can assist by providing exercise counseling and prescriptions for women in midlife, tailored to the specific needs and preferences of those in their care (Dishman, 1991; Fogel & Woods, 1995; King et al., 1992).

Weight Control

Most women who lose weight regain it over time (Foreyt & Goodrick, 1991), and most women gain weight with age, often starting around the time of menopause (Heymsfield et al., 1994). Women's changing role patterns may promote or constrain their ability to practice the personal nutrition care they desire (Devine & Olson, 1992), and they may develop their own personalized norms regarding what they should weigh without regard for cultural pressures to be thin or professional criteria for weight management (Allan, 1988). To be effective, health care providers must address these contextual factors as they pertain to an individual's life. Among women who successfully lose weight, relapse prevention in the form of self-monitoring, stimulus control, contingency management, and social support assists in managing temptation to overeat and handling relapses constructively (Foreyt & Goodrick, 1991). Continuing attendance at a peer social support group provides important external social controls, as does support from health care or program providers (Foreyt & Goodrick, 1991). Maintaining patterns of regular exercise is also important for weight control (Foreyt & Goodrick, 1991).

Selected Issues for Women During Midlife: Hormone Replacement Therapy

A great deal of emphasis has been placed on the role of HRT in alleviating vasomotor and vaginal symptoms, preventing coronary heart disease, and promoting bone health. There are several controversies, however, over its effects and uses. Women need to be clearly informed about these so they can assess the benefits of HRT against its risks.

The rationale for HRT is that hormone shifts during the menopausal transition are the major cause of symptom development and increased health risks. Women taking hormones have fewer vasomotor symptoms than women taking placebos, and both local and systemic estrogen have been successful in treating vaginal symptoms (U.S. Congress, OTA, 1992). Additionally, epidemiologic studies indicate a definite protective effect of estrogen in modifying the occurrence of cardiovascular disease and osteoporosis (Christiansen & Riis, 1990; Stampfer et al., 1991).

Several questions remain regarding HRT. First, HRT is thought to provide protection through alterations in plasma concentrations of lipoprotein. Most studies, however, report the effects of estrogen alone; fewer give evidence of the effects of progestin, which is added to prevent endometrial hyperplasia associated with endometrial cancer. The cardiovascular effects of progestin are unclear. Clinical trials have reported that progestin may blunt estrogen's favorable increase of high-density lipoprotein (Walsh et al., 1990). Conversely, Nabulsi et al. (1993) found that the use of estrogen combined with progestin appeared to be associated with a better cardiovascular risk profile than the use of estrogen alone.

Second, concerns remain regarding the effect of exogenous hormones on the breast. Five meta-analyses have examined the literature in this area (Armstrong, 1988; Dupont & Page, 1991; Grady & Ernster, 1991; Sillero-Arenas, Delgado-Rodriguez, Rodrigues-Canteras, Bueno-Cavanillas, & Galvez-Vargas, 1992; Steinberg et al., 1990). None found an association between breast cancer and use of estrogen at any time in a woman's life. However, as Grady and Rubin (1993) point out, the median duration of estrogen replacement therapy is generally only about 2 years; women are often reluctant to comply with a long-term HRT regimen. Reviewing the meta-analyses for implications relating to long-term effects, Grady and Rubin (1993) found that four of the five studies suggested a 23% to 30% increase in breast cancer risk for long-term users of HRT.

Third, HRT is not appropriate for some women. Contraindications to estrogen use include stroke, breast cancer, acute liver disease, pancreatic disease, chronic thrombophlebitis, chronic impaired liver function, recent myocardial infarction, endometrial adenocarcinoma, other estrogen-dependent tumors, gallbladder disease, recent thromboembolic event, and undiagnosed vaginal bleeding (U.S. Congress, OTA, 1992). The only currently approved indications for HRT are for the alleviation of hot flashes and urogenital symptoms and the prevention of osteoporosis and cardiovascular disease in high-risk women.

A variety of different routes of administration, dosages, and treatment regimens may be used for HRT, including oral tablets, transdermal patches, and vaginal creams. For women who have an intact uterus, estrogen is combined with progestin to prevent endometrial overgrowth and irregular bleeding and to decrease the risk of endometrial cancer associated with the unopposed delivery of estrogen. The usual starting dose of oral estrogen is 0.625 mg conjugated estrogens, which is the dose approved by the Food and Drug Administration for both treatment and prevention of osteoporosis. It can be taken either cyclically from calendar day 1 to day 25 or continuously. Progestin 10 mg can be taken on day 14 through day 25 of the cyclic estrogen regimen or from day 1 through day 12 of the continuous estrogen regimen. A third method of delivery is to give combined estrogen with 2.5 mg progestin continuously. This method has the advantage of not having the premenstrual symptom-like side effects of higher dosages (Youngkin, 1990).

The estrogen patch is applied twice a week on dry, hairless skin on the trunk or upper arm. It should not be placed on the breasts because of their sensitivity. Because the estrogen is delivered directly into the systemic circulation, a lower dose (0.05 mg) than with oral administration relieves menopausal symptoms. Like oral estrogen, transdermal estrogen provides beneficial protective effects on the cardiovascular system and bone, although the effects are less immediate; however, unlike oral estrogen, transdermal estrogen does not have adverse gastrointestinal or hypertensive effects (Scharbo-Dehaan, 1994). The estrogen patch is combined with oral progestin therapy when the uterus is present (Youngkin, 1990). The transdermal patch is more costly than oral therapy.

Dyspareunia, pruritus, and decreased vaginal lubrication may be successfully treated with vaginal creams containing estrogen. Premarin cream 0.3 mg does not increase systemic levels of estrogen although a vaginal effect has been documented (Scharbo-Dehaan, 1994). After a loading dose of 2 g daily for 1 to 2 weeks is given, 2 g once or twice a week allows for maintenance.

Hormone replacement therapy is presently the dominant medical treatment for health symptoms and risks related to the menopause, including cardiovascular disease and osteoporosis. Using HRT is not without risks of its own, however, and it is not appropriate or acceptable for all women. Also, studies indicate that most women on HRT take it only sporadically (U.S. Congress, OTA, 1992). Particularly for the risks of cardiovascular disease and osteoporosis, and perhaps for health symptoms management, exercise and a calcium-rich diet might be effective alternatives for or adjuncts to HRT.

Conclusions

The physical and psychosocial changes women experience during midlife, including the menopause and advent of the postparental years, make midlife a time when health needs change and the potential for lasting, effective health promotion increases. With perhaps fewer demands on their time and less responsibility to care for others, women at midlife can turn to a renewed self-care and the more successful maintenance of health promotion behaviors. Gilligan (1982) has proposed that transitions at midlife involve changes in the understandings of the activities of care, so that helping women to care for themselves in new ways as a result of their developmental changes may be the optimum strategy for promoting the health of women in midlife. Health care providers sensitive to these changes can encourage and support women in their efforts to increase their physical activity, practice personal nutritional care and more effective stress management, and enjoy their sexuality. Using targeted assessments of the stages of change, providers can teach self-regulation skills and relapse prevention tailored to the needs of individual women to assist them in enhancing their self-care. As the prime of life (Fogel & Woods, 1995; Mitchell & Helson, 1990), midlife may be the ideal time for doing this, not only to enhance well-being and health during the middle years, but also as preparation for healthful aging.

References

Allan, J. D. (1988). Knowing what to weigh: Women's self-care activities related to weight. *Advances in Nursing Science, 11*(1), 47-60.

American Heart Association. (1991). *1992 Heart and stroke facts.* Dallas, TX: Author.

Armstrong, B. (1988). Estrogen therapy after the menopause—boon or bane? *Medical Journal of Australia, 148,* 213-214.

Avioli, L. V. (1991). Significance of osteoporosis: A growing international health care problem. *Calcified Tissue International, 49*(Suppl.), S5-S7.

Avis, N. E., & McKinlay, S. M. (1991). A longitudinal analysis of women's attitudes toward the menopause: Results from the Massachusetts Women's Health Study. *Maturitas, 13,* 65-79.

Bachmann, G. A. (1993). Sexual function in the perimenopause. *Obstetrics and Gynecology Clinics of North America, 20,* 379-389.

Barnett, R. C., Marshall, N. L., & Singer, J. D. (1992). Job experiences over time, multiple roles, and women's mental health: A longitudinal study. *Journal of Personality and Social Psychology, 62,* 634-644.

Baranowski, T., Bouchard, C., Bar-Or, O., Bricker, T., et al. (1992). Assessment, prevalence, and cardiovascular benefits of physical activity and fitness in youth. *Medicine and Science in Sports and Exercise, 24*(Suppl.), S237-S247.

Blair, S. N., Kohl, H. W., Paffenbarger, R. S., Clark, D. G., Cooper, K. H., & Gibbons, L. W. (1989). Physical fitness and all-cause mortality: A prospective study of healthy men and women. *Journal of the American Medical Association, 262,* 2395-2401.

Busch, C. M., Zonderman, A. B., & Costa, P. T., Jr. (1994). Menopausal transition and psychological distress in a nationally representative sample: Is menopause associated with psychological distress? *Journal of Aging and Health, 6,* 209-228.

Centers for Disease Control and Prevention. (1993). Prevalence of sedentary lifestyle: Behavioral risk factor surveillance system, United States, 1991. *Morbidity and Mortality Weekly Report, 42,* 576-579.

Choi, P. Y. L., Van Horn, J. D., Picker, D. E., & Roberts, H. I. (1993). Mood changes in women after an aerobics class: A preliminary study. *Health Care for Women International, 14,* 167-177.

Christiansen, C., & Riis, B. J. (1990). Five years with continuous combined oestrogen/progestogen therapy: Effects on calcium metabolism, lipoproteins, and bleeding pattern. *British Journal of Obstetrics and Gynaecology, 97,* 1087-1092.

Cox, C. L. (1982). An interaction model of client health behavior: Theoretical prescription for nursing. *Advances in Nursing Science, 5,* 41-56.

Dalsky, G. P., Stocke, K. S., Ehsani, A. A., Slatopolsky, E., Lee, W. C., Birge, S. J., Jr. (1988). Weight-bearing exercise training and lumbar bone mineral content in postmenopausal women. *Annals of Internal Medicine, 108,* 824-828.

Dan, A., & Wilbur, J. (1990). Foreword: Women's health. *Family & Community Health,* 13, vi-vii.

Dan, A., Wilbur, J., Hedricks, C., O'Connor, E., & Holm, K. (1990). Lifelong physical activity in midlife and older women. *Psychology of Women Quarterly, 14,* 537-542.

Dennerstein, L., Smith, A. M. A., Morse, C., Burger, H., Green, A., Hopper, J., & Ryan, M. (1993). Menopausal symptoms in Australian women. *Medical Journal of Australia, 159,* 232-236.

Dequeker, J., Nijs, J., Verstraeten, N. A., Guesens, P., & Gevers, G. (1987). Genetic determinants of bone mineral content at the spine and radius: A twin study. *Bone, 8,* 207-209.

Devine, C. M., & Olson, C. M. (1992). Women's perceptions about the way social roles promote or constrain personal nutrition care. *Women & Health, 19,* 79-95.

Dishman, R. K. (1991). Increasing and maintaining exercise and physical activity. *Behavior Therapy, 22,* 345-378.

Duffy, M. E. (1988). Determinants of health promotion in midlife women. *Nursing Research, 37,* 358-362.

DuPont, W. D., & Page, D. L. (1991). Menopausal estrogen replacement therapy and breast cancer. *Archives of Internal Medicine, 151,* 67-72.

Engeland, G. M., Kuller, L. H., Matthews, K. A., et al. (1990). Hormone replacement therapy and lipoprotein changes during early menopause. *Obstetrics and Gynecology, 76,* 5.

Erikson, E. H. (1982). *The life cycle completed.* New York: Norton.

Erlik, Y., Meldrum, D. R., & Judd, H. L. (1982). Estrogen levels in postmenopausal women with hot flashes. *Obstetrics and Gynecology, 59,* 403-407.

Fogel, C. I., & Woods, N. F. (1995). Midlife women's health. In C. I. Fogel & N. F. Woods (Eds.), *Women's health care: A comprehensive handbook* (pp. 79-100). Thousand Oaks, CA: Sage.

Folkman, S., & Lazarus, R. (1988). *Ways of Coping Questionnaire.* Palo Alto, CA: Consulting Psychologists Press.

Foreyt, J. P., & Goodrick, G. K. (1991). Factors common to successful therapy for the obese patient. *Medicine and Science in Sports and Exercise, 23,* 292-297.

Gilligan, C. (1982). Adult development and women's development: Arrangements for a marriage. In J. Z. Giele (Ed.), *Women in the middle years: Current knowledge and directions for research and policy* (pp. 89-114). New York: John Wiley & Sons.

Gillis, A., & Perry, A. (1991). The relationships between physical activity and health-promoting behaviours in mid-life women. *Journal of Advanced Nursing, 16,* 299-310.

Gizis, F. C. (1992). Nutrition in women across the life span. *Nursing Clinics of North America, 27,* 971-982.

Gordon, T., Kannel, W. B., Hjortland, M. C., & McNamara, P. M. (1978). Menopause and coronary heart disease: The Framingham study. *Annals of Internal Medicine, 89,* 157-161.

Grady, D., & Ernster, V. (1991). Does postmenopausal hormone therapy cause breast cancer? *American Journal of Epidemiology, 134,* 1396-1400.

Grady, D., & Rubin, S. (1993). The postmenopausal estrogen/breast cancer controversy [Letter]. *Journal of the American Medical Association, 269,* 990.

Hammar, M., Berg, G., & Lindgren, R. (1990). Does physical exercise influence the frequency of postmenopausal hot flushes? *Acta Obstetricia et Gynecologica Scandinavica, 69,* 409-412.

Hartweg, D. L. (1993). Self-care actions of healthy middle-aged women to promote well-being. *Nursing Research, 42,* 221-227.

Haskell, W. L., Leon, A. S., Caspersen, C. J., Froelicher, V. F., Hagberg, J. M., Harlan, W., Holloszy, J. O., Regensteiner, J. G., Thompson, P. D., Washburn, R. A., & Wilson, P. W. F. (1992). Cardiovascular benefits and assessments of physical activity and physical fitness in adults. *Medicine and Science in Sports and Exercise, 24*(Suppl. 6), S201-S220.

Hatcher, R. A., Trussell, J., Stewart, F., Stewart, G. K., Kowal, D., Guest, F., Cates, W., Jr., & Policar, M. S. (1994). *Contraceptive technology* (16th rev. ed.). New York: Irvington Publishers.

Heber, D., McCarthy, W. J., Ashley, J., & Byerly, L. O. (1989). Weight reduction for breast cancer prevention by restriction of dietary fat and calories: Rationale, mechanisms, and interventions. *Nutrition, 5*(3), 149-154.

Heymsfield, S. B., Gallagher, D., Poehlman, E. T., Wolper, C., et al. (1994). Menopausal changes in body composition and energy expenditure. *Experimental Gerontology, 29,* 377-389.

Holmes, T., & Rahe, R. (1967). The Social Readjustment Rating Scale. *Journal of Psychosocial Research, 10,* 213-217.

Hopper, J. L., & Seeman, E. (1994). The bone density of female twins discordant for tobacco use. *New England Journal of Medicine, 330,* 387-392.

Hoyer, W. J., & Rybash, J. M. (1994). Characterizing adult cognitive development. *Journal of Adult Development, 1,* 7-12.

Jarrett, M. E., & Lethbridge, D. J. (1990). The contraceptive needs of midlife women. *Nurse Practitioner, 15* (12), 34-39.

Kanner, A. D., Coyne, J. C., Schaefer, C., & Lazarus, R. S. (1981). Comparison of two modes of stress measurement: Daily hassles and uplifts versus major life events. *Journal of Behavioral Medicine, 4,* 1-39.

Kaufert, P. A., Gilbert, P., & Hassard, T. (1988). Researching the symptoms of menopause: An exercise in methodology. *Maturitas, 10,* 117-131.

King, A. C., Blair, S. N., Bild, D. E., Dishman, R. K., Dubbert, P. M., Marcus, B. H., Oldridge, N. B., Paffenbarger, R. S., Powell, K. E., & Yeager, K. K. (1992). Determinants of physical activity and interventions in adults. *Medicine and Science in Sports and Exercise, 24* (Suppl. 6), S221-S236.

King, A. C., Haskell, W. L., Taylor, C. B., Kraemer, H. C., & DeBusk, R. F. (1991). Group- vs. home-based exercise training in healthy older men and women: A community-based clinical trial. *Journal of the American Medical Association, 266,* 1535-1542.

Manderino, M. A., & Brown, M. C. (1992). A practical, step-by-step approach to stress management for women. *Nurse Practitioner, 17,* 18-28.

Marlatt, G. A., & Gordon, J. R. (1985). *Relapse prevention.* New York: Guilford Press.

Matthews, K. A., Wing, R. R., Kuller, L. H., Meilahn, E. N., Kelsey, S. F., Costello, E. J., & Caggiula, A. W. (1990). Influences of natural menopause on psychological characteristics and symptoms of middle-aged healthy women. *Journal of Consulting and Clinical Psychology, 58,* 345-351.

McAdams, D. P., de St. Aubin, E., & Logan, R. L. (1993). Generativity among young, midlife, and older adults. *Psychology and Aging, 8,* 221-230.

McElmurry, B. J., & Huddleston, D. S. (1991). Self-care and menopause: Critical review of research. *Health Care for Women International, 12,* 15-26.

McKinlay, S. M., Brambilla, D. J., & Posner, J. G. (1992). The normal menopause transition. *Maturitas, 14,* 103-115.

Miller, A., Wilbur, J., & Montgomery, A. (1996). Psychological well-being and perceived quality of social roles in midlife women. (Submitted)

Mitchell, V., & Helson, R. (1990). Women's prime of life: Is it the 50's? *Psychology of Women Quarterly, 14,* 451-470.

Monti, D., Troiano, L., Tropea, F., Grassilli, E., Cossarizza, A., Barozzi, D., Pelloni, M. C., Tamassia, M. G., Bellomo, G., & Franceschi, C. (1992). Apoptosis-programmed cell death: A role in the aging process? *American Journal of Clinical Nutrition 55* (Suppl.), 1208S-1215S.

Murray, R. B., & Zentner, J. P. (1993). *Nursing assessment and health promotion: Strategies through the life span* (5th ed.). Norwalk, CT: Appleton & Lange.

Nabulsi, A. A., Folsom, A. R., White, A., Patsch, W., Heiss, G., Wu, K. K., & Szklo, M. (1993). Association of hormone-replacement-therapy with various cardiovascular risk factors in post-menopausal women. *New England Journal of Medicine, 328,* 1069-1075.

Neugarten, B. L. (1968). The awareness of middle age. In B. L. Neugarten (Ed.), *Middle age and aging: A reader in social psychology* (pp. 93-98). Chicago: University of Chicago.

Notelovitz, M. (1990). Exercise and health maintenance in menopausal women. *Annals of the New York Academy of Sciences, 592,* 204-220.

Orem, D. E. (1991). *Nursing: Concepts of practice* (4th ed.). St. Louis: Mosby-Yearbook.

Pate, R. R., Pratt, M., Blair, S. N., Haskell, W. L., Macera, C. A., et al. (1995). Physical activity and public health: A recommendation from the Centers for Disease Control and Prevention and the American College of Sports Medicine. *Journal of the American Medical Association, 273,* 402-407.

Pender, N. J. (1987). *Health promotion in nursing practice* (2nd ed.). Norwalk, CT: Appleton & Lange.

Pollock, M. L., & Wilmore, J. H. (1990). *Exercise in health and disease* (2nd ed.). Philadelphia: W. B. Saunders.

Prochaska, J. O., & DiClemente, C. C. (1985). Common processes of self-change in smoking, weight control, and psychological distress. In S. Shiffman & T. Wills (Eds.) *Coping and substance use* (pp. 345-364). Orlando, FL: Academic Press.

Pruzansky, M. E., Turano, M., Luckey, M., & Senie, R. (1987). Low body weight as a risk factor for hip fracture in both black and white women. *Journal of Orthopaedic Research, 7,* 192-197.

Raglin, J. S. (1990). Exercise and mental health: Beneficial and detrimental effects. *Sports Medicine, 9,* 323-329.

RDA Subcommittee. (1989). *Recommended dietary allowances.* Washington, DC: National Academy of Sciences.

Rich, E. R. (1991). *Personal health management program: Stress management.* New York: Pace University, Lienhard School of Nursing, University Health Care Unit, Center for Nursing Research and Clinical Practice.

Riggs, B. L., & Melton, L. J., III. (1986). Involutional osteoporosis. *New England Journal of Medicine, 314,* 1676-1686.

Rimer, B. K. (1990). Perspective on intrapersonal theory in health education and health behavior. In K. Glanz, F. M. Lewis, & B. K. Rimer (Eds.), *Health behavior and health education: Theory, research, and practice* (pp. 140-157). San Francisco: Jossey-Bass.

Rosenberg, I. (1991). Nutrition and aging. In G. E. Gaull, F. N. Kotsonis, & M. A. Mackey (Eds.), *Nutrition in the '90s.* New York: Marcel Dekker.

Scharbo-Dehaan, M. (1994). Management strategies for hormonal replacement therapy. *Nurse Practitioner, 19* (12), 47-48, 50-52, 55-56.

Sherman, B. M., Wallace, R. B., Bean, J. A., Change, Y., & Schlabaugh, L. (1981). The relationship of menopausal hot flushes to medical and reproductive experience. *Journal of Gerontology, 36,* 306-309.

Sherwin, B. B. (1994). Sex hormones and psychological functioning in postmenopausal women. *Experimental Gerontology, 29,* 423-430.

Sillero-Arenas, M., Delgado-Rodriguez, M., Rodrigues-Canteras, R., Bueno-Cavanillas, A., & Galvez-Vargas, R. (1992). Menopausal hormone replacement therapy and breast cancer: A meta-analysis. *Obstetrics and Gynecology, 79,* 286-294.

Silverman, S. L., & Madison, R. E. (1988). Decreased incidence of hip fracture in Hispanics, Asians, and blacks: California hospital discharge data. *American Journal of Public Health, 78,* 1482-1483.

Smith, E. L., Gilligan, C., McAdam, M., Ensign, C. P., & Smith, P. E. (1989). Deterring bone loss by exercise intervention in premenopausal and postmenopausal women. *Calcified Tissue International, 44,* 312-321.

Stampfer, M. J., Colditz, G. A., & Willett, W. C. (1990). Menopause and heart disease: A review. *Annals of the New York Academy of Sciences, 6,* 193-203.

Stampfer, M. J., Colditz, G. A., Willett, W. C., Manson, J. E., Rosner, B., Speizer, F. E., & Hennekens, C. H. (1991). Postmenopausal estrogen therapy and cardiovascular disease: Ten-year follow-up from the Nurses' Health Study. *New England Journal of Medicine, 325,* 756-762.

Steinberg, K., Thacker, S., Smith, S., Stroup, D., Zack, M., Flanders, D., & Berkelman, R. (1990). A meta-analysis of the effect of estrogen replacement therapy on the risk of breast cancer. *Journal of the American Medical Association, 265,* 1985-1990.

Thorneycroft, I. H. (1993). Contraception in women older than 40 years of age. *Obstetrics and Gynecology Clinics of North America, 20,* 273-278.

Trussell, J., & Vaughan, B. (1991). *Selected results concerning sexual behavior and contraceptive use from the 1988 National Survey of Family Growth and the 1988 National Survey of Adolescent Males* (Working Paper #91-12). Princeton, NJ: Office of Population Research, Princeton University.

U.S. Congress. Office of Technology Assessment. (1992). *The menopause, hormone therapy, and women's health* (OTA-BP-BA-88). Washington, DC: U.S. Government Printing Office.

U.S. Departments of Agriculture and Health and Human Services. (1990). *Nutrition and your health: Dietary guidelines for Americans* (3rd ed.). Washington, DC: U.S. Government Printing Office.

U.S. Department of Health and Human Services. (1991). *Healthy people 2000: National health promotion and disease prevention objectives* (DHHS Publication No. PHS 91-50212). Washington, DC: U.S. Government Printing Office.

U.S. Department of Health and Human Services. Public Health Service. (1994). *Clinician's handbook of clinical preventive services.* Washington, DC: U.S. Government Printing Office.

Waldron, I., & Jacobs, J. A. (1989). Effects of multiple roles on women's health—Evidence from a national longitudinal study. *Women & Health, 15,* 3-19.

Walsh, B. W., Schiff, I., Rosner, B., Greenberg, L., Raunikar, V., & Sacks, F. M. (1990). Effects of postmenopausal estrogen replacement on the concentrations and metabolism of plasma lipoproteins. *New England Journal of Medicine, 325,* 1196-1204.

Wardlaw, G. (1988). The effects of diet and life-style on bone mass in women. *Journal of the American Dietetic Association, 88,* 17-22.

Wilbur, J., Dan, A. J., Montgomery, A., & Holm, K. (1994). Aerobic fitness and body mass protect against bone loss in healthy midlife women. *Menopause: The Journal of the North American Menopause Society, 1,* 181-190.

Wilbur, J., Holm, K., & Dan, A. (1992). The relationship of energy expenditure to physical and psychological symptoms in women at midlife. *Nursing Outlook, 40,* 269-276.

Wilbur, J., Holm, K., & Dan, A. (1993). A quantitative survey to measure energy expenditure in midlife women. *Journal of Nursing Measurement, 1,* 29-40.

Wilbur, J., Miller, A., & Montgomery A. (1995). The influence of demographic characteristics, menopausal status, and symptoms on women's attitudes toward menopause. *Women and Health, 23* (3), 19–39.

Wilbur, J., Miller, A., & Montgomery A. (1995, June). *Menopausal status, body composition and symptoms in midlife women.* Paper presented at the Society for Menstrual Cycle Research Conference, Montreal, Canada.

Women's Bureau. (1992, November). *The status of working women: A statistical profile of midlife women aged 35-54.* Washington, DC: U.S. Department of Labor, Office of the Secretary, Women's Bureau.

Youngkin, E. Q. (1990). Estrogen replacement therapy and the Estraderm transdermal system. *Nurse Practitioner, 15* (5), 19-20, 22-24, 26, 31.

Youngkin, E. Q., & Davis, M. S. (1994). *Women's health: A primary care clinical guide.* Norwalk, CT: Appleton & Lange.

CHAPTER 5

Preventive Health Issues: The Perimenopausal to Mature Years (45–64)

Nancy Fugate Woods
Ellen Sullivan Mitchell

Introduction

Women in midlife comprise a rapidly growing segment of the U.S. population. As the baby boomers age, this large cohort has drawn increasing attention to health in anticipation of the cost for their health care as they grow older. Increased life expectancy for women warrants attention to prevention of disease and morbidity in their later years. Women born during the decade after World War II will have an average life expectancy of 69 to 73 years, with an estimated 70 to 74 years for Caucasian women and 61 to 66 years for African American women and other women of color. Estimates that nearly half of these women will live one-third of their lives after they experience menopause at about age 51 are thus plausible (U.S. Bureau of the Census, 1975).

Women have benefited from improved living conditions and treatment of infectious diseases, as have men, but the reduction in maternal mortality has given women a longevity advantage of nearly 7 years over men. Women's longer lifespan may be simultaneously advantageous and disadvantageous because their increasing years often include an increased likelihood of experiencing diseases related to aging.

This chapter reviews the major causes of mortality and morbidity for midlife (ages 45–64) and older women as a basis for considering prevention of disease during midlife. The chapter begins with a discussion of defining characteristics of midlife. A review of mortality and morbidity statistics for women during midlife and old age follows. The chapter concludes with an examination of the ways women can help prevent morbidity and mortality in their middle and older years through preventive self-care activities and the use of preventive clinical services.

Defining Characteristics of Midlife

The defining characteristics of midlife have blurred as women's roles in society have changed. Early works about midlife grounded the definition in the change in women's roles from mothering and homemaking to being employed outside the home after their children had grown. Some used menopause as a marker for midlife, linking this part of life to the end of reproductive function. Still others used age ranges, such as 45 to 64, as a boundary for this part of life (Brooks-Gunn & Kirsch, 1984). Regardless of the definition used to bound midlife, it is important to appreciate the sociopolitical situations in which an age cohort of women arrive at midlife. Each cohort of women has experienced the early part of their lifespan in a historically unique fashion, so each birth cohort is likely to have a unique perspective from which to view the world as well as some unique health problems and exposure to health services. Because many health statistics are calculated based on the age band of 45 to 64 years for midlife, this age-based definition of midlife is used in this chapter.

Causes of Morbidity and Mortality

Midlife is often the period of life during which women experience their first chronic illness. Many of the causes of morbidity during this part of the lifespan portend future problems that may account for causes of death as women age. Indeed, heart disease, cancer, and stroke together account for 67% of all women's deaths (National Center for Health Statistics, 1992).

Leading causes of death in order of their incidence for women aged 45 to 54 years include malignant neoplasms, heart disease, cerebrovascular disease, accidents, liver disease, suicide, chronic obstructive pulmonary disease (COPD), diabetes, pneumonia, and homicide. For women 55 to 64 years old, leading causes of death include malignant neoplasms, heart disease, cerebrovascular disease, COPD, pneumonia, diabetes, liver disease, accidents, suicide, and homicide (National Center for Health Statistics 1993c).

As mortality is postponed by women's increasing lifespan, morbidity becomes compressed into the later years of life. Nonetheless, morbidity, particularly that due to chronic illness, frequently occurs during the middle years. During midlife, more than 10% of women experience each of the following chronic conditions: arthritis, hypertension, chronic sinusitis, skeletal deformity or orthopedic impairment, and heart disease. A smaller but significant proportion, over 5%, experience hearing impairment, chronic bronchitis, hemorrhoids, asthma, and diabetes. From 1% to 3% of women in midlife experience visual impairment, cataracts, ulcer, abdominal hernia, and emphysema (National Center for Health Statistics, 1993a). Women experience more disability as they age than do men. They have 33% more days of limited activity and 37% more days when they are bedridden than do men (National Center for Health Statistics, 1993b).

Women 45 to 64 years of age are hospitalized most frequently for heart disease, malignant neoplasms, cholelithiasis, benign neoplasms, psychoses, and diabetes. The most common procedures women undergo are hysterectomy, oophorectomy and salpingo-oophorectomy, cardiac catheterization, cholecystectomy, excision or destruction of intervertebral disc and spinal fusion, diagnostic dilation and curettage of the uterus, and biopsies of the integumentary system. (National Center for Health Statistics, 1993b).

Although some risk factors for disease, such as age, cannot be changed, many can be altered. Altering these risk factors depends on motivation and ability to change behavior. Modifying one's lifestyle requires not only individual but also group and community efforts.

When all causes of death and morbidity are considered, a few risk factors are associated with many diseases and these can be modified during midlife through individual and social actions. Three of the most important risk factors for diseases that account for morbidity and mortality during the middle and older years are smoking, the quality of dietary intake, and sedentary lifestyle. Smoking is associated with lung cancer, coronary artery disease (CAD), cerebrovascular disease, peripheral vascular disease, cervical cancer, hypertension, osteoporosis, a variety of respiratory diseases (eg, COPD), and injuries due to fires. Diets high in animal fat and low in fruits and vegetables are linked to colon cancer as well as obesity and sedentary lifestyle (Giovannucci et al., 1995; Manson et al., 1990; Thun et al., 1992). Other dietary risk factors include a low calcium intake associated with osteoporosis. In addition, recent evidence suggests that body mass index and weight gain are associated with diabetes mellitus in women (Colditz, Willett, Rotnitzky, & Manson, 1995), which in itself is a risk factor in women for CAD (Barrett-Connor, Cohn, Wingard, & Edelstein, 1991). Obesity is also linked to risk of CAD in women (Manson et al., 1990).

Primary Prevention Strategies

Avoiding or stopping risky behaviors linked to health problems constitute primary prevention efforts. Seeking early detection of disease by using clinical preventive services represents secondary prevention, and pursuing activities to prevent complications of existing disease involves tertiary prevention efforts. Because women have traditionally assumed responsibility for their families, their efforts at prevention for themselves will also benefit their families. Health behaviors with the greatest effects on lowering the incidence of death and disease include smoking cessation, dietary modification, maintenance of ideal weight, and regular exercise.

Smoking Cessation

Smoking cessation is one of the most important behavioral changes a woman can make to improve her health and prevent disease. Nearly 25% of women smoke during midlife, with a larger proportion of Native American (28%) and Puerto Rican (30%) than Caucasian women doing so. Older women are likely to be heavier smokers and are also less likely to quit smoking than younger women (Centers for Disease Control and Prevention [CDC], 1991). Women who are poor and less well educated are more likely to smoke than their wealthier and better educated counterparts.

Quitting smoking for 10 years reduces women's risk of lung cancer by 30% to 50% (CDC, 1990). Women who stop smoking reduce their risk of cardiovascular disease mortality by 24% within 2 years of quitting and approach the risk of those who never smoked for both total cancer and heart disease mortality after 10 to 14 years of abstinence (Kawachi et al., 1993). The risk of stroke declines substantially within

2 to 4 years after cessation of smoking regardless of age at starting and the number of cigarettes smoked (Kawachi et al., 1993). These important facts make smoking cessation a significant preventive effort.

Understanding why women smoke is critical to targeting smoking cessation programs. Waldron's (1991) extensive review of gender differences in smoking led her to conclude that women smoke to control their weight and to reduce stress and negative moods. For example, women use cigarette smoking to regulate moods and cope with the stresses of relentless child care in the context of strained financial resources (Romans, McNoe, Herbison, Walton, & Mullen, 1993). Increasing social acceptance of women smoking and advertising to recruit women smokers have created a normative shift supportive of women smokers. Together, changing norms about women smoking and women's own uses of smoking for managing weight and stress help account for gender differences in starting and stopping smoking.

The U.S. Preventive Services Task Force (1989) recommended that all patients who smoked cigarettes, pipes, or cigars or who used smokeless tobacco receive tobacco use counseling and that some may benefit from treatment with nicotine gum as an adjunct to counseling. The Task Force concluded that the most effective smoking cessation programs were multimodal programs that included counseling by physicians and nonphysicians plus providing reinforcement over a longer period of time in conjunction with nicotine supplement. Aspects of smoking cessation counseling recommended by the Task Force included direct face-to-face advice and suggestions provided in a brief, unambiguous, and informative statement on the need to stop using tobacco. Reviewing the short- and long-term health, social, and economic benefits of quitting and fostering the smoker's belief in the ability to stop were also seen as important. Recommendations included:

- addressing the person's concerns and barriers to stopping, such as age, social environment, nicotine dependence, and general health
- obtaining a specific quit date
- preparing them for withdrawal symptoms
- providing reassurance to those who had relapsed before long-term smoking cessation was achieved after they had made several unsuccessful attempts to quit

Scheduled reinforcement, including support visits or follow-up telephone calls, especially during the first 4 to 8 weeks, made cessation more effective. Providing self-help packages available from voluntary organizations in most communities to aid smokers who quit on their own was also helpful. Referral to community programs through local hospitals, health departments, community health centers, work sites, commercial services, and voluntary organizations was also recommended. Finally, prescription of nicotine gum was recommended as an adjunct to counseling, thought to facilitate cessation by relieving withdrawal symptoms. Smokers should be counseled to stop smoking completely before using nicotine gum and instructed to chew it slowly and intermittently over 20 to 30 minutes to aid absorption through the buccal mucosa. Gum should be used for 4 to 6 months as needed (U.S. Preventive Services Task Force, 1989). More recently transdermal nicotine is recommended as an alternative to nicotine gum to use with smoking cessation counseling. The patch is better tolerated than the gum except for transient mild skin irritation in 50% to 60% of those who use it. On the horizon are newer nicotine formulations such as a nasal spray and a nicotine inhaler (Medical Letter, 1995).

Other factors that help smoking cessation are work sites with no-smoking policies. In one study 53% of women employees reduced their smoking as a result of such a policy (Kinne, Kristal, White, & Hunt, 1993).

Exploration of why women do not use smoking cessation programs revealed several barriers as exemplified in a study of African American women living in Chicago public housing (Lacey et al., 1993). These barriers included:

- managing their lives in highly stressful environments
- major isolation within their environments
- smoking as a pleasure attainable with limited financial resources
- perceived minimal health risk related to smoking
- commonality of smoking within their communities
- scarcity of information about the process of cessation
- belief that all that was needed was self-determination

Although these reasons were derived from a population of women with limited resources, some may be applicable to women whose life circumstances reflect greater social privilege. Individual efforts to quit smoking often are impeded by withdrawal symptoms, problems related to weight gain after smoking cessation, difficulty acquiring prescriptions such as nicotine gum or the nicotine patch, and membership in a social network or work setting where smoking occurs. However, even in no-smoking workplaces, women in low status jobs and with little control over their work had difficulty stopping smoking (Hibbard, 1993).

Women's experiences with relapse after participation in smoking cessation programs are related to a variety of factors. Sixty-two percent of women participating in a multicomponent 8-week cessation program for women completed the program and over half had stopped smoking for 6 months after completion of the program. Factors influencing successful program outcome included their history of asthma, smoking status of the woman's mother when she was a child, eating patterns including weekly consumption of chocolate and candy, and number of children the woman had at home (Jensen & Coambs, 1994). Evidence that personal health status, family drug history, current lifestyle, and social environments influenced program outcome is consistent with findings from other studies.

Physiologic response to nicotine is also likely to influence smoking cessation success. Women with greater systolic blood pressure reactivity to cognitive stress experienced a shorter time to relapse (Swan, Ward, Jack, & Javitz, 1993). Nicotine dose seems to affect women's experience of weight gain after smoking cessation, with higher doses in the patch being related to weight loss rather than to weight gain (Leischow, Sachs, Bostrom, & Hansen, 1992).

The social context in which a woman lives and works also can be supportive or nonsupportive of her smoking cessation efforts. Living with a smoking spouse or working in an environment in which many people smoke makes it difficult to quit. Education for prevention and smoking cessation is increasingly being provided in workplaces and with community reinforcement. Women who have been able to stop smoking can be particularly influential in encouraging others to model their behavior rather than succumbing to advertisements that use women's bodies to sell tobacco.

Modifying Dietary Intake

Modifying dietary intake, like smoking cessation, requires a lifestyle change. As a result of the complexity of changing dietary intake patterns, women's efforts to institute such changes are often unsuccessful. Interventions that are multimodal and focus on the individual woman and her social environment are most likely to be successful.

As women age, metabolic rates decrease. Coupled with decreasing exercise levels, the changing metabolic rate requires a downward adjustment in caloric intake for weight maintenance. At midlife, women should select foods for high nutrient content with low or moderate caloric content. One example is drinking skim milk instead of whole milk. The U.S. Preventive Services Task Force (1989) recommended that clinicians provide counseling regarding dietary intake of calories, fat (especially saturated), cholesterol, complex carbohydrates (starches), fiber, and sodium.

Calcium

Requirements for calcium have been reevaluated recently because of evidence that a woman's risk of osteoporosis increases in midlife. Their increased risk is based on dietary surveys that reveal women's usual daily intake of calcium is less than half the amount needed to maintain bone mass. Recent recommendations are 1000 mg/d for women from age 25 until menopause, 1200 mg daily for women from puberty to age 25 and postmenopausal women taking estrogen, and 1500 mg/d for postmenopausal women not taking estrogen (Bilezikian & Silverberg, 1992). In addition to increasing calcium intake, women should be aware that high-protein diets and a high caffeine intake increase renal calcium excretion and induce acidosis that stimulates bone resorption.

Fiber and Fluid

Fluid intake should include eight to ten 8-ounce glasses of water per day to meet metabolic needs and temperature regulation. With aging, the gastrointestinal tract becomes less efficient. Increasing fluid and fiber content helps prevent constipation. The role of fiber intake in decreasing the rate of colorectal cancer, minimizing glucose intolerance, facilitating weight reduction, limiting development of lipid disorders, and preventing diverticular disease is gaining increased attention (U.S. Preventive Task Force, 1989). Recent studies indicate that a high-fiber diet in premenopausal women produced a decrease in both estradiol and sex hormone-binding globulin (SHBG) levels (Goldin et al., 1994).

Fat Intake

Most studies of dietary fat reduction have been done with men and have emphasized the benefits for lipid metabolism. However, studies of women regarding lipids and CAD indicate that high-density lipoprotein (HDL) cholesterol is a strong predictor (Kannel, 1987). To date, the role of fat reduction and HDL level is unclear. Currently, the consequences of a low-fat diet for reducing cancer risk, including breast and colon cancer, are being studied.

Studies reported to date indicate that women can make dramatic reduction in dietary fat intake and maintain the change. The Women's Health Trial Vanguard Study (Henderson et al., 1990; Insull et al., 1990) randomized 303 women, aged 45 to 69, who were at increased risk for breast cancer to an intensive dietary modification intervention or control group. Women in the intervention group met in small groups of approximately eight each with a nutritionist for 8 sessions each week, 4 sessions bimonthly, and subsequently monthly sessions. The nutritionist acted as an educator, facilitator, and diet counselor using behavioral as well as nutritional sciences to guide the intervention. Each woman developed her own individual and flexible plan to achieve the dietary goal, which was a reduction of calories from fat to 20%. Processes of food selection, preparation of foods, and portion size selection were included in the intervention. Women kept 4-day food records as a basis for evaluating the effectiveness of the intervention. Women in the intervention group reduced the percent of calories from fat from 39% to 20% at 6 months, 21.6% at 12 months, and 22.6% at 24 months. The women who did not receive the intervention consumed 39% of calories from fat before the intervention and 37% at the end of the study. Women in the treatment group reduced their cholesterol intake by 50% and increased their carbohydrate intake. A second study of 1700 women confirmed the results with a streamlined intervention process (Henderson et al., 1992). Of interest was that 73 postmenopausal women from this study who were not taking hormone replacement therapy reduced their total cholesterol by 12 mg/dL, with a reduction in low-density lipoprotein (LDL), not HDL, and lost 3.4 kg of weight after 10 to 22 weeks of intervention. At follow-up after 1 year, fat intake had increased by only 1.4%. Another outcome was the reduction of plasma estradiol by 17% among postmenopausal women, thought to be an important link to the effects of dietary fat on cancer. Fat, particularly polyunsaturated and short chain fatty acids, may increase hormone concentrations by interfering with binding of gonadal steroids to binding proteins, such as SHBG (Prentice et al., 1990).

A recent study of dietary factors in relation to serum gonadal hormone concentrations in 325 healthy Massachusetts women aged 50 to 60 who had a normal menstrual period within the previous year revealed that neither total fat intake nor fat components of the diet influenced hormone concentrations (London, Willett, Longcope, & McKinlay, 1991). In contrast, when dietary intake of fat and fiber were studied in premenopausal women under controlled dietary conditions, change to a low-fat (20–25% of calories from fat) condition significantly decreased estrone, estrone sulfate, testosterone, androstenedione, and SHBG. In another study changing dietary fat intake alone decreased androstenedione levels (Goldin et al., 1994).

The U.S. Preventive Services Task Force (1989) recommends reducing dietary fat to less than 30% of caloric intake. Dietary modifications should include increased amounts of whole grain foods and cereals, vegetables and fruits, and complex carbohydrates and fiber. These have a lower average caloric density and are preferred for maintaining caloric balance and healthful body weight (Fogel & Woods, 1995; U.S.

Preventive Services Task Force, 1989). These guidelines are being tested in the Women's Health Initiative (WHI), which was started in 1993. This multisite, random-ized, controlled clinical investigation will follow postmenopausal women ages 50 to 79 for a period of 8 to 10 years. In addition to an observational component to esti-mate the risk of several diseases and identify new risk factors, the WHI prevention trial will test consequences of dietary modification as well as hormone therapy (es-trogen and estrogen and progestin). (Office of Research on Women's Health, 1992.)

Alcohol Intake

The health consequences of excessive alcohol intake are well understood. Nonetheless, the link of more moderate intake to disease in women remains con-troversial. The proposed link to breast cancer in women requires further study. In the interim, some counsel women not to exceed more than an ounce of alcohol in-take per day. The Massachusetts study of midlife women revealed that alcohol in-take was not associated with estrogen or gonadotropin levels (London et al., 1991). A controlled dietary study of menstruating women demonstrated that alcohol con-sumption was associated with increased levels of several hormones, including de-hydroepiandrosterone sulfate in the follicular phase; plasma estrone and estradiol levels in the periovulatory phase; and estrone, estradiol, and estriol levels during the luteal phase. This may account for the link between alcohol consumption and increased breast cancer risk (Reichman et al., 1993). To add to the controversy, Garg, Wagener, and Madans (1993) found a 40% decreased risk of ischemic heart disease in women who consumed between one-half and two alcoholic beverages a day. More evidence is needed before recommendations can be made because it is known that women are at greater risk than men for damaging effects from alco-hol consumption. Women have higher blood alcohol levels than men when they consume equal amounts of alcohol because women do not metabolize alcohol as effectively as men (Frezza et al., 1990).

Engaging in Regular Exercise

The U.S. Preventive Services Task Force (1989) recommends counseling about reg-ular physical activity tailored to the person's health status and lifestyle. Among women in midlife, reasons for lower levels of exercise span family, work, and en-ergy levels. Women with a sedentary lifestyle are at increased risk of weight gain, muscle atrophy, increased stress response, and sleep problems. In addition, there is interest in the relationship between exercise habits and CAD, high blood pres-sure, non–insulin-dependent diabetes mellitus, colon cancer, HDL cholesterol lev-els, and osteoporosis. Exercise has been associated with improved affect and with decreased depression and anxiety (U.S. Preventive Services Task Force, 1989). The amount of exercise may be more important to health than the intensity. Regular ac-tivity is associated with higher HDL levels, whereas extremely intense activity can actually decrease HDL concentrations (Taylor & Ward, 1993). A study of 507 midlife women found that those who reported higher levels of activity at baseline had less weight gain 3 years later. In addition, women who increased their activity during the 3 years had the smallest increases in weight and had the smallest decreases in HDL-C and HDL$_2$-C. Changes in their lipid concentrations due to activity were independent of changes in body weight (Owens et al., 1992). African American women participating in the same study reported significantly less physical activity than the Caucasian women and had higher blood pressure and poorer glucose tolerance levels as well as greater body mass index and abdominal fat distribution (Wing et al., 1989).

Aerobic conditioning and muscle training are aspects of an exercise program that may benefit women during midlife. Aerobic exercise can improve cardiovascular endurance, reduce risk of cardiovascular disease, and prevent or minimize age-related increases in body fat. Resistance training can increase muscle strength and may increase bone density. Links of specific types and amounts of exercise to bone mineral content remain uncertain (Simkin, Ayalon, & Leitcher, 1987).

A 6-month home-based aerobic exercise training program improved perceptions of satisfaction with shape and appearance, fitness, and weight among midlife women as well as men. In addition, maximal oxygen uptake improved significantly. Weight did not change significantly (King et al., 1989). In another study, women participated in a 12-week exercise program of aerobic exercise (walking and jogging at prescribed exercise intensity) or nonaerobic strength and flexibility training. Women in the aerobic exercise group experienced significant decreases in their heart rates and increases in peak maximal oxygen uptake and time on treadmill after completing the program. Aerobic exercise for the postmenopausal but not the premenopausal women was associated with significantly lower blood pressure levels and an attenuation of blood pressure reactivity in comparison to strength training. Aerobic exercise seemed to attenuate psychophysiologic responses to low-to-moderate level stressors but not to more intense stressors in this study (Blumenthal et al., 1991).

Various exercise forms including brisk walking, stationary cycling, bicycling, jogging, running, or swimming can be incorporated into a low-impact aerobic program. Exercising to refreshment and relaxation rather than to exhaustion is important in making an exercise habit enjoyable. Specific recommendations about the intensity, frequency, and duration of exercise vary with the source. Most experts recommend exercising three to four times per week for 15 to 45 minutes minimum. Recently the Centers for Disease Control and Prevention recommended that every U.S. adult accumulate 30 minutes or more of moderate to intense physical activity daily (Pate et al., 1995). The intensity can be assessed in many ways, but the most direct is achieving and maintaining a pulse rate as computed below:

Pulse rate = (220 − age) × 70%

Starting at a modest level of exertion and time and ultimately increasing the regimen to 30 to 45 minutes per time and to greater levels of exertion are recommended (Cahill, 1995).

Dangers of exercise have yet to be evaluated carefully for women. Risks of osteoarthritis in the hips and knees and risk of sudden death in people who begin a vigorous exercise program after being sedentary are among those not yet evaluated for women in midlife. For women who do not have specific health problems, moderate exercise is likely to have more benefit than risk. Women with health problems need advice about limitations for exercise.

In addition to stopping smoking, modifying dietary intake, and developing exercise programs, obtaining adequate rest and sleep and learning stress management techniques may help prevent disease. These aspects are discussed elsewhere in this text.

Secondary Prevention Strategies

Using health services to prevent disease is an important adjunct to a woman's own efforts at preventing disease. The following services have important consequences for women's health:

- clinical breast examination and mammography for breast cancer
- Pap smear screening for cervical cancer
- blood pressure screening for hypertension

In addition, use of hormone therapy for primary and secondary prevention of osteoporosis and cardiovascular disease by postmenopausal women is currently being investigated. Because many early detection strategies are still being evaluated, the frequency with which they are recommended remains controversial. Unfortunately, the limitations on frequency may serve poorly the women who need the screening most—the poor and uninsured. Nonetheless, policy decisions about third-party reimbursement for services such as mammography remains a barrier for many women obtaining access to screening.

Three expert panels have evaluated a range of preventive services for their use: the U.S. Preventive Services Task Force (1989), the Canadian Task Force on the Periodic Health Examination (Eddy, 1991), and the American College of Physicians (Hayward, Steinberg, Forde, Roizen, & Roach, 1991). In addition the American Cancer Society (Mettlin & Dodd, 1991) and the American College of Obstetricians and Gynecologists (1989) have published similar guidelines. Areas of concurrence by at least two of the groups are outlined in Table 5–1. Screening recommendations refer to routine use with low-risk, asymptomatic women.

Clinical Breast Examination and Mammography

Breast cancer is of great concern to women because of its prevalence and life-threatening consequences. Unfortunately the recent disagreement in recommendations for frequency of screening for women younger than age 50 has caused confusion about the use of mammography.

All three expert panels recommend annual clinical breast examination after women reach age 40. The U.S. Preventive Services Task Force recommends mammography screening every year for women beginning at age 50 and concluding at age 75 unless pathology has been detected. For women at high risk because of a family history of premenopausally diagnosed breast cancer in first-degree relatives, they advise beginning regular clinical breast examinations and mammography at an earlier age (eg, at age 35). The American Cancer Society and the National Cancer Institute recommend monthly breast self-examination (BSE) and regular clinical examination of the breast for all women. The American Cancer Society also recom-

Table 5-1. Areas of Agreement for Screening for Women by U.S. Preventive Services Task Force, Canadian Task Force on the Periodic Health Examination, and American College of Physicians Task Force

Clinical breast exam	Annually for women over age 40 y
Mammography	Annually for women after age 50 y
Pap smears	Every 1–3 y for sexually active women after they begin sexual activity or by age 18; for women at average risk, every 3 y after 3 consecutive normal Paps
Blood pressure	Once every 1–2 y
Nonfasting cholesterol	Every 5 y
Stool for occult blood	Annually after age 50 y

Source: Canadian Task Force on the Periodic Health Examination. The periodic health examination: 2. 1987 update. *Canadian Medical Association Journal*, 138, 618–626.

mends for all women with average risk baseline mammography between ages 35 and 40, followed by annual or biennial mammograms from ages 40 to 49, and annual mammograms beginning at age 50. Other groups recommend annual clinical breast examinations for all women starting at age 40 but do not recommend beginning yearly mammography until age 50. These groups base this recommendation on the results of an assessment in Canada that has been challenged by U.S. scientists.

The U.S. Preventive Services Task Force recommends that clinicians refer women to mammographers who use low-dose equipment and adhere to high standards of quality control. Mammography facilities must be certified.

Pap Smears for Cervical Cancer Screening

Pap smears are recommended for all women who have been or who are sexually active. They should begin with onset of sexual activity or at age 18 years, whichever is earlier, and be repeated every 1 to 3 years at the discretion of the care provider after three consecutive normal tests. The frequency should be based on risk factors such as onset of sexual intercourse before age 16, history of multiple sexual partners, history of abnormal Pap tests, and low socioeconomic status. Laboratories with adequate quality control measures should be used to interpret results of the tests. Follow-up of test results should be ensured (U.S. Preventive Services Task Force, 1989).

Blood Pressure Screening

Blood pressure screening for women with normal blood pressure and low risk for hypertension is recommended every 1 to 2 years. Although women can obtain blood pressure measurements themselves, they need to be certain the equipment they are using is accurate, especially equipment in public places. In addition, women need to seek care for elevation in blood pressure. Measurements at least every 2 years are recommended if the blood pressure was below 85 mm Hg and 140 mm Hg diastolic and systolic, respectively. If the last diastolic reading was 85 to 89 mm Hg, screening should occur annually. Hypertension should not be diagnosed on the basis of a single visit, but elevated readings should be confirmed on more than one reading at each of three separate visits (U.S. Preventive Services Task Force, 1989).

Hormone Therapy

As the baby boomers approach menopause, use of hormones (estrogen alone or estrogen with a progestin) by middle-aged and older women has generated renewed scientific interest for its potential value in primary and secondary prevention of osteoporosis and heart disease. Although estrogen was first approved for use by postmenopausal women during the 1940s, the prevalence of estrogen use did not increase substantially until the 1960s when clinicians prescribed it for relief of menopausal hot flashes and urogenital symptoms. During the early 1970s, evidence of an increased incidence of endometrial cancer associated with estrogen therapy and worries about possible associations with increased risk of vascular disease (as had occurred with use of oral contraceptives) led to a decrease in prescription of estrogen therapy (Bush, 1991). In the 1980s, a progestin was added to prescriptions of estrogen therapy to reduce the risk of endometrial cancer (Hemminki, Kennedy, Baum, & McKinlay, 1988). In 1986, the Food and Drug Administration approved use of postmenopausal estrogen for the prevention and management of osteoporosis based on evidence supporting the effectiveness of estrogen in reducing hip and vertebral fractures (Weiss, Ure, Ballard, Williams, & Daling, 1980). Evidence linking use of estrogen therapy to a reduction in the incidence of heart disease has introduced yet another indication for hormone therapy—the prevention of heart disease by use of estrogen or estrogen/progestin therapy (Bush et al., 1987).

Despite the promise of new evidence for protective effects of estrogen and combined hormone therapy, caution pervades discussion of recommendations for its use. The American College of Physicians (ACP) recently published guidelines in which they advocated careful and separate consideration of benefits of short-term use of hormone therapy for managing menopausal symptoms and use of hormone therapy for disease prevention (ACP, 1992). The ACP advises a limited course of therapy (1–5 years) for women seeking relief from symptoms such as hot flashes associated with menopause. In the absence of data from randomized clinical trials to provide definitive estimates of benefits and risks, the ACP recommends that women of all races should consider preventive hormone therapy. Those who have had a hysterectomy are likely to benefit from estrogen therapy and have no need for combined hormone therapy (estrogen and a progestin). Women who have CAD or who are at increased risk of CAD are likely to benefit from hormone therapy and should receive combined therapy if they have a uterus unless careful endometrial monitoring is performed (eg, endometrial biopsies, aspirations). Risks of hormone therapy may outweigh benefits for women at increased risk of breast cancer. The ACP guidelines conclude that "for other women, the best course of action is not clear" (ACP, 1992, p. 1038).

The guidelines, based on a review of the most recent data available regarding the risks and benefits of hormone therapy for postmenopausal women with respect to endometrial cancer, breast cancer, CAD, osteoporosis, and stroke, reflect

the following potential benefits and risks (Grady et al., 1992). Estrogen alone reduces the risk of heart disease by about 35%, but it was not possible to estimate
the risk reduction associated with using estrogen in combination with progestin at
the time of the review. Reduced risk of osteoporotic fractures is evident for hip
fractures (by about 25%) and vertebral fractures (by about 50%). Reduced risk of
hip and vertebral fractures for women using estrogen and a progestin could not
be estimated. Increased life expectancy was probable for women using estrogen
alone, but estimated to be not as great for women using estrogen and a progestin
if protection from heart disease is shown to be less than that for women using estrogen alone. Recent evidence from the Postmenopausal Estrogen/Progestin
Interventions (PEPI) study suggests that adding progestin does not increase the
risk factors for CAD more than that when no hormones are used. Potential risks of
estrogen use include endometrial cancer associated with estrogen alone (an eight-
fold increase for women using estrogen for 10–20 years), but risk does not seem
to be increased for women using estrogen and a progestin. Evidence for an increased risk of breast cancer is inconsistent for women using estrogen alone for
less than 5 years. Risk is estimated not to increase until women had used estrogen
for 10 to 20 years, and then by about 25%. Unpredictable endometrial bleeding
lasting 6 to 8 months occurs in some women using estrogen and progestin, and
endometrial evaluation is necessary yearly among women with a uterus using estrogen alone and for women using estrogen and progestin if heavy or prolonged
or frequent or persistent unexplained bleeding occurs. There is a 20% lifetime risk
of hysterectomy for endometrial hyperplasia or cancer due to estrogen alone but
probably no increase in risk for women using estrogen and a progestin (Grady et
al., 1992).

Although information about the benefits and risks of long-term use of estrogen
or combined hormone therapy await further research, data currently available indicate benefits for symptom management for women with menopausal hot flashes,
night sweats, and urogenital symptoms; enhancing bone health and reducing the
risk of osteoporosis; and reducing the risk of heart disease. The increased monitoring by a health professional may also contribute to the early detection of other
treatable diseases, thereby having a net positive effect on women's health. Possible
risks associated with use of estrogen or combined hormone therapy include increased risk of endometrial cancer in women who have a uterus and who are using
estrogen alone, increased risk of breast cancer, resumption of menses or spotting
related to progestin therapy, increased risk of gallbladder disease, growth of uterine fibroids, and the necessity to adhere to a medication regimen for an extended
period of one's life (Grady et al., 1992).

At the time of this writing, two large clinical trials, the PEPI study and the
Women's Health Initiative Trial are both underway. The PEPI trial results have
begun to inform women and professionals about the possible benefits for reducing
cardiovascular disease risk by examining the effects of estrogen and progestin on
LDL and HDL cholesterol levels and other risk factors. The trial included 875
healthy postmenopausal women aged 45 to 64 years who had no known con-
traindication to hormone therapy. They were randomized to placebo, conjugated
equine estrogen (CEE), 0.625 mg, CEE 0.625 mg plus cyclic medroxyprogesterone

acetate (MPA) 10 mg/d for 12 days a month, CEE 0.625 mg plus consecutive MPA 2.5 mg/d; or CEE 0.625 mg plus cyclic micronized progesterone (MP) 200 mg/d for 12 days a month. Estrogen alone or in combination with a progestin improved lipoproteins and lowered fibrinogen levels without adverse effects on postchallenge insulin or blood pressure. Unopposed estrogen was the optimal regimen for elevating HDL-C concentration. A high rate of endometrial hyperplasia occurred in the groups that used unopposed estrogen, restricting recommendations for its use to women without a uterus. In women who have a uterus, CEE with cyclic MP had the most favorable effect on HDL-C and with no excess increased risk of endometrial hyperplasia. MPA had no detrimental effects on lipids compared with the risk for those not taking hormones (Writing Group for the PEPI Trial, 1995).

The Women's Health Initiative will assess the long-term consequences of hormone therapy in postmenopausal women for heart disease, osteoporosis, and breast cancer. (In addition, the use of a low-fat diet and calcium and vitamin D supplementation will be compared with the effects of hormone therapy on several disease end points.)

Although the long-term consequences of hormone therapy for postmenopausal women remain to be assessed through clinical trials such as the Women's Health Initiative, completed studies have indicated that hormone therapies offer both benefit and risk to women using them. As a result, many women face making the decision to adopt hormone therapy with incomplete information. As a result of exclusion from long-term clinical trials, women have information about the short-term risks and benefits, largely gleaned from retrospective studies, with their problematic bias in selection of who used and did not use hormones, and with an absence of information about long-term risks and benefits gained from clinical trials comparing consequences of using estrogen alone with combined hormone therapy.

Additional trials are underway in which hormone therapy (estrogen alone or estrogen with a progestin) are being studied for their secondary prevention effects. One example is the Heart Estrogen-Progestin Replacement Study (HERS) in which hormone therapy is being tested for its ability to prevent recurrent cardiac events in women who have had a myocardial infarction.

Despite the flurry of research activity directed at investigating the health consequences of hormone therapy, to date only one research team has studied how women decide to adopt hormone therapy. Results of one study indicated that although health professionals tend to emphasize risk reduction effects of using hormones, women were concerned about the immediate effects of estrogen on symptoms they perceived as distressing (Rothert et al., 1990). In a later study of women's decisions to use estrogen or combined hormone therapy to alleviate menopausal symptoms, again based on hypothetical cases, women's decision patterns sorted into four distinct groups. One group of women based their decision to take hormones on whether their hot flashes were severe. A second would use hormones if hot flashes were severe, but also would consider the risk of osteoporosis and cancer in making their decision. A third group was most influenced by the unpleasant effects of adding progestin to the hormone therapy because they did not want to resume menses or spotting. The fourth considered health risks, particularly the risk of cancer. These groups were distinguished by several factors: educational level, perceived stress, and attitudes toward menopause and use of medications. Women in the second group had the most formal education and higher stress levels and were more likely to use vitamins to control menopausal symptoms. Women in the third group had the most positive attitudes toward menopause. In all cases, prediction of willingness to take estrogen was related to the perception that hormone treatment might be helpful in controlling menopausal symptoms and knowledge about menopause and its effects on women. Expectations that menopause would be difficult were related to lower likelihood of taking hormone therapy. Current comfort level, as indicated by hot flashes, was an overriding concern in women's decisions (Schmitt et al., 1991).

Studies of women who actually were given prescriptions for hormone therapy reveal that women use hormones sporadically. Women's primary reason for stopping treatment was their fear of cancer (Ravnikar, 1987). Results of another recent survey indicated that women using estrogen were more likely to be aware that lower estrogen levels were associated with osteoporosis, perceived that menopause was a medical condition, believed the natural approaches to managing menopausal symptoms were less preferable, received care from a gynecologist, and believed women should take hormones for hot flashes. Women using estrogen were also more than twice as likely to have had a hysterectomy and to have a Pap smear at least every 2 years. Those not using estrogen were more likely to have had relatives with uterine cancer. Women rated having menstrual periods again as the most unfavorable aspect of hormone use (Ferguson, Hoegh, & Johnson, 1989).

Understanding women's beliefs about hormone therapy and their actual practices would be incomplete without considering the social and historical context in which these occur. Women who were part of the baby-boom birth cohort are now attempting to sift through the available information about hormone therapy. Some remember the 1960s encouragement to remain "feminine forever" by using estrogens. Most will remember the 1970s news reports linking estrogen therapy to an increased incidence of endometrial cancer. Some find the current attempt to assess the benefits and risks of hormone therapy yet another attempt to 'medicalize' menopause. Some women are waiting for additional results of the PEPI trial to become available before deciding about therapy. Results of the Women's Health Initiative study will not be available for another decade. Because of all the publicity about osteoporosis and heart disease and the possible healthful effects of using hormones, women who once asked: "What is the risk of using hormone therapies?" are now asking "What is the risk of not using hormone therapies?" Answers to their questions may have to await the completion of research projects such as the Women's Health Initiative study.

References

American College of Obstetricians and Gynecologists. Committee on Professional Standards. (1989). Report of task force on routine cancer screening. In *Standards for Obstetric-Gynecologic Services* (pp. 97-104). Washington, DC: Author.

American College of Physicians. (1992). Guidelines for counseling postmenopausal women about preventive hormone therapy. *Annals of Internal Medicine, 117* (12), 1038-104.

Barrett-Connor, E. L., Cohn, B. A., Wingard, D. L., & Edelstein, S. L. (1991). Why is diabetes mellitus a stronger risk factor for fatal ischemic heart disease in women than in men? The Rancho Bernardo study. *Journal of the American Medical Association, 265,* 267-631.

Bilezikian, J. & Silverberg, S. (1992). Osteoporosis: A practical approach to the perimenopausal woman. *Journal of Women's Health, 1*(1), 21-27.

Brooks-Gunn, J., & Kirsch, B. (1984). Life events and the boundaries of midlife for women. In G. Baruch & J. Brooks-Gunn (Eds.), *Women in Midlife* (pp. 11-30). New York: Plenum Press.

Bush, T. (1991). Feminine forever revisited: Menopausal hormone therapy in the 1990's. *Journal of Women's Health, 1,* 1-4.

Bush, T. L., Barrett-Connor, E., Cowan, L. D., Criqui, M. H., Wallace, R. B., Suchindran, C. M., Tyroler, H. A., Rifkind, B. M. (1987). Cardiovascular mortality and noncontraceptive use of estrogen in women: Results from the Lipid Research Clinics Program Follow-up Study. *Circulation, 75,* 1102-1109.

Cahill, C. (1995). Exercise. In C. Fogel & N. Woods (Eds.), *Women's health: A comprehensive handbook* (pp. 261-280). Thousand Oaks, CA: Sage.

Centers for Disease Control. (1990). Trends in lung cancer incidence and mortality—United States, 1980–1987. *Morbidity and Mortality Weekly Report 39*(8), 875-883.

Centers for Disease Control. (1991). Cigarette smoking among reproductive aged women—Behavioral risk factors surveillance system, 10\989. *Morbidity and Mortality Weekly Report 40* (42), 719-723.

Colditz, G. A., Willett, W. C., Rotnitzky, A., & Manson, J. E. (1995). Weight gain as a risk factor for clinical diabetes mellitus in women. *Annals of Internal Medicine, 122,* 481-486.

Eddy, D. (Ed.). (1991). *Common screening tests.* Philadelphia: American College of Physicians.

Ferguson, K. J., Hoegh, C., & Johnson, S. (1989). Estrogen replacement therapy: A survey of women's knowledge and attitudes. *Archives of Internal Medicine, 149,* 133-136.

Fogel, C., & Woods, N. (1995). Midlife women's health. In C. Fogel & N. Woods (Eds.), *Women's health: A comprehensive handbook* (pp. 79-100). Thousand Oaks, CA: Sage.

Frezza, M., di Padova, C., Pozzato, G., Terpin, M., Baraona, E., & Lieber, C. S. (1990). High blood alcohol levels in women. The role of decreased gastric alcohol dehydrogenase activity and first-pass metabolism. *New England Journal of Medicine, 322,* 95-99.

Garg, R., Wagener, D. K., & Madans, J. H. (1993). Alcohol consumption and risk of ischemic heart disease in women. *Archives of Internal Medicine, 153* (10), 1211–1216.

Giovannucci, E., & Willet, W. C. (1994). Dietary factors and risk of colon cancer. *Annals of Medicine 26* (6), 443–452.

Goldin, B. R., Woods, M. N., Spiegelman, D. L., Longcope, C., Morrill-La Brode, A., Dwyer, J. T., Gualtieri, L. J., Hertzmakr, E., & Gorbach, S. L. (1994). The effect of dietary fat and fiber on serum estrogen concentrations in premenopausal women under controlled dietary conditions. *Cancer, 74,* 1125-1131.

Grady, D., Rubin, S., Petitti, D., Fox, C., Black, D., Ettinger, B., Ernster, V., & Cummings, S. (1992). Hormone therapy to prevent disease and prolong life in postmenopausal women. *Annals of Internal Medicine, 117* (12), 1016-1037.

Hayward, R. S., Steinberg, E., Forde, D., Roizen, M., & Roach, K. (1991). Preventive care guidelines: 1991. *Annals of Internal Medicine, 114,* 758-783. (Erratum, *Annals of Internal Medicine* [1991] *115,* 332).

Hemminki, E. Kennedy, D., Baum, C., & McKinlay, M. (1988). Prescribing of noncontraceptive estrogens and progestins in the United States, 1974-1986. *American Journal of Public Health, 78,* 1479-1481.

Henderson, M. M., Insull, W., Jr., Moskowitz, M., Goldman, S., & Woods, M. N. (1992). Maintenance of a low-fat diet: follow-up of the Women's Health Trial. *Cancer Epidemiology, Biomarkers and Prevention, 1*(4), 315-323.

Henderson, M. M., Kushi, L. H., Thompson, D. J., Gorbach, S. L., Clifford, C. K., Insull, W., Jr., Moskowitz, M., & Thompson, R. S. (1990). Feasibility of a randomized trial of a low-fat diet for the prevention of breast cancer: Dietary compliance in the Women's Health Trial Vanguard Study. *Preventive Medicine, 19*(2), 115-133.

Hibbard, J. H. (1993). Social roles as predictors of cessation in a cohort of women smokers. *Women and Health, 20,* 71-80.

Insull, W., Jr., Henderson, M., Prentice, R., Thompson, B. D., Clifford, C., Goldman, S., Gorbach, S., Moskowitz, M., Thompson, R., & Woods, M. (1990). Results of a randomized feasibility study of a low-fat diet. *Archives of Internal Medicine, 150*(2), 421-427.

Jensen, P. M., & Coambs, R. B. (1994). Health and behavioral predictors of success in an intensive smoking cessation program for women. *Women and Health, 21*(1), 57-72.

Kannel, W. B. (1987). Metabolic risk factors for coronary artery disease in women: Perspective from the Framingham Study. *American Heart Journal, 114,* 413-419.

Kawachi, I., Colditz, G., Stampfer, M., Willett, W., Manson, J., Rosner, B., Speizer, F., & Hennekens, C. (1993). Smoking cessation and decreased risk of stroke in women. *Journal of the American Medical Association, 269*(2), 232-236.

Kinne, S., Kristal, A., White, E., & Hunt, J. (1993). Work-site smoking policies: Their population impact in Washington State. *American Journal of Public Health, 83*(7), 1031-1033.

Knopp, R. H., Zhu, X., & Bonet, B. (1994). Effects of estrogens on lipoprotein metabolism and cardiovascular disease in women. *Atherosclerosis, 110* (Suppl.), 83–91.

Lacey, L., Manfredi, C., Balch, G., Warnecke, R., Allen, K., & Edwards, C. (1993). Social support in smoking cessation among black women in Chicago public housing. *Public Health Reports, 108* (3), 387-394.

Leischow, S. J., Sachs, D. D., Bostrom, A. G., & Hansen, M. D. (1992). Effects of differing nicotine-replacement doses on weight gain after smoking cessation. *Archives of Family Medicine, 1*(2), 233-237.

London, S., Willett, W., Longcope, C., & McKinlay, S. (1991). Alcohol and other dietary factors in relation to serum hormone concentrations in women at climacteric. *American Journal of Clinical Nutrition, 53,* 166-171.

Manson, J. E., Colditz, G. A, Stampfer, M. J., Willett, W. C., Rosner, B., Monson, R. R., Speizer, F. E., & Hennekens, C. H. (1990). A prospective study of obesity and risk of coronary heart disease in women. *New England Journal of Medicine, 322,* 882-889.

Medical Letter on Drugs and Therapeutics. (1995). Use of nicotine to stop smoking, *37,* 6-8.

Mettlin, C., & Dodd, G. D. (1991). The American Cancer Society guidelines for the cancer related checkup: An update. *CA: A Cancer Journal for Clinicians, 41,* 279-282.

National Center for Health Statistics. (1992). Advance report of final mortality statistics, 1990. *Monthly Vital Statistics Report, 41* (7). Hyattsville, MD: Author.

National Center for Health Statistics. (1993a). Advance report of final mortality statistics, 1991. *Monthly Vital Statistics Report, 42* (2). Hyattsville, MD: Author.

National Center for Health Statistics (1993b). *Current estimates from the National Health Interview Survey, 1992* (Series 10). Hyattsville, MD: Author.

National Center for Health Statistics (1993c). *Health in the United States and prevention profile, 1992.* Hyattsville, MD: Author.

Office of Research on Women's Health. (1992). *Report of the National Institutes of Health: Opportunities for research on women's health* (NIH Publication No. 92-3457). Bethesda, MD: Author.

Pate, R. R., Pratt, M., Blair, S. N., Haskell, W. L., Macera, C. A., Bouchard, C., Buchner, D., Ettinger, W., Heath, G. W., King, A. C., et al. (1995). Physical activity and public health. *Journal of the American Medical Association, 273,* 402-407.

Prentice, R., Thompson, D., Clifford, C., Gorbach, S., Goldin, B., & Byar, D. (1990). Dietary fat reduction and plasma estradiol concentration in healthy postmenopausal women. *Journal of the National Cancer Institute, 82,* 129-134.

Ravnikar, V. A. (1987). Compliance with hormone therapy. *American Journal of Obstetrics and Gynecology, 156,* 1332-1334.

Reichman, M. E., Judd, J. T., Longcope, C., Schatzkin, A., Clevidence, B. A., Nair, P. P., Campbell, W. S., & Taylor, P. R. (1993). Effects of alcohol consumption on plasma and urinary hormone concentrations in premenopausal women. *Journal of the National Cancer Institute, 85,* 722-727.

Romans, S. E., McNoe, B. M., Herbison, G. P., Walton, V. A., & Mullen, P. E. (1993). Cigarette smoking and psychiatric morbidity in women. *Australian and New Zealand Journal of Psychiatry, 27* (3), 399-404.

Rothert, M., Rover, D., Holmen, M., Schmitt, N., Talarczyk, G., Knoll, J., & Gogate, J. (1990). Women's use of information regarding hormone replacement therapy. *Research in Nursing and Health, 13,* 355-366.

Sheridan, D., & Winogrand, I. (1987). *The preventive approach to patient care.* New York, Elsevier.

Schmitt, N., Gogate, J., Rothert, M., Rovner, D., Holmes, M., Talarczyk, G., Given, B., & Kroll, J. (1991). Capturing and clustering women's judgment policies: The case of hormonal therapy for menopause. *Journal of Gerontology, Psychological Sciences, 46* (3), 92-101.

Simkin, A., Ayalon, J., & Leitcher, I. (1987). Increased trabecular bone density due to bone-loading exercises in postmenopausal osteoporetic women. *Calcified Tissue International, 40* (2), 59-63.

Swan, G. E., Ward, M. M., Jack, L. M., Javitz, H. S. (1993). Cardiovascular reactivity as a predictor of relapse in male and female smokers. *Health Psychology 12*(6), 451-458.

Taylor, P. A. & Ward, A. (1993). Women, high-density lipoprotein cholesterol and exercise. *Archives of Internal Medicine, 153,* 1178-1184.

Thun, M. J., Calle, E. E., Namboodiri, M. N., Flanders, W. D., Coates, R. J., Byers, T., et al. (1992). Risk factors for fatal colon cancer in a large prospective study. *Journal National Cancer Institute, 84,* 1491-1500.

U.S. Bureau of the Census. (1975). *Historical statistics of the United States. Colonial times to 1970. Part 1.* Washington, DC: U.S. Government Printing Office.

U.S. Preventive Services Task Force. (1989). *Guide to clinical preventive services: Report of the U.S. Preventive Services Task Force.* Baltimore: Williams & Wilkins.

Waldron, I. (1991). Patterns and causes of gender differences in smoking. *Social Science and Medicine, 32*(9), 989-1005.

Weiss, N. S., Ure, C. L., Ballard, J. H., Williams, A. R., & Daling J. R. (1980). Decreased risk of fractures of the hip and lower forearm with postmenopausal use of estrogen. *New England Journal of Medicine, 303,* 1195-1198.

Writing Group for the PEPI Trial. (1995). Effects of estrogen or estrogen/progestin regimens on heart disease risk factors in postmenopausal women. The Postmenopausal Estrogen/Progestin Interventions (PEPI) Trial. *Journal of the American Medical Association, 273*(3), 199-208.

CHAPTER 6

Health Promotion: The Mature Years (64 and Older)

Lucille Davis
Mary Maryland

Introduction

This chapter discusses health issues of older women (64 and older) from a health promotion perspective, including cultural, family, and socioeconomic factors and how these factors affect the health of older women.

The Demography and Feminization of Aging

The graying of America has transformed our society. Although our society has been aging steadily in the last century, the pace of aging has accelerated as reflected in a dramatic increase in the numbers and percentage of the aged population. Since 1980, the number of people 65 has increased 21% (5.3 million) compared to 8% for the remainder of the population. In 1989, 6000 people in the United States turned 65 every day (Harper, 1992). The growth of the "old-old" (85 years and older) is even more dramatic with this population projected to reach over 5 million by the year 2000 (U.S. Senate Special Committee on Aging, 1988).

The aging population exhibits ethnic and racial differences. For example, although African Americans die younger than their Caucasian counterparts, as a result of the "crossover phenomenon," (Wing, Manton, Stallard, Haines, & Tyroles, 1985), African Americans outlive their Caucasian counterparts after the age of 75 and African American women outlive African American men and their Caucasian female and male counterparts. Theoretically, the latter phenomenon is due to survival of the fittest of the African Americans and "earlier susceptibility to illness and violent death" (Harper, 1992).

The feminization of aging is evident because women continue to outlive men (and as noted above, especially African American women). The life expectancy for women is 78.3 compared to 71.4 for men (Sapp & Bliesmer, 1995). Women comprise 59% of all people over 65 and 72% of people over 85 (Office of Technology Assessment, 1992). The demographic profile of older women has major implications for many of society's institutions including schools, health care agencies, and families. There are at least four areas of concern for older women; most older women are:

- concentrated in the older age group, especially among the old-old
- widowed, live alone, do not have a spouse to care for them
- in poor health (Sapp & Bliesmer, 1995)

Health Promotion and the Aged

The graying of society coupled with the epidemiologic transition (shift from infectious diseases to chronic diseases as leading causes of death) has stimulated greater interest in health promotion. Although the effectiveness of health promotion has been documented, researchers and clinicians have given little attention to health promotion and the elderly. However, with more people living into the ninth and tenth decade of life, there has been a new focus on the elderly as noted in national reports, *Healthy People 2000* (U.S. Public Health Service, 1991) and forums such as the 1995 White House Mini Conference on Aging. Some clinicians have suggested that health promotion services for the elderly are limited because of negative attitudes toward aging. Because the elderly have been systematically excluded from preventive programs, data about effectiveness of these programs are limited. Current data show that health promotions programs (eg, exercise programs) are effective in improving elders' health physical and psychosocial health (Dychtwald, 1986).

According to Pender (1987), health promotion includes self-initiated actions and perceptions that maintain or enhance self-actualization, self-fulfillment, and personal health or wellness. Health promotion programs for the elderly focus on strengths and abilities and seek to maximize personal empowerment, independence, and autonomy. Some studies report that many older people routinely engage in health promotion activities (eg, exercise, relaxation, nutrition, and self-discipline) more than younger people (Schafer, 1989; Walker, 1989).

Health Status

Chronological age does not predict health status. Sapp and Bliesmer (1995) cite John Heinz, former chairman of the U.S. Senate Special Committee on Aging, who spoke eloquently about the heterogeneity of the elderly population:

> Growing old, while an inevitable process for all of us, has no common denominator when it comes to health. The image of a grayed and crippled, frail older American is just as much a stereotype as that of a robust and active one; neither captures the range of health status found in this segment of our Nation's population (U.S. Senate Special Committee on Aging, 1986).

Personal definitions of health change with age and are linked to older persons' decisions about health, including participation in health promotive and preventive programs.

Traditional definitions of health (eg, absence of disease) are not appropriate for the elderly, many of whom are living with chronic illnesses. In this age group, emphasis is on functional health and psychosocial dimensions (Miller, 1995) and includes concepts such as "feeling good," or being able to do things that are personally important. From an aging perspective, health is a complex dynamic interactional process that involves functional and psychosocial factors (Walker, 1988).

Health Promotion and Older Women

Later life has become the longest phase of women's lives. Because women can expect to live one third of their lives after menopause (Dougherty & Knutesen, 1995), it is important that women learn to develop healthy lifestyles early in life. Adoption of health-promoting behaviors earlier in life, including the "prime of life" or middle years, can prevent or delay chronic illnesses in later life, such as cardiovascular disease, diabetes, and gynecologic problems. A life course perspective is especially significant for older minority women because they are at greater risk than nonminority for poor health in old age. They have experienced a lifetime of accumulated deficits (eg, environmental risks, poor health care, and discrimination), making them a high-risk population in relation to morbidity and mortality (Harper, 1992).

Former U.S. Surgeon General, C. Everett Koop (1988), in paraphrasing an old saying, "an ounce of prevention is worth more than a pound of cure," asserted that good health in later life is largely the result of personal habits (good diet, regular exercise, and a general healthy lifestyle) and environmental factors (safety, public order, and decent housing). Although medical science has made significant progress in the treatment of diseases, women continue to experience high rates of preventable disability and death. Specifically, cardiovascular disease, one of the leading causes of death among older women, is preventable. Other illnesses such as breast and uterine cancer can be successfully treated if diagnosed in early stages.

Many of the illnesses women have in later life are not inevitable and are modifiable. As Harper (1992) suggests, "the aging process is not genetically hard-wired and biologically determined" (p. 227). Aging is not synonymous with disease or illness and is a social, political, and economic process. Over a decade ago, Fries and Crapo (1981) suggested that a "disease-free aging" is not unrealistic and that postponement of chronic disease is possible and consistent with current health gains in the elderly population. Many of the health problems older women experience are linked to poor health practices, some of which begin in early life, such as poor dietary habits and a sedentary lifestyle. Recently, interest has increased in assessing the damaging effects of the latter behaviors because of the role they play in predisposing women to cardiovascular disease and cancer, which are the leading causes of death among older women (National Center for Health Statistics, 1995). The challenge for care providers and policymakers is to identify ways to facilitate healthy lifestyles by providing support and incentives for women in general and older women in particular.

Health Promotion Behaviors and Older Women

Health promotion for older women includes behaviors that strive to achieve the highest level of overall wellness. Health-promoting activities are becoming increasingly popular. Display 6-1 summarizes some of these activities.

DISPLAY 6-1
Health Promoting Activities for the Older Adult

Blood presure checks

Safe driving courses

Stop smoking classes

Flu shots

Immunizations

Hearing screeings

Vision screenings

Aerobic exercises such as walking, aerobics, or aquatics

Stress reduction activities

Nutritional education

General health educaiton classes

Screenings for early detection of cancer, such as skin and breast cancer

Classes about seasonal health issues such as hypothermia, heart related illness and colds and flu

(Adapted from Miller, C. A. [1995]. Nursing care of the older adult [2nd ed.]. Philadelphia: Lippincott.)

Some health problems responsible for increased morbidity and mortality among older women include osteoporosis, cardiovascular disease, diabetes, and cervical and breast cancer. Specific health promotion behaviors can prevent or delay the onset of these illnesses and prevent complications. Risk factors linked to them can be reduced by two major health-promoting behaviors—exercise and diet. These are lifestyle behaviors that can be controlled, to a large extent, by older women themselves. The following section discusses these illnesses in relation to health-promoting behaviors.

Osteoporosis

Osteoporosis is a preventable and common health problem among older women. Despite the prevalence of osteoporosis among older women, a recent Harris poll found that over half (62%) of older women were not familiar with osteoporosis and did not know about the importance of exercise and calcium supplements as health-promoting and preventive measures (Leader, 1990). Health care workers can help promote health through patient education that focuses on exercise and nutritional needs in relation to osteoporosis.

Cardiovascular Disease and Diabetes

In the case of cardiovascular disease and diabetes in older women, it is important to consider the role of exercise and diet in health promotion. Although women should practice healthy behaviors such as exercise at younger ages, evidence shows that older women can benefit from low to moderate physical activity when practiced on a regular basis. Benefits include improved cardiopulmonary functioning, weight control, and improved mood and cognition (Lewis & Campanelli, 1990). In relation to dietary behaviors, many older women may not know how their nutritional needs change as a result of aging. Also, with normal aging there is a decline in lean body mass and an increase in body fat. Although calorie intake may vary according to basal metabolism, physical activity levels, and occupation, older women should adjust their food intake to prevent overweight because weight control is important in preventing and reducing risks associated with chronic illnesses such as cardiovascular disease, hypertension, and non–insulin-dependent diabetes. Essentially, exercise and dietary behaviors, if practiced throughout early and middle years, can delay or prevent chronicity and frailty among older women.

Health-promoting behaviors become important when the woman has experienced a health problem such as a stroke. The goal then is to restore her to a level of wellness or health within the constraints of the disability and to prevent further complications. Disability can be reduced after a chronic problem has developed by structuring the person's physical and psychological environment. Rehabilitation efforts must begin early. Typically, therapy for stroke patients is targeted at strengthening muscle groups in an effort to recapture motor function, achieve greater independence, and maximize the ability to perform activities of daily living. In addition to recovering motor function, it is important to consider rehabilitation for the improvement of sensory function (DeLisa & Gans, 1993). Formal and informal supports may be needed to promote self-esteem, diminish depression, and help set realistic goals because it is difficult to make radical and multiple changes. Many older women live alone with limited resources and may need to develop new coping skills to deal with the impact of the illness, often within a limited social network. Living with a chronic illness involves learning to balance a number of factors such as medications, diet, and exercise, along with making personal and environmental changes.

Cancer

Cervical and breast cancer are the most prevalent cancers among older women (National Cancer Institute, 1990). Health-promoting behaviors involve regular physical examinations that include mammograms and Pap smears. Unfortunately, older women and some physicians believe that such procedures are not necessary because the woman is "too old." For breast and cervical cancer, this lack of attention for older women can be seen in the following statistics:

1. In women over 60, only 16% have ever had a mammogram.
2. In the population over age 65, there is little or no Pap smear screening.
3. Older women do not receive routine care or see a obstetrician or gynecologist (Dougherty & Knutesen, 1995).

Early detection and prompt treatment can reduce complications and prevent premature death.

Cultural Context of Older Women and Health

Older women's health beliefs, practices, and behaviors are shaped by culture and ethnicity that include race, religion, and language. Recognition by health providers and policymakers of the increasing ethnic diversity among the elderly is becoming more important. This diversity will continue as reflected in the fact that more than 20% of all persons over 65 will be non-Caucasian by the year 2050 (Meyers, 1990). In fact, it is projected that by the turn of the century the average United States resident will be able to trace his or her ancestry to Africa, Asia, the Pacific Islands, the Latino countries, or the Arab world rather than to European roots (Tripp-Reimer, Johnson, & Hayden et al., 1995). Unfortunately, there are few data on health care practices and health promotion strategies and programs that reflect the diversity of populations in this country. This is true across the lifespan and particularly for older women.

In many ethnic groups, older women are frequently seen as healers. Often they use nontraditional health practices such as folk practices, ethnic healers, and indigenous lay health care systems. In many cases, older women may use traditional medicine in conjunction with folk practices or as a supplement to prescribed medical regimens (Davis & McGadney, 1993). Health promotion educational materials and programs should be designed and implemented within a cultural context (eg, self-care manuals for African American elders, [Davis, McGadney, & Perri, 1990]). Health care recommendations for health promotion are more likely to be successful if the women can integrate their beliefs and values (some of which may not be harmful) into an individualized culturally sensitive health plan. For example, noncompliance is likely if a woman is given nutritional counseling that does not include her traditional foods; or if a treatment is prescribed that is in conflict with cultural beliefs (eg, taking only half of a prescribed medicine because it is "too strong or hot" [Tripp-Reimer et al., 1995]). It is important to avoid cultural stereotyping and remember that all cultural and ethnic groups are heterogeneous and reflect a range of diversity in beliefs and values. Although ethnic affiliation may provide a context, interventions must be individualized.

Socioeconomic Context of Older Women and Health

Older women are more likely to live in poverty, especially minority older women. Older women make up the majority of the elderly poor (71.2%), and are more likely to be poor compared to older men (Fowls, 1993). In addition, they are likely to be widowed, often losing income and having resources consumed by medical and funeral costs (Davis, 1988). Poverty has a negative impact on health because it may limit access to health care as well as to the resources required to maintain a healthy lifestyle. The potency of poverty was noted in a recent study by Okie (1991) in which it was found that, although people showed differences in vulnerability to different cancers, poverty was the strongest (in comparison with heredity and culture) influence on cancer rates. Poverty exerted the greatest effect because it reduced access to health care and education and determined where the women lived.

The social roles older women have held in society have had a significant influence on their economic status and ability to gain access to health care. Although all older women (99%) have Medicare, they do not necessarily have access to the health care services they need. More importantly, Medicare supports the traditional focus on treatment rather than prevention. Preventive services are especially important for low income and minority women because they are a high-risk group for diseases that preventive tests could detect. Because women have a greater life expectancy than men, undetected illnesses have a significant chance of compromising health in later life (Cude, 1995). Women with Medicare supplement insurance are more likely to use preventive screening services; however, older men are more likely to have such insurance (Cude, 1995).

Unfortunately, negative attitudes by health care providers have the potential for interfering with older women's access to and motivation to seek preventive health care. The health care system continues to be infected by cultural values and stereotypes about older women, which places this population at double risk for discriminatory practices. Therefore, limited health resources are less likely to be made available to older women, especially those who are poor and require additional resources.

Family Context and Health of Older Women

As a social system, the family fulfills important basic functions for its members, including boundary maintenance, resource attainment, and communication. The health and well-being of older women can be significantly influenced by the health of the family. Family functions can determine health behaviors and preventive activities. The life cycle of the family as illustrated by Duvall's (1977) classical developmental family model presents new challenges and opportunities for older women. According to Duvall (1977), the family cycle and family developmental tasks are defined as:

> [a] sequence of characteristic stages beginning with family formation and continuing through the life of the family through its dissolution . . . . Developmental tasks are growth responsibilities that arise in the life of a family, achievement of which leads to success with later tasks (pp. 137-138).

An important developmental task for the aging family involves supporting and caring for older family members. Assessment of the aging family as a social system is important to identify strengths, resources, and needs, particularly in relation to its older members. The process of family assessment focuses on three main areas. First, assessing the family's use of health services is essential because the cost of routine care can drain financial resources. Asking about the number and reasons for health care visits or the lack of visits can show how family priorities affect health of older family members. Second, determining the family's perception of illness and health can provide clues about the use of nontraditional home remedies as well as health services, including preventive health services. Third, because older women's health choices may be delegated to family members, it is important to understand how responsible family members negotiate and advocate for older women to ensure the availability of appropriate health services.

Social Issues

Social changes, including the changing family structure, have affected the health of older women. One of the most profound social changes affecting families has been the return or continuation of women in the work force along with the responsibility of caring for aged family members. Because women continue to be the major caregivers, many middle-aged and older women are "women in the middle" (Brody, 1985). The result of this new caregiving role usually involves a disruption of lifestyle accompanied by increased stress and lack of attention to personal health needs. With increased longevity, it is becoming more common for a woman in her sixties to be caring for a 90-year-old mother as well as an aging spouse. In other situations, older widows may feel depressed because of the loss of a spouse or other relatives and friends. From a health promotion perspective, older women may require additional informal and formal support and services. Women who are caregivers may need respite care so that coping skills can be strengthened.

Models for Improving Health Promotion Behaviors of Older Women

There are several models that can guide programs and efforts to encourage health promotive and preventive behaviors among older women. The three models that will be discussed are: the PEN model (Airhihenbuwa, 1992), the Health Belief Model (HBM) (Maiman & Becker, 1974) and the Transtheoretical Model of Change (Prochaska & DiClemente, 1983).

PEN Model

The PEN model, which has been used with African Americans, consists of three components central to health for promotion for older women: 1) health education; 2) educational diagnosis of health behaviors, and 3) cultural appropriateness of health behaviors. The acronym refers to:

- (P) person, which stresses the importance of personal empowerment
- (E) extended family, which addresses the significance of the family context of health education and health beliefs
- (N) neighborhood, which identifies the importance of community involvement in designing and implementing health promotion programs

In applying the PEN model to older women, (P) or person empowerment points to the importance of promoting self-responsibility in older women by encouraging them to become educated about their own bodies, how they function, and how to detect early signs of disease or health problems. The more informed older women are about their bodies and how to take care of themselves, the more confident they will feel about advocating for health services. Because older women have grown up in an era when health care providers (especially doctors) were seen as "knowing best," they may not feel comfortable in assuming assertive roles in their health care. Therefore, professionals involved in their care must be sensitive to the degree of self-responsibility older women are willing to assume. It is safe to predict that future cohorts of older women will be more knowledgeable and assertive about their health care.

In relation to (E), extended family, the increasing prevalence of multigenerational families indicates the extended family will be an important context for promoting health behaviors. The family history and experience with health providers and treatment modalities affects the aging family's expectations and motivation regarding older womens' participation in health programs and services. Support from the extended family network (eg, communication, transportation, financial) and cultural norms will influence how older women are perceived in the family, particularly in relation to the priority of their health needs.

Finally, (N) refers to the neighborhood or community context; older women's health can be enhanced by mobilizing community resources. For example, professionals involved in caring for older women can mobilize self-help groups where older women can share concerns and use the group as a resource in addressing common health and aging issues. A positive outcome of group intervention is the role modeling that can occur as they see peers who are coping successfully with similar problems. The quality of life in old age can be enriched through personal relationships and can even increase longevity. For example, there is evidence that older people who maintain strong bonds with family, friends, and neighbors have lowered death and illness rates (Connidis & Davies, 1990).

The community can facilitate primary prevention for older women by helping them and their families become more aware of options and resources and involving them in formal and informal community and political groups to support social and legislative changes to strengthen the continuum of health care and services. PEN is a culturally sensitive model; it suggests that health care providers and others involved in the care of older women appreciate the cultural and social roots of health beliefs and practices and identify how they reinforce negative or positive health behaviors of persons, families, and neighborhoods. The latter information can be used to develop strategies for promoting positive health practices, changing negative practices, and planning health promotion programs (Airhihenbuwa, 1992). More importantly, it is essential to include family and community members so that such programs are culturally relevant and age specific for older individuals and their families.

The Health Belief Model

The HBM, developed to explain why people do not participate in preventive care, is built on the premise that a person's behavior depends on the value that the person places on a particular outcome and the individual's estimate of the likelihood that a given action will result in that outcome (Maiman & Becker, 1974). The HBM suggests that it is important to evaluate preexisting beliefs (which may not be known by the provider) regarding diseases and symptoms as well as attitudes and beliefs about efficacy of health care services; beliefs about efficacy are especially true for preventive care that involves participating in routine screening for asymptomatic diseases (eg, routine mammograms). The HBM is limited because valid scales have not ben developed for chronic illness (Redeker, 1988) and the model has not included adequate samples of older populations.

Transtheoretical Model of Change

This model was originally used in research on addiction. The model focuses on the stages of change that people move through in changing behavior and suggests that change can be looked at on a continuum. Five stages are hypothesized, as follows:

1. Precontemplation—the person does not recognize that he or she has a problem.
2. Contemplation—the person begins to recognize that a problem exists.
3. Preparation—the person prepares to take action to treat the problem.
4. Action—the person actually obtains help for the problem.
5. Maintenance—the last stage, where the person is involved in maintaining the positive change.

This model has not focused on health behaviors and the elderly; however, pilot studies have shown that it can be used with the elderly and health promotion behaviors (Barke & Nicholas, 1990). Presently, a project using this model is underway (Improving Exercise and Dietary Behaviors of Black Elders) as part of a National Institute on Aging (NIA) funded Center for Health Promotion With Minority Elders (CHIME) (Prohaska, 1993–1996). This is a promising model for health promotion because it suggests that programs and strategies need to be tailored so that they are specific to a person's stage of change. That is, a health promotion program for a person in the first stage, precontemplation, would be very different from that for a person in the last stage, maintenance. The model also allows professionals to develop programs for people who have dropped out of programs (recyclers) and want to start a program again. This model can be used with older women to identify the stage of change they are currently in regarding a health behavior (eg, exercise) and then design a program to move them to the next stage.

Policy Context of Health Promotion of Older Women

Relevant policies that address the health promotion needs of older women were recently articulated in a conference sponsored by the National Osteoporosis Foundation. The conference was designed as a mini White House conference on aging and resulted in several resolutions that can support a national agenda for older women's health (National Osteoporosis Foundation, 1995). Some of the policies germane to this chapter are as follows:

1. Develop public and private partnerships to educate health care consumers and providers on health promotion and disease prevention behaviors across the life cycle and incentives that encourage and recognize health promoting behaviors.
2. Educate care providers (and others involved in care of older women) to understand and provide a full range of preventive services to women across the lifespan, with particular attention to underserved and special populations.
3. Provide services with consideration of access issues and of mandated third-party coverage for preventive services identified in *Healthy People 2000.*
4. Develop a national initiative to ensure access to screening and early detection tests.

Summary

The health of older women will not significantly improve until some of the major obstacles are removed, such as lack of financial resources, access, and fragmented care. More importantly, negative attitudes related to gender, age, and race can adversely affect the quality and quantity of health services and care, particularly health promotion and preventive care provided to older women. In discussing health issues and problems related to health care for African American elders, Harper (1992) articulates a perspective that is equally important for older women; she argues for a "public strategy, a combined approach of consensus building, 'universality' and efficient 'targeting'" (p. 212). Society can no longer afford to have a "color-coded" (Harper, 1992) or gender-coded health system. There is no doubt that future cohorts of older women will be more knowledgeable and assertive and demand a health system that is more comprehensive and nondiscriminatory than the current one.

As we move into the 21st century, society must increase its efforts to improve the health of one segment of society, namely older women, and realize that by doing so the quality of life for all people will improve.

References

Airhihenbuwa, C. O. (1992). Health promotion and disease preventive strategies for African Americans: A conceptual mode. In R. L. Braithworth & S. E. Tayor (Eds.). *Health issues in the black community*. San Francisco: Jossey-Bass.

Barke, C. R., & Nicholas, D. R. (1990). Physical changes in older adults: The stages of change. *Journal of Applied Gerontology, 9* (2), 216-223.

Brody, E. (1985). Parent care as a normative family stress. *Gerontologist, 25,* 19-29.

Connidis, L. A., & Davies (1990). Confidants and companions in later life; the place fief family and friends. *Journal of Gerontology; Social Sciences, 45*(4), 141-150.

Cude, B. (1995). Medicare, medigap and other insurance issues. *Health needs of older women: Now and into the 21st century.* Mini White House Conference on Aging. National Osteoporosis Foundation.

Davis, K. (1988). *Testimony to the U.S. House of Representatives Select Committee on Aging.* Hearing on quality of life for older women: Older women alone. Washington DC: U.S. Government Printing Office.

Davis, L., & McGadney, B. (1993). Self-care practices of black elders. In C. M. Barresi & D. E. Stull (Eds.) *Ethnic elderly and long term care.* New York: Springer.

Davis, L., & McGadney, B., & Perri, P. (1990). Self-care for black elders with hypertension, diabetes and arthritis. Lisle, IL: Tucker Publishing.

DeLisa, J. A., & Gans, B. M. (1993). *Rehabilitation medicine: Principles and practice* (2nd ed.). Philadelphia: Lippincott.

Dougherty, J.D., & Knuteson (1995). The female reproductive system and its problems in the elderly. In Stanley, M. and Beare, P.G. (ed.). *Gerontological Nursing*. Philadelphia:Davis.

Duvall, E. M. (1977). *Marriage and family development.* Philadelphia: Lippincott.

Fowls, D. G. (Ed.). (1993). *A profile of older Americans: 1993.* Washington, DC: American Association of Retired Persons.

Fries, J. F., & Crapo, P. (1981). *Vitality and aging.* San Francisco: Freeman.

Harper, M. (Ed.) (1992). Elderly issues in the African American community. In R. L. Braithwaite & S. E. Taylor (Eds.). *Health issues in the black community.* San Francisco: Jossey-Bass.

Koop, E.C. (1988). *Surgeon General's workshop health promotion and aging proceedings.* U.S. Public Health Service.

Leader, S. (1990). *Health needs of older women: Now and into the 21st century. Screening and early detection.* National Osteoporosis Foundation.

Lewis, C. B., & Campanelli, L. C. (1990). *Health promotion and exercise for older adults.* Rockville, MD: Aspen.

Maiman, L. A., & Becker, M. H. (1974). The health belief model. In Becker, M. H. (Ed.). *The health belief model and personal health behavior.* Thorofare, NJ: Slack.

Meyer, G. C. (1990). Demography of aging. In R. H. Binstock & L. K. George (Eds.). *Aging and social sciences.* New York: Academic Press.

Miller, C. A. (1992). *Nursing care of older adults.* Glenview, IL: Little Brown.

National Cancer Institute (1990). *Cancer statistics review (1973-1987).* (NIH Publication, No. 90-2789). Washington, D.C.: Author.

National Center for Health Statistics. (1995). *Births, marriages, divorces and deaths for August 1994* (Monthly Vital Statistics Report *43*, p. 8). Hyattsville, MD: U.S. Public Health Service.

National Osteoporosis Foundation. (1995). *Health needs of older women: Now and into the 21st century.* White House Mini Conference on Aging.

Office of Technology Assessment. (1992). *The menopause, hormone therapy and women's health* (OTA-BP-88). Washington DC: Author.

Okie, S. (1991). Study links cancer and poverty: Blacks higher rates are tied to income. *Washington Post,* April 17, pp. A1, A6.

Pender, N. J. (1987). *Health promotion in nursing practice* (2nd ed.). Norwalk CT: Appleton and Lander.

Prochaska, J. O., & DiClemente, C. C. (1982). Transtheoretical therapy: Toward a more integrative model of change. *Psychotherapy: Theory, Research and Practice, 19,* 276-288.

Prohaska, T. (1993-1996). Center for health promotion with minority elders. (Grant No. NIA AG12042). Washington, DC: National Institute on Aging.

Redeker, N. S. (1988). Health beliefs and adherence in chronic illness. *Image* (20), 31-38.

Sapp, M. & Bliesmer, (1995). A health promotion/protection approach to meeting elders' health-care needs through public policy and standards of care. In M. Stanley & G. Beare (eds.). *Gerontological nursing.* Philadelphia: Davis.

Schafer, S. L. (1989). Aggressive approach to promoting health responsibility. *Journal of Gerontological Nursing* (15), 22-28.

Tripp-Reimer, T., Johnson, R., & Hayden, R. (1995). Cultural dimensions in gerontological nursing. In M. Stanley & P. L. Beare (Eds.), *Gerontological nursing.* Philadelphia: Davis.

U.S. Public Health Service. (1990). *Healthy people 2000: National health promotion and disease prevention objectives.* Washington DC: U.S. Government Printing Office.

U.S. Senate Special Committee on Aging. (1986). *The health status and health care needs of older Americans* (Senate Committee Publication No. 87-6635). Washington, DC: U.S. Government Printing Office.

U.S. Senate Committee on Aging in America. (1988). *Trends and Projections.* Washington, DC: U.S. Department of Health and Human Services.

Walker, S. N. (1988). Health-promoting lifestyles of older adults: comparison with young and middle aged adults; correlates and patterns. *Advances in Nursing Science* (11), 76-89.

Wing, S., Manton, K. G., Stallard, E., Haines, C. G., & Tyroles, H. A. (1985). The black/white mortality crossover: Investigation in a community-based study. *Journal of Gerontology, 40*(2), 78-84.

Bibliography

Rakowski, W. (1994). The definition and measurement of prevention, preventive health care and health promotion. *Generations, 18*(1), 18-23.

Stanley, M., & Beare, P. (1995). Preface. *Gerontological nursing.* Philadelphia: Davis.

CHAPTER 7

Preventive Health Issues: The Mature Years (64 and Older)

Deborah Rohm Young
Abby C. King

Introduction

Mature women ideally can look forward to one of the most independent times of life. Many have finished their child-rearing responsibilities, have retired from the work force, and face a future in which they can focus on their special interests and enjoy relaxed time with their family and friends. At times, however, these women are burdened with unexpected pitfalls—a diagnosis of chronic disease or severe illness or the loss of their spouse can play a significant part in determining the quality of their later years. Preventive health measures that are either maintained from earlier years or adopted during their mature years can provide women with a buffer to avoid chronic diseases or lessen their impact. This chapter presents preventive health strategies appropriate for women aged 64 and older that may be beneficial in limiting the extent of disability associated with unexpected health challenges.

Older women are at risk for many diseases, including coronary heart disease (CHD), cancer, osteoporosis, diabetes, hypertension, and arthritis. Most of these diseases are afflictions that are chronic in nature and will persist throughout their remaining years; however, some may actually be life-threatening. CHD is the leading cause of death in women over the age of 65, with death from cancer falling second (U.S. Department of Health and Human Services, 1993b). Bone loss that is associated with aging accelerates after menopause, which can result in osteoporosis and vertebral and hip fractures for many elderly women (Snow-Harter & Marcus, 1991). Complications after hip fracture account for greater morbidity and mortality than any other osteoporotic-related fracture (Jensen & Tondevold, 1979). Non–insulin-dependent diabetes mellitus, hypertension, and arthritis are diseases that are not generally life-threatening when adequately controlled but are related to quality of life issues. Choosing healthful lifestyle behaviors, participating in preventive screenings, and visiting their physician for regular checkups are measures women can take to either prevent the onset of these diseases or hasten their diagnosis and treatment, thereby limiting their impact.

Definitions of Preventive Health Measures

Good health for older adults encompasses more than just absence of disease or symptoms. It includes being able to function in a manner acceptable to both one-self and society, to respond effectively to environmental stresses, and to maintain good quality of life (Walker, 1989). Preventive health can be classified into three general types: primary, secondary, and tertiary prevention (Leavell & Clark, 1965). Primary prevention includes measures that are enacted to provide protection against contracting a disease. Examples of primary prevention include immunizations and certain lifestyle behaviors, such as engaging in regular physical activity, following a low-fat diet or avoiding the habit of smoking cigarettes. Secondary prevention comprises activities related to early diagnosis and treatment to delay the onset of a disease, such as screenings for cancers and other diseases. This type of prevention is relevant to populations who are at increased risk for certain diseases. Finally, tertiary prevention is enacted to slow the progression of a disease and provide for optimal quality of life and function while living with a disease. Examples of tertiary prevention include cardiovascular rehabilitation after an acute coronary event, strength training after a radical mastectomy, and exercises to maintain function in an arthritic joint. Preventive health measures that are suitable for older women include all of the prevention concepts. However, because the principal outcomes of prevention for older individuals have traditionally been to maximize functional independence, avoid unnecessary disability, and enhance quality of life after disease onset (Walker, 1989), most of the preventive health efforts targeted at older adults have been secondary and tertiary prevention strategies.

Age-Related Activities

Physical Activity

Participating in regular physical activity is a preventive health practice that can be of great value for older women. Women who regularly participate in physical activity:

- have lower rates of CHD, stroke, diabetes, obesity, and hypertension (Hagberg, 1994)
- are less likely to develop some forms of cancer (Lee, 1994)
- tend to maintain their bone mass (Snow-Harter & Marcus, 1991)
- may have less functional impairment due to arthritic conditions (Hicks, 1990)
- may be able to maintain good physical functioning that will allow them to remain independent (Branch, 1985)
- may experience an overall sense of well-being (Hill, Storandt, & Malley, 1993)

Unfortunately, adults over the age of 64 tend not to participate in regular physical activity—nearly 62% of older adults are completely sedentary, and women over the age of 55 are more likely to be sedentary than similarly aged men (Centers for Disease Control and Prevention [CDC], 1993). The following section presents some of the relevant investigations outlining the benefits of regular physical activity for older women in terms of primary, secondary, and tertiary prevention health strategies.

Physical Activity and Cardiovascular Disease

Few studies examining the association between physical inactivity and incidence of cardiovascular disease have included women as subjects; however, the few studies that have generally found that physical inactivity is a risk factor for CHD and stroke of a magnitude similar to that for men. Analyses from the Framingham Cardiovascular Disease Study found that women who were more physically active had significantly lower rates of death from CHD. This association disappeared, however, when controlling for the effects of age because the older women were more likely to be sedentary compared to the younger women (Kannel & Sorlie, 1979). A 12-year follow-up of Swedish women found that low levels of physical activity were related to higher incidence of total mortality, stroke, and myocardial infarction independent of the effects of age, although the association between physical activity and myocardial infarction did not remain significant after adjustment for other known risk factors (Lapidus & Bengtsson, 1986). However, another investigation found significant associations between low physical activity at work and increased risk of total mortality, stroke, and myocardial infarction after controlling for risk factors (Salonen, Puska, & Tuomilehto, 1982). Moreover, Blair et al. (1989) found reduced all-cause mortality for women at higher levels of physical fitness (a product of regular physical activity), which was particularly pronounced for women categorized in the 50 to 59– and the over 60–year-old age groups. Further analyses suggested that the lower mortality rates were due to lower death rates for cardiovascular disease and cancer rather than other causes of death (Blair et al., 1989). These few studies, as well as others (Brunner, Manelis, Modan, & Levin, 1974; Magnus, Matroos, & Strackee, 1979), suggest that high levels of physical activity may be associated with lower incidence of cardiovascular disease, although more studies that include women clearly need to be conducted. Because women generally experience CHD at an older age than men, the follow-up period to determine cardiovascular end points for women may have been insufficient, and the beneficial effects of regular physical activity may actually be underestimated in women (Douglas et al., 1992). Nevertheless, these data suggest that women who have been regularly active throughout their lives (a primary prevention strategy) experience a lower incidence of cardiovascular disease. This appears to be particularly applicable to older women who are at increased risk of CHD and stroke.

Physical Activity and Selected Risk Factors for Cardiovascular Disease.

A regular physical activity program may be particularly beneficial for older women who are at increased risk for cardiovascular disease. In a cross-sectional study, Kohrt, Malley, Dalsky, and Holloszy (1992) found that older women (mean age 62 years) who were endurance trained had a significantly lower percent of body fat, lower skinfold thicknesses, and less adipose tissue in their upper, central body regions compared to similarly aged sedentary women. Moreover, an endurance exercise training program was associated with overall weight loss in women between the ages of 60 and 70 years, with a preferential loss of weight found in the central body regions (Kohrt, Obert, & Holloszy, 1992). Beneficial changes in regional fat distribution are particularly important for older women. Abdominal obesity is associated with increased risk of myocardial infarction, stroke, diabetes mellitus, and death (Despres et al., 1990; Lapidus & Bengtsson, 1988), as well as metabolic disorders that are associated with insulin resistance, glucose intolerance, and unfavorable lipoprotein profiles (Despres et al., 1990). Additionally, aging is associated with an accumulation of adipose tissue in the abdominal region for both women and men (Durnin & Womersley, 1974). Women with high adipose tissue distribution in the abdominal region have a similar CHD risk to men, indicating that much of the differential in rates of CHD between men and women may be explained by gender differences in regional fat distribution (Larsson et al., 1992; Wingard, 1990).

Level of physical activity is also associated with lipoprotein profiles in older women. Women between the ages of 50 and 89 years who reported regular exercise had significantly greater high-density lipoprotein (HDL) cholesterol levels compared with women who did not exercise regularly—a finding that persisted after adjusting for age, alcohol use, cigarette use, estrogen use, and waist/hip ratio (Reaven, McPhillips, Barrett-Connor, & Criqui, 1990). Kohrt et al. (1992) found significant decreases in total cholesterol and triglyceride levels after a 9- to 12-month exercise training program of older adults. Data were not evaluated for each gender separately, however, thereby limiting the study's implications for older women. After a community-based sample completed 2 years of exercise training, King, Haskell, Young, Oka, and Stefanick (1995) found that older women and men had significant increases in HDL cholesterol levels compared to baseline levels. These findings suggest that improvements in HDL cholesterol can occur in older adults, but it may take a longer time for the effects to be realized (King et al., 1995).

Physical Activity and Cancer

Data from long-term, prospective studies suggest that regular physical activity may be protective for some types of cancers. Physical inactivity is associated with increased risk of colon cancer in some populations of women (Slattery, Schumacher, Smith, West, & Abd-Elghany, 1988; Vena, Graham, Zielezny, Brasure, & Swanson, 1987; Wu, Paganini-Hill, Ross, & Henderson, 1987), but other studies have not found an association (Albanes, Blair, & Taylor, 1989; Ballard-Barbash et al., 1990). These negative findings may be due to lower involvement in vigorous physical activity for women compared to men in the cohorts under study or low incidence rates of colon cancer among women (Ballard-Barbash et al., 1990). Rates of breast cancer have been found to be lower in:

- postmenopausal women who were classified as being more physically active (Albanes et al., 1989)
- women working in occupations whose job titles were classified as high active (Vena et al., 1987)
- women who were former college athletes (Frisch et al., 1987)

Data regarding the association between physical activity and breast cancer, however, currently are insufficient to conclude that physical activity has a protective effect on this type of cancer (Sternfeld, 1992). Although several studies have suggested that physical activity may be associated with lower rates of other types of cancer in women (Albanes et al., 1989; Frisch et al., 1987), findings are as yet inconclusive and further prospective studies are needed.

Physical Activity, Bone Loss, Osteoporosis, and Fractures

Evidence suggests that bone mineral content increases in response to the application of mechanical stress (Snow-Harter & Marcus, 1991); therefore, weight-bearing physical activity can potentially maintain bone mineral content or, at a minimum, slow the rate of bone loss postmenopausal women experience. Grove and Londeree (1992) compared the effects of low-impact versus high-impact exercise on bone mineral density in the lumbar vertebrae in early postmenopausal women (mean age 56 years). They found that after a 1-year training program, bone mineral density was maintained in both exercise groups although it significantly declined in the nonexercising control group (Grove & Londeree, 1992). This finding suggests that low-impact physical activity (defined as imparting force less than 1.5 times body weight and including activities such as slow and fast walking and the Charleston dance) may be as beneficial as high-impact activities that carry an added risk of musculoskeletal injuries. Data from other investigations suggest that maintenance of bone mineral density appears to be site specific; that is, weight-bearing activity such as walking is likely to maintain bone density in areas that are stressed from the activity (ie, the spine), but will not in nonspecific areas (ie, the radius) (Snow-Harter & Marcus, 1991).

Bone loss to the point of changes in the trabecular microarchitecture and increased vulnerability to fracture defines the condition of osteoporosis (Snow-Harter & Marcus, 1991). The efficacy of physical activity in the treatment and prevention of osteoporosis has not yet been determined (1991). Because data suggest that bone mineral density may be maintained with weight-bearing or load-generating exercise, it is thought that with regular exercise the clinical manifestation of bone loss, osteoporosis, may be forestalled. Controlled, randomized, clinical trials in women diagnosed with osteoporosis need to be conducted to determine if and what types of physical activity can improve bone mineral density.

Several observational studies suggest that regular physical activity is associated with lower rates of fractures in older adults. Jaglal, Kreiger, and Darlington (1993) found that previous levels of physical activity, as well as recent moderate physical activity, were associated with lower risk of hip fracture in postmenopausal women. In another case-control study, recent weight-bearing activity was also associated with reduced risk of hip fracture in older adults (Cooper, Barker, & Wickham, 1988). Moreover, a prospective investigation found that regular physical activity was protective from overall fracture risk in adults with a mean age of 73 years (Sorock et al., 1988). It is not known from these findings if the association between physical activity and reduced risk of fracture is due to greater bone mineral density, improved balance, or improved muscle strength. However, because of the high risk of morbidity and mortality from hip fractures in older women, incorporating a regular physical activity routine into one's life may be a prudent preventive health measure.

Physical Activity and Non–Insulin-Dependent Diabetes Mellitus

Several reports suggest that a lifetime of regular physical activity is associated with reduced incidence of non–insulin-dependent diabetes mellitus in men (Burchfiel et al., 1995; Helmrich, Ragland, Leung, & Paffenbarger, 1991; Manson et al., 1992), and at least one report suggests that these findings extend to women (Frisch, Wyshak, Albright, Albright, & Schiff, 1986). Glucose intolerance (a precursor to a diabetes diagnosis) increases with age although it is not known if this effect is truly due to age or is confounded by age-associated changes in obesity, level of physical activity, and general health (Laws & Reaven, 1991). Several investigations of older adults found that regular exercise improves the physiologic control of glucose metabolism (Hollenbeck, Haskell, Rosenthal, & Reaven, 1984; Tonino, 1989). Seven consecutive days of physical activity had a beneficial effect on insulin response to an oral glucose challenge in sedentary adults aged 60 to 80 (Cononie, Goldberg, Rogus, & Hagberg, 1994). The beneficial effect of physical activity on glucose tolerance appears to be directly related to the last bout of exercise (Laws & Reaven, 1991), so, from primary and secondary preventive health standpoints, exercise must be performed regularly to maintain or achieve normal glucose tolerance.

Physical Activity and Hypertension

Moderate-intensity physical activity is thought to decrease systolic and diastolic blood pressure in older, hypertensive women. A population-based, cross-sectional investigation of women aged 50 to 89 found that both systolic and diastolic blood pressures were lower at higher physical activity intensity levels across all age groups (Reaven, Barrett-Connor, & Edelstein, 1991). Moreover, rates of hypertension were lower for women who engaged in activity of any intensity compared to their sedentary counterparts (Reaven et al., 1991). Three months of endurance exercise training of hypertensive women aged 70 to 79 and men at moderate intensities resulted in significantly lower systolic and diastolic pressures compared to sedentary and resistance training groups (Cononie et al., 1991). These results, as well as others (Hagberg, Montain, Martin, & Ehsani, 1989; Roman, Camuzzi, Villalon, & Klenner, 1981), have led to the current position that exercise training at moderate intensities (40–70% maximal oxygen uptake) may elicit similar blood pressure reductions as higher intensity exercise (American College of Sports Medicine [ACSM], 1993). The beneficial effect of moderate-intensity physical activity may be particularly important in elderly hypertensive populations, for whom risks of acute myocardial infarction and musculoskeletal injuries are reduced with lower intensity training (ACSM, 1993).

Physical Activity and Arthritis

The role of physical activity for the older adult diagnosed with rheumatoid arthritis is one that falls into the category of tertiary prevention. The goals of exercise are to maintain and increase strength, maintain or improve range of motion of the affected joint, and decrease pain (Hicks, 1990). A physical activity program that incorporates range of motion, stretching, strengthening, and endurance exercises is considered an important component of the overall management of patients with rheumatoid arthritis (Hicks, 1990). Due to the nature of the disease and the specific needs of each patient afflicted with rheumatoid arthritis, the design and management of any physical activity program should be conducted by a health care professional.

Physical Activity and Physical Function

The ability to maintain good function and live independently are primary objectives of preventive health measures for the older adult (Walker, 1989). Evidence suggests that regular physical activity may protect against functional decline. Evaluating data from the Longitudinal Study of Aging, Mor et al. (1989) found that women and men between the ages of 70 and 74 who reported regular exercise and who sometimes walked a mile were more likely to report being able to carry 25 lb, walk ¼ mile, climb 10 steps, and do heavy housework after 2 years of follow-up compared to older adults who did not report regular exercise. Frequent involvement in activities such as walking, gardening, and vigorous exercise was associated with maintaining mobility (defined as being able to walk up and down stairs and walk ½ mile) after 4 years of follow-up of representative, community-dwelling women and men aged 65 years and older (LaCroix, Guralnick, Berkman, Wallace, & Satterfield, 1993). Other investigations have also found that physical activity is associated with reduced risk of functional decline (Branch, 1985; Simonsick et al., 1993). The benefit of physical activity, however, seems to be restricted to current physical activity because Simonsick et al. (1993) found that although a low physical activity level was predictive of functional decline at 3 years of follow-up, it was no longer predictive at 6 years. Further, in a 21-year follow-up of the Framingham cohort, baseline physical activity level did not predict physical disability (Pinsky, Leaverton, & Stokes, 1987). Results from these prospective studies provide good evidence for maintaining a physically active lifestyle to decrease the risk of loss of physical function.

The relationship between strength and physical function is of importance to older adults. Some of the loss of function in the elderly can be attributed to age-related loss of strength (Buchner & deLateur, 1991). It is vital, therefore, to include activities designed to maintain and improve muscular strength in a well-rounded physical activity program for older women. Recent studies suggest that older women who enrolled in resistance training exercise trials benefited with increased muscular strength without a substantial risk of injury and seemed to enjoy this form of exercise (Nichols, Omizo, Peterson, & Nelson, 1993; Pyka, Lindenberger, Charette, & Marcus, 1994).

Physical Activity and Psychological Well-being

Another benefit of regular physical activity is a possible improvement in the psychological health of the older adult. A 1-year endurance training program of older adults (mean age 64 years) was associated with significant improvement in morale (defined as general well-being and positive future outlook) from pre- to post-testing compared to the sedentary control group (Hill et al., 1993). Overall well-being also was improved in older women and men after a 4-month exercise training program, and one index of well-being was significantly improved relative to an attention-only control group (Gitlin et al., 1992). In a group of adults between the ages of 50 and 65, King, Taylor, and Haskell (1993) found that subjects randomized to a 1-year exercise training program had significant reductions in perceived stress and anxiety relative to controls. Similar results were found for subjects randomized into lower and higher intensity formats, suggesting that physical activity at moderate-intensity levels may be sufficient to achieve positive mental health benefits (King et al., 1993). Two population-based investigations found that physical inactivity was an independent risk factor for future depressive symptoms in women (Camacho, Roberts, Lazarus, Kaplan, & Cohen, 1991; Farmer et al., 1988). All of the subjects in the studies reviewed above were from psychologically healthy populations, suggesting that physical activity may be useful as a primary prevention strategy. There are, however, investigations that have not found exercise training to be associated with improvement in psychological outcomes, and insufficient numbers of well-controlled investigations have been performed to conclude that physical activity leads to enhanced mental health in older populations (Brown, 1992).

Few studies have been performed examining the effects of physical activity on psychological outcomes in older individuals with suboptimal mental health. The results of at least one study with 30 community-dwelling moderately depressed elderly suggest that a walking program may, at least in the short term, have a positive effect on both psychological and somatic symptoms of depression (McNeil, LeBlanc, & Joyner, 1991). A social contact only program resulted in effects on psychological symptoms only (McNeil et al., 1991). Further research examining the effect of physical activity in older adults with symptoms of mental health disorders is needed to determine if physical activity can also play a part in secondary and tertiary prevention strategies.

Health Screenings

Regular health screenings are important for secondary health prevention efforts regarding early detection and treatment of certain cancers for which older women are at increased risk. Regular mammograms and clinical breast examinations are the best way of detecting early breast cancers (Rimer, 1992). Yearly mammograms are recommended for women aged 50 to 75 to increase detection of early stage cancers (National Cancer Institute, 1986). Women over the age of 65, however, are less likely to have ever had a mammogram compared with their younger counterparts (Dawson & Thompson, 1990). Common reasons that women listed for not having had a mammogram included not thinking about it, believing that it was not necessary because they were not experiencing a problem, and lack of physician's recommendation (Dawson & Thompson, 1990). Underutilization of this important preventive health measure as well as controversies and misconceptions about who should be receiving regular mammograms signify the importance of education as well as the development of strategies aimed at attaining optimal utilization.

Regular Pap smears to screen for premalignant or early cancerous conditions of the cervix are another important secondary preventive health measure for older women. With early detection available from Pap smears, the cure rate of cervical cancer is over 85% (Older Women's League, 1988). Similar to the situation for mammogram utilization, women over the age of 60 are less likely to have annual Pap smears compared with younger women. One reason for this is that older women are out of their childbearing years and do not receive the routine Pap smears that accompany prenatal care. However, women over the age of 65 have a 50% greater risk of dying from cervical cancer compared with younger women (National Cancer Institute, 1989). These facts clearly identify the need for mature women to undergo regular screening procedures to detect pre- or early cancerous conditions.

Nutrition

As a woman approaches advanced years, she increases her risk for poor nutritional status. Independent community-dwelling individuals who are impoverished, are isolated, have inappropriate dietary practices, or experience untoward drug interactions are likely to have inadequate nutrition (Davis, Murphy, & Neuhaus, 1988). Both insufficient food intake and overconsumption of calories put older women at increased risk. Women and men with low incomes may prioritize other expenses over food purchases, thereby restricting food access and limiting food choices. Irregularity of type and quantity of food consumption can lead to inadequate vitamin and mineral consumption, increasing an individual's risk for cognitive impairments and depression (caused by inadequacy of vitamins B_{12}, folate, and pyridoxine [Rosenberg & Miller, 1992]). In contrast, chronic overconsumption that leads to obesity increases a woman's risk of hypertension, diabetes mellitus, and CHD (Bjorntorp, 1988). Use of medications, as well as medication interactions, can have an impact on nutrient absorption, metabolism, utilization, and excretion (White, 1994). These factors, which are relevant to many older women, can increase the risk of poor nutrition and its resulting complications.

Preventive health practices aimed at maintaining good nutritional status can be enacted with a conscious effort by the woman at risk. Numerous prepared meals available in grocery stores can enable her to eat from a wide variety of foods to ensure adequate vitamin and mineral intake. If her appetite is decreased and she is at risk of inadequate energy intake, a woman can increase her caloric intake by regularly consuming one of the readily available high-calorie nutrient supplements. If a women is using medications, she can consult her health care professional about potential effects the medication(s) may have on her nutritional status and the optimal methods for minimizing these impacts. Finally, for women who find themselves without sufficient income for adequate food purchases or are disinterested in meal planning, efforts should be made to link them up with nutrition programs in the community or Meals-on-Wheels or similar home food service delivery programs.

In addition to an individual's plan to eat healthfully, efforts can be enacted by the community to ensure that nutritionally adequate meals are consumed by the elderly. Educational programs highlighting the need for high-quality diets and literature emphasizing easy-to-prepare meals with high nutrient quality can be made available in grocery stores as well as senior centers. Transportation can be provided to senior centers to enable those who need assistance to attend group meals. With the combined effort of the elderly individual and the community, negative consequences of inadequate nutritional status can be minimized.

Smoking Cessation

One is never too old to stop smoking. Former smokers between the ages of 65 and 74 who quit smoking 1 to 5 years previously had similar risks of CHD compared to lifelong nonsmokers (Smith, 1988). Women are more likely than men to smoke for reasons relating to tension reduction and weight control; therefore, smoking cessation efforts designed specifically for women should emphasize alternative strategies for successfully coping with these issues (Ockene, 1993). Older women who are current smokers should continue to seek out individual or group programs and strategies to enable them to discontinue this unhealthful habit.

Estrogen Replacement Therapy

Postmenopausal women should discuss the benefits and risks of estrogen replacement therapy with their health care professionals. Estrogen can be prescribed in combination with progestin or may be given unopposed, may be prescribed in varying doses and durations, and may be administered in a variety of forms, including pills, patches, and creams. The decision to initiate estrogen therapy, and in what form, dosage, and duration, should be made with a physician who is familiar with the woman's personal health risks. Replacement estrogen maintains bone mass and reduces the risk of fracture in postmenopausal women and is a superior strategy for prevention of osteoporosis compared to weight-bearing physical activity (Snow-Harter & Marcus, 1991). However, these benefits last only as long as a woman takes estrogen—once estrogen use is discontinued, bone loss resumes at a rate similar to that found in postmenopausal women who were never treated with estrogen (Lindsay et al., 1978). Use of estrogen is also thought to reduce a woman's risk of CHD (Speroff, 1993), although the definitive investigation regarding this issue is just now underway (U.S. Department of Health and Human Services, 1993a). There are, however, risks associated with long-term estrogen replacement therapy, which include possible increased risk of breast (Colditz et al., 1990) and endometrial cancers (Paganini-Hill, Ross, & Henderson, 1989) in some groups of women. A woman considering use of estrogen therapy should discuss this matter with her physician to determine if the benefits outweigh the risks for her personal risk profile.

Selected Issues: Unexpected Roles of Mature Women

Widows

Three out of every four wives will become widows over the course of their lives (U.S. Bureau of the Census, 1990). Bereavement is a possible cause of disease in the elderly and may also be associated with physical changes that are often associated with the normal aging process (Barrett, 1985). Moreover, social changes, which include changes in eating behaviors and meal preparation, are more likely with the loss of one's husband. Rosenbloom and Whittington (1993) examined the effects of bereavement on eating behaviors and nutrient intake in recent widows over the age of 60 and found that their mealtimes were less enjoyable, their appetites were poorer, and they were more likely to have unintentionally lost weight. Compared to their married peers, they were less likely to take vitamin and mineral supplements and, in general, were placing themselves at greater risk for nutrient deficiencies and poor nutritional status (Rosenbloom & Whittington, 1993). Although poverty was not a factor in the Rosenbloom and Whittington (1993) investigation, widows in the nation's population are more likely to be impoverished compared to their same-aged married peers, influencing their ability to purchase adequate supplies of nutritious food and compounding their risk for poor nutritional status.

Preventive measures can be taken to diminish the impact of this traumatic event. Women who are faced with the imminent loss of a spouse can cultivate other social networks so support is available when needed. Many communities have ongoing services that provide for the specific needs of those who have recently been widowed and have programs available to assist with grief resolution. A woman who has been widowed should be encouraged to take advantage of the resources available to her and ask for assistance when it is needed to maintain her health and cope with her new social status.

Caregivers

Another unexpected role in which older women may find themselves is that of a caregiver for a chronically ill spouse or relative. It is estimated that more than 2.2 million Americans provide regular unpaid assistance to over 1.2 million noninstitutionalized elderly persons with disabilities (Stone, Cafferata, & Sangl, 1987). Over 70% of these family caregivers are women, with adult daughters and wives assuming this role in similar percentages (Stone et al., 1987). Family caregiving has been associated with a variety of unfavorable social conditions and psychological states, including social isolation (Haley, Levine, Brown, Berry, & Hughes, 1987) and depression (Dura, Stukenberg, Kiecolt-Glaser, 1990; Haley et al., 1987). Caregivers may also experience an increased vulnerability to physical illness (Chenoweth & Spencer, 1986; Stone et al., 1987), as well as disruptions in immune function (Kiecolt-Glaser et al., 1987). A spouse is one's major source of social support, but a spouse caregiver may be reluctant to ask for support for fear that it may be burdensome and counterproductive in light of the care receiver's chronic illness (Revenson, 1994). Another source of caregiver burden is the diminished ability to do required chores and other daily activities necessary for daily living. By not having her own social, psychological, and physical needs met, the caregiver is at risk of adverse outcomes.

Seeking support from family and friends is a valuable coping resource available to caregivers. Support from individuals other than one's spouse can not only alleviate some of the burden of providing care, but also may provide an outlet to vent frustrations and concerns regarding the stress of living with a chronically ill spouse or relative (Revenson, 1994). In addition, participation in moderate levels of physical activity may be a means for health enhancement as well as a strategy for controlling the stress involved in caregiving.

Strategies for Maintenance of Behaviors

Regular Physical Activity

Barriers to Physical Activity

Although physical activity provides numerous preventive health benefits to the older woman, most women over the age of 65 are either underactive or completely sedentary (Caspersen, Christenson, & Pollard, 1986; CDC, 1993). Identifying relevant barriers to physical activity and providing strategies to minimize these barriers are necessary to increase the physical activity patterns of mature women. Some potent barriers that today's older women face are those of unpleasant (or lack of) early experiences with exercise, prior social norms that discouraged physical activity for girls and women, and the notion that physical stress is "work" and not an activity that is to be enjoyed (O'Brien & Vertinsky, 1991). Clearly, to encourage physical activity in older women, activity must be perceived as pleasant and enjoyable.

Perceptions regarding lack of time available for physical activity also may be a barrier for older women (Fitzgerald, Singleton, Neale, Prasad, & Hess, 1994). Lack of time is one of the most commonly cited reasons adults give for not regularly engaging in physical activity (King et al., 1992). Those who are physically active also consider time to be a barrier to activity, indicating that a general lack of interest or commitment, rather than lack of time, may be a predisposing factor to inactivity (King et al., 1992). However, some older women overestimate the amount of time necessary to achieve aerobic fitness, suggesting the need for messages targeted to older adults that provide basic knowledge about appropriate physical activity and address misconceptions (Fitzgerald et al., 1994).

Senior women may believe that they are facing undue risks if they increase their physical activity level. They may have concerns related to the likelihood of serious injury or sudden death from physical exertion (O'Brien & Vertinsky, 1991). Although engaging in exercise transiently increases the risk of sudden cardiac death in persons with CHD, the absolute incidence of sudden cardiac death while engaging in physical activity is low (Thompson & Fahrenbach, 1994). Specific data are not available for women, but rates have been calculated as approximately 6 to 7 deaths per 100,000 exercising men (Thompson & Fahrenbach, 1994).

Exercise does increase the risk of musculoskeletal injuries, but some data suggest that risk is higher only when older adults are engaging in high-impact physical activity compared to low-impact physical activity. In a walk/jog training group of women and men with a mean age of 72 years, 43% of the subjects (9 of 21) sustained a musculoskeletal injury during the 26-week program; however, eight of the nine injuries occurred after the group increased the intensity of training by including jogging in the training program (Pollock et al., 1991). Moreover, all 6 women who jogged as part of their training were injured (Pollock et al., 1991). Another study examined high- versus moderate-intensity walking in the elderly and found the incidence of musculoskeletal injury was only 14%, and the number of injuries was similar for the two training intensities (Carroll et al., 1992). In a clinical exercise trial of adults aged 50 to 65, King, Haskell, Taylor, Kraemer, and DeBusk (1991) also found no significant differences in rates of activity-related injuries in subjects randomized to high- or low-intensity exercise programs. Carroll et al. (1992) surmised that the higher impact forces associated with jogging and not the exercise intensity itself are responsible for most activity-related injuries in older adults.

Physical Activity Adherence and Programming Issues

Some of the personal, environmental, and social factors associated with exercise adherence for adults in general are also relevant to older adults' participation and adherence rates. Richter, Macera, Williams, and Koerber (1993) interviewed randomly selected elderly adults (mean age 76) living in a retirement center that had planned exercise programs and found participation rates were very low, although 75% of those interviewed were aware of the programs. After further questioning the respondents about why they did not attend the classes, they found that the respondents thought the class times were not optimal and the intensity of the classes was inappropriate (either too vigorous or not vigorous enough). Furthermore, 62% of the respondents reported that they currently exercised on a regular basis and 53% thought that they were more active than their same-aged peers (Richter et al., 1993). These findings substantiate previous investigations relating to exercise nonparticipation or dropout, namely: the programs were not convenient and did not consist of enjoyable activities (King et al., 1992). Moreover, because most of the respondents indicated that they exercised regularly, although they did not attend the classes, the results support the notion that adults generally prefer home-based exercise as opposed to classes (King et al., 1991; King, Taylor, Haskell, & DeBusk, 1990).

The previous two sections identified issues that are tied to older women's physical activity participation. These issues are important in planning optimal programs and strategies relevant to older women so that misconceptions, unfounded fears, or components of the program itself do not prevent participation. Physical activity programs that are designed to attract older women should include educational messages that dispel myths regarding the risks of exercise and provide opportunities for types of activities that older women enjoy. Inclusion of an initial target or focus group in the early phase of planning is recommended to ensure that specific needs relevant to the group are met (Richter et al., 1993).

Appropriate Physical Activity for Older Women

To achieve many of the health benefits of physical activity described previously, a well-rounded physical activity program that includes endurance, strength, flexibility, and balance components is recommended. It is not necessary, and may in fact be counterproductive (based on findings from Pollock et al., 1991), to engage in very strenuous activities such as jogging. Rather, activities that are aerobic and rhythmic in nature, use large muscle groups such as the legs, arms, and torso, can be performed comfortably for 30 minutes, and are associated with a moderate increase in heart rate and breathing are generally sufficient for endurance training for elderly adults. Examples of activities that can provide increased endurance, particularly for the previously sedentary woman, include walking, hiking, bicycling, gardening, and swimming or water exercises. Recent guidelines published by the CDC and the ACSM suggest that activity of this type should be carried out on most days of the week (Pate et al., 1993). Similarly, although it is important for older women to maintain or increase muscular strength, it is not necessary for them to join the local gym and begin "pumping iron." Although some older women find resistance training enjoyable (Nichols et al., 1993; Pyka et al., 1994), most would probably be intimidated in that type of an environment. There are other methods to maintain or increase strength; for example, a woman can carry hand weights and pump her arms when she goes for her daily walk, she can reach above her head to pull items off of a kitchen shelf, and can lift food cans in a repetitive manner. To maintain or increase muscular strength, it is recommended that adults engage in 8 to 12 repetitions of strengthening activities that condition the major muscle groups at least twice per week (ACSM, 1990). Finally, it is preferable to perform flexibility and balance activities both before and after aerobic physical activity. Before the activity, some light stretching and calisthenics will help divert blood flow from the truncal region and into leg muscles where it will be needed. After the activity, when one's muscles are fully warmed, extended stretching exercises are recommended. A well-rounded physical activity program that includes all of these components is likely one of the best preventive health measures that the mature woman can use.

Health Screenings

Barriers and Facilitators of Screenings

Although regular mammograms and Pap smears are important components of preventive health for older women, many women do not participate in these screenings. In addition to the barriers to mammography previously cited, some women resist mammograms because of fears of radiation, fear of finding an abnormality, concerns about pain or discomfort associated with the procedure, difficulty in scheduling an appointment because of work and family responsibilities and location of the screening site. The cost of the procedure may also be a concern, particularly for low-income women (Rimer, 1992). Barriers to having regular Pap smears include misunderstandings of the importance of regular screenings, fear of embarrassment owing to the nature of the procedure, and lack of prenatal care during pregnancies (Peters, Bear, & Thomas, 1989). Some unique factors are associated with women who do receive screenings. Women who receive a recommendation or referral from their physician, get regular checkups, visit gynecologic specialists, have better health status in general, and perceive themselves to be vulnerable to breast cancer (because of the presence of risk factors) are more likely to have received a mammogram (Rimer, 1992). Most factors associated with cervical cancer screenings are linked to visits with a health care professional for family planning and prenatal checkups (Peters et al., 1989), often leaving postmenopausal women with limited opportunities for screening.

Strategies for increasing use of mammograms and Pap smears among older women include:

- increasing the knowledge base of older women so they understand that, because of their age, they are at risk for breast and cervical cancer
- reducing the costs associated with the procedures
- providing easy access to screening

Rimer et al. (1992) found that inviting women over the age of 65 to participate in mammography screening and an educational seminar, providing cost subsidies, and providing a mobile van for screening were strategies significantly more effective in encouraging women to have a mammogram compared with only providing cost subsidies. Because much of the impetus to have regular screening for cervical cancer is eliminated when women reach postmenopausal status, women of all ages must be educated to understand that Pap smears are a necessary preventive health measure throughout the lifespan. Health care provider education and encouragement to continue providing necessary screenings to older women are needed as well.

Summary

The mature woman has a variety of preventive health options available to her to maintain optimal health and well-being. Some of these options require action on her part, however. Regular physical activity can provide ample benefits to the older woman (as well as to children and adults of all ages), but a personal commitment must be made to participate in the activity. For some preventive health measures, such as health screenings and hormone replacement therapy, the woman needs to consult with her health care professional to receive benefits. Finally, a woman may have to reach out into the community to find what services and programs are available that meet her needs, as well as seek out assistance from family and friends, if necessary. Health professionals can facilitate this process by using a proactive, public health approach to the dissemination of preventive health measures, rather than relying on the traditional "disease model" approach for this target group. Only by applying a wide variety of approaches that include the contributions and resources of older women, communities, and health care professionals will older women be able to fully realize the benefits that can accrue from preventive health practices.

Acknowledgment

This work was supported in part by a grant from the American Heart Association, Hawaii Affiliate, awarded to Dr. Young and PHS Grant #AG-00440 from the National Institute on Aging awarded to Dr. King.

References

Albanes, D., Blair, A., & Taylor, P. R. (1989). Physical activity and risk of cancer in the NHANES I population. *American Journal of Public Health, 79,* 744-750.

American College of Sports Medicine Position Stand. (1990). The recommended quantity and quality of exercise for developing and maintain cardiorespiratory and muscular fitness in healthy adults. *Medicine and Science in Sports and Exercise, 22,* 265-274.

American College of Sports Medicine Position Stand. (1993). Physical activity, physical fitness, and hypertension. *Medicine and Science in Sports and Exercise, 25,* i-x.

Ballard-Barbash, R., Schatzkin, A., Albanes, D., Schiffman, M. H., Kreger, B. E., Kannel, W. B., Anderson, K. M., & Hhelsel, W. E. (1990). Physical activity and risk of large bowel cancer in the Framingham study. *Cancer Research, 50,* 3610-3613.

Barrett, V. W. (1985). The elderly, death, and bereavement planning. In O. S. Margolis, H. C. Raether, A. H. Kutscher, S. C. Klagbrun, E. Marcus, V. R. Pine, & D. J. Cherico (Eds.), *Loss, grief, and bereavement.* New York: Praeger Special Studies.

Bjorntorp, P. (1988). The associations between obesity, adipose tissue distribution and disease. *Acta Medica Scandinavica Supplement, 723,* 121-134.

Blair, S. N., Kohl, H. W., III, Paffenbarger, R. S., Jr., Clark, D. G., Cooper, K. H., & Gibbons, L. W. (1989). Physical fitness and all-cause mortality: A prospective study of healthy men and women. *Journal of the American Medical Association, 262,* 2395-2401.

Branch, L. G. (1985). Health practices and incident disability among the elderly. *American Journal of Public Health, 75,* 1436-1439.

Brown, D. R. (1992). Physical activity, ageing, and psychological well-being. *Canadian Journal of Sport Sciences, 17,* 185-193.

Brunner, D., Manelis, G., Modan, M., & Levin, S. (1974). Physical activity at work and the incidence of myocardial infarction, angina pectoris and death due to ischemic heart disease: An epidemiological study in Isreali collective settlements (kibbutzim). *Journal of Chronic Diseases, 27,* 217-223.

Buchner, D. M., & deLateur. (1991). The importance of skeletal muscle strength to physical function in older adults. *Annals of Behavioral Medicine, 13,* 91-98.

Burchfiel, C. M., Sharp, D. S., Curb, J. D., Rodriguez, B. L., Hwang, L.-J., Marcus, E. B., & Yano, K. (1995). Physical activity and incidence of diabetes: the Honolulu Heart Program. *American Journal of Epidemiology, 141,* 360–368.

Camacho, T. C., Roberts, R. E., Lazarus, N. B., Kaplan, G. A., & Cohen, R. D. (1991). Physical activity and depression: Evidence from the Alameda County study. *American Journal of Epidemiology, 134,* 220-231.

Carroll, J. F., Pollock, M. L., Graves, J. E., Leggett, S. H., Spitler, D. L., & Lowenthal, D. T. (1992). Incidence of injury during moderate- and high-intensity walking training in the elderly. *Journal of Gerontology, 47,* M61-M66.

Caspersen, C. J., Christenson, G. M., & Pollard, R. A. (1986). Status of the 1990 physical fitness and exercise objectives—evidence from NHIS 1985. *Public Health Reports, 101,* 587-592.

Centers for Disease Control and Prevention. (1993). Prevalence of sedentary lifestyle: Behavioral risk factor surveillance system, United States, 1991. *Morbidity and Mortality Weekly Report, 42,* 576-579.

Chenoweth, B., & Spencer, B. (1986). Dementia: The experience of family caregivers. *Gerontologist, 27,* 201-208.

Colditz, G. A., Stampfer, M. J., Willett, W. C., Hennekens, C. H., Rosner, B., & Speizer, F. E. (1990). Prospective study of estrogen replacement therapy and risk of breast cancer in postmenopausal women. *Journal of the American Medical Association, 264,* 2648-2653.

Cononie, C. C., Goldberg, A. P., Rogus, E., & Hagberg, J. M. (1994). Seven consecutive days of exercise lowers plasma insulin responses to an oral glucose challenge in sedentary elderly. *Journal of the American Geriatrics Society, 42,* 394-398.

Cononie, C. C., Graves, J. E., Pollock M. L., Phillips, M. I., Sumners, C., & Hagberg, J. M. (1991). Effect of exercise training on blood pressure in 70- to 79-yr-old men and women. *Medicine and Science in Sports and Exercise, 23,* 505-511.

Cooper, C., Barker, D. J. P., & Wickham, C. (1988). Physical activity, muscle strength, and calcium intake in fracture of the proximal femur in Britain. *British Medical Journal, 297,* 1443-1446.

Davis, M. A., Murphy, S. P., & Neuhaus, J. M. (1988). Living arrangements and eating behaviors of older adults in the United States. *Journal of Gerontology, 43,* S96-S98.

Dawson, D. A., & Thompson, G. B. (1990). Breast cancer risk factors and screening: United States, 1987. (DHHS Publication No. PHS 90-1500, pp. 1-33). Hyattsville, MD: U.S. Department of Health and Human Services.

Despres, J.-P., Moorjani, S., Lupien, P. J., Tremblay, A., Nadeau, A., & Bouchard, C. (1990). Regional distribution of body fat, plasma lipoproteins, and cardiovascular disease. *Arteriosclerosis, 10,* 497-511.

Douglas, P. S., Clarkson, T. B., Flowers, N. C., Hajjar, K. A., Horton, E., Klocke, F. J., LaRosa, J., & Shively, C. (1992). Exercise and atherosclerotic heart disease in women. *Medicine and Science in Sports and Exercise, 24,* S266-S276.

Dura, J. R., Stukenberg, K. W., & Kiecolt-Glaser, J. K. (1990). Chronic stress and depressive disorders in older adults. *Journal of Abnormal Psychology, 99,* 284-290.

Durnin, J. V., & Womersley, J. (1974). Body fat assessed from total body density and its estimation from skinfold thickness; measurements on 481 men and women aged from 16 to 72 years. *British Journal of Nutrition, 32,* 77-97.

Farmer, M. E., Locke, B. Z., Moscicki, E. K., Dannenberg, A. L., Larson, D. B., & Radloff, L. S. (1988). Physical activity and depressive symptoms: the NHANES I epidemiologic follow-up survey. *American Journal of Epidemiology, 128,* 1340-1351.

Fitzgerald, J. T., Singleton, S. P., Neale, A. V., Prasad, A. S., & Hess, J. W. (1994). Activity levels, fitness status, exercise knowledge, and exercise beliefs among healthy older African American and white women. *Journal of Aging and Health, 6,* 296-313.

Frisch, R. E., Wyshak, G., Albright, N. L., Albright, T. E., Schiff, I., Witschi, J., & Marguglio, M. (1987). Lower lifetime occurrence of breast cancer and cancers of the reproductive system among former college athletes. *American Journal of Clinical Nutrition, 45,* 328-335.

Frisch, R. E., Wyshak, G., Albright, T. E., Albright, N. L., & Schiff, I. (1986). Lower prevalence of diabetes in female former college athletes compared with nonathletes. *Diabetes, 35,* 1101-1105.

Gitlin, L. N., Lawton, M. P., Windsor-Landsberg, L. A., Kleban, M. H., Sands, L. P., & Posner, J. (1992). In search of psychological benefits: Exercise in healthy older adults. *Journal of Aging and Health, 4,* 174-192.

Grove, K. A., & Londeree, B. R. (1992). Bone density in postmenopausal women: High impact vs low impact exercise. *Medicine and Science in Sports and Exercise, 24,* 1190-1194.

Hagberg, J. M. (1994) Physical activity, fitness, health, and aging. In C. Bouchard, R. J. Shephard, & T. Stephens. (Eds.), *Physical activity, fitness, and health: International proceedings and consensus statement* (pp. 993-1006). Champaign, IL: Human Kinetics Publishers.

Hagberg, J. M., Montain, S. J., Martin, W. H., & Ehsani, A. A. (1989). Effect of exercise training on 60-69 year old persons with essential hypertension. *American Journal of Cardiology, 64,* 348-353.

Haley, W. E., Levine, E. G., Brown, S. L., Berry, J. W., & Hughes, G. H. (1987). Psychological, social and health consequences of caring for a relative with senile dementia. *Journal of the American Geriatrics Society, 35,* 405-411.

Helmrich, S. P., Ragland, D. R., Leung, R. W., & Paffenbarger, R. S., Jr. (1991). Physical activity and reduced occurrence of non-insulin-dependent diabetes mellitus. *New England Journal of Medicine, 325,* 147-152.

Hicks, J. E. (1990). Exercise in patients with inflammatory arthritis and connective tissue disease. *Rheumatic Disease Clinics of North America, 16,* 845-870.

Hill, R. D., Storandt, M., & Malley, M. (1993). The impact of long-term exercise training on psychological function in older adults. *Journal of Gerontology: Psychological Sciences, 48,* P12-P17.

Hollenbeck, C. B., Haskell, W., Rosenthal, M., & Reaven, G. M. (1984). Effect of habitual physical activity on regulation of insulin-stimulated glucose disposal in older males. *Journal of the American Geriatrics Society, 33,* 273-277.

Jaglal, S. B., Kreiger, N., & Darlington, G. (1993). Past and recent physical activity and risk of hip fracture. *American Journal of Epidemiology, 138,* 107-118.

Jensen, J. S., & Tondevold, E. Mortality after hip fractures. (1979). *Acta Orthopaedic Scandinavia, 50,* 16 -167.

Kannel, W. B., & Sorlie, P. (1979). Some health benefits of physical activity: The Framingham study. *Archives of Internal Medicine, 139,* 857-861.

Kiecolt-Glaser, J. K., Glaser, R., Shuttleworth, E. C., Dyer, C. S., Ogrocki, P., & Speicher, C. E. (1987). Chronic stress and immunity in family caregivers of Alzheimer's disease victims. *Psychosomatic Medicine, 49,* 523-535.

King, A. C., Blair, S. N., Bild, D. E., Dishman, R. K., Dubbert, P. M., Marcus, B. H., Oldridge, N. B., Paffenbarger, R. S., Jr., Powell, K. E., & Yeager, K. K. (1992). Determinants of physical activity and interventions in adults. *Medicine and Science in Sports and Exercise, 24,* S221-S236.

King, A. C., Haskell, W. L., Taylor, C. B., Kraemer, H. C., & DeBusk, R. F. (1991). Group- vs home-based exercise training in healthy older men and women: A community-based clinical trial. *Journal of the American Medical Association, 26,* 1535-1542.

King, A. C., Haskell, W. L., Young, D. R., Oka, R. K., & Stefanick, M. L. (1995). Long-term effects of varying intensities and formats of physical activity on participation rates, fitness, and lipoproteins in men and women aged 50-65 years. *Circulation, 91,* 2596–2604.

King, A. C., Taylor, C. B., & Haskell, W. L. (1993). The effects of differing intensities and formats of twelve months of exercise training on psychological outcomes in older adults. *Health Psychology, 12,* 292-300.

King, A. C., Taylor, C. B., Haskell, W. L., & DeBusk, R. F. (1990). Identifying strategies for increasing employee physical activity levels: Findings from the Stanford/Lockheed exercise survey. *Health Education Quarterly, 17,* 269-285.

Kohrt, W. M., Malley, M. T., Dalsky, G. P., & Holloszy, J. O. (1992). Body composition of healthy sedentary and trained, young and older men and women. *Medicine and Science in Sports and Exercise, 24,* 832-837.

Kohrt, W. M., Obert, K. A., & Holloszy, J. O. (1992). Exercise training improves fat distribution patterns in 60- to 70-year-old men and women. *Journal of Gerontology: Medical Sciences, 47,* M99-M105.

LaCroix, A. Z., Guralnick, J. M., Berkman, L. F., Wallace, R. B., & Satterfield, S. (1993). Maintaining mobility in late life: II. Smoking, alcohol consumption, physical activity, and body mass index. *American Journal of Epidemiology, 137,* 858-869.

Lapidus, L., & Bengtsson, C. (1986). Socioeconomic factors and physical activity in relation to cardiovascular disease and death. A 12 year follow up of participants in a population study of women in Gothenberg, Sweden. *British Heart Journal, 55,* 295-301.

Lapidus, L., & Bengtsson, C. (1988). Regional obesity as a health hazard in women—a prospective study. *Acta Medica Scandinavica Supplement, 723,* 53-59.

Larsson, B., Bengtsson, C., Bjorntorp, P., Lapidus, L., Sjostrom, L., Svardsudd, K., Tibblin, G., Wedel, H., Welin, L., & Wilhelmsen, L. (1992). Is abdominal body fat distribution a major explanation for the sex difference in the incidence of myocardial infarction? *American Journal of Epidemiology, 135,* 266-273.

Laws, A., & Reaven, G. M. (1991). Physical activity, glucose tolerance, and diabetes in older adults. *Annals of Behavioral Medicine, 13,* 125-132.

Leavell, H., & Clark, A. (1965). *Preventive medicine for doctors in the community.* New York: McGraw-Hill.

Lee, I.-M. (1994). Physical activity, fitness, and cancer. In C. Bouchard, R. J. Shephard, & T. Stephens. (Eds.), *Physical activity, fitness, and health: International proceedings and consensus statement* (pp. 814-831). Champaign, IL: Human Kinetics Publishers.

Lindsay, R., Hart, D. M., MacLean, A., Clark, A. C., Kraszewski, A., & Garwood, J. (1978). Bone response to termination of estrogen treatment. *Lancet, 1,* 1325-1327/

Magnus, K., Matroos, A., & Strackee, J. (1979). Walking, cycling or gardening, with or without seasonal interruption, in relation to acute coronary events. *American Journal of Epidemiology, 110,* 724-733.

Manson, J. E., Nathan, D. M., Krolewski, A. S., Stampfer, M. J., Willett, W. C., & Hennekens, C. H. (1992). A prospective study of exercise and incidence of diabetes among US male physicians. *Journal of the American Medical Association, 268,* 63-67.

McNeil, J. K., LeBlanc, E. M., & Joyner, M. (1991). The effect of exercise on depressive symptoms in the moderately depressed elderly. *Psychology and Aging, 6,* 487-488.

Mor, V., Murphy, J., Masterson-Allen, S., Willey, C., Razmpour, A., Jackson, M. E., Greer, D., & Katz, S. (1989). Risk of functional decline among well elders. *Journal of Clinical Epidemiology, 42,* 895-904.

National Cancer Institute. (1986). Cancer control objectives for the nation: 1985-2000. *NCI Monographs, 2,* 27-32.

National Cancer Institute. (1989). *Annual cancer statistics review, including cancer trends: 1950-1985.* Bethesda, MD: Author.

Nichols, J. F., Omizo, D. K., Peterson, K. K., & Nelson, K. P. (1993). Efficacy of heavy-resistance training for active women over sixty: Muscular strength, body composition, and program adherence. *Journal of the American Geriatrics Society, 41,* 205-210.

O'Brien, S. J., & Vertinsky, P. A. (1991). Unfit survivors: Exercise as a resource for aging women. *The Gerontologist, 31,* 347-357.

Ockene, J. K. (1993). Smoking among women across the life span: Prevalence, interventions, and implications for cessation research. *Annals of Behavioral Medicine, 15,* 135-148.

Older Women's League. (1988). The picture of health for midlife and older women in America. *Women and Health, 14,* 53-74.

Paganini-Hill, A., Ross, R. K., & Henderson, B. E. (1989). Endometrial cancer and patterns of use of oestrogen replacement therapy: a cohort study. *British Medical Journal, 297,* 519.

Pate, R.R., Pratt, M, Blair, S.N., Haskell, W.C., Macera, C.A. et al., (1995). Physical activity and public health: A recommendation from the Centers for Disease Control and Prevention and the American College of Sports Medicine. *Journal of the American Medical Association, 273,* 402-40.

Peters, R. K., Bear, M. B., & Thomas, D. (1989). Barriers to screening for cancer of the cervix. *Preventive Medicine, 18,* 133-146.

Pinsky, J. L., Leaverton, P. E., & Stokes, J., III. (1987). Predictors of good function: The Framingham study. *Journal of Chronic Diseases, 40,* 159S-167S.

Pollock, M. L., Carroll, J. F., Graves, J. E., Leggett, S. H., Braith, R. W., Limacher, M., & Hagberg, J. M. (1991). Injuries and adherence to walk/jog and resistance training programs in the elderly. *Medicine and Science in Sports and Exercise, 23,* 1194-1200.

Pyka, G., Lindenberger, E., Charette, S., & Marcus, R. (1994). Muscle strength and fiber adaptations to a year-long resistance training program in elderly men and women. *Journal of Gerontology, 49,* M22-M27.

Reaven, P. D., Barrett-Connor, E., & Edelstein, S. (1991). Relation between leisure-time physical activity and blood pressure in older women. *Circulation, 83,* 559-565.

Reaven, P. D., McPhillips, J. B., Barrett-Connor, E. L., & Criqui, M. H. (1990). Leisure time exercise and lipid and lipoprotein levels in an older population. *Journal of the American Geriatrics Society, 38,* 847-854.

Revenson, T. A. (1994). Social support and marital coping with chronic illness. *Annals of Behavioral Medicine, 16,* 122-130.

Richter, D. L., Macera, C. A., Williams, H., & Koerber, M. (1993). Disincentive to participation in planned exercise activities among older adults. *Health Values, 17,* 51-55.

Rimer, B. K. (1992). Understanding the acceptance of mammography by women. *Annals of Internal Medicine, 14,* 197-203.

Rimer, B. K., Resch, N., King, E., Ross, E., Lerman, C., Boyce, A., Kessler, H., & Engstrom, P. F. (1992). Multistrategy health education program to increase mammography use among women ages 65 and older. *Public Health Reports, 107,* 369-380.

Roman, O., Camuzzi, A. L., Villalon, E., & Klenner, C. (1981). Physical training program in arterial hypertension: A long-term prospective follow-up. *Cardiology, 67,* 230-243.

Rosenberg, I. H., & Miller, J. W. (1992). Nutritional factors in physical and cognitive functions of elderly people. *American Journal of Clinical Nutrition, 55,* 1237S-1243S.

Rosenbloom, C. A., & Whittington, F. J. (1993). The effects of bereavement on eating behaviors and nutrient intakes in elderly widowed persons. *Journal of Gerontology, 48,* S223-S229.

Salonen, J. T., Puska, P., & Tuomilehto, J. (1982). Physical activity and risk of myocardial infarction, cerebral stroke and death. A longitudinal study in Eastern Finland. *American Journal of Epidemiology, 115,* 526-537.

Simonsick, E. M., Lafferty, M. E., Phillips, C. L., Mendes deLeon, C. F., Kasl, S. V., Seeman, T. E., Fillenbaum, G., Hebert, P., & Lemke, J. (1993). Risk due to inactivity in physically capable older adults. *American Journal of Public Health, 83,* 1443-1450.

Slattery, M. L., Schumacher, M. C., Smith, K. R., West, D. W., & Abd-Elghany, N. (1988). Physical activity, diet, and risk of colon cancer in Utah. *American Journal of Epidemiology, 128,* 989-999.

Smith, D. L. (1988). Health promotion for older adults. *Health Values, 12,* 46-51.

Snow-Harter, C., & Marcus, R. (1991). Exercise, bone mineral density, and osteoporosis. *Exercise and Sports Science Reviews, 19,* 351-388.

Sorock, G. S., Bush, T. L., Golden, A. L., Fried, L. P., Breuer, B., & Hale, W. E. (1988). Physical activity and fracture risk in a free-living elderly cohort. *Journal of Gerontology, 5,* M134-M139.

Speroff, L. (1993). Menopause and hormone replacement therapy. *Clinics in Geriatric Medicine, 9,* 33-55.

Sternfeld, B. (1992). Cancer and the protective effect of physical activity: The epidemiological evidence. *Medicine and Science in Sports and Exercise, 24,* 1195-1209.

Stone, R., Cafferata, G. L., & Sangl, J. (1987). Caregivers of the frail elderly: A national profile. *The Gerontologist, 27,* 616-626.

Thompson, P. D., & Fahrenbach, M. C. (1994). Risks of exercising: Cardiovascular including sudden cardiac death. In C. Bouchard, R. J. Shephard, & T. Stephens (Eds.), *Physical activity, fitness, and health: International proceedings and consensus statement* (pp. 1019-1028). Champaign, IL: Human Kinetics Publishers.

Tonino, R. P. (1989). Effect of physical training on the insulin resistance of aging. *American Journal of Physiology, 256,* E352-E355.

U.S. Bureau of the Census. (1990). *Statistical abstract of the United States: 1988* (108th ed.). Washington, DC: U.S. Government Printing Office.

U.S. Department of Health and Human Services. (1993a). 16 national centers selected for women's health research studies. *Public Health Reports, 108,* 520-521.

U.S. Department of Health and Human Services. (1993b). *Vital statistics of the United States, 1989. Vol. II, Mortality, Part A.* (DHHS publication No. PHS 93-1101). Hyattsville, MD: Author

Vena, J. E., Graham, S., Zielezny, M., Brasure, J., & Swanson, M. K. (1987). Occupational exercise and risk of cancer. *American Journal of Clinical Nutrition, 45,* 318-327.

Walker S. N. (1989). Health promotion for older adults: Directions for research. *American Journal of Health Promotion, 3,* 47-52.

White, J. V. (1994). Risk factors for poor nutritional status. *Primary Care, 21,* 19-31.

Wingard, D. L. (1990). Sex differences and coronary heart disease: A case of comparing apples and pears? *Circulation, 81,* 1710-1712.

Wu, A. H., Paganini-Hill, A., Ross, R. K., & Henderson, B. E. (1987). Alcohol, physical activity, and other risk factors for colorectal cancer: A prospective study. *British Journal of Cancer, 55,* 687-694.

UNIT 3

Systems and Other Health-Related Concerns

CHAPTER 8

Coronary Heart Disease

Karyn Holm
Janet Scherubel

Introduction

Coronary heart disease is now acknowledged as an important cause of mortality in women. The National Institutes of Health (NIH) and the American Heart Association (AHA) have taken leadership roles to ensure that clinicians and researchers are aware of this number one killer of women. The initiatives began in the 1980s with the NIH and the AHA hosting invitational conferences to address the issues. Since this time, clinicians and researchers have become increasingly aware of the need to direct their attention to the manifestations of coronary heart disease in women, with the emphasis on prevention.

We know that women are living longer than men and that coronary disease is more common in older women. We also know that the current emphasis on decreasing the cost of health care without decreasing quality has important implications for the approach to issues of coronary disease in women. Because women are older when they experience symptoms, they will usually have more advanced coronary disease. They will also be more likely to have more coexisting disease. An important concern is whether women who are typically older when they experience symptoms are being diagnosed correctly and, on diagnosis, if they are receiving comparable care.

Epidemiology

Current projections are that by 2030 there will be 60 million Americans over the age of 65 years with 70% of all deaths beyond 75 years a consequence of coronary heart disease (Kannel & Volkanas, 1992). Throughout the world, women outlive men in advanced societies where women are not dying from diseases caused by poor nutrition, contaminated water, and complications of childbirth. The reasons for this are largely unknown. Therefore longevity, particularly in women, is a contemporary phenomenon. One of the consequences of this is that more absolute numbers of women will die from coronary heart disease.

Contributory Factors

Many attribute heart disease in women to estrogen decline associated with menopause. Figure 8–1 uses data from the National Center for Health Statistics (Holm & Penckofer, 1992) to make comparisons of the percentage of male and female deaths due to ischemic heart disease. A higher percentage of men experience heart disease at midlife. For women, heart disease increases linearly with age, with women catching up to men a number of years after menopause.

Some regions in the United States show higher heart disease rates for women than others. If one examines the age-adjusted death rates per 100,000 population for total cardiovascular disease by state, it is clear that mortality due to coronary disease is higher in some states than in others. The reason for this is not entirely clear. Socioeconomic status may have an impact. For example, lower socioeconomic status is often linked to factors such as social isolation, social support or lack of it, coping styles, job stress and strain, and anger and hostility. These factors may actually potentiate coronary disease. An equally important factor is that many persons of low socioeconomic status do not have the same access to health care as those of the middle class (Kaplan & Keil, 1993).

Lower occupational standing, lower income, and poorer education are important determinants. Recently, experts have noted that overall coronary heart disease rates are more strongly related to education than income in both men and women, with better educated people having lower coronary risk (Luepker et al., 1993).

The Influence of Risk Factors

Risk factors for coronary heart disease are classified as nonmodifiable and modifiable. Nonmodifiable risk factors are those we can do nothing about and include

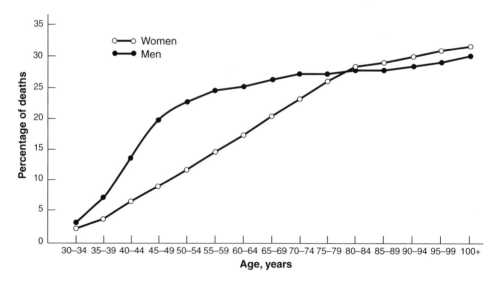

Figure 8-1. Myocardial ischemia (Adapted from Holm, K., & Penckofer, S. [1992]. Cardiovascular risk factors in women. Journal of Myocardial Ischemia, *4(1), 25-46).*

age, family history, gender, and race. Modifiable risk factors, listed in Display 8–1, are hypertension (risk increases with increased blood pressure), cigarette smoking (rates higher in women), hyperlipidemia (women seem more susceptible), obesity (women are more susceptible at later years), physical inactivity (for both genders at all ages), diabetes (seems more important in women), and menopause (heart disease rates in women escalate well after menopause). Of late, pregnancy is being recognized as a potential factor in the development of heart disease. Oral contraceptives are also now considered as a possible risk factor.

Age

Heart disease rates increase with increasing age, a fact known for a number of years. More people die from coronary heart disease at older ages than at younger ages. With women now living longer than men, it is women who will be more susceptible at older ages. However, preventive health behaviors can begin early in life.

Family History

Family history of coronary disease is considered by many to be the most potent risk factor. Evidence indicates that at younger ages, death from coronary heart disease is influenced by genetic factors in both men and women. However, with advancing age, the genetic effect may not be as important (Marenberg, Risch, Berkman, Floderus, & de Faire, 1994). At the present time it is not possible to change genetic predisposition to heart disease. However, it may be that some of the familial tendency toward coronary disease is a function of learned lifestyle behaviors that can be modified.

Gender

Because traditional thinking was that coronary disease was a disease of men, gender became entrenched in the minds of researchers and clinicians as an important risk factor. Now we know that coronary disease is not restricted by gender; it is more commonly manifested in men at younger ages and in both genders at older ages. Because women now live longer than men, more absolute numbers of women will die from coronary heart disease.

DISPLAY 8-1
Modifiable Risk Factors

1. Hypertension	6. Physical inactivity
2. Smoking	7. Menopause
3. Hyperlipidemia	8. Pregnancy
4. Diabetes	9. Oral contraceptives
5. Obesity	

Race

Investigators have suggested that racial differences may be responsible for coronary heart disease rates, with African American women being at greater risk than Caucasian women. A disturbing trend is that over the past decade, life expectancy for African Americans has declined and is now lower than for Caucasians. According to the AHA (1994), the death rate for Caucasian women was 22% lower than for African American women. Notably coronary disease has been cited as the cause of this phenomenon (Pappas, 1994). This may be in part a result of the higher rates of hypertension in African American women. Another primary reason is that Caucasian women have greater access to health care than women of color. Race is often used synonymously with social class, but underlying living circumstances must be considered.

Hypertension

Hypertension is defined as systolic pressure equal to or above 140 mm Hg and diastolic pressure equal to or above 90 mm Hg. High blood pressure is thought by some to be the strongest predictor for coronary disease. Besides increasing the likelihood of heart attack and stroke, hypertension can result in damage to the eyes and kidneys. Contemporary data suggest that a woman with documented hypertension is many times more likely to be diagnosed with heart disease. It has also been suggested that a 10 mm Hg increase in systolic blood pressure in women may result in a 20% to 30% increase in coronary disease risk (Bush, 1990).

Smoking

Women continue to smoke more than men, with smoking rates being higher in the less educated (Wenger, Speroff, & Packard, 1993). This is occurring despite all of the antismoking efforts and legislation over the past decade. The reason for this is thought to be the high rates of smoking in teenage women. Current projections indicate that although overall smoking rates will decrease by the year 2000, women will continue to smoke more than men (Holm, Penckofer, Keresztes, Biordi & Chandler, 1993).

Research has shown that the relative risk of myocardial infarction among current smokers as compared with women who never smoked is over threefold. However, most of this increase in risk will dissipate in 2 to 3 years after cessation (Rosenberg, Palmer, & Shapiro, 1990). Smoking cessation may be more difficult for women. The primary reason for this is the weight gain often associated with smoking cessation.

Antismoking activities began as early as the beginning of this century. We are all familiar with the successful efforts in this country to reduce smoking rates. Legislation forbidding smoking in public places has had a noteworthy impact on smoking behaviors.

Hyperlipidemia

Current recommendations are that total serum cholesterol should be less than 200 mg/dL. Elevated serum lipid levels in women have been linked to advancing age. More than 50% of women aged 55 to 64 have serum cholesterol levels above

240 mg/dL. When the serum cholesterol level is greater than 200 mg/dL, a lipoprotein analysis is needed. The two primary types of lipoproteins are high-density lipoproteins (HDLs) and low-density lipoproteins (LDLs). HDLs transport cholesterol out of the cardiovascular system for excretion; LDLs transport cholesterol to the arteries where it is deposited. Therefore, the HDLs are known as the good cholesterol and the LDLs as the bad cholesterol. An important consideration is the ratio of total cholesterol to HDLs. When this ratio is greater than 4.5, a woman is said to be at increased risk for coronary disease (Holm et al., 1993).

Diabetes

For men and women, diabetes is an independent risk factor for coronary disease and is related to increased mortality from coronary disease. Perhaps diabetes may be more important in women than in men. In diabetic women, coronary disease mortality is four to six times that of women without diabetes. In diabetic men, coronary disease mortality is two to three times that of men without diabetes (Jones & Gotto, 1994). The reason for this is not clearly understood. It is known that those with diabetes have a greater tendency to have other risk factors such as hypertension, central obesity, and hyperlipidemia. Perhaps insulin resistance is key to aggravating these other risk factors.

Obesity

Although obesity is often said to be a women's issue, recent evidence demonstrates that the prevalence of overweight among U.S. adults has increased markedly over the past decade (Kuczmarski, Fiegel, Campbell, & Johnson, 1994). The statistics are alarming. Over the past decade, weight has increased 8% with an average body weight increase of 3.6 kg for both genders. Overweight is defined by most as 20% above ideal weight and obesity as 30% or more above ideal weight. Controlling for cigarette smoking, which can influence body weight, it has been noted that even mild (10%) to moderate (20%) overweight increases the risk of coronary disease in midlife women (Manson et al., 1990). In the United States, at least 30% of women are obese (Sempos et al., 1993). Other observations suggest that obesity is highly related to social class, with women in lower social classes more likely to be obese.

The influence of culture is a major consideration. For example, African American women may engage less frequently in dieting behaviors, and therefore may be less inclined to think that being overweight is a problem (Stevens, Kumanyika, & Keil, 1994). Another important consideration is the location of body fat. Excessive abdominal fat (a waist-to-hip ratio > 0.8), creating an apple-shaped appearance, has been shown to be an indicator of increased coronary risk. Conversely, women who carry the majority of their weight in their hips and thighs, often producing a pear-shaped appearance, are said to have lower coronary risk.

Physical Inactivity

According to the Centers for Disease Control and Prevention (1993), the proportion of those who engage in moderate physical activity five or more times per week increased only slightly, from 22% in 1987 to 24% in 1991. This is even with the increased emphasis on being and staying physically active. We know that in both men and women physical fitness is linked to lower coronary disease rates; therefore, efforts must be made to improve activity levels in both men and women.

Menopause

It is not until at least a decade after cessation of menstruation that heart disease rates in women peak. Most women have experienced menopause by age 55, yet heart disease rates do not escalate until women are well into their sixties (Holm, Penckofer, and Chandler, 1995). Perhaps the key question is whether or not the postmenopausal delay in heart disease rates in women is the consequence of the decline in estrogen experienced at menopause. The question remains whether menopause is itself a risk factor for coronary disease.

Pregnancy

Whether pregnancy is an independent risk factor for coronary heart disease is still unclear. When analyzing data from the Framingham Heart Study and data from the National Health and Nutrition Examination Survey National Epidemiologic Follow-up Study, investigators noted that rates of coronary heart disease were statistically greater among women with multiple pregnancies (six or more) than among women who had never been pregnant (Ness et al., 1993). Adjustments for other risk factors such as obesity did not change the rates of coronary disease. A number of mechanisms such as insulin resistance and redistribution of body fat with pregnancy have been suggested; further study is needed to verify whether it is number of pregnancies alone that precipitates the increased risk. There is also the issue of postpartum cardiomyopathy and accompanying heart failure that is associated with a mortality of rate 50% to 85%. Postpartum cardiomyopathy is suspected when heart failure occurs in the last month of pregnancy without previously known heart disease risk (Wenger et al., 1993).

Oral Contraceptives

The hormones used in oral contraceptives have been linked to the development of heart disease. Wynn (1992) points out that lipid metabolism, carbohydrate metabolism, and the hemostatic system are all influenced by higher dose contraceptives. More information is needed concerning the lower dose preparations and associated risk of coronary heart disease.

Symptoms, Disease Patterns, and Responses to Disease

The usual pattern and progression of coronary disease begins with the experience of angina, then progresses to tissue ischemia and necrosis with myocardial infarction, and then to heart failure when the left ventricle fails to pump oxygenated blood.

Angina

Angina pain typically begins in the chest and radiates to the left arm. The pain is often intense and described as crushing or burning. Although it most often occurs with exertion as during exercise, with emotional stress, or with exposure to severe temperatures, it can also occur after a heavy meal, or, in severe cases, at rest. Angina can have serious consequences if it is not relieved by rest or nitroglycerin. This description of angina is based on clinical experience with men although typical angina can also be experienced by women.

Approximately 50% of women with anginal pain do not present with objective evidence of ischemia as indicated by normal coronary arteriograms. This leads many to think that angina in women is not serious (Eaker et al., 1993). Women who do not experience typical angina may have episodes of silent ischemia, that is, ischemia without typical symptoms of angina. These women may experience vague symptoms such as fatigue, shortness of breath, abdominal pain, nausea, or vomiting. Relating such symptoms to ischemia is difficult. However, women should be questioned about how they respond to exercise, stress, extremes in temperature, and heavy meals.

Ischemia

Myocardial ischemia occurs when blood flow in the coronary arteries is temporarily disrupted. With ischemia, tissue injury but not tissue death occurs. Myocardial infarction is permanent with resulting tissue necrosis and is a consequence of complete obstruction of one or more of the coronary arteries (see Fig. 8–1).

Myocardial Infarction

Myocardial infarction is more common in men at younger ages and women at older ages. Current estimates are that at 65 years and older, women experience a 10% greater mortality from myocardial infarction (AHA, 1994). However, women rarely experience myocardial infarction as the initial manifestation of coronary heart disease.

The most common cause of complete coronary obstruction and subsequent myocardial infarction is thrombosis, which represents the final stage of a number of complex interrelationships involving coronary atherosclerosis, vasomotor tone, and platelet activation.

Total obstruction of a coronary artery rapidly progresses to tissue necrosis in 4 to 6 hours. The amount of irreversible damage is the most important determinant of left ventricular function, which then becomes the most important indicator of morbidity and mortality. Age at onset of myocardial infarction is an important consideration for men and women. Older patients often do not experience typical symptoms such as radiating chest pain. Women are older when they experience myocardial infarction, leading to the conclusion that many of the symptoms experienced by women may be a function of age rather than gender (Hendel, 1990).

Diagnosis of coronary disease in women is difficult. The most common diagnostic test for documenting the likely cause of chest pain is the exercise test. Again, some women with coronary disease will have vague symptoms and therefore will not be identified as candidates for an exercise test. Even when women are identified as having probable coronary disease, they may experience difficulties with the exercise test itself. Because women are older when they seek diagnosis, they may have difficulty completing the test. Today's older women are not used to exercising and will likely be afraid to exert themselves to a percentage of maximal heart rate. Low fitness levels and coexisting diseases such as arthritis and osteoporosis compound the problem.

Reinfarction, which results in doubling of the mortality rate, is slightly more common in women. In the Framingham study at the 30-year follow-up, the reinfarction rate was 25% in women and 22% in men (Kannel & Abbott, 1987). Following myocardial infarction in women, adherence to treatment is an important predictor of mortality. Those who do not adhere to treatment regimens are at greatest risk (Gallagher, Viscoli, & Horwitz 1993).

Fewer women than men are identified as candidates for elective coronary artery bypass surgery (Becker, Corrao, & Alpert, 1988) or for coronary artery bypass surgery after myocardial infarction (McClellan, McNeil, & Newhouse, 1994). For elderly patients, at least half of whom are women, the survival benefits associated with greater use of catheterization and coronary bypass surgery are minimal. Late referrals for surgical intervention may increase the operative mortality seen in women after bypass surgery (Kahn et al., 1990).

Delay in seeking treatment when acute symptoms occur can lead to death. Spouse or family intervention is often key. Older women with a history of angina and congestive heart failure delay longer (Meischke, Eisenberg, & Larsen, 1993). Other gender-related differences recently noted included the confounding influence of race and socioeconomic status (Moser & Dracup 1993). Poorer women and women of color may not seek treatment because they do not have the resources.

Why are some women so much more hesitant than men to seek treatment? First, women who are apt to experience symptoms are more likely to be older and alone because they have outlived their spouses. Therefore, their social support networks may be limited. Second, even in women who have had experience with angina and chest pain, past experience with other kinds of pain in their lives (menstrual cramps, childbirth) has taught them that if they wait long enough the pain will subside. Third, women may not recognize the signs of myocardial infarction because no one has pointed out the meaning of their symptoms. Finally, even if women do recognize that the pain they are experiencing may be a myocardial infarction, they deny it, and their families often participate in the denial. Even with a media campaign designed to minimize delay time, the interval between onset of symptoms and seeking treatment remained somewhat the same (from 3 hours to 2 hours, 20 minutes) (Blohm, Hartford, Karlson, Karlsson, & Herlitz, 1994).

Heart Failure

Heart failure is becoming increasingly common as we now are saving more and more individuals from death due to myocardial infarction. The elderly and African Americans are most susceptible (Lenfant, 1994). Researchers have noted in animal studies that progressive death of individual cardiac cells occurs with aging. Death of individual cells creates a greater workload on the remaining cells, which is compounded when hypertension or myocardial infarction is superimposed on the process. This helps us understand why older people have a greater prevalence of heart failure. Heart failure occurs when left ventricular function fails. Characteristics of heart failure include signs and symptoms of volume overload such as shortness of breath, rales, and edema and symptoms of inadequate perfusion of tissues such as fatigue or poor exercise tolerance (Public Health Service, 1994b).

A history of myocardial infarction is generally recognized as the most common precursor to the development of congestive heart failure. Women have been shown to have a greater incidence of heart failure after myocardial infarction. Not only are women older at the onset of heart failure but they have coronary risk factors that seem to be highly related to the development of heart failure. For example, there seems to be a strong relationship between heart failure and diabetes in women with the presence of diabetes tending to potentiate the heart failure process. In an 18-year follow-up, diabetes was noted as an important variable in the development of heart failure in men and women; however, the prevalence of diabetes was greater in women (Kimmelstiel & Goldberg, 1990). Therefore, the best intervention for heart failure is the early detection of significant precursors to heart failure such as diabetes, hypertension, and hyperlipidemia (Lenfant, 1994).

Relevance Across the Lifespan

Generally with coronary disease it is difficult to separate the influences of a long-term disease process from the influences of aging (Holm & Kirchhoff, 1983). There are many related questions. For example, does deposition of arterial plaque represent normal aging? Is the atherosclerotic process the result of risk factors acting over time? Finally, is it possible to live without ever developing atherosclerosis? Contemporary wisdom is that the atherosclerosis process begins in childhood and continues until death. Most experts will agree that vascular changes associated with atherosclerosis are a consequence of multiple factors, the most important being age and coronary risk factors. Recently, there has been a growing awareness of the influence of genetic factors on the development of the disease process.

Throughout life, attention must be paid to prevention. All of the modifiable risk factors should be considered. In the childhood and adolescent years, school site programs are developing across the country. When children are exposed to heart healthy habits early in life, the expectation is that these habits will remain in adulthood. Pregnancy also presents special concerns relative to coronary disease. There is need for prenatal care with a focus on instituting heart healthy habits for the baby.

The aging woman must recognize that the years after menopause are the years when vulnerability to coronary disease escalates. Psychosocial factors are important. For example, the aging woman is likely to have outlived friends and family and therefore be living alone. Perhaps church or community organizations can help women in interpreting symptoms or in following a diet or exercise program.

Clinical, Therapeutic, and Behavioral Interventions

Primary prevention of coronary heart disease in women should receive greater attention. This means establishing strong patterns of health behaviors early in life.

Pregnant women can receive information about how to begin instituting healthy heart behaviors as their babies enter childhood. For school-age children, parents and teachers can learn about the importance of diet and physical activity. Intervention should occur at many levels. Constant information provided by a number of sources is in order. The individual clinician, the teachers of children, and the media all have responsibility, but it must begin with the clinician who is the primary educator of children, parents, teachers, and the media. The issue is how to convey information that is understood and accepted, information that becomes part of each child's lifestyle. Clinicians must be role models, practicing the health behaviors they espouse. This means that credibility begins with their own health behaviors. Clinicians, in turn, show parents and teachers how to do likewise. Role model behaviors should be practiced by all who relate to children and adolescents.

A heart healthy lifestyle includes attention to diet, physical activity, and weight control. At menopause, consideration can be given to hormone therapy after careful evaluation of the risks and benefits of therapy for each woman.

Diet

The basic components of a healthy diet must be conveyed. This includes limiting fat intake to 30% or less of total calories. The kind of fat is important. Saturated fats, solid at room temperature, are the least desirable; polyunsaturated fat, which is liquid at room temperature, is most desirable. Specific information about dietary fats is shown in Table 8–1. Tips for decreasing fat content in the diet are highlighted in Display 8–2.

The new labeling on food products can be helpful in achieving dietary goals. As seen in Figure 8–2, the new nutritional label provides useful information about nutrients. Of particular importance to women are fiber, calcium, and fat content. Even more important than actual amount of nutrients is the relative proportion of nutrients, especially proportion of calories from fat.

Dietary fiber is another consideration. Overall, relative risk for ischemic heart disease in both men and women increases when dietary fiber is low. The goal must be to increase fiber in everyone's diet. High-fiber foods, found in fruits and vegetables, are a healthy addition to anyone's diet. Because caffeine has been linked to coronary disease, heavy (four or more cups per day) caffeine consumption should be discouraged.

Women most often have the responsibility for meal planning, grocery shopping, and food preparation. All of these nutrition management responsibilities are crucial to the heart health of family members. To do the best job possible, women should be encouraged to set a good example for their children in both words and actions. Making healthy food choices at the grocery store and in preparing family meals is reinforcing to offspring and spouses.

Table 8-1. Source of Dietary Fats and Influence on Blood Lipids

Type	Description	Source
Monounsaturated	Positive effects raise HDL	Olive, peanut, sesame, nut oils and canola oil
Polyunsaturated	Can decrease cholesterol but maintains levels of HDL	Soybean, corn, cotton seed, safflower, sunflower oil; red meat; poultry skin; lard; butter; cheese; coconut oil
Saturated	Raise both HDL and LDL	Red meat, poultry skin, lard, butter, cheese, coconut oil
Trans fatty acids	Raise LDL and lower HDL	Hydrogenated vegetable oils such as margarines and shortenings

Physical Activity

Physical activity should be encouraged at all ages. In our sedentary society, with its heavy reliance on the automobile, enthusiasm for spectator sports, and love of television, there seems to be little opportunity for exercise. However, we must show women how to create opportunities to be physically active. This presents a challenge. The view that exercise must somehow be separate from our usual daily routines has evolved with our affluence. We must stress to young women that being physically active is a necessary part of any health program. For those with natural athletic ability, participating in sports and other activities will come naturally. However, most will have to learn that although they may not make the tennis or softball team, their activity goals should be based on self-improvement. This must be stressed because often physical education teachers pay more attention to those who have natural ability as opposed to the majority who must learn to be physically active. For older women, who were young adults before the fitness craze of the 1960s, learning about and being physically active will be a new experience.

DISPLAY 8-2
Dietary Modifications to Reduce Fat

1. Use skim milk and nonfat yogurt.
2. Eat more fish and poultry.
3. Eat more complex carbohydrates such as pasta, whole grain bread, and potatoes.
4. Use egg whites or egg substitutes instead of egg yolks.
5. Avoid high-cholesterol organ meats such as liver, kidney, brain, and sweetbreads.
6. Boil, steam, broil, roast, or bake food, instead of frying.
7. Use nonfat salad dressings.
8. Flavor food with herbs and seasonings instead of fat-laden sauces.

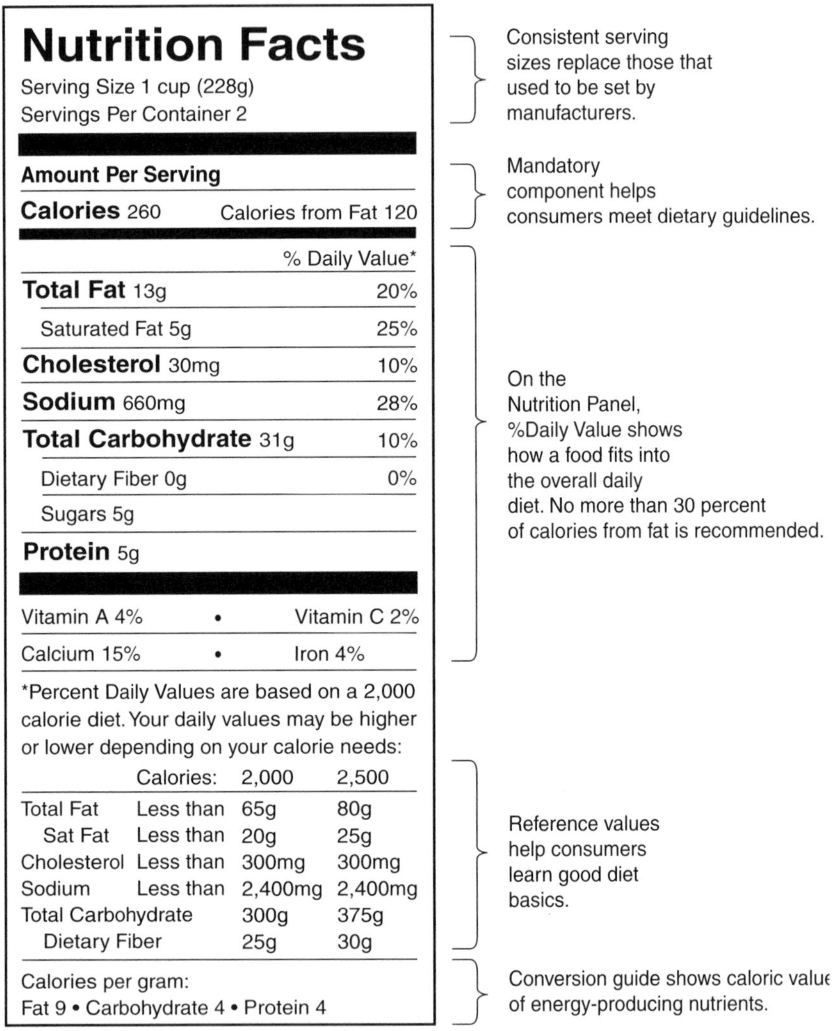
Nutrition Facts
Serving Size 1 cup (228g)
Servings Per Container 2
Amount Per Serving
Calories 260 Calories from Fat 120
% Daily Value*
Total Fat 13g 20%
Saturated Fat 5g 25%
Cholesterol 30mg 10%
Sodium 660mg 28%
Total Carbohydrate 31g 10%
Dietary Fiber 0g 0%
Sugars 5g
Protein 5g
Vitamin A 4% • Vitamin C 2%
Calcium 15% • Iron 4%
*Percent Daily Values are based on a 2,000 calorie diet. Your daily values may be higher or lower depending on your calorie needs:
Calories: 2,000 2,500
Total Fat Less than 65g 80g
Sat Fat Less than 20g 25g
Cholesterol Less than 300mg 300mg
Sodium Less than 2,400mg 2,400mg
Total Carbohydrate 300g 375g
Dietary Fiber 25g 30g
Calories per gram:
Fat 9 • Carbohydrate 4 • Protein 4
Consistent serving sizes replace those that used to be set by manufacturers.
Mandatory component helps consumers meet dietary guidelines.
On the Nutrition Panel, %Daily Value shows how a food fits into the overall daily diet. No more than 30 percent of calories from fat is recommended.
Reference values help consumers learn good diet basics.
Conversion guide shows caloric valu of energy-producing nutrients.

Figure 8-2. 1994 nutrition label format. Nutrients required on nutrition panel are those most important to the health of today's consumers, most of whom need to worry about getting too much of certain items (fat, for example), rather than too few vitamins or minerals, as in the past. (Adapted from Eschleman, M. (1996). Introduction to nutrition therapy. *Philadelphia: Lippincott-Raven Publishers)*

Certainly the media can be helpful, as well as nationwide efforts stressing the importance of physical activity, but older women may have a difficult time identifying with an issue they consider for younger people only. Our efforts must be directed toward teaching older women that physical activity is important for heart health as well as for overall health.

Weight Control

Contemporary thinking is that excess body weight is a function of an imbalance between dietary intake and energy expended. When energy is not used, fat storage is the result. Although this is a commonly held notion, heredity does play a role. As care providers, we should realize that a woman who is having difficulty with weight control may be fighting heredity. Someone who has overweight parents has a greater chance of being overweight. Recent data indicate that heredity accounts for approximately 10% to 30% of weight variance (Hamilton, Kolotkin, Cogburn, Moore, & Watterson, 1990). This means that changes in lifestyle, particularly diet and physical activity, can play a significant role in maintaining proper weight.

Obesity is an important risk factor for coronary heart disease. Weight control can help to modify other important risk factors. Hypertension, adult-onset diabetes, and cholesterol are all aggravated by increased body weight. Excess body weight results in an additional workload on the heart. Weight loss will decrease their impact.

Weight management is an important component of prevention. Most people who are engaged in some form of weight management are women. Recent data indicate that at least two-thirds of people who lose weight on weight reduction programs gain back at minimum the weight they have lost. Many gain back even more. Therefore, attention must be directed toward realistic goals as well as toward other components of successful weight loss programs (Display 8–3). Women seem to be the most vulnerable because they store fat more quickly and lose fat more slowly. However, many women are successful. The traits that have been observed in women who have successfully maintained a significant weight loss are listed in Display 8–4.

Hormone Therapy

Since after World War II, when estrogen became available in pill form, estrogen has been used to alleviate symptoms of menopause, such as hot flashes and vaginal dryness. Hormone therapy to reduce coronary risk is now commonly prescribed for women at menopause (Holm, Penckofer, Chandler, 1995). Some now advocate that women begin taking hormones in the form of low-dose birth control pills at an earlier age. Yet, healthy skepticism is in order because hormone therapy is not for everyone, particularly those with a family or personal history of cancer.

Hormone therapy exerts its favorable effect by decreasing LDLs and increasing HDLs. This helps restore lipids to premenopausal levels. This effect occurs when estrogen is used without progesterone. However, when progesterone is added to

DISPLAY 8-3
Components of an Effective Weight Management Program

1. Identify reasonable weight loss goals.	4. Balance diet with physical activity.
2. Understand that there is no quick fix.	5. Read food labels.
3. Focus on healthy food choices.	

DISPLAY 8-4
Traits of Those Who Successfully Maintain Weight Loss

- Adopt a balanced diet, low in fat.
- Exercise at least three times per week.
- Self-monitor weight.
- Use alternative methods to cope with stress.
- View themselves as thin.
- Focus on health rather than a scale weight.
- Have adequate support systems.
- Continue contact with a health care provider.
- Believe they can maintain their weight.

Adapted from Antinoro, L. (1994). Prevention of weight gain in obese patients who have lost weight. *Heart Disease and Stroke, 3*(5), 233–235

the regimen (combination therapy), most commonly to lessen the risk of endometrial cancer, the favorable effect on lipids is not as great. Generally, with combination therapy, LDLs are elevated and HDLs remain the same. Recently, in the Postmenopausal Estrogen/Progestin Interventions (PEPI) Trial, investigators reported that estrogen does not lose its beneficial effects when combined with progesterone (Working Group for the PEPI Trial, 1995). In this multicenter study, LDL cholesterol was reduced with estrogen alone and with combination therapy. Elevation of HDLs occurred as expected with estrogen alone, and only when a specific preparation of progesterone was used in combination therapy. Further, triglyceride levels, which also tend to increase at menopause, remained at high levels. This requires further investigation.

Hormone therapy also aids in the prevention of bone loss. The textbook portrait of the woman most at risk for developing osteoporosis is the light-skinned, slim, small-boned Caucasian woman who smokes and has a family history of osteoporosis. At menopause when bone loss escalates, this woman will benefit from hormone therapy because estrogen will prevent accelerated loss. Combination therapy, however, is still being evaluated for its effect on bone loss at menopause. The risk of breast cancer in women using both estrogen alone and estrogen in combination with progesterone is still a threat. There are as many studies showing risk of breast cancer as there are demonstrating no additional risk.

Even with the documented health benefits of hormone therapy, many women choose not to take hormones or if they do begin taking hormones, they choose to discontinue therapy. One estimate is that the average duration of hormone therapy is approximately 9 months (O'Leary-Cobb, 1994). This is despite the persuasion from clinicians and media of the benefits of therapy. Why this is so is not clear. Perhaps women are reluctant to discuss the issues with their care providers while at the same time have many unanswered questions. Women must realize that their questions and concerns are important. Clinicians must be ready to help women receive the information they need to make a decision.

When women seek advice about hormone therapy, they should also be given information about associated discomforts. For example, estrogen when given alone causes bleeding that resembles monthly periods. With combination therapy, some women may experience withdrawal bleeding that may last for months. Women should also be told that they may gain weight and retain fluid. Other less publicized side effects include changes in carbohydrate metabolism, increased blood clotting, gallbladder disease, and aggravation of existing fibroid tumors.

For all risk factors, preventive health behaviors will lower relative risk by at least one-third to one-half. Each modifiable risk factor should be considered. Targeted interventions for specific risk factors may be needed. For example, to prevent hypertension in women, the National Heart, Lung and Blood Institute's Working Group on Primary Prevention of Hypertension offers the recommendations shown in Display 8–5.

Implications and Research

Much remains to be learned. As we enter the era of health reform with managed care, the focus will be on keeping women well and out of the health care system. Thus, the question is: Who will be responsible for determining women's coronary risk? First, women must learn to be responsible for their own health. An important overriding issue is that women must learn to be intelligent consumers of health care and be partners with their care providers. All women should be instructed to keep records of their health and family history. Women should be educated in asking questions. Display 8–6 provides questions women should be advised to ask their health care providers. Communication is imperative if women are to keep their special concerns at the forefront. However, it must not be forgotten that communication is reciprocal and ongoing.

We have too little information about how risk factors for coronary disease respond to simple cost-effective interventions such as being physically active throughout life. We have too little information about how we can help women to be and to remain physically active. Therefore, testing incentives and interven-

DISPLAY 8-5
Preventing Hypertension in Women

- Increase physical activity and reduce calorie intake for weight loss.
- Keep alcohol intake under two drinks per day.
- Participate in moderate-intensity, low-resistance, dynamic exercise, such as walking, cycling, or dancing.
- Restrict sodium chloride (salt) intake for the general population of no more than 6 gd.

DISPLAY 8-6
Questions for Women to Ask Health Care Providers

---

1. What is important in my family and personal health history?
2. How do you view menopause, as a normal process or as a deficiency state?
3. Should I take hormones? When should I begin?
4. What recommendations do you have for weight management?
5. How would you suggest that I incorporate physical activity into my lifestyle?

---

tions that address these goals should be a high priority. In our automated, computerized society, finding opportunities to be physically active has become increasingly difficult. Identifying opportunities for physical activity within the structure of everyday life is a challenge. Physical education within school systems must be maintained. Teaching young people to chart their own preferences for physical activity is also needed. Perhaps creating structural and policy changes in the workplace, as was the case with smoking, is necessary. It may be that policies within heart-healthy organizations, such as eliminating elevator service to the first through fourth floors, creating fitness centers at the workplace, and allowing women an hour per day to exercise, can make a difference. To ensure the success of any change in emphasis on physical activity, research efforts must aim to identify what will motivate women to be physically active and maintain healthy levels of physical activity throughout life. The link between diet and physical activity also deserves increased attention. Further, addressing whether women who become physically active at midlife are different from those who have been active throughout life is an important goal.

For clinicians, attention should be given to risk factor education, maximizing each interaction with patients as an opportunity to convey information. There should be opportunities to discuss risk modification and to provide fact sheets and brochures. Volunteering to provide blood pressure screenings in the community may also prove effective. Being part of the local heart association speakers' bureau, can provide an opportunity to convey information to large groups of healthy women.

Definitive answers about heart disease in women are many years coming. This alone presents an opportunity for researchers and clinicians to work together to define research questions and test interventions aimed at primary, secondary, and tertiary prevention. Partnerships between researchers and clinicians have never been more important. The fight against heart disease in women can be won. The first steps have been taken over recent years. We have identified that coronary disease in women is a reality. We are aware that women have difficulties with diagnosis and treatment because of a number of factors. We must also be aware that emphasis on prevention must occur from birth to old age. For all women, physical activity, diet, and weight control are key. When women seek health care for any reason, the opportunity to emphasize heart health must not be ignored.

Acknowledgment

The authors acknowledge Sue Penckofer, PhD, RN, Associate Professor Medical-Surgical Nursing, Niehoff School of Nursing, for her assistance with this manuscript.

References

American Heart Association. (1994). *Heart and stroke facts: 1994 statistical supplement.* Dallas, TX: Author.

Antinoro, L. (1994). Prevention of weight gain in obese patients who have lost weight. *Heart Disease and Stroke, 3*(4), 233-235.

Becker, R. C., Corrao, J. M., & Alpert, J. S. (1988). Review: Coronary artery bypass surgery in women. *Clinical Cardiology, 11,* 443-448.

Blohm, M., Hartford, M., Karlson, B. W., Karlsson, T., & Herlitz, J. (1994). A media campaign aiming at reducing delay times and increasing the use of ambulance in AMI. *American Journal of Emergency Medicine, 12*(3), 315-318.

Bush, T. L. (1990) The epidemiology of cardiovascular disease in postmenopausal women. *Annals of the New York Academy Sciences, 592,* 263-271.

Centers for Disease Control and Prevention. (1993). Prevention of sedentary lifestyle—risk factor surveillance system. *MMWR,* (4), 576–579.

Eaker, E. D., Chesebro, J. H., Sacks, F. M., Wenger, N. K., Whisnant, J. P., & Winston, M. (1993). Cardiovascular disease in women: AHA medical/scientific statement. *Circulation, 88* (4), Part I, 1999-2009.

Gallagher, E. J., Viscoli, C. M., & Horwitz, R. I. (1993). The relationship of treatment adherence to the risk of death after myocardial infarction in women. *Journal of the American Medical Association, 270*(6), 742-744.

Hamilton, M., Kolotkin, R. L., Cogburn, D. F., Moore, D. T., & Watterson, K. (1990). *The Duke University Medical Center book of diet and fitness* (pp. 3-18). New York: Fawcett Columbine.

Hendel, R. C. (1990). Myocardial infarction in women. *Cardiology, 77* (Suppl. 2), 43-57.

Holm, K., & Kirchhoff, K. Exercise and aging. *Heart and Lung, 13*(5), 519-524.

Holm, K., & Penckofer, S. (1992). Cardiovascular risk factors in women. *Journal of Myocardial Ischemia, 4*(1), 25-46.

Holm, K., Penckofer, S., and Chandler, P. J. Deciding on hormone replacement therapy. *American Journal of Nursing, 1995, 95*(8), 57–59.

Holm, K., Penckofer, S., Keresztes, P., Biordi, D., & Chandler, P. (1993). Coronary artery disease in women: Assessment, diagnosis, intervention, and strategies for life style change. *NACOG: Issues in Women Health, 4*(2), 272-285.

Jones, P. H., & Gotto, A. M. (1994). Prevention of coronary heart disease in 1994: Evidence for intervention. *Heart Disease and Stroke, 3*(6), 290-296.

Kahn, S., Nessim, S., Gray, R., Czer, L., Chaux, A., & Matloff, J. (1990). Increased mortality of women in coronary artery bypass surgery: Evidence for referral bias. *Annals of Internal Medicine, 112,* 561-567.

Kannel, W. B., & Abbott, R. D. (1987). Incidence and prognosis of myocardial infarction in women: The Framingham study. In E. D. Eaker, B. Packard, & N. K. Wenger (Eds.), *Coronary heart disease in women: Proceedings NIH workshop* (pp. 208-214). New York: Publisher.

Kannel, W. B., & Vokonas, P. S. (1992). Demographics of the prevalence, incidence, and management of coronary heart disease in the elderly and in women. *Annals of Epidemiology, 2*(1/2), 5-14.

Kaplan, G. A., & Keil, J. E. (1993). Socioeconomic factors and cardiovascular disease: A review of the literature. *Circulation, 88*(4), 1973-1998.

Kimmelstiel, C., & Goldberg, R. J. (1990) Congestive heart failure in women: Focus on heart failure due to coronary artery disease and diabetes. *Cardiology, 77* (Suppl. 2), 71-79.

Kuczmarski, R. J., Fiegel, K. M., Campbell, S. M., & Johnson, C. L. (1994). Increasing prevalence of overweight among US adults. *Journal of the American Medical Association, 272*(3), 205-211.

Lenfant, C. (1994). Report of the task force on research in heart failure. *Circulation, 90*(3), 1118-1123.

Luepker, R. V., Rosamond, W. D., Murphy, R., Sprafka, J. M., Folsom, A. R., McGovern, P. G., & Blackburn, H. (1993). Socioeconomic status and coronary heart disease risk factor trends: The Minnesota heart survey. *Circulation, 88,* Part I, 2172-2179.

Manson, J., Colditz, G., Stampfer, M., Willett, W., Rosner, B. Monson, R., Speizer, F., & Hennekens, C. (1990). A prospective study of obesity and risk of coronary heart disease in women. *New England Journal of Medicine, 322* (13), 882-889.

Marenberg, M. E., Risch, N., Berkman, L. F., Floderus, B., & de Faire, U. (1994). Genetic susceptibility to death from coronary heart disease in a study of twins. *New England Journal of Medicine, 330*(15), 1041-1046.

McClellan, M., McNeil, B. J., & Newhouse, J. P. (1994). Does more intensive treatment of acute myocardial infarction in the elderly reduce mortality? *Journal of the American Medical Association, 272*(11), 859-866.

Meischke, H., Eisenberg, M. S., & Larsen, M. P. (1993). Prehospital delay interval for patients who use emergency medical services: The effect of heart-related medical conditions and demographic variables. *Annals of Emergency Medicine, 22,* 1597-1601.

Moser, D. K., & Dracup, K. (1993). Gender differences in treatment-seeking delay in acute myocardial infarction. *Progress in Cardiovascular Nursing, 8*(1), 6-12.

Ness, R. B., Harris, T., Cobb, J., Flegal, K. M., Kelsey, J. L., Balanger, A., Stunkard, A. J., & D'Agostino, R. B. (1993). Number of pregnancies and the subsequent risk of cardiovascular disease. *New England Journal of Medicine, 328*(21), 1528-1533.

O'Leary-Cobb, J. (1994). Why women choose not to take hormone therapy. *Women's Health Forum, 3*(3), 1-3.

Pappas, G. (1994). Elucidating the relationships between race, socioeconomic status, and health. *American Journal of Public Health, 84,* 892-893.

Public Health Service, Agency for Health Care Policy and Research. (1994a). *Clinical practice guideline, Number 10: Diagnosing and managing unstable angina.* Rockville, MD: Author.

Public Health Service, Agency for Health Care Policy and Research. (1994b). *Clinical practice guideline, Number 11: Heart failure: Evaluation and care of patients with left-ventricular systolic dysfunction.* Rockville, MD: Author.

Rosenberg, L., Palmer, J. R., & Shapiro, S. (1990) Decline in the risk of myocardial infarction among women who stop smoking. *New England Journal of Medicine, 322*(4), 213-217.

Sempos, C. T., Cleeman, J. I., Carroll, M. D., Johnson, C. L., Bachorik, P. S., Gordon, D. I., Burt, V. I., Bretel, R. R., Brown, C. D., Lippel, K., & Fifkind, B. M. (1993). Prevalence of high blood cholesterol among US adults: An update based on guidelines from the second report of the National Cholesterol Education Program adult treatment panel. *Journal of the American Medical Association, 269* (23), 3009-3014.

Stevens, J., Kumanyika, S. K., & Keil, J. E. (1994). Attitudes toward body size and dieting: Differences between elderly black and white women. *American Journal of Public Health, 84,* 1322-1325.

Wenger, N. K., Speroff, L., & Packard, B. (1993). Cardiovascular health and disease in women. *New England Journal of Medicine, 329,* 247-256.

Working Group for the PEPI Trial. (1995). Effects of estrogen or estrogen/progestin regimens on heart disease risk factors in postmenopausal women. *Journal of the American Medical Association, 273*(3), 199-208.

Wynn, V. (1992) Oral contraceptives and coronary heart disease. *Journal of Reproductive Medicine, 36*(3), 219-225.

Bibliography

Coronary heart disease. (1994). *Harvard Women's Health Watch, 1*(6), 1.

Ell, K., Haywood, L. J., Sobel, E., deGuzman, M., Blumfield, D., & Ning, J. P. (1994). Acute chest pain in African Americans: Factors in the delay in seeking emergency care. *American Journal of Public Health, 84*(6), 965-970.

Erlik, Y., et al.(1982). Estrogen levels in postmenopausal women with hot flashes. *Journal of the American College of Obstetricians and Gynecologists, 59*(4), 403-407.

Goldman, L., & Torteson, A. (1991). Uncertainty about postmenopausal estrogen. *New England Journal of Medicine, 325*(11), 800-802.

Grady, D., et al.(1992). Hormone therapy to prevent disease and prolong life in postmenopausal women. *Annals of Internal Medicine, 117*(12), 1016-1037.

Helfant, R. H. (1993). *Women take heart* (pp. 17-191). New York: Putnam.

Judelson, D. R. (1994). CHD in women: There is a difference. CME Network, Loyola University Medical Center, Maywood, IL.

Khaw, K., & Barrett-Connor, E. (1987). Dietary fiber and reduced ischemic heart disease mortality rates in men and women: A 12-year prospective study. *American Journal of Epidemiology, 126*(6), 1093-1102.

Kronenberg, F. (1993). Giving hot flashes the cold shoulder-without drugs. *Menopause Management, II*(4), 20-27.

O'Hare, J. A., & Abuaisha, P. B. (1993). Delay and hospitalization with acute myocardial infarction. *Irish Journal of Medical Science, 161*(2), 37-39.

Prevalence of adults with no known major risk factors for coronary heart disease-behavioral risk factor surveillance system, 1992. (1994). *Morbidity and Mortality Weekly Report, 43*(4) 61-69.

The pill until menopause? (1994). *Harvard Women's Health Watch, 1*(7), 1.

Vecchia, C., Gentile, A., Negri, E., Parazzini, F., & Frannceschi, S. (1989). Coffee consumption and myocardial infarction in women. *American Journal of Epidemiology, 130*(3), 481-485.

Weight reduction and management: Long term strategies for success. (1994). *National Women's Health Report, 16*(1), 1.5.

CHAPTER 9

Vascular Disease

Karin Coyne
Judith Hsia

Introduction

Vascular disorders are diseases of blood vessels other than the coronary arteries; thus, they encompass cerebral, aortic, and peripheral vascular diseases. Noncardiac vascular disorders currently affect over 5.2 million Americans and are the primary cause of serious disability in the United States (American Heart Association [AHA], 1995). Vascular disorders are acquired through a wide range of pathophysiologic bases including atherosclerosis, inflammatory vasculitides, connective tissue abnormalities, and thrombosis. A number of congenital vascular abnormalities also affect women and have particular significance because of the risk of genetic transmission from affected women to their offspring. This chapter provides an overview of the disease entities, risk factors, disease patterns, current therapies and interventions, relevance across the lifespan, and a summary with future research and policy implications. Cerebrovascular disease, which is the third leading cause of death among women, is discussed first followed by diseases of the aorta and peripheral vascular disorders.

Cerebrovascular Disorders

Clinical Manifestations

Cerebrovascular disorders affect both large vessels such as the common and internal carotid arteries and small arteries supplying the brain. Clinical manifestations of cerebrovascular disease span the spectrum from asymptomatic carotid stenosis through transient ischemic attack to completed stroke. Incidence rates for the range of cerebrovascular disorders are presented in Table 9–1.

Disease Patterns

By definition, asymptomatic carotid stenosis lacks symptoms. Patients are usually identified when carotid ultrasound is performed to evaluate an asymptomatic carotid bruit. Improvements in carotid ultrasound technology have facilitated evaluation of asymptomatic populations for prevalence of carotid atherosclerosis. Women are more prone to have asymptomatic carotid bruits than men; however, men are more likely to have carotid stenosis (Ford et al., 1986).

The fact that carotid stenosis is asymptomatic belies the severity of the disease. Chambers and Norris (1986) noted that the severity of carotid stenosis is a signifi-

Table 9-1. Incidence of Cerebrovascular Disease in Women

Authors	Age Range	Disease Severity	Incidence (per study population)
Asymptomatic Carotid Disease			
O'Leary et al., 1992 (n = 2906)	65+	Stenosis: mild (1–49%)	60%
		moderate (50–74%)	4%
		severe (>75%)	1.1%
Bonithon-Kopp et al., 1993 (n = 308)	45–54	Thickening of carotid wall	34%
		Presence of plaque	7%
Transient Ischemic Attacks			**Incidence**
Dennis, Bamford, Sandercock,	45–64		.26
& Warlow, 1989 (n = 105,000 men	55–64		.63
and women—incidences only	65–74		.90
related to female rates only)	75–84		2.29
	≥85		2.87
Babikian, Kase, & Wolf, 1994	65–74		.76
(Framingham study)			
Stroke			**(per 1000)**
Broderick, Phillips, Whisnanat,	15–85+		1.10
O'Fallon, & Bergstralh, 1989			
Rochester, MN			

cant predictor of future neurologic events. Unfortunately, increasing severity of carotid stenosis does not parlay into the appearance of symptoms. Among the 18 carotid occlusions noted by Chambers and Norris, 8 (44%) were asymptomatic. In the Asymptomatic Carotid Atherosclerosis Study, Brott et al. (1994) found 15% of their population to have evidence of cerebral infarction by computed tomographic (CT) scanning with no clinical history of stroke.

A transient ischemic attack (TIA) is a focal neurologic deficit, that is, a symptom complex consistent with stroke, which resolves completely within 24 hours. The incidence of TIA is relatively equal among men and women and appears to be relatively low (see Table 9–1). Unfortunately, due to the transient nature, a significant proportion of TIAs go unreported. This may have deleterious effects; Hopkins (1993) asserts that 30% of people with TIA will have a stroke within the next few years.

Transient ischemic attacks are embolic in origin, caused by a showering of blood clot or ulcerated atherosclerotic plaque into the brain's circulation, blocking the blood supply to an area of the brain. The full range of focal neurologic findings may be observed in TIAs, including transient blindness in one eye (amaurosis fugax), weakness, tingling or numbness of the face or an extremity, behavioral abnormalities, and transient loss of speech. Brain imaging with CT scanning or magnetic resonance imaging (MRI) may demonstrate residual anatomic changes despite complete clinical recovery.

Strokes are caused by damage to brain tissue, either by depriving it of blood supply or by bleeding into the brain, and can be embolic, atherothrombotic, hemorrhagic, or a subarachnoid hemorrhage. Embolic strokes are sudden in onset with the deficit being most severe at onset. In contrast, a progression of symptoms is common in atherothrombotic strokes. Lacunar infarcts, a subset of atherothrombotic strokes, are small infarcts caused by occlusion of small perforating vessels originating from the major cerebral arteries (ie, the anterior, middle, and posterior cerebral and basilar arteries). Hemorrhagic strokes have a sudden onset and can be reliably ascertained either by CT scanning or MRI. Subarachnoid hemorrhage, which results from rupture of a previously asymptomatic congenital aneurysm of the cerebral circulation, arteriovenous malformation, or atherosclerosis appears to be more common in women than in men (Hopkins, 1993; Wong, Giuliani, & Haley, 1990). Clinical manifestations of cerebral infarction reflect the function of the area of brain damaged by oxygen and nutrient deprivation. For example, loss of blood supply to areas responsible for motor function results in hemiparesis. For reasons not entirely clear, women tend to have a higher extension and recurrence rate than men (Hopkins, 1993).

The AHA (1995) estimates half a million strokes occur annually in the United States with approximately 22% resulting in deaths. As has been the case for coronary heart disease, mortality from stroke fell during the past three decades. In the United States, mortality among women has fallen 5.2% annually, compared with a reduction in mortality of 5.7% each year in men (Bonita, Stewart, & Beaglehole, 1990; McGovern et al., 1992). Some of the mortality improvement is attributed to increased survival after stroke; however, the overall incidence is lower as well (Broderick et al., 1989). The prevalence of stroke survivors has increased; consequently, stroke is currently the most frequent cause of chronic serious disability.

Strokes are much more frequent among African American women than among Caucasians at all ages (Kittner, White, Losonczy, Wolf, & Hebel, 1990); relative risk of stroke for African American women compared to Caucasian women during a 10-year follow-up study was 5.8 for women aged 35 to 44, 3.3 for women aged 45 to 54, 3.0 for women aged 55 to 64, and 1.3 for women aged 65 to 74. The likelihood of fatal stroke was also greater for African Americans than Caucasians, particularly among younger women. Relative risk of stroke death was three times greater for African American women aged 45 to 59 and 1.68 times greater for women 60 to 74 years old (Howard et al., 1994). In contrast, fatal strokes were less common among Hispanic women; relative risk was 0.76 for women aged 60 to 74 and 0.47 for women 75 years or older compared with Caucasians. Native Americans appear to have an even lower risk of stroke death (Kattapong & Becker, 1993).

Recovery after stroke is better among younger patients and those with smaller strokes. Aside from physical disabilities, having a stroke has psychological, social, and economic effects on patients and their families. Depression after stroke occurs in 20% to 63% of patients and can last for a number of years (Sandin, Cifu, & Noll, 1994). Emotionalism, feelings of loss of control, anxiety, denial, and anger have also been reported as psychological consequences of stroke (House, Dennis, Molyneux, Warlow, & Hawton, 1989; Sandin, Cifu, & Noll, 1994). Social consequences after stroke include social isolation, dependency, economic strain (and possibly loss of employment opportunities), and family disruption. Sandin, Cifu, and Noll (1994) claimed that women who are highly educated suffer the greatest social isolation. The economic aftermath of stroke is high. Costs for hospitalization and nursing home services were estimated at $15.7 billion for 1995 (AHA, 1995). Costs related to personal income loss and personal medical expenditures related to stroke are currently not known.

There is a lack of research in the area of quality of life after stroke, which is appalling given the number of stroke survivors and the lack of knowledge of factors that may improve their quality of life. The knowledge gained from such research could have a significant impact on stroke outcome decisions and is urgently needed.

Risk Factors

Risk factors associated with the spectrum of cerebrovascular disease include increased age, diabetes, hypertension, cigarette smoking, total and low-density lipoprotein cholesterol, triglycerides, and left ventricular mass (which is increased in hypertensives) (Bikkina et al., 1994; Bonithan-Kopp et al., 1993; Colditz et al., 1988; O'Leary et al, 1992; Shinton & Beevers, 1989; Tell et al., 1994; Thompson, Greenberg, & Meade, 1989). Although diabetes and hypertension are more prevalent among African Americans, these risk factors account for only half the excess stroke risk among African American women (Kittner et al., 1990). Unfortunately, the remaining excess stroke risk for African American women remains elusive.

Risk factors associated with TIA and atherothrombotic stroke include hypercoagulable states, family history of stroke, atrial fibrillation, cardiomyopathy, and mitral valve prolapse (Folsom, Prineas, Kaye, & Munger, 1990; Langer & Criqui, 1993; Sandok & Guiliani, 1982; Wong et al., 1990). Atrial fibrillation is a potent risk factor for brain embolism, the frequency of which has been estimated at 6% per year (Ezekowitz et al., 1992; Peterson, Boysen, Godtfredsen, Anderson, & Anderson, 1989). Other predisposing heart abnormalities include interatrial shunt, atrial or ventricular thrombus, atrial septal aneurysm, spontaneous echo contrast, or atherosclerotic disease of the aorta (Commess et al., 1994; Ezekowitz et al., 1992).

Other risk factors that have been associated specifically with stroke in women include hemoglobin levels of greater than 14 g (Kannel, Gordan, & Wolf, 1972), lack of physical activity (Lindenstrom, Boysen, & Nyboe, 1993), decreased cognitive function, decreased functional status, and decreased bone density (Browner et al., 1993). Migraines have been associated with ischemic stroke in women younger than 45 (Bogousslavsky, Regli, van Melle, Payot, & Uske, 1988; Rothrock, Walicke, Swenson, Lyden, & Logan, 1988; Tzourio et al., 1995).

A risk factor that has been and remains controversial is the use of oral contraceptives. Although Realini and Goldzieher (1985) noted deficiencies in past research findings in their meta-analysis on this subject, they could find little support for an association between stroke and oral contraceptive use. With the advent of lower dose contraceptives (< 50 μg estrogen), the risk of stroke (if present) was expected to become nonexistent. Despite the decrease in estrogen doses, Thorogood, Mann, Murphy, and Vessey (1992) found an increase in risk for subarachnoid hemorrhage. Lidegaard (1993) also noted an increased risk of stroke with oral contraceptive use despite exclusive use of low-dose estrogens. Ironically, Longstreth, Nelson, Koepsell, and van Belle (1994) found a reduced risk for subarachnoid hemorrhage in women taking low-dose contraceptives. Thus, whether the use of low-dose oral contraceptives increases the risk of stroke in women remains to be resolved and warrants further investigation.

In concordance with the concern over oral contraceptives and stroke risk is the concern of postmenopausal estrogen use and stroke risk. Paganini-Hill, Ross, and Henderson (1988) found a protective effect from postmenopausal estrogen use, whereas Wilson, Garrison, and Castelli (1985) found no benefits and noted an increased risk of cerebrovascular disease with postmenopausal estrogen use. The meta-analysis by Grady et al. (1992) showed no increase in risk for stroke with postmenopausal estrogen use. Consequently, this issue remains controversial.

Therapies and Interventions

Given the increased risk of stroke in patients with asymptomatic carotid disease and TIA, the therapeutic goal is the prevention of stroke. It is thought that preventive measures, predominantly risk factor modification, have been effective in reducing the prevalence of and mortality from stroke in the United States. Patients with TIA or asymptomatic carotid disease should be informed of the future risks and encouraged to focus on secondary prevention efforts. Secondary prevention includes risk factor modification with such programs as smoking cessation, dietary education (low fat, low cholesterol), weight loss and exercise programs, and, when applicable, educational programs on controlling diabetes mellitus and hypertension. Although the above preventive efforts are frequently endorsed by clinicians, no clinical trials have been conducted to assess the efficacy of these preventive measures in women.

Recommendations regarding the value of carotid endarterectomy, an operation in which the carotid plaque is surgically removed, in both asymptomatic patients with significant carotid narrowing and symptomatic patients (ie, TIA) have remained in flux during the past decade. Three clinical trials (CASANOVA Study Group, 1991; Hobson et al., 1993; Mayo Asymptomatic Carotid Endarterectomy Study Group, 1991) have randomized patients to either medical treatment or carotid endarterectomy for asymptomatic carotid stenosis. All produced negative results, indicating that endarterectomy for asymptomatic carotid stenosis does not provide better outcomes than medical treatment alone. Importantly, among the 1012 patients enrolled in the three trials, only 17% were women; gender-specific analyses were not conducted in any of the trials. Consequently, little research has been done to evaluate the long-term outcomes for women with asymptomatic carotid disease.

For patients with TIA, the North American Symptomatic Carotid Endarterectomy Trial Collaborators (1991) and the European Carotid Surgery Trialists' Collaborative Group (1991) found carotid endarterectomy to be more beneficial than medical therapy alone for patients with carotid stenosis greater than 70%. Of these two studies, approximately 31% were women with no gender-specific analysis. A third study (Mayberg et al., 1991) enrolled only men and noted no difference in stroke rate for patients with greater than 50% stenosis; benefits were shown if the outcomes included the incidence of TIA in the analysis. The lack of long-term outcome data in women will be remedied by the ongoing Women's Health Initiative, an NIH-funded study of 160,000 postmenopausal women.

Aside from carotid endarterectomy, other interventions aimed at preventing stroke in patients with TIA involve the prevention of recurrent embolization from carotid or aortic plaque or the heart. Because chronic atrial fibrillation is a potent risk factor for stroke, treatment for this condition is essential. For patients who cannot be converted to and maintained in sinus rhythm, long-term anticoagulation with warfarin has been effective in decreasing the incidence of stroke (Boston Area Anticoagulation Trial for Atrial Fibrillation Investigators, 1990; Ezekowitz et al., 1992; Peterson et al., 1989). Anticoagulation is also appropriate for patients with spontaneous echo contrast or left ventricular thrombus detected by echocardiography. Those with predisposing structural heart abnormalities such as atrial or ventricular septal defects should have these defects surgically closed.

For patients with TIA who are not in atrial fibrillation, aspirin has traditionally been recommended. The SALT Collaborative Group (1991) and the Dutch TIA Trial Group (1991) claimed aspirin doses from 30 to 1500 mg daily were effective in reducing overall risk of stroke by 35%. The combined population was approximately 35% women, but no gender-specific analyses were performed. Interestingly, a gender- specific analysis was performed by the UK-TIA Study Group (1988), which revealed no risk reduction for women taking aspirin. In a further investigation into possible gender differences of aspirin's efficacy, Spranger, Aspey, and Harrison (1989) found that testosterone influenced aspirin's inhibition of platelet aggregation, whereas estradiol did not. In a meta-analysis of five trials, the Atrial Fibrillation Investigators (1994) noted that aspirin decreased the risk of stroke in men by 44% but decreased the risk in women by 23%. The research suggests that the antithrombotic effect of aspirin may not be the same in women as it is in men. This also poignantly demonstrates the need for gender-specific analyses in clinical trials.

Sivenius, Riekkinen, Kilpelainen, Laakso, and Penttila (1991) studied the combined effect of aspirin and dipyridamole versus placebo in 590 women and found a 50% risk reduction for the treatment group. The combination of antithrombotic therapies to prevent stroke in women with TIA warrants further investigation.

A thorough discussion on the treatment regimens for the acute phase of a stroke (which varies according to the stroke etiology) is beyond the scope of this chapter. Briefly, once a stroke is suspected, cerebral imaging, either CT scanning or MRI, is performed to assess stroke size, brain swelling, and presence of bleeding. Depending on stroke etiology, treatment can incorporate thrombolytics, heparin anticoagulation, hypertension control, mechanical hyperventilation, corticosteroids, calcium channel blockers, glutamate antagonists, and surgical intervention (Camerlingo et al., 1994; Duke, Bloch, Turpie, Trebilcock, & Bayer, 1986; Noll & Roth, 1994; Wardlaw & Warlow, 1992).

Although the long-term benefit of stroke rehabilitation has not been demonstrated in a randomized trial setting, rehabilitation remains the standard of care. Dombovy, Sandok, and Basford (1986) question the efficacy and appropriateness of stroke rehabilitation for all patients when spontaneous recovery accounts for the majority of improvement in functional capacity at 30 days for an estimated 65% of patients (Hopkins, 1993). Perhaps a means of identifying patients in greatest need of rehabilitation would be beneficial given the current era of cost containment.

Unfortunately, there is little research in the area of stroke outcomes and virtually none with a focus on women or a gender subgroup analysis.

Relevance Across the Lifespan

The prevalence of stroke increases with age in women, paralleling the prevalence of carotid atherosclerosis, TIAs, and atrial fibrillation. In contrast, subarachnoid hemorrhage is as frequent in young adults as in the elderly.

The reported incidence of stroke in pregnancy has ranged from 1/1666 to 1/26,099 (Wiebers & Whisnant, 1985); age did not seem to affect risk in pregnant women. The risk associated with oral contraceptives and hormone replacement therapy in postmenopausal women needs to be clearly defined.

Because strokes in women tend to occur later in life than in men, many women are without caretakers after discharge and become nursing home residents. Langer and Criqui (1993) noted that 76% of nursing home admissions after stroke are women. Mayo et al. (1989) noted that men were discharged to home significantly more often than women primarily because of the presence of a caretaker at home (usually a spouse). Certainly, long-term care after a stroke is an issue more women are confronted with than men.

Aortic Disorders

The aorta arises at the base of the heart and serves as a conduit from the left ventricle to end organs. The thoracic aorta is that portion of the aorta within the chest and is divided into the ascending, transverse, and descending thoracic aorta. The portion of the aorta below the diaphragm is the abdominal aorta. Major branches from the aorta include the brachiocephalic, left common carotid, and left subclavian branches off the transverse aorta, and the celiac, gastroepiploic, mesenteric, and renal arteries arising from the abdominal aorta, which supply the gastrointestinal tract and kidneys. The aorta bifurcates to form the common iliac arteries supplying the legs.

Aortic disease can be categorized as congenital or acquired. Congenital aortic disorders include coarctation of the aorta and inherited connective tissue diseases affecting aortic structure. Acquired aortic diseases include aortic aneurysm and dissection as well as aortic vasculitides.

Congenital Aortic Disorders

Two categories of congenital aortic disorders are coarctation of the aorta and connective tissue diseases affecting aortic wall structure. In coarctation of the aorta, the transverse aorta is narrowed at its junction with the descending aorta, obstructing blood flow to the abdominal aorta. Coarctation of the aorta was reported in 50 of 132,993 live births in Finland from 1982 to 1983, an incidence of about 1/2500. Coarctation is more often identified among Caucasians than other ethnic groups (Tikkanen & Heinionen, 1993). Although two times more frequent in men, coarctation of the aorta is the fifth most common congenital anomaly and thus frequently occurs in women as well.

The most common inherited connective tissue diseases affecting the aorta are Marfan syndrome and Ehlers-Danlos syndrome subtype IV. In both syndromes, patients form abnormal connective tissue, impairing the structural integrity of the aortic wall. Marfan syndrome is reported in about 1/10,000 births in all ethnic groups (Godfrey, 1993). Ehlers-Danlos syndrome is a heterogeneous group of conditions caused by abnormal collagen formation causing hyperelastic joints and fragile skin. Ten subtypes of Ehlers-Danlos syndrome with different genetic collagen defects have been identified (Byers, 1994), but only subtype IV significantly affects blood vessels. The frequency of Ehlers-Danlos syndrome is not known, but the incidence of type IV is thought to be between 1/100,000 and 1/1,000,000 (Tilstra & Byers, 1994). Both Marfan and Ehlers-Danlos syndromes are equally prevalent in women and men.

Disease Patterns

Coarctation of the aorta occurs in association with chromosomal anomalies such as trisomy and Turner's syndrome. The latter syndrome occurs in 1 of every 2500 women born and is caused by the presence of a single X chromosome rather than the usual XX karyotype. About 5% of women with Turner's syndrome have coarctation of the aorta. Coarctation also occurs in conjunction with other congenital heart abnormalities, particularly bicuspid aortic valve and patent ductus arteriosus. Coarctation can also be an isolated finding, occurring independently of aortic valve and chromosomal anomalies. Maternal toxin exposure has not been identified as a risk factor for coarctation (Tikkanen & Heinionen, 1993).

Coarctation of the aorta is usually identified during infancy to childhood because of a loud murmur, hypertension, and unequal blood pressures in the two arms or in the arms and legs. The presence and severity of coarctation and any associated congenital cardiac anomalies can be readily confirmed by echocardiography.

Marfan syndrome is inherited in 60% to 80% of cases, with new genetic mutations accounting for the remainder. The genetic abnormality responsible for Marfan syndrome has been identified on chromosome 15 in the gene for fibrillin, a glycoprotein component of elastic tissues (Lee et al., 1991). Marfan syndrome includes abnormalities of the skeleton (excessive limb length, scoliosis, and anterior chest deformity), eye (retinal detachment, subluxation of lenses), and cardiovascular system (valvular and aortic abnormalities). Structural cardiovascular abnormalities may be identified by echocardiography. About 80% of patients with Marfan syndrome will have aortic root dilatation (Roman, Rosen, Kramer-Fox, & Devereux, 1993). Aortic dissection or rupture, which may occur even in nondilated aortas, is the leading cause of death in patients with Marfan syndrome.

Ehlers-Danlos syndrome is inherited with an autosomal dominant pattern. The genetic defect in type IV Ehlers-Danlos syndrome has been identified as an abnormality in type III collagen synthesis, secretion, and structure (Tsipouras et al, 1986). Ehlers-Danlos syndrome type IV is characterized by thin, translucent skin, easy bruising, arterial rupture, and obstetric-gynecologic dysfunction (Sorokin, Johnson, Rogowski, Richardson, & Evans, 1994). Echocardiography will identify cardiac valvular and aortic abnormalities in patients with type IV Ehlers-Danlos syndrome.

Therapies and Interventions

In patients with coarctation, the aorta can either be dilated by balloon angioplasty or surgically repaired. Restenosis occurs in a proportion of patients using either of these treatment approaches. Johnson, Canter, Strauss, and Spray (1993) found the restenosis (re-coarctation) rate for infants treated with balloon angioplasty to be 57%, whereas the rate after surgical repair was 14%. Interestingly, Mendelson et al. (1994) found a 7.3% restenosis rate in children older than 12 months treated with balloon angioplasty. Unfortunately, gender subgroup analyses were not performed in either study. Clearly, long-term outcomes for varying interventions need to be evaluated. Patients with hemodynamically significant coarctation should take antibiotic prophylaxis for dental or other invasive procedures.

Patients with Marfan syndrome should have serial echocardiographic follow-up of aortic root dimension. β-Adrenergic blockers should be prescribed to reduce sheer forces in the aorta, and strenuous physical activity should be curtailed. Prophylactic aortic surgery is usually done to prevent rupture once the aorta reaches 60 mm in diameter (Godfrey, 1993). Individuals with Marfan or Ehlers-Danlos syndrome who have valvular insufficiency should take antibiotic prophylaxis for dental or invasive procedures.

Relevance Across the Lifespan

In women with coarctation of the aorta (particularly with an abdominal aortic coarctation), placental blood flow may be inadequate during pregnancy due to aortic obstruction. Aortic rupture and dissection have been reported with maternal mortality approaching 4% (Dizon-Townson, Magee, Twickler, & Cox, 1995). Additionally, women with coarctation are more likely to have offspring with congenital heart disease. Genetic counseling and, if desired and available, fetal echocardiography at about 16 weeks' gestation are appropriate.

Because inheritance of Marfan syndrome is autosomal dominant, affected women have a 50:50 chance of transmitting the disease to their offspring. Further, among women with Marfan syndrome, the risk of spontaneous abortion, aortic rupture, or aortic dissection is augmented by pregnancy. Although the average life expectancy with Marfan syndrome is shortened to 44 years, the median life expectancy (the age at which 50% of patients are expected to be alive) for women is 74 years. Women do have a slightly more favorable prognosis than men, with the median life expectancy of men being 70 years (Silverman et al., 1995). Recent improvements and careful management of Marfan syndrome are expected to continue to improve survival.

The overall mean age of death for women with type IV Ehlers-Danlos syndrome is in the early thirties (Pepin, Superti-Furga, & Byers, 1992). Ehlers-Danlos syndrome, particularly subtype IV, is associated with significant obstetric risk caused by uterine rupture or spontaneous, catastrophic arterial rupture (Rudd, Nimrod, Holbrook, & Byers, 1983). Among women who become pregnant, maternal mortality has been estimated at 25% (Sorokin et al., 1994). For women with this syndrome, the risks of pregnancy should be fully discussed once childbearing potential is reached.

Early diagnosis and careful management are important in women with congenital aortic disorders because of the impact of these disorders on childbearing potential and the risks involved with pregnancy. Early treatment and management extend life expectancy.

Acquired Aortic Disorders

The two most common acquired structural abnormalities of the aorta are aortic aneurysm and aortic dissection. An aneurysm is a localized bulging of a blood vessel in which all three vessel wall layers, that is, the intima, media and adventitia, remain intact. Where the vessel wall becomes thin, the risk of aortic rupture is increased.

Abdominal aortic aneurysms (AAAs) account for 75% of atherosclerotic aortic aneurysms and caused 14,982 deaths in 1988, 34% of which were in women (Ernst, 1993). AAAs increase in frequency with age and are more common in patients with a family history of aortic aneurysm. In a study of patients with the familial trait of AAA, Darling et al. (1989) found a significantly higher incidence of aneurysm ruptures in women than men (30.1% versus 16.9%, p < 0.03). This is significant given that Ernst (1993) speculates that the mortality from rupture may exceed 90% (inclusive of prehospital deaths).

Scott, Wilson, Ashton, and Kay (1993) screened 8944 volunteers, aged 65 to 80 years, for ultrasound evidence of AAA, 56% of whom were women. Aortic diameters exceeding 3 cm were defined as aneurysmal and were detected in 7.4% of men, compared with 1.2% of women, thus suggesting that AAA is less common in women. Thoracic aneurysms may be atherosclerotic but are more commonly due to inherited connective tissue disorders (ie, Marfan syndrome). The prevalence of thoracic aneurysms in the population at large is not known.

Aortic dissection is the most common acute aortic disease, with a prevalence of 5 to 10 cases per million patients (Anagnostopoulos, Prabhakar, & Kittle, 1972) with about one-third of the dissections occurring in women. Predisposing factors for aortic dissection include hypertension and Marfan syndrome. Although pregnancy has been reported as a risk factor for aortic dissection (Roberts, 1981), this association remains controversial (Oskoui & Lindsay, 1994).

Disease Patterns

Currently, by far the most common cause of aortic aneurysm is atherosclerosis. Cohen and Hallett (1994) proposed a multifactorial scenario regarding the atherosclerotic changes that occur, including:

- a genetic increase in elastase
- increased serum proteolytic enzyme delivery to the aortic wall by neutrophils and smooth muscle cells participating in the atherosclerotic process
- subsequent weakening of the aortic wall with dilatation
- increased collagenase activity further reducing the strength of the aortic wall and predisposing to rupture

Abdominal aortic aneurysms are usually detected as asymptomatic, pulsatile abdominal masses. Aneurysm size is readily quantified by abdominal ultrasound, and surgical repair is recommended for aneurysms exceeding 5 cm in diameter. In Minnesota, the 8-year risk of rupture for aneurysms 3.5 to 4.9 cm in diameter was 5% compared with 25% for aneurysms 5 cm or larger (Nevitt, Ballard, & Hallett, 1989).

Thoracic aneurysms are more frequently symptomatic because of compression of intrathoracic structures, leading to cough, hoarseness, stridor, hemoptysis, and obstructive pneumonia. Diagnosis of thoracic aneurysms may be confirmed by MRI or CT scanning or by transesophageal echocardiography.

Aortic dissection is a dramatic event, presenting with severe, knifelike back or chest pain, hypotension and, at times, a sensation of impending doom. Upper extremity pulses may be absent, and congestive heart failure may result from acute aortic valve insufficiency. Because the pleura and pericardium enwrap the ascending aorta, aortic rupture can lead to pleural and pericardial effusions. If the dissection extends into the carotid arteries, localizing neurologic signs may be present. Aortic dissection is associated with hypertension, aortic aneurysm, congenital malformation of the aortic valve (Roberts & Roberts, 1991) and, possibly, pregnancy.

In aortic dissection, the intima of the aortic wall is torn, permitting immediate egress of blood under arterial pressure into the media. Seventy percent of patients have intimal tears that occur in the ascending aorta (most commonly in the right lateral wall where blood strikes the aorta on ejection from the left ventricle), 10% occur in the arch, and 20% occur distal to the origin of the left subclavian artery. Within seconds after the tear, systolic pressure forces blood through the tear into the aortic wall, dissecting along the length of the aorta and producing a false lumen. Transesophageal echocardiography identifies a reentry tear from the false lumen back into the true lumen in a minority of patients. The dissecting channel is in the outer half of the aortic media, so the outer wall is very thin, predisposing to rupture. Rupture into the pericardium is common because the parietal pericardium is attached to the ascending aorta just proximal to the origin of the brachiocephalic artery. Tears in the arch rupture into the mediastinum, the descending aorta into pleura, and the abdominal aorta into the retroperitoneum.

Therapies and Interventions

Once identified, AAAs less than 5 cm should be followed with serial ultrasound studies. In a longitudinal study, Nevitt et al. (1989) found that 76% of aneurysms increased an average of 0.21 cm in diameter per year and that the risk of rupture was less than the risk of surgery for patients with aneurysms less than 5 cm in diameter. AAAs greater than 5 cm in diameter should be repaired. Surgical repair is recommended for thoracic aneurysms producing symptoms or for asymptomatic aneurysms exceeding 7 cm in diameter because of the increased risk of rupture (Collins, Coster, Cohn, & Van de Vanter, 1983).

When aortic dissection is suspected, the patient should urgently be transported to an emergency room. Diagnosis should be confirmed by the most quickly available modality, be it transesophageal echocardiography, CT scanning, or contrast radiography. The drawback to MRI in this setting is the prohibition against metal in the scanner, which precludes continuous monitoring of these patients who are often unstable.

For dissections involving the ascending aorta and aortic arch, stabilizing measures should be initiated, including β-adrenergic blockade to reduce sheer forces in the aorta, and emergent surgical repair undertaken. Although a life-threatening occurrence, with current therapy, long-term survival has reached 66% at 5 years (Crawford, Svensson, Coselli, Safi, & Hess, 1988). For dissections involving the left subclavian and extending distally, conservative management has yielded better outcomes than surgical intervention. Thus, blood pressure should be controlled and sheer forces reduced with a β-adrenergic blocker such as labetalol (Grubb, Sirio, & Zelis, 1987).

Relevance Across the Lifespan

Abdominal aortic aneurysm is a disease of older women. In contrast, thoracic aneurysms occur in younger individuals, particularly those with connective tissue disorders. Aortic dissection in women with hypertension usually occurs in the fifth to seventh decades of life (Marsalese et al., 1989). In contrast, aortic dissection associated with pregnancy or Marfan syndrome occurs in a much younger population (Nolte et al., 1995).

In view of the life-threatening nature of aortic aneurysm and dissection, early diagnosis and prompt, appropriate treatment are essential. Women with preexisting aortic disorders may be particularly predisposed to catastrophic aortic events while pregnant. Risks of pregnancy should be discussed once childbearing potential is reached.

Aortic Vasculitides

Inflammatory diseases that result from immune complex deposits or cell-mediated reactions in the arterial wall and affect the aorta are Takayasu's arteritis and giant cell arteritis. Takayasu's arteritis (or "pulseless disease") is a nonatherosclerotic aortic disease involving the aorta and other large vessels that occurs predominantly in women under the age of 40. Giant cell arteritis, also known as temporal arteritis, is a large vessel granulomatous vasculitis that primarily affects women over age 55. The etiologies of both Takayasu's arteritis and giant cell arteritis are unknown.

The prevalence of these large vessel vasculitides in the population is not known. As the name suggests, Takayasu's arteritis is particularly prevalent in Asians, but it occurs in other ethnic groups as well. Giant cell arteritis is more common in African American women (Gonzalez, Varner, Lisse, Daniels, & Hokanson, 1989).

Disease Patterns

Takayasu's arteritis often presents with nonspecific systemic symptoms such as fever, weight loss, myalgias, arthralgias, and anorexia. Subsequently, occlusive arterial disease will be manifested with claudication, that is, exercise-induced muscle cramps, bruits, and absent pulses, affecting the arms more frequently than the legs. Laboratory abnormalities include an elevated erythrocyte sedimentation rate, elevated white blood cell count, anemia, and hypergammaglobulinemia (Pariser, 1994).

Like Takayasu's disease, giant cell arteritis presents with systemic symptoms with localized symptoms relating to the affected arteries. Frequently, headaches localized to the temporal or occipital artery distribution may develop along with jaw claudication and visual deficits caused by involvement of the vessels supplying the brain. Tenderness of the affected arteries may be apparent. The erythrocyte sedimentation rate is always greatly elevated often over 100 mm/h (Salvarani, Gabriel, O'Fallon, & Hunder, 1995).

Therapies and Interventions

Upper extremity ischemia and stroke may result from undiagnosed or untreated Takayasu's arteritis, whereas blindness may result from untreated giant cell arteritis; thus, aggressive medical therapy is warranted. Both Takayasu's arteritis and giant cell arteritis are treated primarily with glucocorticoids. Giant cell arteritis, in particular, usually requires high-dose corticosteroid therapy (Buchbinder & Detsky, 1992).

Relevance Across the Lifespan

Women of all ages commonly report nonspecific symptoms such as weight loss, malaise, and achiness, which may be difficult to evaluate. Takayasu's disease typically affects young women, whereas giant cell arteritis affects the elderly. The sequelae of these disorders can be severe, even life-threatening; thus, accurate diagnoses are imperative to ensure aggressive medical therapy to prevent future disability.

Peripheral Vascular Disorders

Peripheral arterial and venous diseases are common in older adults and are responsible for significant morbidity and mortality. Arterial disease may be atherosclerotic or nonatherosclerotic in origin. Venous disorders include inflammation and thrombosis.

Peripheral Arterial Disease

Peripheral arterial disease (PAD) most commonly involves the larger arteries of the leg, that is, the iliac, femoral, and popliteal arteries, although subclavian stenoses can occur. PAD is an independent risk factor for cardiovascular morbidity and mortality in both men and women (Criqui et al., 1992; Eagle et al., 1994; Smith, Shipley, & Rose, 1990). The prevalence rates (Table 9–2) are similar in both men and women; however, there is a strong association with PAD and increasing age (Balkau, Vray, & Eschwege, 1994; Criqui et al., 1985). It is important to note that prevalence rates are highly dependent on the population studied and the means by which vascular disease is diagnosed.

Perhaps one of the most challenging problems with PAD is in its diagnosis; consequently, it is believed to be underdiagnosed (Balkau et al., 1994). With the increased risk of cardiovascular mortality and morbidity, early identification and diagnosis (before symptom onset) would certainly be advantageous to patient outcomes. The most popular method in diagnosing PAD (and certainly the easiest for epidemiologic studies) is the Rose questionnaire that simply ascertains whether or not the patient has been experiencing symptoms of PAD (ie, leg pain). (Unfortunately, the Rose questionnaire excludes all asymptomatic patients.) Table 9–2 shows the range of prevalence rates (0.6–14.1%) based on the Rose questionnaire, which differ dramatically from the prevalence rates based on the ankle-arm index (11.4–28%). (The ankle-arm index is the ratio of ankle systolic blood pressure to arm systolic blood pressure; normal is above 1.0 [Newman et al., 1993].) There is no consensus on what the best method is to identify patients with PAD. One study (Feigelson, Criqui, Froneck, Langer, & Molgaard, 1994) compared different survey methods and found that measuring the post-tibial flow with a Doppler flowmeter was the most accurate means to detect large vessel PAD in an asymptomatic population.

Disease Patterns

The symptomatic spectrum of severity for PAD ranges from intermittent claudication to ischemic leg pain to acute arterial occlusion. Intermittent claudication, the harbinger of PAD and the peripheral vascular equivalent to angina, is a crampy pain in the affected extremity, brought on by exertion and relieved by rest. In contrast, ischemic leg pain at rest is constant, often worse at night, and may be relieved by dependent positioning. Acute arterial occlusion presents with sudden onset of a cold, painful, pulseless foot. Both ischemic rest pain and acute arterial occlusion require more urgent intervention than intermittent claudication.

In patients with suspected peripheral vascular disease, cardiovascular risk factors (ie, smoking history, hypertension, diabetes mellitus, and hypercholesterolemia) should be carefully assessed. In patients with peripheral vascular disease, but no symptoms referable to the heart, half will have coronary artery disease. The extent to which patients with PAD should be screened for occult coronary disease remains controversial (Baron et al., 1994; Poldermans et al., 1993).

Peripheral vascular disease may be confirmed by ultrasound and Doppler studies. If revascularization is planned because of threatened limb loss or refractory symptoms, either traditional radiographic arteriography or magnetic resonance angiography is needed (Cambria et al., 1993; Carpenter et al., 1993).

Table 9-2. Incidence of Peripheral Arterial Disease in Women

Authors	Age Range	Rose questionnaire	Arm-Ankle Index
Criqui et al., 1985	<60	5.6%	
n = 624 (338 women)	≥70	33.8%	
Hale, Marks, May, Moore, & Stewart, 1988	≥65	14.1%	
n = 1704 (1083 women)			
Kannel & McGee, 1985* Framingham Study	35–84	3.6/1000	
n = 5209 (? women)			
Newman et al., 1993	≥65	2%	11.4%
n = 5084 (2870 women)			
Newman, Sutton-Tyrrell, Rutan, Locher,	≥60	6.4%	28%
& Kuller, 1993		(total sample)	(women only)
n = 187 (105 women)			
Reunanen, Takkunen, & Aromaa, 1982	30–59	1.8%	
n = 110,962 (5224 women)			

*The Framingham study was the only study to find a significant difference in incidence rates between genders.

Risk Factors

Peripheral arterial disease is generally atherosclerotic in origin and rarely occurs in women without the presence of advanced age, diabetes mellitus, or cigarette smoking. Krupski (1991) found that over 90% of patients with PAD were either current smokers or had a smoking history. Other cardiovascular risk factors such as hypertension, diabetes mellitus, and hyperlipidemia also contribute to the risk of PAD with diabetes being particularly associated with small vessel disease. Orchard et al. (1990) observed that women with a 25-year plus duration of insulin-dependent diabetes have a prevalence rate of PAD three times higher than that of men with a 25-year plus duration of insulin-dependent diabetes (30% versus 11%, $p = .003$). Other possible contributions to arterial ischemia include vasospasm, platelet deposition, and inflammation (Bertiglia, Colantuoni, Coppini, & Intaglietta, 1991; Heyns et al., 1982; Neumann et al., 1990).

Therapies and Interventions

The primary goal for patients with intermittent claudication is to improve their exercise performance and functional capacity (Hiatt et al., 1995). The goal for patients with acute arterial occlusion and chronic leg ischemia, on the other hand, is to avoid disability. Both conditions require immediate medical attention that may involve emergent arteriography, thrombolytics, anticoagulation, or thrombectomy.

Initial management for chronic arterial insufficiency without rest pain is conservative, with good control of hypertension, diabetes, and hyperlipidemia. Patients must stop smoking. Modest exercise training is sometimes helpful, enabling muscles to make efficient use of blood flow that is available. Most patients will improve with conservative management. If pain at rest is reported or persistent claudication after a trial of conservative management, patients should be referred for revascularization, either by percutaneous angioplasty or bypass grafting (AHA Consensus Document, 1991). Balloon angioplasty is appropriate for patients with segmental iliac, femoral, or popliteal stenoses; primary success rates exceed 75% with a wide range of restenosis rates reported (Doubilet & Abrams, 1984; Johnston et al., 1987). Results from surgical revascularization are comparable (Wilson, Wolf, & Cross, 1989). In a review of hospital discharge diagnoses in Maryland, Tunis, Bass, and Steinberg (1991) noted that 41% of peripheral angioplasty and peripheral bypass operations were performed on women, whereas a significantly higher proportion of women (49%, p<.0001) undergo limb amputation for PAD. The reason for this difference is not known.

Relevance Across the Lifespan

Peripheral arterial disease increases in frequency with age with diabetics being the exception to this relationship. The issue of smoking and risk of PAD is particularly acute among women. Approximately 25% of women smoke with some particular groups of women smoking more (eg, 46.6 % of waitresses smoke) (Nelson et al., 1994). Smoking initiation rates have fallen among women aged 14 to 24 but have nearly tripled among girls 10 to 14 years of age (Gilpin, Lee,

Evans, & Pierce, 1994). African Americans have a higher prevalence of smoking than other ethnic groups and African American women are less likely to stop smoking than Caucasian women (Stotts, Glynn, & Baquet, 1994). Clearly, women of all ages need to be targeted for educational programs on the health risks of smoking because it is such a significant factor in the development of vascular disease in women.

Peripheral Venous Disease

Veins contain about 70% of the blood volume. In the arms and legs, veins are characterized as deep or superficial with venous connectors carrying blood between the deep and superficial venous systems. Multiple valves along the length of veins prevent retrograde flow as blood is propelled back to the heart by skeletal muscle contraction. Disorders of the veins include varicose veins and venous thrombophlebitis, which is categorized by location as either superficial or deep.

Disease Patterns

The most prevalent venous disorder is varicose veins, thought to occur in at least 10% to 20% of women, which is twice the rate experienced by men (Diminck, Kaplan, & Salmeron, 1993). Varicose veins usually cause no symptoms although some patients report aching legs after prolonged standing. The incidence of superficial venous phlebitis is not known. Superficial phlebitis is identified by the presence of a tender, warm, red chord along the saphenous vein.

Characteristic physical findings of deep venous thrombophlebitis include localized warmth, redness, tenderness, and swelling of the extremity. Tenderness over the superficial femoral or common femoral veins is more suggestive of proximal venous thrombosis. Physical findings are not highly specific, so that further testing is usually necessary for diagnosis.

The true incidence of deep venous thrombosis (DVT) is not known, but it may be substantial. The clinical diagnosis for venous thromboembolism is neither sensitive nor specific, which creates innumerable difficulties in obtaining true incidences of venous thrombosis. In the population-based Worcester DVT study, the annual incidence of deep venous thrombophlebitis was 48 cases per 100,000 women (Anderson et al., 1991), a significantly lower rate than men.

Risk Factors

Venous stasis caused by pregnancy, obesity, or prolonged standing contributes to the formation of enlarged, tortuous vessels characteristic of varicose veins. Superficial phlebitis commonly occurs as a consequence of indwelling intravenous catheters and is more common in women with varicose veins.

Risk factors for DVT include age, obesity, malignancy, lower extremity fractures, congestive heart failure, chronic obstructive pulmonary disease, hypercoagulable state, obesity, trauma, and surgery. Most women have multiple risk factors. The prevalence of DVT after gynecologic surgery ranges from 4.3% to 34.6% (Zelop, 1993) with the risk of venous thrombosis increasing with the age of the patient, length of surgery, and immobilization. Bonnar (1985) has attributed as many as 40% of deaths after pelvic surgery to venous thrombosis and pulmonary embolism. Although Helmrich, Rosenberg, Kaufman, Strom, & Shapiro (1987) found that the use of oral contraceptives at all doses (including < 50 µg estrogen) increased the risk for venous thrombosis, Gertsman et al. (1991) found that risk for venous thrombosis increased with the dose of estrogen (ie, doses with > 50 µg estrogen had a 1.5 times higher risk than doses < 50 µg). This increased risk appears to dissipate once oral contraceptive usage is discontinued.

Therapies and Interventions

Management of varicose veins is conservative. Patients are encouraged to elevate their legs, avoid prolonged standing, and wear support stockings. Surgical ligation and removal of varicose veins is often performed for cosmetic reasons and is indicated for patients with persistent, severe symptoms or with recurrent superficial phlebitis. Superficial phlebitis can usually be managed conservatively with analgesics or anti-inflammatory agents, heat, and elevation. Recurrent inflammation of varicose veins may ultimately require their surgical removal.

In contrast to superficial phlebitis, deep venous thrombophlebitis requires prompt diagnosis and specific treatment to prevent propagation and embolization of clot. Physical findings are not highly specific, so patients in whom venous thrombosis is suspected should be anticoagulated pending noninvasive testing (ie, impedance plethysmography, two-dimensional ultrasound [duplex] scanning, or venography, which is the gold standard). Once proximal deep venous thrombophlebitis has been confirmed, women should receive intravenous heparin, with subsequent transition to warfarin. Pregnant women, who cannot take warfarin, may be transitioned to subcutaneous heparin.

Clearly prophylaxis against DVT is preferable to treatment after the problem has arisen. The efficacy of mechanical prophylaxis using either compression stockings or intermittent pneumatic compression is well established (Zelop, 1993). A variety of pharmacologic regimens for prophylaxis against venous thrombosis have been recommended, including low-dose warfarin and intravenous or subcutaneous heparin. The suitability of any of these approaches depends on the patient and clinical setting.

Relevance Across the Lifespan

The incidence of varicose veins and deep venous thrombophlebitis increases with age for both men and women. Pregnant women should not be treated for deep venous thrombophlebitis with warfarin because the drug is teratogenic; thus, consideration of pregnancy in women of childbearing potential is worthwhile before warfarin therapy is instituted. Venous disorders are particularly prevalent among the elderly, a population in which women outnumber men. Public awareness of these and other vascular disorders will lead to earlier medical attention and appropriate treatment.

Summary

The prevalence of noncardiac vascular disease in women is significant. Unfortunately, the vast majority of research in this area has been on men with generalizations made to women, thereby negating any gender differences that may exist as biologic, psychological, or social factors. Yet, it is apparent that gender differences do exist given current morbidity and mortality rates that show men are affected with vascular disease at an earlier age than women. Certainly, the further investigation of gender differences may offer insight into the etiologic processes of vascular disorders.

Future research recommendations are listed in Display 9–1. The knowledge gained is essential for future policy-making decisions regarding treatment choices and clinical and long-term outcomes, particularly in a future of limited resources. It is imperative that future policy decisions be based on sound scientific research.

Policy Issues

The United States has a growing elderly population who will be at risk for developing vascular disorders, particularly cerebrovascular and peripheral vascular diseases, which are the primary cause of serious disability today. Undoubtedly, the

DISPLAY 9-1
Research Recommendations

- Gender-specific analyses need to be incorporated into all clinical trials. Treatment effects should not be assumed to be equal between men and women.
- Existing data bases from clinical trials and registries should be compiled and reviewed. This is especially beneficial for disease entities with lower prevalence rates such as Marfan syndrome and aortic aneurysms.
- Long-term outcomes for the previously discussed vascular disorders need to be studied. What interventions produce the best long-term outcomes at the least cost? What are the effects of current interventions on the patient's quality of life?
- The efficacy of stroke rehabilitation must be researched. Perhaps other resources (ie, community programs, adult day-care facilities) could provide rehabilitative services at a lower cost and equal benefit.
- What are the effects of primary and secondary prevention efforts in women?
- A reliable and easy-to-use method to diagnose peripheral arterial disease needs to be devised. What is the best method of screening large populations at risk?
- The economic, social, and psychological consequences of stroke and peripheral arterial disease on elderly women need to be identified. How is their quality of life affected? How do these long-term consequences affect health care costs and delivery?
- Social and psychological factors that predispose women to vascular disorders have not been researched. Do they exist?

number who will be disabled from vascular disorders will greatly increase. An aggressive approach is needed to undertake research with a focus on women in this area, particularly in regards to long-term care. The time for this undertaking is now.

References

American Heart Association. (1991). Consensus document. *Circulation, 84*(IV), 1-26.

American Heart Association. (1995). *Heart and stroke facts.* Dallas, TX: Author.

Anagnostopoulos, C. E., Prabhakar, M. J., & Kittle, C. F. (1972). Aortic dissections and dissecting aneurysms. *American Journal of Cardiology, 30,* 263-273.

Anderson, F. A., Wheeler, H. B., Goldberg, R. J., Hosmer, D. W., Patwardhan, N. A., Jovanovic, B., Forcier, A., & Dalen, J. E. (1991). A population-based perspective of the hospital incidence and case-fatality rates of deep-vein thrombosis and pulmonary embolism. *Archives of Internal Medicine, 151,* 933-938.

Atrial Fibrillation Investigators. (1994). Risk factors for stroke and efficacy of antithrombotic therapy in atrial fibrillation. Analysis of pooled data from five randomized controlled trials. *Archives of Internal Medicine, 154,* 1449-1457.

Babikian, V. L., Kase, C. S., & Wolf, P. A. (1994). Cerebrovascular disease in the elderly. In M. L. Albert & E. J. Knoefel (Eds.), *Clinical neurology of aging* (pp. 549). New York: Oxford University Press.

Balkau, B., Vray, M., & Eschwege, E. (1994). Epidemiology of peripheral arterial disease. *Journal of Cardiovascular Pharmacology, 23*(Suppl. 3), S8-S16.

Baron, J. F., Mundler, O., Bertrand, M., Vicaut, E., Barre, E., Godet, G., Samama, C.M., Coriat, P., Kieffer, E., & Viars, P. (1994). Dipyridamole-thallium scintigraphy and gated radionuclide angiography to assess cardiac risk before abdominal aortic surgery. *New England Journal of Medicine, 330,* 663-669.

Bertiglia, S., Colantuoni, A., Coppini, G., & Intaglietta, M. (1991). Hypoxia- or hyperoxia-induced changes in arteriolar vasomotion in skeletal muscle microcirculation. *American Journal of Physiology, 24,* H362-371.

Bikkina, M., Levy D., Evans, J. C., Larson, M. G., Benjamin, E. J., Wolf, P. A., & Castelli, W. P. (1994). Left ventricular mass and risk of stroke in an elderly cohort: The Framingham heart study. *Journal of the American Medical Association, 272,* 33-36.

Bogousslavsky, J., Regli, F., van Melle, G., Payot, M., & Uske, A. (1988). Migraine stroke. *Neurology, 38,* 223-227.

Bonita, R., Stewart, A., & Beaglehole, R. (1990). International trends in stroke mortality: 1970-85. *Stroke, 21,* 989-992.

Bonithan-Kopp, C., Jouven, X., Taquet, A., Touboul, P. J., Guize, L., & Scarabin, P. Y. (1993). Early carotid atherosclerosis in healthy middle-aged women. *Stroke, 24,* 1837-1843.

Bonnar, J. (1985). Venous thromboembolism and gynecologic surgery. *Clinical Obstetrics and Gynecology, 28*(2), 432-446.

Boston Area Anticoagulation Trial for Atrial Fibrillation Investigators. (1990). The effect of low-dose warfarin on the risk of stroke in patients with nonrheumatic atrial fibrillation. *New England Journal of Medicine, 232,* 1505-1511.

Broderick, J. P., Phillips, S. J., Whisnant, J. P., O'Fallon, W. M., & Bergstralh, E. J. (1989). Incidence rates of stroke in the eighties: The end of the decline in stroke? *Stroke, 20,* 577-582.

Brott, T., Tomsick, T., Feinberg, W., Johnson, C., Biller, J., Broderick, J., Kelly, M., Frey, J., Schwartz, S., Blum, C., Nelson, J. J., Chambless, L., Toole, J., for the Asymptomatic Carotid Atherosclerosis Study Investigators. (1994). Baseline silent cerebral infarction in the asymptomatic carotid atherosclerosis study. *Stroke, 25,* 1122-1129.

Browner, W. S, Pressman, A. R., Nevitt, M. C., Cauley, J. A., Cummings, S. R., for the Study of Osteoporotic Fractures Research Group. (1993). Association between low bone density and stroke in elderly women. *Stroke, 24,* 940-946.

Buchbinder, R., & Detsky, A. S. (1992). Management of suspected giant cell arteritis: A decision analysis: *Journal of Rheumatology, 19,* 1220-1228.

Byers, P. H. (1994). Ehlers-Danlos syndrome: Recent advances and current understanding of the clinical and genetic heterogeneity. *Journal of Investigational Dermatology, 103,* 47S-52S.

Cambria, R. P., Yucel, E. K., Brewster, D. C., L'Italien, G., Gutler, J. P., LaMuraglia, G. M., Kaufman, J. A., Waltman, A. C., & Abbott, W. M. (1993). The potential for lower extremity revascularization without contrast arteriography: Experiences with magnetic resonance angiography. *Journal of Vascular Surgery, 17,* 1050-1056.

Camerlingo, M., Casto, L., Censori, B., Ferraro, B., Gazzaniga, G. C., Cesana, B., Marroli, B. (1994). Immediate anticoagulation with heparin for first ever ischemic strokes in the carotid artery territories observed within five hours of onset. *Archives of Neurology, 51*(5), 462-467.

Carpenter, J. P., Owen, R. S., Holland G. A., Baum, R. A., Barker, C. F., Perloff, L. J., Golden, M. A., & Cope, C. (1994). Magnetic resonance angiography of the aorta, iliac, and femoral arteries. *Surgery, 116,* 17-23.

CASANOVA Study Group. (1991). Carotid surgery versus medical therapy in asymptomatic carotid stenosis. *Stroke, 22,* 1229-1235.

Chambers, B. R., & Norris, J. W. (1986). Outcome in patients with asymptomatic neck bruits. *New England Journal of Medicine, 315,* 860-865.

Cohen, J. R., & Hallett, J. W. (1994). Pathophysiology of arterial aneurysm development. In D. E. Strandness & A. Van Breda (Eds.), *Vascular diseases: Surgical and interventional therapy* (pp. 559-564). New York: Churchill Livingstone.

Colditz, G. A., Bonita, R., Stampfer, M. J., Willett, W. C., Rosner, B., Speizer, F. E., & Hennekens, C. H. (1988). Cigarette smoking and risk of stroke in middle-aged women. *New England Journal of Medicine, 318,* 937-941.

Collins, J. J., Coster, J. K., Cohn, L. H., & Van de Vanter, S. H. (1983). Common aortic aneurysms: When to intervene. *Journal of Cardiovascular Medicine, 8,* 245.

Commess, K. A., DeRook, F. A., Beach, K. W., Lytle, N. J., Golby, A. J., & Albers, G. W. (1994). Transesophageal echocardiography and carotid ultrasound in patients with cerebral ischemia: Prevalence of findings and recurrent stroke risk. *Journal of American College of Cardiology, 23,* 1598-1603.

Crawford, E. S., Svensson, L. G., Coselli, J. S., Safi, H. J., & Hess, K. R. (1988). Aortic dissection and dissecting aortic aneurysms. *Annals of Surgery, 208*(3), 254-273.

Criqui, M. H., Froneck, A., Barrett-Connor, E., Klauber, M. R., Gabriel, A., & Goodman, D. (1985). The prevalence of peripheral arterial disease in a defined population. *Circulation, 71*(3), 510-515.

Criqui, M. H., Langer, R. D., Froneck, A., Feigelson, H. S., Klauber, M. R., McCann, T. J., & Browner, D. (1992). Mortality over a period of 10 years in patients with peripheral arterial disease. *New England Journal of Medicine, 326,* 381-386.

Darling, R. C., Brewster, D. C., Darling R. C., LaMuraglia, G. M., Moncure, A. C., Cambria, R. P., & Abbott, W. M. (1989). Are familial abdominal aortic aneurysms different? *Journal of Vascular Surgery, 10,* 39-43.

Dennis, M. S., Bamford, J. M., Sandercock, P. G., & Warlow, C. P. (1989). Incidence of transient ischemic attacks in Oxfordshire, England. *Stroke, 20,* 333-339.

Diminck, M., Kaplan, S., & Salmeron, J. (1993). Peripheral vascular disease. In L. S. Lilly (Ed.), *Pathophysiology of heart disease* (pp. 239-254). Philadelphia: Lea & Febiger.

Dizon-Townson, D., Magee, K. P., Twickler, D. M., & Cox, S. M. (1995). Coarctation of the abdominal aorta in pregnancy: Diagnosis by magnetic resonance imaging. *Obstetrics and Gynecology, 85*(5), 817-819.

Dombovy, M. L., Sandok, B. A., & Basford, J. R. (1986). Rehabilitation for stroke: A review. *Stroke, 17*(3), 363-369.

Doubilet, P., & Abrams, H. L. (1984). The cost of underutilization: Percutaneous transluminal angioplasty for peripheral vascular disease. *New England Journal of Medicine, 310,* 95-102.

Duke, R. J., Bloch, R. F., Turpie, A. G., Trebilcock, R., & Bayer, N. (1986). Intravenous heparin for the prevention of stroke progression in acute partial stable stroke. *Annals of Internal Medicine, 105*(6), 825-828.

Dutch TIA Trial Study Group. (1991). A comparison of two doses of aspirin (30 mg vs. 283 mg a day) in patients after a transient ischemic attack or minor ischemic stroke. *New England Journal of Medicine, 325,* 1261-1266.

Eagle, K. A., Rihal, C. S., Foster, E. D., Mickel, M. C., Gersh, B. J., for the Coronary Artery Surgery Study (CASS) Investigators. (1994). Long-term survival in patients with coronary artery disease: Importance of peripheral vascular disease. *Journal of American College of Cardiology, 23,* 1091-1095.

Ernst, C. B. (1993). Abdominal aortic aneurysm. *New England Journal of Medicine, 326,* 1167-1172.

European Carotid Surgery Trials' Collaborative Group. (1991). MRC European Carotid Surgery Trial: Interim results for symptomatic patients with severe (70-99%) or with mild (0-29%) carotid stenosis. *Lancet, 337,* 1235-1243.

Ezekowitz, M. D., Bridgeres, S. L., James, K. E., Carliner, N. H., Colling, C. L., Gormick, C. C., Krause-Steinrauf, H., Kurtzke, J. F., Nazarian, S. M., Radford, M. J., Rickles, F. R., Shabetai, R., Deykin, D., for the Veterans Affairs Stroke Prevention in Nonrheumatic Atrial Fibrillation Investigators. (1992). Warfarin in the prevention of stroke associated with nonrheumatic atrial fibrillation. *New England Journal of Medicine, 327,* 1406-1412.

Feigelson, H. S., Criqui, M. H., Froneck, A., Langer, R. D., & Molgaard, C. A. (1994). Screening for peripheral arterial disease: The sensitivity, specificity, and predictive value of noninvasive tests in a defined population. *American Journal of Epidemiology, 140,* 526-534.

Folsom, A. R., Prineas, R. J., Kaye, S. A., & Munger, R. G. (1990). Incidence of hypertension and stroke in relation to body fat distribution and other risk factors in older women. *Stroke, 21,* 701-706.

Ford, C. S., Howard, V. J., Howard, G., Frye, J. L., Toole, J. F., & McKinney, W. M. (1986). The sex difference in manifestations of carotid bifurcation disease. *Stroke, 17*(5), 877-881.

Gertsman, B. B., Piper, J. M., Tomita, D. K., Ferguson, W. J., Stadel, B. V., & Lundin, F. E. (1991). Oral contraceptive estrogen dose and the risk of deep venous thromboembolic disease. *American Journal of Epidemiology, 133,* 32-37.

Gilpin, E. A., Lee, L., Evans, N., & Pierce, J. P. (1994). Smoking initiation rates in adults and minors: United States, 1944-1988. *American Journal of Epidemiology, 140,* 535-543.

Godfrey, M. (1993). The Marfan syndrome. In P. Beighton (Ed.), *McKusick's heritable disorders of connective tissue* (5th ed.). St. Louis: Mosby.

Gonzalez, E. B., Varner, W. T., Lisse, J. R., Daniels, J. C., & Hokanson, J. A. (1989). Giant-cell arteritis in the southern United States: An 11-year retrospective study from the Texas Gulf Coast. *Archives of Internal Medicine, 149*(7), 1561-1565.

Grady, D., Rubin, S. M., Petitti, D. B., Fox, C. S., Black, D., Ettinger, B., Ernster, V. L., & Cummings, S. R. (1992). Hormone therapy to prevent disease and prolong life in postmenopausal women. *Annals of Internal Medicine, 117*(12), 1016-1037.

Grubb, B. P., Sirio, C., & Zelis, R. (1987). Intravenous labetalol in aortic aneurysm dissection. *Journal of the American Medical Association, 258*(1), 78-79.

Hale, W. E., Marks, R. G., May, F. E., Moore, M. T., & Stewart, R. B. (1988). Epidemiology of intermittent claudication: Evaluation of risk factors. *Age and Aging, 17,* 57-60.

Helmrich, S. P., Rosenberg, L., Kaufman, D. W., Strom, B., & Shapiro, S. (1987). Venous thromboembolism in relation to oral contraceptive use. *Obstetrics and Gynecology, 69,* 91-95.

Heyns, A. D., Lotter, M. G., Badenhorst, P. N., Pieters, H., Nel, C. J., & Minnaar, P. C. (1982). Kinetics and fate of indium III oxine-labeled platelets in patients with aortic aneurysms. *Archives of Surgery, 117,* 1170-1174.

Hiatt, W. R., Hirsh, A. T., Regensteiner, J. G., Brass, E. P., & the Vascular Clinical Trialists. (1995). Clinical trials for claudication. *Circulation, 92,* 614-621.

Hobson, R. W., Weiss, D. G., Fields, W. S., Goldstone, J., Moore, W. S., Towne, J. B., Wright, C. B., and the Veterans Affairs Cooperative Study Group. (1993). Efficacy of carotid endarterectomy for asymptomatic carotid stenosis. *New England Journal of Medicine, 328,* 221-227.

Hopkins, A. (1993). *Clinical neurology. A modern approach.* Oxford: Oxford University Press.

House, A., Dennis, M., Molyneux, A., Warlow, C., & Hawton, K. (1989). Emotionalism after stroke. *British Medical Journal, 298,* 991-994.

Howard, G., Anderson, R., Sorlie, P., Andrews, V., Backlund, E., & Burke, G. L. (1994). Ethnic differences in stroke mortality between non-Hispanic whites, Hispanic whites, and blacks. *Stroke, 25,* 2120-2125.

Johnson, M. C., Canter, C. E., Strauss, A. W., & Spray, T. L. (1993). Repair of coarctation in infancy: Comparison of surgical and balloon angioplasty. *American Heart Journal, 125*(2, Pt. 1), 464-468.

Johnston, W., Rae, M., Hogg-Johnston, S. A., Colapinto, R. F., Walker, P. M., Baird, R. J., Sniderman, K. W., & Kalman, P. (1987). Five-year results of a prospective study of percutaneous transluminal angioplasty. *Annals of Surgery, 206,* 403-413.

Kannel, W. B., Gordon, T., & Wolf, P. A. (1972). Hemoglobin and the risk of cerebral infarction: The Framingham study. *Stroke, 3,* 409-420.

Kannel, W. B., & McGee, D. L. (1985). Update on some epidemiologic features of intermittent claudication: The Framingham study. *Journal American Geriatrics Society, 33,* 13-18.

Kattapong, V. J., & Becker, T. M. (1993). Ethnic differences in mortality from cerebrovascular disease among New Mexico's Hispanics, Native Americans, and non-Hispanic whites, 1958-87. *Ethnic Disease, 3,* 75-82.

Kittner, S. J., White, L. R., Losonczy, K. G., Wolf, P. A., & Hebel, J. R. (1990). Black-white differences in stroke incidence in a national sample. *Journal of the American Medical Association, 264,* 1267-1270.

Krupski, W. C. (1991). The peripheral vascular consequences of smoking. *Annals of Vascular Surgery, 5,* 291-304.

Langer, R. D., & Criqui, M. H. (1993). Stroke and peripheral vascular disease. In P. S. Douglas (Ed.), *Cardiovascular health and disease in women* (pp. 137-149). Philadelphia: Saunders.

Lee, B., Godfrey, M., Hori, H., Mattei, M. G., Sarfarazi, M., Tsipouras, P., Ramirez, F., & Hollister, D. W. (1991). Linkage of Marfan syndrome and a phenotypically related disorder to two different fibrillin genes. *Nature, 352,* 330-334.

Lidegaard, O. (1993). Oral contraception and risk of cerebral thromboembolic attack: Results of a case-control study. *British Medical Journal, 306,* 956-963.

Lindenstrom, E., Boysen, G., & Nyboe, J. (1993). Lifestyle factors and risk of cerebrovascular disease in women. *Stroke, 24,* 1468-1472.

Longstreth, W. T., Nelson, L. M., Koepsell, T. D., & van Belle, G. (1994). Subarachnoid hemorrhage and hormonal factors in women. *Annals of Internal Medicine, 121,* 168-173.

Marsalese, D. L., Moodie, D. S., Vacante, M., Lytle, B. W., Gill, C., Sterba, R., Cosgrove, D. M., Passalacqua, M., Goormastic, M., & Kovacs, A. (1989). Marfan's syndrome: Natural history and long-term follow-up of cardiovascular involvement. *Journal of the American College of Cardiology, 14,* 422-428.

Mayberg, M. R., Wilson, S. E., Yatsu, F., Weiss, D. G., Messina, L., Hershey, L. A., Colling, C., Eskridge, J., Deykin, D., & Winn, W. R. (1991). Carotid endarterectomy and prevention of cerebral ischemia in symptomatic carotid stenosis. *Journal of the American Medical Association, 266,* 3289-94.

Mayo Asymptomatic Carotid Endarterectomy Study Group. (1991). Results of a randomized controlled trial of carotid endarterectomy for asymptomatic carotid stenosis. *Mayo Clinic Proceedings, 67,* 513-518.

Mayo, N. E., Hendlisz, J., Goldberg, M. S., Korner-Bitensky, N., Becker, R., & Coopersmith, H. (1989). Destinations of stroke patients discharged form the Montreal area acute-care hospitals. *Stroke, 20,* 351-356.

Mendelsohn, A. M., Lloyd, T. R., Crowley, D. C., Sandhu, S. K., Kocis, K. C., & Beekman, R. H. (1994). Late follow-up of balloon angioplasty in children with a native coarctation of the aorta. *American Journal of Cardiology, 74,* 696-700.

McGovern, P. G., Burke, G. L., Sprafka, J. M., Xue, S., Folsom, A. R., & Blackburn, H. (1992). Trends in mortality, morbidity and risk-factor levels for stroke from 1960 through 1990: The Minnesota heart survey. *Journal of American Medical Association, 268,* 753-759.

Nelson, D. E., Emont, S. L., Brackbill, R. M., Cameron, L. L., Peddicord, J., & Fiore, M. C. (1994). Cigarette smoking prevalence by occupation in the United States: A comparison between 1978 to 80 and 1978-90. *Journal of Occupational Medicine, 36,* 516-524.

Neumann, F. J., Waas, W., Diehm C., Weiss, T., Haupt, H. M., Zimmerman, R., Tillmanns, H., & Kubler, W. (1990). Activation and decreased deformability of neutrophils after intermittent claudication. *Circulation, 82,* 922-929.

Nevitt, M. P., Ballard, D. J., & Hallett, J. W. (1989). Prognosis of abdominal aortic aneurysms. *New England Journal of Medicine, 321,* 1009-1014.

Newman, A. B., Siscovick, D. S., Manolio, T. A., Polack, J., Fried L. P., Borhani, N. O., & Wolfson, S. K., for the Cardiovascular Health Study (CHS) Collaborative Research Group. (1993). Ankle-arm index as a marker of atherosclerosis in the cardiovascular health study. *Circulation, 88,* 837-845.

Newman, A. B., Sutton-Tyrrell, K., Rutan, G. H., Locher, J., & Kuller, L. H. (1993). Lower extremity arterial disease in elderly subjects with systolic hypertension. *Journal of Clinical Epidemiology, 44*(1), 15-20.

Noll, S. F., & Roth, E. J. (1994). Stroke rehabilitation: Epidemiologic aspects and acute management. *Archives of Physical and Medical Rehabilitation, 75,* S38-S41.

Nolte, J. E., Rutherford, R. B., Nawaz, S., Rosenberger, A., Speers, W. C., & Krupski, W. C. (1995). Arterial dissections associated with pregnancy. *Journal of Vascular Surgery, 21*(3), 515-520.

North American Symptomatic Carotid Endarterectomy Trial Collaborators. (1991). Beneficial effect of carotid endarterectomy in symptomatic patients with high-grade carotid stenosis. *New England Journal of Medicine, 325,* 445-453.

O'Leary, D. H., Polack, J. F., Kronmal, R. A., Kittner, S. J., Bond, G., Wolfson, S. K., Bommer, W., Price, T. R., Gardin, J. M., & Savage, P. J. (1992). Distribution and correlates of sonographically detected carotid artery disease in the cardiovascular health study. *Stroke, 23,* 1752-1760.

Orchard, T. J., Dorman, J. S., Maser, R. E., Becker, D. J., Drash, A. L., Ellis, D., LaPorte, R. E., & Kuller, L. H. (1990). Prevalence of complications in IDDM by sex and duration. *Diabetes, 39,* 1116-1124.

Oskoui, R., & Lindsay, J. (1994). Aortic dissection in women < 40 years of age and the unimportance of pregnancy. *American Journal of Cardiology, 73,* 821-823.

Paganini-Hill, A., Ross, R. K., & Henderson, B. E. (1988). Postmenopausal estrogen treatment and stroke: A prospective study. *British Medical Journal, 297,* 519-522.

Pariser, K. M. (1994). Takayasu's arteritis. *Current Opinions in Cardiology, 9,* 575-580.

Pepin, M. G., Superti-Furga, A., & Byers, P. H. (1992). Natural history of Ehlers-Danlos syndrome type IV (EDS type IV): Review of 137 cases. *American Journal of Human Genetics, 51,* A44.

Peterson, P., Boysen, G., Godtfredsen, J., Anderson, E. D., & Anderson, B. (1989). Placebo-controlled, randomized trial of warfarin and aspirin for prevention of thromboembolic complications in chronic atrial fibrillation. *Lancet, 1*(8631), 175-179.

Poldermans, D., Fioetti, P. M., Forster, T., Thomson, I. R., Boersma, E., El-Said, E. M., du Boisna, J. J., Roelandt, T. C., & van Urk, H. (1993). Dobutamine stress echocardiography for assessment of perioperative cardiac risk in patients undergoing major vascular surgery. *Circulation, 87,* 1506-1512.

Realini, J. P., & Goldzieher, J. W. (1985). Oral contraceptives and cardiovascular disease: A critique of the epidemiologic studies. *American Journal of Obstetrics and Gynecology, 152,* 729-798.

Reunanen, A., Takkunen, H., & Aromaa, A. (1982). Prevalence of intermittent claudication and its effect on mortality. *Acta Medica Scandinavica, 211,* 249-256.

Roberts, C. S., & Roberts W. C. (1991). Dissection of the aorta associated with congenital malformation of the aortic valve. *Journal of American College of Cardiology, 17,* 712-716.

Roberts, W. C. (1981). Aortic dissection: Anatomy, consequences, and causes. *American Heart Journal, 101,* 195-214.

Roman, M. J., Rosen, S. E., Kramer-Fox, R., & Devereux, R. B. (1993). Prognostic significance of the pattern of aortic root dilation in the Marfan syndrome. *Journal of American College of Cardiology, 22,* 1470-1476.

Rothrock, J. F., Walicke, P., Swenson, M. R., Lyden, P. D., & Logan, W. R. (1988). Migrainous stroke. *Archives of Neurology, 45,* 63-67.

Rudd, N. L., Nimrod, C., Holbrook, K., & Byers, P. H. (1983). Pregnancy complications in type IV Ehlers-Danlos syndrome. *The Lancet, 1,* 50-53.

SALT Collaborative Group. (1991). Swedish aspirin low-dose trial (SALT) of 75 mg aspirin as secondary prophylaxis after cerebrovascular ischaemia events. *Lancet, 338,* 1345-1349.

Salvarani, C., Gabriel, S. E., O'Fallon, W. M., Hunder, G. C. (1995). The incidence of giant cell arteritis in Olmstead County, Minnesota: Apparent fluctuations in a cyclic pattern. *Annals of Internal Medicine, 123,* 192-194.

Sandin, K. J., Cifu, D. X., & Noll, S. F. (1994). Stroke rehabilitation: Psychologic and social implications. *Archives of Physical Medicine and Rehabilitation, 75,* S52-S55.

Sandok, B. A., & Giuliani, E. R. (1982). Cerebral ischemic events in patients with mitral valve prolapse. *Stroke, 13*(4), 448-450.

Scott, R. P., Wilson, N. M., Ashton, H. A., & Kay, D. N. (1993). Is surgery necessary for abdominal aortic aneurysm less than 6 cm in diameter? *Lancet, 342,* 1395-1396.

Shinton, R., & Beevers, G. (1989). Meta-analysis of relation between cigarette smoking and stroke. *British Medical Journal, 298,* 789-794.

Silverman, D. I., Burton, K. J., Gray, J., Bosner, M. S., Kouchoukos, N. T., Roman, M. J., Boxer, M., Devereux, R. B., & Tsipouras, P. (1995). Life expectancy in the Marfan syndrome. *American Journal of Cardiology, 75,* 157-160.

Sivenius, J., Riekkinen, P. J., Kilpelainen, H., Laakso, M., & Penttila, I. (1991). Antiplatelet therapy is effective in the prevention of stroke or death in women: Subgroup analysis of the European stroke prevention study (ESPS). *Acta Neurologica Scandinavica, 84,* 286-290.

Smith, G. D., Shipley, M J., & Rose, G. (1990). Intermittent claudication, heart disease risk factors, and mortality: The Whitehall study. *Circulation, 82,* 1925-1931.

Sorokin, Y., Johnson, M. P., Rogowski, N., Richardson, D. A., & Evans, M. I. (1994). Obstetric and gynecologic dysfunction in the Ehlers-Danlos syndrome. *Journal of Reproductive Medicine, 39,* 281-284.

Spranger, M., Aspey, B. S., & Harrison, M. J. (1989). Sex difference in antithrombotic effect of aspirin. *Stroke, 20,* 34-37.

Stotts, R. S., Glynn, T. J., & Baquet, C. R. (1994). Smoking cessation among blacks. *Journal of Health Care in the Poor and Underserved, 2,* 207-219.

Tell, G. S., Polack, J. F., Ward, B. J., Kittner, S., J., Savage, P. J., Robbins, J., and the Cardiovascular Health Study Collaborative Research Group. (1994). Relation of smoking with carotid artery wall thickness and stenosis in older adults. *Circulation, 90,* 2905-2908.

Thompson, S. G., Greenberg, G., & Meade, T. W. (1989). Risk factors for stroke and myocardial infarction in women in the United Kingdom as assessed in general practice: A case-controlled study. *British Heart Journal, 61,* 402-409.

Thorogood, M., Mann, J., Murphy, M., & Vessey, M. (1992). Fatal stroke and use of oral contraceptives: Findings from a case-control study. *American Journal of Epidemiology, 136,* 35-45.

Tikkanen, J., & Heinionen, O. P. (1993). Risk factors for coarctation of the aorta. *Teratology, 47,* 565-572.

Tilstra, D. J., & Byers, P. H. (1994). Molecular basis of hereditary disorders of connective tissue. *Annual Review of Medicine, 45,* 149-63.

Tsipouras, P., Byers, P. H., Schwartz, R. C., Chu, M. L., Weil, D., Cassidy, S. B., & Ramirez, F. (1986). Ehlers-Danlos syndrome type IV: Cosegregation of the phenotype to a COL3A1 allele of type III procollagen. *Human Genetics, 74,* 41-44.

Tunis, S. R., Bass, E. B., & Steinberg, E. P. (1991). The use of angioplasty, bypass surgery, and amputation in the management of peripheral vascular disease. *New England Journal of Medicine, 325,* 556-562.

Tzourio, C., Tehindrazanarivelo, A., Iglesias, S., Aplerovitch, A., Chedru, F., d'Anglejan-Chatillon, J., & Bousser, M. G. (1995). Case-control study of migraine and risk of ischaemic stroke in young women. *British Medical Journal, 310,* 830-833.

UK-TIA Study Group. (1988). United Kingdom transient ischaemic attack (UK-TIA) aspirin trial: Interim results. *British Medical Journal, 296,* 316-320.

Wardlaw, J. M., & Warlow, C. P. (1992). Thrombolysis in acute ischemic stroke: Does it work? *Stroke, 23,* 1826-1839.

Wiebers, D. O., & Whisnant, J. P. (1985). The incidence of stroke among pregnant women in Rochester, Minn, 1955-1979. *Journal of American Medical Association, 254,* 3055-3057.

Wilson, P. W., Garrison, R. J., & Castelli, W. P. (1985). Postmenopausal estrogen use, cigarette smoking, and cardiovascular morbidity in women over 50. *New England Journal Medicine, 313,* 1038-1043.

Wilson, S. E., Wolf, G. L., & Cross, A. P. (1989). Percutaneous transluminal angioplasty versus operation for peripheral arteriosclerosis: Report of a prospective randomized trial in a selected group of patients. *Journal of Vascular Surgery, 9,* 1-9.

Wong, M. C., Giuliani M. J., & Haley, E. C. (1990). Cerebrovascular disease and stroke in women. *Cardiology, 77*(Suppl. 2), 80-90.

Zelop, C. M. (1993). Gynecology. In S. Z. Goldhaber (Ed.), *Prevention of venous thromboembolism* (pp. 405-424). New York: Marcel Dekker.

CHAPTER 10

Reproductive, Gynecologic, and Urinary Tract Conditions and Disorders

Phyllis W. Sharps

Introduction

During a woman's lifespan she is most likely to have some concerns related to her reproductive, gynecologic, or urinary tract health. Any woman who participates in an intimate heterosexual relationship or believes she has the potential to participate in such a relationship will think about managing her own fertility. Her thoughts are often related to the control of fertility or postponing, delaying, or spacing pregnancies. In some cases a woman and her partner are confronted with an infertility condition. Other women are faced with diseases and dysfunction of the reproductive organs or the urinary tract that have an impact on their lifestyles. Uterine dysfunction and diseases of other reproductive organs may have an impact on fertility, intimate sexual relationships, and overall quality of life. Urinary stress incontinence (USI), a common disorder of the urinary tract, may have significant impact on a woman's lifestyle.

This chapter focuses on the management of fertility and includes a discussion of pregnancy, contraceptive choices, abortion, and infertility. Two common reproductive health conditions, uterine dysfunction and polycystic ovary (PCO) syndrome, are also addressed. Urinary incontinence is discussed. The causes, symptoms, diagnosis, and therapeutic interventions for each condition are described. Finally, the implications for practice and directions for future research are outlined.

Fertility Health Concerns

Generally, from the onset of puberty until the completion of menopause, most women will devote much thought to a variety of issues related to fertility. Such thoughts often center around controlling fertility; becoming pregnant; delaying, spacing, or terminating pregnancies; or the inability to achieve a desired pregnancy. Decisions about fertility affect the woman and her partner. Choices and decisions related to fertility are often influenced by a woman's values and attitudes, her religious background, her family and friends, her partner, and societal values. Almost all women will encounter specific fertility health concerns related to infertility, contraception, or pregnancy.

Controlling Fertility: Birth Control and Contraception

Artifacts and records from ancient civilizations indicate that men and woman have always desired to control fertility. Today, any woman who engages in or has the potential to engage in an intimate heterosexual relationship will be concerned with contraceptive methods during her childbearing years (Caufield, 1994). The family planning movement in the United States was led by Margaret Sanger, a nurse, when she introduced the diaphragm (Lynaugh, 1991). Today, women have several options for the control of fertility.

The terms birth control and contraception are often used interchangeably; however, they each describe a different aspect of fertility control. *Birth control* refers to all procedures that prevent the birth of a baby. Therefore, birth control includes all contraceptive methods, sterilization, intrauterine devices (IUDs), and abortion procedures. *Contraception* is a more specific term referring to any method that prevents the fertilization of the ovum (Alexander & LaRosa, 1994). This chapter discusses the most common birth control methods.

Nationally, 60% of women aged 15 to 44 years (considered the reproductive age) use a method of birth control. The most frequently selected methods are oral contraceptives, female sterilization, and condoms. The IUD is selected less frequently.

The ideal contraceptive method should be easy to use, accessible, affordable, and 100% safe and effective. In addition to these factors, a woman's decision may be influenced by many other factors (Alexander & La Rosa, 1994; Youngkin & Davis, 1994), which are listed in Display 10–1. Unfortunately, many couples make their decision about birth control methods in haste or leave birth control or contraception to chance.

Table 10–1 summarizes the most commonly used birth control methods in the United States. The table also describes the effectiveness of each method in terms of failure rates. The method failure rate is considered to be the number of accidental pregnancies in the first year of use when a couple uses the method consistently and correctly. For example, a failure rate of 10% means 10 of 100 women using the method will become pregnant. The user failure rate, which refers to inaccuracies in the client's use of a method, should also be considered (Heath, 1993).

DISPLAY 10-1
Factors Influencing Choice of Contraceptive Method

- sexual lifestyle
- number of partners and frequency of coitus
- marital or relationship status
- cultural and religious beliefs
- motivation of woman and her partner
- degree of comfort with one's body
- lactation status
- cost
- effectiveness
- safety
- access to health care
- convenience
- temporary or permanent nature of the method
- previous experience
- educational and cognitive status
- confidence in the method

Table 10-1. Birth Control Methods

Method	Mode of Prevention
Chance	
Spermicides	Nonoxynol 9 immobilizes sperm
Withdrawal	Prevents sperm entering vagina
Barrier Methods	
Cervical cap	Vaginal barrier prevents sperm entering cervix; spermicide kills sperm
Diaphragm	Vaginal barrier prevents sperm entering cervix; spermicides kill sperm
Condom	Barrier; prevents sperm entering vagina
Fertility Awareness Methods	
Calendar	Prevent sperm from entering vagina during fertile periods
Ovulation method Symptothermal Postovulation	
IUD	Unknown; thought to affect fertilization, implantation, and endometrium
Progesteasert Copper T380A	
Pills	Suppress ovulation; alters tubal transport; mucous changes, inhibit implantation
Combined Progestin only	Suppress ovulation, cervical mucous changes, altered tubal transport, endometrial changes
Progestin implants	
Norplant	Long-acting progestin (levonorgestrel)
Depo-Provera	Long-acting progestin
Female sterilization	Fallopian tubes are cut and tied; prevents ovum moving to uterus
Male sterilization	Vas deferens cut and tied; prevents sperm mixing into ejaculate

*The percent of women experiencing an accidental pregnancy in the first year of use (failure rate).
†Lowest expected failure rate.
‡The lowest reported percent of women experiencing an accidental pregnancy in the first year of use.
Sources: Alexander & LaRose (1994); Caulfield (1994); Hatcher et al. (1990); Trussel et al. (1990).

How Administered	Failure Rate*	Comments
	85	
Inserted into vagina before intercourse	21	Must use with each intercourse
Withdraw penis before ejaculation	18	Sperm are in semen
Inserted vaginally; rubber cap fits over cervix	18	Fitted by nurse or physician; used with spermicides
Inserted vaginally before intercourse	18	Fitted by nurse or physician; used with spermicides; can be used during lactation
Latex sheath placed on erect penis before ejaculation	12	
Couples avoid intercourse during fertile periods	9[†]	Requires commitment from both partners
	3[†]	
	2[†]	
	1[†]	
Inserted vaginally into uterus	0.9[‡]	Must be inserted by nurse or physician; client should check for placement
	0.5[‡]	
Oral (by mouth), 21 or 28 days daily	0.0[‡]	
Oral (28 or 42 day) packs	1.1[‡]	
6 Silastic capsules surgically implanted on inner side of upper arms	0.04	Provides 5 y of protection
Intramuscular injection		Provides 90 d of protection
Surgical procedure vaginally or abdominally	0.4	Permanent procedure
Surgical procedure; through scrotum	0.15	Permanent procedure

Contraceptive Methods

Contraceptive methods can be classified in several ways: type of method, chemical component of the method, or the continuity of use of the method. The contraceptive methods reviewed are classified according to the continuity of use. Contraceptive methods can be used as episodic, continual, or permanent methods (Heath, 1993).

Episodic Methods

Episodic methods are used only during coitus. These include spermicides, condoms (male and female), diaphragms, and cervical caps.

Recently, with the increase in acquired immunodeficiency syndrome (AIDS), these methods have received renewed attention. The episodic methods provide protection against AIDS and other sexually transmitted diseases (STDs) (Hatcher, et al. 1994; Heath, 1994).

These methods prevent pregnancy by forming a mechanical or chemical barrier that prevents the sperm from coming in contact with the ovum. The male and female condoms, the diaphragm, and the cervical cap make a mechanical barrier to the sperm; spermicides form a chemical barrier. Spermicides may come in the form of vaginal foams, creams, or gels. The chemical agent in the spermicides is nonoxynol 9, which immobilizes and kills the sperm. The spermicides are also used with the diaphragm, thus increasing the effectiveness of these methods.

Advantages of these methods are that, with the exception of the cervical cap and the diaphragm, they can be purchased over the counter without prescriptions. The methods are easy to learn to use and have few systemic effects. They are safe for lactating women, women over age 35, and cigarette smokers.

These methods have few disadvantages. The diaphragm and the cervical cap must be fitted by a physician or nurse practitioner and must be refitted after childbirth or a weight loss or gain of 15 to 20 pounds (Carsaro & Lichtman, 1990). Other problems may be related to allergic reactions to the rubber of the diaphragm, cervical cap, or condoms; allergy to spermicides; recurrent urinary tract infection with the diaphragm; or the increased risk for toxic shock syndrome with the cervical cap. Sometimes couples complain of the perceived messiness, the taste, the expense, the need for privacy and touching the genitalia, and the interruption of the intimate act related to the use of these methods (Carsaro & Lichtman, 1990). Table 10–1 summarizes the barrier methods.

Continual Methods

These methods include oral contraceptive pills (OCPs), levonorgestrel (Norplant) implants, intramuscular progesterone (Depo-Provera), and IUDs. These methods prevent pregnancy by providing a continual release of estrogen or progestin (OCPs) or progestin only (mini-pills, Norplant, Depo-Provera, progesterone IUD) or by causing a local inflammatory response in the uterine wall (IUD) (Heath, 1994). Some methods have been used by women in the United States for more than

30 years (OCPs), whereas other methods have only been available for use since 1990 (Norplant) or 1992 (Depo-Provera) (McKay & Evans, 1994). About 19% of women of reproductive age use OCPs (Alexander & LaRosa, 1994).

Pregnancy is prevented by the effects of estrogen or progestin. The pituitary (gonadotrophin-releasing) hormone and ovarian (follicle-stimulating) hormone (FSH), and the luteinizing hormone (LH) are suppressed, thus preventing ovulation. Also, ovum/tubal transport is altered, the primary mode in which the progestin-only methods (mini-pills, Norplant, Depo-Provera, IUD) prevent pregnancy. The cervical mucus thickens, which inhibits sperm motility and its ability to reach the fallopian tubes. Implantation is inhibited by the alteration of the endometrium and uterine secretions (Clarke, 1990a, 1990b; Youngkin & Davis, 1994).

Most women find these methods convenient and effective. The methods are not associated with interrupting the sex act, which also increases their effectiveness. OCPs are safest for nonsmoking women under the age of 35. The mini-pills (lower dose progestin only) can be safely used during lactation and by women over age 35. Women with a history of thrombophlebitis can also use the mini-pill. The effects are rapidly reversible after the woman stops taking them. These pills have many of the same benefits as OCPs. The Norplant system, Depo-Provera, and IUDs have the advantage of long-term protection. For example, plastic IUDs can stay in place indefinitely; however, it is recommended that copper IUDs be replaced after 8 years. The progesterone IUDs need to be changed yearly (McKay & Evans, 1994). The IUD is relatively inexpensive and requires only annual medical visits. The Norplant system can stay in place for 5 years and the Depo-Provera shots are given every 3 months. Noncontraceptive benefits of the continual methods include lighter menstrual flow, less anemia, and minimal dysmenorrhea (OCP). Other benefits for the continual methods may include lower risk for ovarian and endometrial cancer, lower incidence of endometriosis, lower risk for pelvic inflammatory disease (PID), and lower incidence of benign cysts of the breasts (Heath, 1994; McKay & Evans, 1994). For the progestin-only methods the lower doses result in fewer systemic or major complications related to the ingestion of hormones and a lower rate of ectopic pregnancy. Most women are able to achieve a pregnancy within 12 months after stopping these methods.

The hormones in these methods affect all body systems. Common side effects of OCPs include nausea and vomiting, a 2- to 5-lb weight gain, fatigue, depression, and missed menstrual periods. Many women find the side effects intolerable and will stop using the pill. The pill must be taken every day. Therefore, this method requires a prescription and one to two visits to the health care provider; some women find the cost of the health care and prescriptions prohibitive. Women smokers over age 35 or with or at risk for cancer of the breast, stroke or coronary artery disease, or hypertensive disorders are usually not candidates for the OCP (Heath, 1994;& McKay & Evans, 1994). Women who use IUDs report heavier bleeding and pain and for this reason may discontinue its use (Clarke, 1990a). These continual hormonal methods do not protect against infections by human immunodeficiency virus (HIV) or STDs. The mini-pill has similar disadvantages. Bleeding irregularities may occur with any of the progestin-only methods.

Postcoital Methods

These methods are used to prevent pregnancy after the act of unprotected intercourse. These methods include the morning after pills, the morning after IUD, and menstrual induction. These methods are often considered emergency birth control methods (Alexander & LaRosa, 1994; Caufield, 1994; McKay & Evans, 1994).

High doses of combined oral contraceptives are given within 72 hours of the unprotected intercourse, or sooner . The pills prevent pregnancy as has been described previously. In the United States the drug mifepristone (RU 486) is just being tested for use. However, RU 486 has been used in Europe and is highly effective. RU 486 induces menstruation by preventing implantation and causing sloughing off of the fertilized ovum. The use of RU 486 continues to be extremely controversial in this country. With all of these methods, menstrual bleeding should occur in 2 to 3 weeks.

Permanent Methods

Surgical sterilization offers permanent birth control. In the United States surgical sterilization is the most popular method of birth control among married couples (Alexander & LaRosa, 1994; McKay & Evans, 1994). The usual female procedure is the bilateral tubal ligation. The male procedure is the vasectomy. Although there are some reported successes of reversal of these methods, couples should view these procedures as permanent.

The female sterilization is done by either a laparoscopic or minilaparoscopic surgical procedure. Both procedures involve the destruction or removal of part of the fallopian tubes as a means for prevention of pregnancy. The fallopian tubes are cut and sealed with either cauterization or rings or clips. These procedures effectively prevent the sperm from fertilizing the egg. The procedure is usually done on an outpatient basis; women require about 2 to 3 days of recovery at home.

The male procedure involves cutting or sealing the vas deferens, which interferes with the transport of the sperm to be mixed into the semen. Thus, the ejaculate contains no sperm capable of fertilizing the ovum. The procedure is considered outpatient surgery.

The major benefit of these procedures is that they are safe, permanent methods of birth control. The surgical intervention and postoperative pain are minimal and recovery is rapid. Many couples report improved sexual intimacy after the anxiety related to potential unwanted pregnancies is removed.

There are few disadvantages. However, these procedures do require the involvement of a health care provider to perform the procedures and health insurance or a means to pay for the procedures. Also, there will be a few days of interruption of normal activities until recovery is complete. Finally, the couple must understand that these are permanent procedures.

Fertility Awareness Methods

The fertility awareness methods, also known as natural family planning or periodic abstinence, involve avoiding intercourse during the fertile periods of the menstrual cycle. There has been a renewed interest in these methods by couples who desire a method that they totally control and that avoids the use of chemicals and devices.

The fertility awareness methods use one or a combination of methods to predict ovulation and the period of fertility. The couple avoids pregnancy by avoiding intercourse or unprotected intercourse during the fertile period. The methods that couples use to predict the ovulation and subsequent fertile period are described in Table 10–1. The combination of methods is thought to be the most accurate predictor of ovulation (Caufield, 1994; McKay & Evans, 1994). Additionally, there are over-the-counter chemical kits that a couple can use to determine if ovulation has occurred (Haberman-Cohen, 1993).

The fertility awareness methods increase and encourage communication between partners. Also, a woman gains an increased awareness of her own body and her fertility. Other advantages include no side effects, no interference with normal body functions, no devices or chemicals, low cost, and acceptability to most religious groups. Also, the same methods can be applied to achieving a pregnancy when it is desired (Caufield, 1994; McKay & Evans, 1994).

These methods require a great deal of commitment from both partners as well as time for extensive record-keeping related to predicting the fertile periods. This method has a lower user effectiveness. Some couples find the interference with sexual spontaneity and the prolonged periods of abstinence each month difficult to tolerate (Caufield, 1994; McKay & Evans, 1994).

Elective Abortion

Abortion is the spontaneous or induced expulsion of an embryo or fetus before viability. A *therapeutic abortion* is an induced abortion done to protect the life or health of the mother. An *elective abortion* is also the termination of a pregnancy before fetal viability as a means of contraception (Alexander & LaRosa, 1994; Gant & Cunningham, 1993; McKay & Evans, 1994). The use of abortion as a means of birth control has been and remains controversial in the United States. The 1973 *Roe v. Wade* Supreme Court decision made abortion legal in the United States. However, in 1976 the Supreme Court ruled that Medicaid funding could not be used for abortion procedures. Today, the controversy continues; Medicaid funding can be used in the case of rape and incest, and the states have the authority to limit a woman's right to a legal abortion (Alexander & LaRosa, 1994).

Elective abortion as a birth control method interrupts a pregnancy before the period of fetal viability. The products of conception are removed from the uterus by either surgical or medical procedures. The most common surgical procedure is vacuum (suction) curettage. This is an ambulatory care procedure that can be performed up to the 16th week of gestation. The cervix is dilated before surgery by a variety of dilators, including laminaria. The surgical procedure is performed under local anesthesia. The products of conception are removed by suction evacuation and completion confirmed by curettage (Caufield, 1994; Gant & Cunningham, 1990).

The medical procedures used to induce second trimester abortion consist of a variety of substances, including oxytocin in high doses; hyperosmotic solutions, such as saline, urea, or prostaglandin, injected into the amniotic fluid; and prostaglandins. RU 486, although not approved for use in the United States, has also been used to medically induce abortion. The procedures are eased by dilating the cervix with substances such as laminaria or prostaglandins before starting the induction procedures. The infusion can be done as an inpatient or outpatient procedure. The medical procedures can take 8 to 12 hours (Caufield, 1994; Gant & Cunningham, 1990; Turk, 1990).

An important benefit of abortion is that a woman can terminate an unwanted pregnancy after it has occurred. The legalization of abortion has made procedures safer and has decreased the associated risks of maternal morbidity and mortality. The first trimester abortion procedures require less disruption of daily routines and work schedules, are easier to perform, are more readily available, and cost less than those abortion procedures performed during the second trimester (Caufield, 1994; Turk, 1990).

The major disadvantages of the surgical abortion procedures are similar to those of other surgical procedures. Potential complications include incomplete abortion, surgical lacerations, bleeding, infections, allergic reactions, cardiac arrest, and seizures. Common problems with medical procedures include incomplete abortion, uterine or cervical trauma, bleeding, and infections. Women are at risk for psychological trauma related to the abortion and the loss of the pregnancy (Caufield, 1994; Gant & Cunningham, 1990). The long-term sequelae of repeated abortions on subsequent pregnancies has been studied and the findings are controversial. It is unclear whether repeated abortions increase the rates of fetal loss or preterm labor (McKay & Evans, 1994).

Infertility

Couples who have not been able to achieve a pregnancy after a year of normal unprotected sexual intercourse are considered to be infertile. Additionally, an inability to give birth to a live infant is considered to be an infertile condition. Using these criteria, the incidence of infertility reportedly affects as many as 15% to 20% of all couples (McKay & Evans, 1994; Haberman-Cohen, 1993). A couple's fertility may change over the years of their relationship. A woman who has never been pregnant or a man who has never impregnated a woman is considered to have primary impaired infertility. Secondary impaired infertility is the condition in which a woman has been pregnant at least once and has not been able to conceive again or sustain a pregnancy since the initial pregnancy. Sterility is the condition in which conception is not possible and the cause is unknown (Haberman-Cohen, 1993).

Recent statistics suggest that the incidence of infertility may be increasing (Corfman & Ball, 1994; Hull, 1992). Many explanations have been offered for this trend. Many couples, for a variety of reasons, chose to delay childbearing to an older age, a time when fertility naturally decreases (Potter, 1993). More liberal views toward sexual intimacy have also resulted in women being at greater risk for infections of reproductive organs (eg, PID). Untreated or inadequately treated diseases and infections can leave scar tissue that can impair fertility. Use of substances such as illicit drugs, alcohol, and cigarettes has increased; all have been linked with impaired fertility. Finally, more evidence links environmental toxins with impaired fertility (Haberman-Cohen, 1993).

Several female and male factors must be present for conception to occur. Therefore, infertility must always be considered as a "couple" problem. Both partners must have normally developed and functioning reproductive organs. For both, there must be normal hypothalamic-pituitary-gonadal functioning that results in the production of normal ova and sperm. Deformities and deficiencies in any of these reproductive organs or hormonal functions can result in infertility. The timing of intercourse is critical to ensure that fertilization occurs (Corfman & Ball, 1994).

Causes

Many factors influence a couple's fertility. Stress is a factor that should not be underestimated as a cause for infertility. Psychological stressors that either partner may experience related to work, financial concerns, the marital relationship, or frequent changes in lifestyle can affect fertility. Stress on the autonomic system may result in the increased production of catecholamine, which may result in hormonal imbalances, which in turn may affect ovulation. Some women coping with increased stress may experience an excessive weight gain or loss; excessive weight, as well as underweight, have been associated with anovulation and amenorrhea. Stress can also affect the sympathetic nervous system and result in hormonal balances that adversely influence fertility. The male partner experiencing stress may find that both stress and fatigue may interfere with his sexual performance and his ability to impregnate the woman. Additionally, lack of knowledge or misinformation about sexual activity and its relation to pregnancy may be related to a couple's inability to achieve a desired pregnancy.

Female factors related to infertility include abnormalities of the reproductive organs such as uterine deformities, uterine tumors (fibromyomas), or an incompetent cervix. These conditions may not interfere with the ability to conceive but rather with the woman's ability to maintain the pregnancy. Other causes of infertility for the female partner may be related to the patency of the fallopian tubes, the characteristics of the cervical mucus, lack of menstrual cycles (amenorrhea), nonovulatory menstrual cycles (anovulation), hormonal imbalances, medical conditions (thyroid dysfunctions, diabetes), body weight, endometriosis, and immunologic factors (antisperm antibodies). Occasionally, genetic abnormalities are the cause of infertility.

Male factors for infertility are related to abnormalities of the reproductive organs, use of certain drugs (antihypertensives, antidepressants, tranquilizers, antipsychotics, and illicit drugs), infections, sperm deformities, and either excessive or low sperm counts (Corfman & Ball, 1994).

Evaluation and Diagnosis

A comprehensive fertility evaluation conducted by a team of fertility specialists is critical to identifying the cause of the couple's infertility and subsequently developing the appropriate therapeutic intervention. Initially, a couple may be seen by their usual health care provider. A careful history and physical examination should be conducted at this time. The history should include previous illnesses and surgeries; previous pregnancies; nutrition and exercise habits; and use of alcohol, cigarettes, caffeine, and illicit drugs (Potter, 1990). The couple should be seen together or individually to explore their sexual habits and preferences, as well as sexual knowledge, as it is related to pregnancy. It is usually at this time that the couple's primary health provider can determine if the cause of the infertility is something that he or she has the expertise and resources to treat or if referral to a specialized fertility team is necessary. The specialized fertility team consists of a urologist, gynecologist, endocrinologist, and nurse.

The couple referred to the specialized fertility evaluation team will be involved in intensive diagnostic testing that may be time consuming, of long duration, costly, and stressful for both partners. Diagnostic evaluation for the woman will include laboratory tests to evaluate blood counts, STDs, and hormonal balance. The reproductive structures will be examined by ultrasound and other radiographic tests to evaluate them for normal functioning. For example, hysterosalpingography is a radiographic test used to visualize and evaluate the patency of fallopian tube tissue. Basal body temperature, endometrial biopsies, and hormonal studies are used to detect ovulation. Postcoital testing, sperm agglutination, and sperm immobilization tests are helpful for assessing immunologic compatibility of the cervical mucus and sperm (Haberman-Cohen, 1993; Hull, 1992). The male factors that may be related to the cause of infertility are also evaluated, usually by a urologist. The results from the history, physical examination, and laboratory and diagnostic testing of both partners should identify the cause of infertility. Based on the identified cause, a treatment plan specific to the infertility condition will be implemented.

Therapeutic Interventions

After a couple has had an extensive fertility evaluation and if a treatable cause of the infertility is identified, the prognosis is generally good. There is a 34% chance that the infertile couple will achieve a pregnancy within 6 months and a 76% chance that the couple will achieve a pregnancy within 2 years (McKay & Evans, 1994). The treatment of the infertility is related to the identified cause.

Some conditions of infertility can be treated without surgical interventions. Infertility related to endocrine imbalances (eg, hypo- or hyperthyroidism) responds well to drug therapy to correct the imbalances. Infections of the reproductive organs, such as cervicitis, should be treated with antibiotics. Couples who have an antigen-antibody reaction are encouraged to use condoms for 6 months as a means to decrease the reaction. After 6 months, intercourse is carefully timed to occur at ovulation so that there will be an increased chance for fertilization before the antigen-antibody reaction begins again (McKay & Evans, 1994). Women who are either severely underweight or obese may experience infertility. Therefore, correction of the weight and body fat composition often restores fertility. Women who participate in intense athletic training and who have low body fat should be encouraged to reduce their exercise intensity, which will often increase the body fat to a level compatible for ovulation and subsequent fertility (McKay & Evans, 1994). Underweight women are encouraged to gain weight. When these women are able to regain 90%

to 95% of their body weight, previously low levels of ovarian hormones (FSH and LH) are restored. This will result in lengthening of the menstrual cycle, ovulation, and eventually a pregnancy (Potter, 1990).

Certain diagnostic and surgical procedures may also restore fertility. Sometimes, during the performance of a hysterosalpingogram, the injection of the radiopaque dye may improve the patency of the fallopian tubes. Improving or restoring the patency of the tubes often will facilitate fertilization and the movement of the fertilized ova to the uterus for implantation (Potter, 1990). Surgical procedures to correct or remove ovarian tumors, endometriosis, or blockage of the fallopian tubes may restore fertility. The McDonald cerclage, a surgical procedure used to constrict the cervical os with a suture, is often used for the woman with a history of incompetent cervix. A similar procedure, the Shirodkar cerclage, places a permanent suture around the cervical os. This procedure is ideal for the woman who anticipates future pregnancies. In this case she will be delivered by cesarean section (Cohen-Haberman, 1993).

Drug therapy has been used successfully to stimulate ovulation, when anovulation is the cause of infertility. Clomiphene citrate (Clomid) is the most commonly used fertility drug. Patients are given the drugs daily, with doses increased every 5 days until ovulation occurs. As many as 90% of women will achieve ovulation and the subsequent pregnancy rate is high (McKay & Evans, 1994). The incidence of twinning is higher for women using Clomid. Bromocriptine is used for women who have high levels of prolactin. The drug, a prolactin antagonist, is given in increasing doses until ovulation occurs (Potter, 1990).

Fertility can also be treated with other assisted reproductive technologies. Artificial insemination may be used when sperm counts are low. In vitro fertilization (IVF) and gamete intrafallopian transfer (GIFT) are have been successful in treating infertility. In the IVF procedures, ova are removed and fertilized in a laboratory, and the embryos are replaced into the uterus. During the GIFT procedures, ova and sperm are placed in the fallopian tubes where fertilization occurs as it would naturally. The rate of successful pregnancy appears to be higher for the GIFT procedures compared to the IVF procedures (Potter, 1990). The newer procedures, zygote intrafallopian transfer and tubal embryo transfer, are similar procedures that transvaginally aspirate ooyctes, fertilize them, and replace the zygotes or embryos back into the fallopian tubes via laparoscopy. The success rates vary from 10% to 33% with these procedures (Gant & Cunningham, 1993). All of these technologic advances offer the opportunity for the infertile couple to achieve the desired pregnancy.

Eventually, couples have to make choices about the cost of infertility treatments. The cost of the various diagnostic and intervention procedures can range from $20,000 to $125,000. Often, a couple's medical insurance does not cover the expenses incurred. Moreover, for many couples, the financial burden related to infertility comes at a time when they have the least financial resources (Corfman & Ball, 1994).

Regardless of the intervention used to treat the infertility, supportive counseling will be an important part of the intervention. A diagnosis of infertility, the subsequent evaluation, and the intervention are stressful events for many couples. Emotional support for the couple will be critical as they deal with the possible loss of the parenting role or the loss of a pregnancy. Couples experience a variety of emotional phases as they work through the fertility evaluation and treatment. Initially, there may be surprise that there is impaired fertility. The surprise is followed by denial and then anger. The anger may be directed at self, fertile friends and couples, or even the other partner. Often the couple will isolate themselves from friends and families to avoid what they may perceive as negative pressures, feelings, and attitudes related to their childlessness. Finally, the couple may feel guilt. Perhaps they believe something done at a younger age may have caused the current infertility. Eventually, some couples may have to face the fact that their infertility is permanent. These couples will experience real grief and the health care provider should encourage the expression of their grief (Thomas, 1992). After the grieving period they will have to make adjustments and decisions related to staying childless or adopting. Through all of this the couple will need a health care provider who is nonjudgmental, who provides accurate information, who listens and can advocate for the couple, and who supports the couple's decisions.

Pregnancy

Pregnancy has been described in a variety of ways. Some researchers describe it as a biologic event or a crisis event or a developmental event expressing a woman's fulfillment and self-realization (Fagler & Nicoll, 1990). Others suggest that it is a social event that reflects many of the social conflicts and problems seen in today's society (Balin, 1988). It is a *condition* common to women during their reproductive years. The total period of normal gestation varies between 38 and 42 lunar weeks or 9 calendar months. However it is described, pregnancy involves significant physiologic, psychological, and sociologic changes that have a significant impact on the woman and her partner or other significant family members.

In general, birth rates have remained stable in the United States. However, birth rates vary by age and ethnicity. The age groups experiencing increases in birth rates are teens and women over age 35. African American teens have the highest birth rates, followed by Hispanics, with Caucasian teens having the lowest birth rates. African American women at all ages, except 30 to 34 years, have higher birth rates when compared with Caucasian women. The incidence of births of low-birthweight infants is highest among African American women. The increased numbers of African American teens giving birth and the poverty and lack of resources often experienced by African American women are thought to account for the higher rate of low-birthweight infants (Stevens, 1993).

Changes

Physiologically, every system of a woman's body changes during pregnancy. The breasts enlarge as they prepare for lactation and the abdomen enlarges as the uterus grows to accommodate fetal growth. Often there are increases in the skin's pigmentation, as well as hair and nail growth. Major cardiovascular and respiratory changes occur to accommodate the growing fetus. Women may develop a physiologic anemia as a result of the increase in blood volume. Other cardiovascular changes may result in varicose veins and hemorrhoids. She may also experience periods of difficult breathing as the growing uterus puts pressure on the diaphragm. The gastrointestinal system usually decreases its activity, accounting for constipation or heartburn and indigestion. Urinary frequency and urgency are common as the growing fetus creates pressure on the bladder. The inevitable weight gain is related to the increase in size of the abdomen, breasts, and the growing fetus. Women may also experience more vaginal discharge as the pregnancy progresses, largely as a result of changes in the balance of the hormones of pregnancy. A woman's posture and sense of balance will change, again related to the enlarging uterus and the relaxation of pelvic joints and supporting uterine ligaments (Blackman, 1992).

Various psychological changes accompany pregnancy. Early in the pregnancy a woman may experience ambivalence. Even when a pregnancy is desired and planned, a couple may have some ambivalence. The pregnant woman may experience joy or fear, pride or doubt, anxiety and fear related to the pregnancy and its outcomes, denial, resentment, shock, anger, or excitement (Fagler & Nicoll, 1990). Pregnancy is often characterized by its emotional ups and downs for the woman. Some women may actually experience depression during pregnancy. Often the psychological changes have significant and lifelong effects on the woman (Blackman & Loper, 1992).

Sociologic changes that a woman and her partner experience are often related to cultural and religious beliefs and attitudes about the roles of women, pregnancy, and parenthood (Fagler & Nicoll, 1990). The couple is expected to know about the cultural or religious beliefs and attitudes about pregnancy and subsequent parenting and to incorporate these ideals into their lifestyle. Sometimes younger couples are at odds with older members of the culture, such as parents or in-laws. Frequently the issues are related to the woman's working or not working and the responsibility each partner will have for childrearing and household maintenance (Fagler & Nicoll, 1993).

Evaluation and Diagnosis

Whenever a sexually active women misses a period or has symptoms suggestive of pregnancy, a pregnancy should be expected. Early symptoms that suggest pregnancy include amenorrhea (missed menstrual period), breast tenderness or tingling, urinary frequency or urgency, quickening (feeling the fetus move), fatigue, and weight gain. The accurate diagnosis of pregnancy is based on urine or blood testing and ultrasonography. The blood and urine test detect the presence of human chorionic gonadotropin (hCG), a hormone produced in high levels by the developing placenta during the first 50 to 75 days of gestation. Ultrasonography provides visualization of the developing fetus and other products of the pregnancy (McKay & Evans, 1994).

Therapeutic Interventions

Prenatal Care. Early, continuous, and adequate prenatal care is believed to be critical to optimal pregnancy outcomes. As soon as any woman suspects or knows that she is pregnant prenatal care should begin. A woman may select a medical doctor (obstetrician, family practice specialist) or a certified nurse midwife. During the first 28 weeks of gestation (first 6 calendar months), women are usually seen by their health care practitioner every 4 weeks. From 28 to 36 weeks' gestation (6–8 calendar months) pregnant women are usually seen every 2 weeks. During the final 4 weeks of gestation (9th calendar month), women are usually seen every week until labor (the birth process) begins.

At the initial prenatal visit the practitioner will take an extensive history and physical, which should also include a thorough assessment and examination of reproductive health and organs. Additionally laboratory tests are done to determine blood type and Rh factor and assess for anemia. Other tests are done to screen for infections and diseases such as urinary tract infections, STDs, HIV, and infections of the reproductive organs. Some practitioners suggest that routine screening for tuberculosis should also be included because of the recent increase of these infections. A pregnant health care practitioner should be screened for exposure to hepatitis B. If she is positive, she should be vaccinated during pregnancy (McKay & Evans, 1994). Still other laboratory studies are done to identify potential genetic problems such as Tay-Sachs disease and sickle cell anemia. All the data gathered during the initial visit will assist the practitioner in assessing the general health status of the pregnant woman and identifying current or potential risks (McKay & Evans, 1994).

Health Teaching. Counseling and education of the pregnant woman, her partner, and significant others are critical to healthy outcomes for mother and infant. Pregnant women and their partners frequently have questions, misinformation or misconceptions about what to eat, weight gain, physical discomforts, drug and alcohol use, sexuality, and the impending childbirth process. Any practitioner caring for a pregnant woman needs to make time to answer questions, teach, or make referrals to classes.

Adequate nutrition should be stressed. Inadequate nutrition has been associated with increased risks for miscarriage, anemia, preterm labor, intrauterine growth, low-birthweight infants, and difficulty establishing lactation (Bobak & Jensen, 1993). The diet should be low in fat and high in fiber, with adequate protein and carbohydrates. Often prenatal vitamins and iron are prescribed to ensure adequate mineral and vitamin intake to meet the increased demands caused by the pregnancy and the developing fetus. The diet should be adequate in calories to ensure adequate weight gain for the fetus. The recommended weight gains for pregnant women are based on prepregnancy height and weight status and can range from 15 to 40 lb. The recommended weight gain for normal weight women is 25 to 35 lb; for underweight women, 28 to 40 lb; and for overweight women, 15 to 25 lb (Moore, 1993).

Along with good nutrition, women should be encouraged to continue appropriate moderate exercise. Women should be cautioned that their center of gravity and balance will shift as the fetus grows and the abdomen enlarges. Prenatal aerobic exercise classes and walking generally are considered safe during pregnancy. However, skiing, jogging, and biking are considered high intensity and not recommended during pregnancy (American College of Obstetricians and Gynecologists, 1990; Retts, 1993).

Many pregnant women will experience several physical discomforts during pregnancy. Therefore, the woman and her partner should be advised that various discomforts accompany pregnancy. Some women experience these discomforts as a minor limitation to daily activities, whereas others may find the discomforts extremely disruptive to daily activities. Information about the discomforts of pregnancy, when they are likely to be experienced, and suggestions about how to handle them are appreciated by pregnant women.

Early in the pregnancy many women experience nausea and sometimes vomiting. Many women find that dry crackers and toast are helpful. Other women may need to avoid fatty foods. The nausea usually resolves by the end of 13 weeks' gestation (3 calendar months). The nausea is thought to be related to the increased hormone levels associated with early pregnancy. Breast tenderness is another hormone-related symptom that appears early in pregnancy. Symptoms related to the increasing size and pressure of the uterus include urinary frequency (early and late pregnancy) and varicose veins. Women should be encouraged to empty the bladder frequently and to wear low-heeled shoes and support hose to facilitate circulation and to reduce the discomfort from the varicose veins. Also varicose veins of the rectum may be present and women should be advised that a warm bath or warm water over the buttocks in the shower will be soothing. A high-fiber diet and adequate fluid intake will help to prevent constipation, also common during pregnancy. Avoiding constipation will also lessen the discomfort from hemorrhoids. Heartburn, indigestion, and constipation are related to the slowing of gastrointestinal functions during pregnancy. Women may need to decrease their intake of fatty or spicy foods to avoid discomfort from heartburn or indigestion. Women should be advised to avoid sodium bicarbonate products to treat heartburn or indigestion. Women may also experience increased vaginal secretions during pregnancy, and should be advised to keep undergarments dry and to wear cotton or cotton-crotch undergarments.

Another area of concern for most pregnant women and their partners is the use of substances such as tobacco, drugs and alcohol. Women should be advised about the adverse effects of cocaine, heroin, marijuana, and other illicit drugs on the fetus. They should be cautioned about using over-the-counter drugs. Women should be encouraged to seek the practitioner's advice about the use of nonprescription drugs during pregnancy. Women who use drugs for chronic conditions and diseases such as epilepsy, diabetes, or thyroid disorders will need to be evaluated by their health care provider as well as by other medical specialists. Many of these drugs have been linked to congenital deformities and poor fetal outcomes. The health care provider must present these women with the benefits and risks for continued use during pregnancy so that they can make informed choices about their care. Women should be advised about smoking and fetal outcomes. Smoking has been linked with the birth of low-birthweight infants, increased neonatal deaths of low-birthweight infants, and an increased rate of spontaneous abortions (Floyd, 1993). A safe level of alcohol intake has not been established for pregnancy. However, fetal alcohol syndrome has been found among women who drink heavily during pregnancy.

Neonates with fetal alcohol syndrome have a low birthweight as a result of retarded prenatal growth; malformations of the heart, head, face, and extremities; infantile psychomotor retardation; and mental retardation (Centers for Disease Control and Prevention, 1993).

An area frequently ignored by health care providers is sexuality during pregnancy. Many couples have concerns about expressing sexuality during pregnancy and frequently do not feel comfortable discussing their concerns. Most couples still have a need for sexual intimacy, affection, closeness, and reassurance. Usually, by the third trimester the desire for sexual intercourse decreases. In general, there is no reason to abstain from sexual intercourse. The couple's desires and comfort should dictate sexual activity during pregnancy. However, if there is vaginal bleeding, membrane rupture, history of habitual spontaneous abortion, incompetent cervix, preterm labor, descent of the fetus for the delivery position, or cervical dilation for delivery, couples should be cautioned to refrain from intercourse (Nagey, 1989).

Childbirth Interventions. The childbirth process for most women occurs in the hospital. Some women will choose to deliver at a birthing center or at home. In either case, a woman may select to be delivered by a certified nurse midwife or a medical doctor. Many couples choose this alternative to in-hospital births because they want a more natural birth experience and more involvement of children and family members in the birth event. The safety of home and birth center births has been questioned. However, midwives have physician backup if the woman needs other medical or surgical interventions beyond the midwife's scope of practice. Hospitals have responded to consumer desires for homelike births by creating birthing rooms or birth centers and by relaxing visitation rules in obstetric units. The woman and her family can have a homelike environment within the hospital and all of the medical and surgical resources of the hospital available if needed.

The childbirth process may be assisted by one of several obstetric interventions. These interventions may include intravenous fluids, electronic monitors that provide information about the status of uterine contractions and the fetus (fetal heart rates), and certain drugs to augment existing labor or to start the labor process. These drugs may be given intravenously (oxytocin [Pitocin]) or inserted into the vagina (prostaglandin gel). Frequently, analgesic drugs and regional anesthetics are used to provide relief from the uterine contractions during labor (labor pains) and to lessen the discomfort during the actual expulsion of the fetus through the vagina. The analgesic drugs most commonly used are synthetic narcotics and the most common regional anesthetic used is the epidural. The obstetrician or nurse midwife makes decisions about the use of these agents based on the mother's desires, the status of the mother and the labor, the status of the fetus, and the imminence of delivery. Another common obstetric intervention is the episiotomy, a surgical incision into the perineum to facilitate the delivery of the fetal head and to prevent the uncontrolled tearing of the perineum. The couple may opt for a natural childbirth, using no medications, except perhaps a local anesthetic instilled into the perineum for the repair of the episiotomy.

Some women will need to have a surgical intervention, the cesarean section, for the birth process. More than 900,000 cesarean procedures are performed each year. The rate for cesarean section is estimated to be 25% of all births (Taffel, Placek & Kosary, 1992;

Tighe & Sweezy, 1990), which is an increase of 4% since the 1960s. Conditions likely to require a cesarean section include:

- fetus presenting with the buttocks (breech) or feet in the birth canal
- fetus too large to pass through the birth canal as confirmed by ultrasonography
- fetus showing signs of distress during the labor process
- severe placental bleeding
- other fetal or maternal diseases or conditions that threaten well-being or life or will worsen during the laboring process

Special Populations

Pregnancy for adolescents, women older than 35 years, women with chronic illnesses, working women, and women who experience the loss of a pregnancy offer special challenges for the woman and the health care providers. Teen pregnancy continues to plague this society. In America, 1 million adolescent pregnancies result in approximately 500,000 births and 400,000 induced abortions each year. The Children's Defense Fund (1990) reports that each day 7742 American adolescents initiate sexual activity and 2795 adolescent girls become pregnant. It is a crisis for the girl and her family. Teens have a higher likelihood of receiving inadequate or no prenatal care and therefore are at increased risk for complications of pregnancy and poor maternal and fetal outcomes. The greater crisis is the social consequence for the teenage mother and her infant. Teen mothers are less likely to marry or to stay married and more likely to continue childbearing. They are less likely to continue their education and to have an income that enables them to care for themselves or their children. Therefore, teen mothers are perceived as a burden to local and national government programs.

The older pregnant woman offers a challenge because she is often at risk for more medical complications of pregnancy. She may have more anxiety related to her medical risk status, her abilities to mother, and potential interruptions in her lifestyle related to her career or her relationship with her partner. However, the older woman may possess more psychological maturity and more material resources for motherhood. As many of 50% of all women work during some part of their pregnancy, and 50% of these women work until the final months of their pregnancy. These women often have anxiety about workplace hazards, stopping work, or returning to work. They frequently experience depressive symptoms, guilt, and fatigue during the pregnancy. These women must have adequate prenatal care, adequate rest, and adequate nutrition throughout the pregnancy.

Modern medicine has prolonged and improved the life of women who have chronic medical conditions such as sickle cell anemia, diabetes, or epilepsy, previously thought to be incompatible with pregnancy. Such women need to continue with their usual medical care routines as well as prenatal care. These women need to have a health care provider who understands their chronic condition and can anticipate how the condition will be influenced by pregnancy and vice versa. The care of these women often requires collaboration and cooperation among several specialists to ensure a safe outcome for the mother and infant.

Another special population includes women who lose a fetus, have a stillborn infant, or suffer the death of an infant after birth. These losses are called perinatal losses. One in 5 pregnancies ends in a miscarriage or a spontaneous abortion and 16 in

1000 pregnancies end with a stillborn infant or the death of the infant after birth. These couples experience fear, anger, guilt, sadness, depression, and grief over their loss. They will need the support of their families and friends and intervention from specialists trained in perinatal loss or referral to perinatal loss support groups (Wheeler, Limbo, & Gensch, 1993).

Uterine Dysfunction

Several conditions may cause alteration of uterine function. The most common conditions include dysfunctional uterine bleeding, endometriosis, and uterine myomas (fibroids). This section of the chapter focuses on these three most common conditions.

Dysfunctional Uterine Bleeding

This condition consists of abnormal uterine bleeding with no known pathologic cause. It is most commonly seen among women during puberty and during the perimenopausal period (Brown, 1993).

Causes and Symptoms

The most common cause of dysfunctional uterine bleeding is anovulation. Therefore, it is most frequently seen before the maturation of ovarian function (puberty), as ovarian function declines (perimenopausal), or among obese women or women with PCO syndrome. The anovulatory cycles are characterized by a high level of estrogen instead of the balanced estrogen and progesterone secretions that result in regular shedding of the uterine endometrium and a regular uterine bleeding cycle. These patients present with irregular, prolonged bleeding. The bleeding may follow several patterns that may vary from heavy prolonged bleeding at regular intervals to normal bleeding in irregular cycles to frequent regular bleeding at intervals of less than 21 days (Brown, 1993; McKay & Evans, 1994).

Diagnosis and Therapeutic Interventions

A complete history and several laboratory tests are necessary to assess for pregnancy: hematocrit and hemoglobin to determine the degree of bleeding; status of ovulation and thyroid function; and biopsy of cervical and uterine tissue to diagnose the cause of the bleeding (Bayer & DeCherney, 1993; Brown, 1993; McKay & Evans, 1994).

Treatment has different goals related to the patient's age. For the adolescent woman the goal is stabilization of the endometrium and cessation of the bleeding. Often a low-dose combination OCP is used. The initial treatment is 1 pill four times daily for 5 days. When the pills are stopped, withdrawal bleeding will begin. This is usually followed by continuing the OCP for 6 to 12 months. This treatment does not correct the bleeding, but it allows for the maturation of the ovulatory process (Bayer & DeCherney, 1994; Brown, 1993; Coller, 1991).

Adult women who have no pathologic conditions of the uterine endometrium and no other risk factors may also be treated with low- dose OCPs. Bleeding may also be treated by a dilation and curettage surgical procedure or by intravenous Premarin (a conjugated estrogen). If bleeding persists and a woman has completed childbearing, a hysterectomy may be considered when the dysfunctional bleeding is unresponsive to all other treatments (Bayer & DeCherney, 1993; Brown, 1993; Coller, 1991).

Endometriosis

Endometriosis is another alteration of uterine tissue that is associated with uterine dysfunction. Endometriosis is the condition of functioning uterine tissue that implants outside the uterus. Endometriosis occurs when endometrial cells from the uterus travel through the fallopian tubes and implant themselves on various pelvic structures such as the bladder, rectum, ovaries, the outside surface of the uterus, vulva, and the vagina. It is difficult to determine accurately the incidence of endometriosis, especially in asymptomatic fertile women and adolescents. However, as many as 50% of women seen for pelvic pain, infertility, or pelvic mass are later diagnosed as having endometriosis (Kappila, 1993; McCandace & Heuther, 1990).

Causes and Symptoms

The cause of endometriosis is unknown, but several theories have been proposed. Retrograde menstruation is one theory. This theory suggests that menstrual fluids and tissue are forced through the fallopian tubes and into the abdominal cavity where the endometrial tissue is implanted and continues to grow. Other theories suggest a genetic predisposition, citing family history of endometriosis, or an alteration in the immune system that tolerates the growth of the endometrial implants (McCandace & Heuther, 1990).

Women often are asymptomatic. However, the symptoms that most women experience are related to the changes in the endometrial patches in response to the hormonal cycle. The endometrial patches grow, thicken, and bleed during the hormonal cycle just as the normally functioning uterine tissue. Women with endometriosis usually seek medical help because of dysmenorrhea, adnexal tenderness or mass, or infertility (Kappila, 1993). Symptoms may appear as early as puberty, but generally symptoms first appear after several years of menstrual cycles. The symptoms increase over the years as the endometrial tissue continues to grow (McCandace & Heuther, 1990).

Diagnosis and Therapeutic Interventions

There are no specific laboratory tests for diagnosis of endometriosis; laparoscopy is required for definitive diagnosis. Endometriosis can be classified in four stages from mild (stage I) to extensive (stage IV). Treatment is determined by the severity of the endometriosis. Mild conditions may be treated by the surgical removal of the implants and with the drug danazol. Other women may respond to treatment with OCPs. These drug therapies slow the proliferation of the endometrial tissue. However, drug therapy prolongs the waiting period before pregnancy can be attempted. Women with severe and extensive conditions, and who have also completed childbearing, may consider a complete hysterectomy as the treatment of choice.

Pregnancy is thought to have a positive influence on endometriosis. Women who have had a pregnancy during the early reproductive years are less likely to develop endometriosis. A woman with endometriosis who delays pregnancy may be faced with infertility (McCandace & Heuther, 1990).

Myomas

Uterine myomas (fibroids) are the most common benign neoplasm of the reproductive tract. They are solid tumors of the uterus and are often associated with uterine dysfunction. The incidence of malignant cancer with fibroids is less than 1/500 cases (Brown, 1993). Myomas occur in almost 20% of women over age 30. For unknown reasons, the tumors occur three to nine times more frequently in African American women compared with Caucasian women (Bayer & DeCherney, 1993; Korn, 1993).

Causes and Symptoms

The causes are unclear. However, certain risk factors appear to be related to tumor growth. These factors include African American ethnicity, an estrogen-dominant environment that is a characteristic of nulliparous and obese women, and the presence of insulin-like growth factors (Brown, 1993).

Nonpregnant women with myomas are often asymptomatic. However, the symptoms most often associated with myomas are urinary frequency, irregular and heavy bleeding, and pelvic pain. Large myomas may be associated with infertility. Pregnant women with myomas may be at increased risk for abortion, preterm labor, labor complications, or postpartum hemorrhage (McKay & Evans, 1994).

Diagnosis and Therapeutic Interventions

Blood tests are indicated because anemia may be present when bleeding has been heavy and prolonged. Vaginal ultrasonography and hysterosalpingography confirm the presence, number, and size of these tumors. Pelvic examination is useful to differentiate other pelvic masses or growths from myomas.

Treatment is related to a woman's desire for future pregnancies. If childbearing is complete and if tumors are symptomatic, have grown rapidly, or are large, a subtotal hysterectomy is the treatment of choice. Myomectomy, the removal of the individual tumors with repair of the uterus, is the treatment of choice when a future pregnancy is desired. Patients who have hysterectomies are cured; 20% of women who have myomectomies will require future hysterectomies (Korn, 1993; McKay & Evans, 1994).

Ovarian Dysfunction

Polycystic Ovary Syndrome

Polycystic ovary syndrome, also known as persistent anovulation or Stim-Leventhal syndrome, is an endocrine disorder. It effects 2% to 5% of all women of reproductive age.

PCO syndrome is commonly associated with infertility (Bayer & DeCherney, 1993; McKay & Evans, 1994).

Causes and Symptoms

The causes are unknown. However, certain risk factors appear to be associated with PCO. Obese women appear to have a higher risk for PCO because they often have higher levels of estrone, which is thought to suppress ovarian hormones that are critical to ovulation and subsequent fertility.

The symptoms seen most frequently are consistently high levels of estrogen, androgen, and LH. The high levels of these hormones cause the ovaries to enlarge and develop multiple cysts. Other symptoms are the absence of menstrual periods or abnormal uterine bleeding and infertility (McKay & Evans, 1994).

Diagnosis and Therapeutic Interventions

Definitive diagnosis is made with laparoscopy, which visualizes the thickened ovaries containing multiple cysts. The obese woman is encouraged to lose weight. The weight loss may reduce the conversion of androgens to estrone, which may restore ovulation and fertility. Treatment is often related to the desire for future fertility. If pregnancy is desired, Clomid (clomiphene) or other fertility drugs may be used to stimulate ovulation. If pregnancy is not desired, other drugs (Depo-Provera) are used to ensure regular shedding of the endometrial tissue. A low-dose OCP may be used to provide regular ovarian cycles and contraception. In severe cases of PCO a complete hysterectomy followed by estrogen replacement therapy may be the treatment of choice (McKay & Evans, 1994).

Urinary Dysfunction

Urinary Incontinence

Urinary incontinence is the uncontrolled loss of urine significant enough to cause social or hygienic consequences (Thomas, 1993). The incidence is hard to establish because many women believe it is a natural consequence of childbirth and may not seek medical help. It is estimated that 12 million women suffer from urinary incontinence or 40% of all women. Approximately one-third of all postmenopausal women report urinary incontinence (McKay & Evans, 1994; Thomas, 1993).

The four types of urinary incontinence are:

1. stress incontinence
2. urge incontinence
3. overflow incontinence
4. mixed incontinence

Mixed incontinence, a combination of the first three types, is common in frail elderly women (Bernard, 1994). Stress urinary incontinence (SUI) is most common among women. About 59% to 70% of women with urinary incontinence have SUI, defined as the involuntary loss of urine during activities that increase intra-abdominal pressure such as coughing, sneezing, lifting heavy objects, or exercising (Skoner, Thomas, & Caron, 1994; Thomas, 1993). This section of the chapter focuses on SUI.

Causes and Symptoms

The evidence related to the causes and risk factors is inclusive. Risk factors include damage to the urethral sphincter and pelvic floor muscles during childbirth or changes to the genitourinary tract associated with pregnancy. Other nonobstetric factors include age, menopause, urinary tract infections, gynecologic surgery such as a hysterotomy, and anatomic weakness of the urinary bladder (Skoner et al., 1994).

Symptoms frequently seen are the leakage of a small but variable amount of urine at the time that the stress occurs; leakage even if the bladder has recently been emptied; leakage only in the upright position; and leakage most often caused by laughing, coughing, sneezing, or athletic activity (Skoner et al., 1994).

Diagnosis and Therapeutic Interventions

A careful history is indicated to identify potential risk factors and the urinary pattern. Other diagnostic tests may be indicated to identify deformities or other problems of the genitourinary tract (Bernard, 1994).

Therapeutic interventions useful for SUI include nonsurgical and surgical interventions. Several nonsurgical treatments may be used. Estrogen therapy is often most beneficial for women with SUI. The estrogen is administered intravaginally daily at bedtime for 6 weeks. After the initial course of therapy the estrogen is continued indefinitely as a maintenance dose two to three times weekly. Kegel exercises can also be used to strengthen pelvic floor muscles. Biofeedback therapy and other behavioral modification techniques may also be useful. Several surgical procedures may be used if the nonsurgical treatments do not relieve the SUI. The goal of the surgical procedures is to elevate certain genitourinary structures, which will increase and maintain the intra-abdominal pressure (Bernard, 1994).

Summary

Over the years clinicians and researchers in the field of women's health have increased our knowledge of women's reproductive, gynecologic, and urinary health. Clinicians have a significant role in informing women about self-care strategies that include developing a lifestyle of health-promoting behaviors. Women should be encouraged to seek prompt, appropriate, and adequate treatment for any infection of the reproductive tract. Unusual discharges, bleeding, or sores of the genitalia warrant a visit to the health care provider. Women should be encouraged to maintain a healthy body weight/body fat ratio to ensure ovulatory cycles. Adequate nutrition will help to maintain appropriate body weight/boy fat ratios. Alcohol, caffeine, and nicotine should be used with caution and in moderation because of their link to impaired fertility. Moderate, frequent exercise is beneficial. However, female athletes should be advised that vigorous exercise may impair fertility. Finally, women should continue to have regular health checkups that include reproductive health appraisals.

Future Directions

Future directions for research and policy development should focus on areas such as developing and using less invasive technology for labor and delivery that will increase and improve maternal and fetal well-being and outcomes; making preconceptual and prenatal care available and accessible to all women regardless of their income or risk status; and developing contraceptive technology that will achieve effective contraception without altering a woman's health, that is easily reversible, is low cost, and is easily obtainable by all women. Research needs to continue into the treatment of infertility and its related causes. A woman's health policy agenda should view reproductive, gynecologic, and urinary health across the lifespan. Young girls to older women should be educated about self-help health promotion and disease prevention strategies that will lead to optimal health across the lifespan. The emphasis placed by the National Institutes of Health on women's health issues as more than an extension of men's health should move the women's health research agenda forward into the next century.

References

American College of Obstetricians and Gynecologists. (1990). *Exercise during pregnancy and the postnatal period.* Washington, DC: Author.

Alexander, L. L., & LaRosa, J. H. (1994). *New dimensions in women's health.* Boston: Jones and Bartlett.

Balin, J. (1988). The social dimension of pregnancy and birth. *Qualitative Sociology, 11,* 275-301.

Bayer & DeCherney. (1993). Clinical manifestations and treatment of dysfunctional uterine bleeding. *Journal of the American Medical Association, 269*(14), 1823-1828.

Bernard, M. (1994). Urinary incontinence in elderly females. *Journal of the Oklahoma State Medical Association, 87,* 217-224.

Blackman, S., & Loper, D. (1992). *Maternal, fetal and neonatal physiology: A clinical perspective.* Philadelphia: Saunders.

Bobak, I., & Jensen, M. (1993). *Maternity and gynecologic care: The nurse and the family.* Baltimore: Mosby.

Carsaro, M., & Lichtman, R. (1990). Barrier methods. In R. Lichtman & S. Papera (Eds.), *Gynecology: Well-women care* (pp. 71-90). Norwalk, CT: Appleton & Lange.

Caufield, K. A. (1994). Controlling fertility. In E. Youngkin & M. S. Davis. *Women's health: A primary care clinical guide* (pp. 101-160). Norwalk, CT: Appleton & Lange.

Centers for Disease Control and Prevention. (1993). Fetal alcohol syndrome: United States, 1979-1992. *Morbidity and Mortality Weekly Report, 42,* 339.

Children's Defense Fund. (1990). *S.O.S. America! A children's defense budget.* Washington, DC: Author.

Clarke, H. (1990a). Intrauterine devices. In R. Lichtman & S. Papera (Eds.), *Gynecology: Well-women care* (pp. 109-126). Norwalk, CT: Appleton & Lange.

Clarke, H. (1990b). Oral contraceptives. In R. Lichtman & S. Papera (Eds.), *Gynecology: Well-women care* (pp. 91-108). Norwalk, CT: Appleton & Lange.

Coller, T. (1991). Dysfunctional uterine bleeding and amenorrhea: Differential diagnosis. *Journal of Nurse-Midwifery, 36*(1), 49-62.

Corfman, R., & Ball, G. (1994). Treatment options for infertile couples. *Minnesota Medicine, 77,* 28-32.

Fagler, S., & Nicoll, L. (1990). A framework for the psychological aspects of pregnancy. *NAACOG'S Clinical Issues in Perinatal and Women's Health, 1,* 267.

Floyd, L. R. (1993). A review of smoking in pregnancy: Effects on pregnancy outcomes and cessation efforts. *Annual Review of Public Health, 14,* 379.

Gant, N. F., & Cunningham (1993). *Basic gynecology and obstetrics.* Norwalk, CT: Appleton & Lange.

Haberman-Cohen, J. (1993). Fertility management. In I. Bobak & M. Jensen (Eds.), *Maternity and gynecologic care: The nurse and the family* (pp. 1278-1333). Baltimore: Mosby.

Hatcher, R. A., Trussell, J., Stewart, F., Stewart, G. K., Kowal, D., Guest, F., Cates, W., Jr., & Pilicar, M. S. (1994). *Contraceptive technology* (16th Rev. ed., pp. 191-221). New York: Irvington Publishers.

Heath, C. (1993). Helping patients chose an appropriate contraception. *American Family Physician, 48*(6), 1115-1124.

Hull, M. (1992). Infertility treatment: Relative effectiveness of conventional and assisted conception methods. *Human Reproduction, 7* (6), 785-796.

Kappila, A. (1993). Changing concepts of medical treatment of endometriosis. *Acta Obstetricia et Gynecologica Scandinavica, 72,* 324-332.

Lynaugh, J. (1991). The death of Sadie Sachs...Margaret Sanger. *Nursing Research, 40,* 124-125.

McCandace, K. L., & Heuther, S. (1990). Alterations of the reproductive system. *Pathophysiology: The biologic basis for disease in adults and children* (pp. 691-693). Baltimore: Mosby.

McKay, H. T., & Evans, A. T. (1994). Gynecology and obstetrics. In L. M. Tierney, S. J. McPhee, & M. A. Papadakin (Eds.), *Current medical management and treatment* (pp. 587-639). Norwalk, CT: Appleton & Lange.

Moore, M. C. (1993). Maternal and fetal nutrition. In I. Bobak & M. Jensen (Eds.), *Maternity and gynecologic care: The nurse and the family* (pp. 214-237). Baltimore: Mosby.

Nagey, D. (1989). The content of prenatal care. *Obstetrics and Gynecology, 74,* 516.

Potter, S. (1990). Infertility. In R. Lichtman & S. Papera (Eds.), *Gynecology: Well-women care.* Norwalk, CT: Appleton & Lange.

Retts, (1993). Women and exercise. *The Female Patient, 18,* 59.

Skoner, M., Thompson, W. B., & Caron, V. (1994). Factors associated with the risk of stress urinary incontinence in women. *Nursing Research, 43*(5), 301-306.

Stevens, K. (1993). Perinatal and women's health nursing. In I. Bobak & M. Jensen (Eds.), *Maternity and gynecologic care: The nurse and the family* (pp. 4-17). Baltimore: Mosby.

Taffel, S., Placek, P., & Kosary, C. (1992). U.S. cesarean section rates 1990: An update. *Birth, 19*(1), 21.

Thomas, J. (1992). Supporting parents and professionals when a baby dies. *Care of the Critically Ill, 8,* 172.

Thomas, S. (1993). Gynecologic urology. In J. S. Brown & W. R. Cronbleholme (Eds.), *Handbook of gynecology and obstetrics* (pp. 163-177). Norwalk, CT: Appleton & Lange.

Tighe, D., & Sweezy, S. (1990). The perioperative experience of cesarean birth: Preparation, considerations, and complications. *Journal of Perinatal Neonatal Nursing, 3*(3), 14.

Turk, P. (1990). Abortion. In R. Lichtman & S. Papera (Eds.), *Gynecology: Well-women care* (pp. 451-464). Norwalk, CT: Appleton & Lange.

Wheeler, S., Limbo, R., & Gensch, B. (1993). Loss and grief. In I. Bobak & M. Jensen (Eds.), *Maternity and gynecologic care: The nurse and the family* (pp. 4-17). Baltimore: Mosby.

Bibliography

McDonald, T. L., & Johnson, S. R. (1993). Contraception. In B. J. McElmurry & R. S. Parker (Eds.), *Annual review of women's health.* New York: National League for Nursing Press.

Scalone, M. R. (1990). Natural family planning and fertility awareness. In R. Lichtman & S. Papera (Eds.), *Gynecology: Well-women care* (pp. 59-70). Norwalk, CT: Appleton & Lange.

CHAPTER 11

Cancer

Roma D. Williams

Introduction

This chapter addresses the cancers that occur only or primarily in women and cancers that are now seen with increasing frequency in women. The major sites of cancer for women, in order of occurrence, are breast, lung, colon/rectum, uterus, and ovary. The epidemiology, etiology, and symptoms of these cancers as they relate to women are described. Implications for research and health education are addressed. In addition, the relevance of cancer for women across the lifespan is explored.

Overview of Cancer

About one in three Americans will eventually develop cancer (American Cancer Society [ACS], 1995). In fact, it is estimated that by the year 2000, cancer may be the leading cause of death, moving ahead of cardiovascular disease. The ACS estimates that in 1996 there will be 262,440 deaths among women from cancer for all sites. These deaths represent 47.3% of all cancer deaths. Of the 1,359,150 new cancer cases, 594,850 (43.76%) will occur in women and 764,300 (56.2%) will occur in men (Figs. 11–1 and 11–2).

Major advances in cancer prevention, diagnosis, and treatment have occurred over the past few decades. These improvements have resulted in increasing emphasis being placed on primary and secondary prevention. The goal of primary prevention is risk reduction and the ACS (1995) reports that a substantial number of cancers can be avoided through risk reduction behaviors. Because cancer risks for Americans include exposure through food, environment, and lifestyle, reducing the risk of cancer is possible by modifying one's lifestyle and behavior. Preventive steps women can take include limiting dietary fat, never using tobacco, and using safer sexual practices. Women can also achieve benefits from secondary prevention. The goal of secondary prevention is to discover cancer in its earliest stage when it is most curable. The key to early detection is screening tests to look for signs of cancer in people who are symptom free. For example, the Papanicolaou (Pap) test, a lifesaving screening test, could eradicate cervical cancer if it were used by all women.

Unfortunately, not all women use primary and secondary prevention strategies to avoid or detect cancer. This is particularly true of some segments of the population in which cancer incidence and mortality rates are generally higher (ACS, 1995).

(text continues on page 196)

193

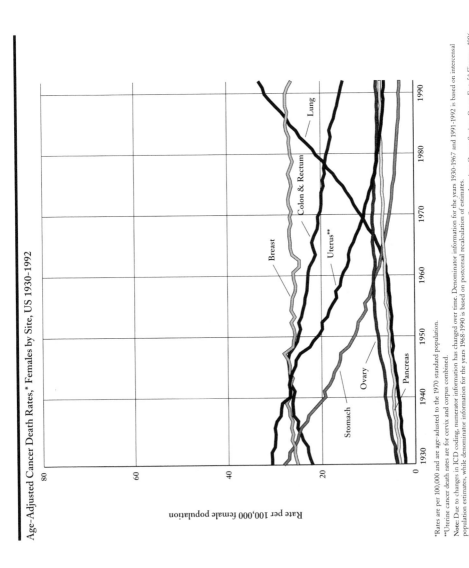

Age-Adjusted Cancer Death Rates,* Females by Site, US 1930-1992

Rate per 100,000 female population

*Rates are per 100,000 and are age-adjusted to the 1970 standard population.
**Uterine cancer death rates are for cervix and corpus combined.
Note: Due to changes in ICD coding, numerator information has changed over time. Denominator information for the years 1930-1967 and 1991-1992 is based on intercensal population estimates, while denominator information for the years 1968-1990 is based on postcensal recalculation of estimates.
Source: Vital Statistics of the United States, 1995

Source: American Cancer Society, *Cancer Facts & Figures—1996.*

Figure 11-1. Age-adjusted cancer death rates, *females by site, United States, 1930-1992. (Used with permission. American Cancer Society, Inc. © 1996.)

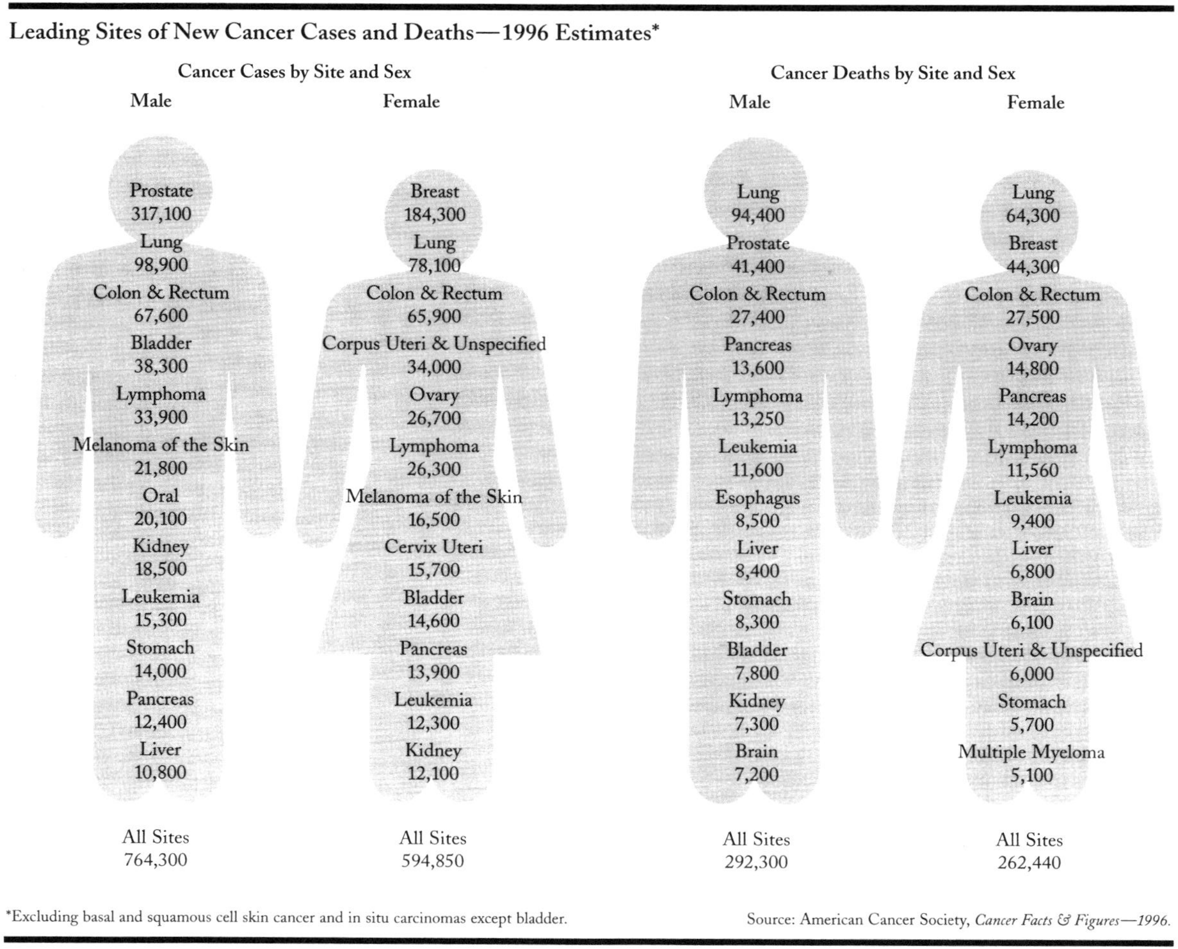

Leading Sites of New Cancer Cases and Deaths—1996 Estimates*

Cancer Cases by Site and Sex

Male

Prostate 317,100
Lung 98,900
Colon & Rectum 67,600
Bladder 38,300
Lymphoma 33,900
Melanoma of the Skin 21,800
Oral 20,100
Kidney 18,500
Leukemia 15,300
Stomach 14,000
Pancreas 12,400
Liver 10,800

All Sites 764,300

Female

Breast 184,300
Lung 78,100
Colon & Rectum 65,900
Corpus Uteri & Unspecified 34,000
Ovary 26,700
Lymphoma 26,300
Melanoma of the Skin 16,500
Cervix Uteri 15,700
Bladder 14,600
Pancreas 13,900
Leukemia 12,300
Kidney 12,100

All Sites 594,850

Cancer Deaths by Site and Sex

Male

Lung 94,400
Prostate 41,400
Colon & Rectum 27,400
Pancreas 13,600
Lymphoma 13,250
Leukemia 11,600
Esophagus 8,500
Liver 8,400
Stomach 8,300
Bladder 7,800
Kidney 7,300
Brain 7,200

All Sites 292,300

Female

Lung 64,300
Breast 44,300
Colon & Rectum 27,500
Ovary 14,800
Pancreas 14,200
Lymphoma 11,560
Leukemia 9,400
Liver 6,800
Brain 6,100
Corpus Uteri & Unspecified 6,000
Stomach 5,700
Multiple Myeloma 5,100

All Sites 262,440

*Excluding basal and squamous cell skin cancer and in situ carcinomas except bladder.

Source: American Cancer Society, *Cancer Facts & Figures—1996.*

Figure 11-2. Leading sites of new cancer cases and deaths—1996 estimates. (Used with permission. American Cancer Society, Inc. © 1996.)

An individual's socioeconomic status, regardless of race, is a major determinant of cancer survival (Mack, McGrath, Pendleton, & Zieber, 1993). Socioeconomic factors, such as lack of health insurance or transportation, can impede access to care and lead to late diagnosis and poor survival. A woman's use of mammography and other screening services is inversely associated with income and educational attainment (Breen & Kessler, 1994; Calle, Flanders, & Thun, 1993). A woman's cultural values and belief systems can affect her attitudes about seeking health care or following screening guidelines (Brown & Williams, 1994; Varricchio, 1995).

Although there is no typical profile for the person with cancer, the incidence of cancer rises with age; most cases affect adults in midlife or older. In fact, more than half of all cancers and 60% of all cancer deaths occur after age 65 (Young, Percy, & Asire, 1981). Table 11–1 reflects the percentage of the population developing invasive cancers at certain ages (ACS, 1995).

At the turn of the century women lived an average of 50 years. With today's longer lifespan comes the increased risk of a woman developing cancer. Unfortunately, older women are less likely to avail themselves of cancer screening (Makuc, Freid, & Parsons, 1994). Health care professionals must make adults aware of their increased risk of developing cancer as they age and encourage recommended primary and secondary prevention strategies.

Table 11-1. Percentage of Population (Probability) Developing Invasive Cancers at Certain Ages

		Birth to 39	40–59	60–79	Ever (Birth to Death)
All sites	Male	1.72 (1 in 58)	7.74 (1 in 13)	34.30 (1 in 3)	44.84 (1 in 2)
	Female	1.92 (1 in 52)	9.33 (1 in 11)	23.22 (1 in 4)	39.26 (1 in 3)
Breast	Female	0.46 (1 in 217)	3.83 (1 in 26)	6.77 (1 in 15)	12.30 (1 in 8)
Colon and	Male	0.06 (1 in 1,667)	0.93 (1 in 108)	4.39 (1 in 23)	6.14 (1 in 16)
rectum	Female	0.05 (1 in 2,000)	0.73 (1 in 137)	3.32 (1 in 30)	5.92 (1 in 17)
Prostate	Male	<1 in 10,000	0.97 (1 in 103)	12.84 (1 in 8)	15.44 (1 in 6)
Lung	Male	0.04 (1 in 2,500)	1.55 (1 in 65)	6.71 (1 in 15)	8.49 (1 in 12)
	Female	0.03 (1 in 3,333)	1.07 (1 in 93)	3.62 (1 in 28)	5.17 (1 in 19)

Note: This chart shows the risks of being diagnosed with the most common cancers over certain age intervals. These risks are calculated for persons free of the specified cancer at the beginning of the age interval. Risk estimates do not assume all persons live to the end of the age interval or to any fixed age. Risk estimates are presented to give an approximate measure of the burden of cancer to society. Measures are based on population level rates and do not take into account individual behaviors and risk factors. For example, lung cancer is rare among nonsmokers or persons not heavily exposed to environmental tobacco smoke, so the risk for a nonsmoking man getting lung cancer in his lifetime is much lower than 8.5%, and it is much higher for a smoker. It is clear that the risk of developing cancer increases with age. For prostate cancer, the risk before age 60 is very low, but between age 60 and 80, 1 in 8 men will be diagnosed with prostate cancer.

Source of data: Applied Research Branch, National Cancer Institute. Used with permission. American Cancer Society, Inc. © 1995.

Breast Cancer

Epidemiology

Each year an estimated 184,000 women learn that they have breast cancer. Breast cancer is the most common form of cancer affecting women at any age. According to the ACS (1996), approximately 45,000 women die each year of breast cancer, making it the second leading cause of cancer deaths in women after lung cancer. It is the leading cause of death for women aged 50 to 54 (ACS, 1995). The incidence rates for women have increased about 2% per year since the 1970s. The recent rise in rates is not clearly understood but is believed to be due to marked increases in mammography utilization (ACS, 1995). Breast cancer is at epidemic proportions in the United States, affecting one in every eight women sometime in their lifetime (ACS, 1996; Feuer et al., 1993).

Etiology, Antecedents, and Risk Factors

According to Strax (1990), gender (ie, female) and age (ie, getting older) are the most important risk factors in the development of breast cancer. About two-thirds of all breast cancer occurs in women aged 50 and older. Other determinants of risk, according to the ACS, include early age at menarche, late age at menopause, never having children or late age at first birth, and high socioeconomic status (ACS, 1994). In 1995, ACS added to this risk factor list higher education and lengthy exposure to cyclic estrogen. Studies on populations migrating from low- to high-risk geographic areas support the role that environmental factors play in the etiology of breast cancer (Pisani, 1992). Recent research has identified a gene responsible for familial breast cancer (ACS, 1995). In addition, family or personal history of breast cancer is associated with an increased risk of developing breast cancer. If a woman's mother or sister has had breast cancer, her risk of breast cancer is two to three times greater than that of the general population. A woman who has had cancer in one breast is at increased risk of up to five times that of the general population for developing the disease in the other breast (Isaacs, 1992). It is important to note that fewer than 25% of women diagnosed with breast cancer meet high-risk characteristics (Robischon, 1988). Only 20% of patients with breast cancer report having a family history of the disease (Isaacs, 1993). According to the ACS (1995), most women who develop breast cancer have one or more risk factors for breast cancer; however, the risks are at such a low level that they only partially explain the high frequency of the disease.

Antecedents

A woman's breast tissue changes throughout her lifetime. Most of these changes are benign and occur with the menstrual cycle. A common form of benign breast disease is known as chronic cystic mastopathy, also known as fibrocystic disease or fibrocystic complex, chronic cystic changes, and cystic hyperplasia (Powell & Stelling, 1994). There are, however, certain categories of fibrocystic complex that represent an increased risk for invasive breast carcinoma. The categories that have a slightly increased risk for invasive breast carcinoma, moderately increased risk, and significantly increased risk are, respectively, the proliferative without atypia (20% of cases), the proliferative with atypia (7% of cases), and carcinoma in situ (3% of cases) (Deckers & Ricci, 1992). Important to these women are surveillance techniques that include breast self-examination (BSE), clinical breast examination (CBE), mammogram, ultrasound tests, aspiration of cysts, and biopsies of lumps that persist after aspiration.

Symptoms, Disease Patterns, and Responses to Disease

Signs and symptoms include breast changes that persist such as a lump, thickening or swelling, dimpling, skin irritation, distortion, retraction, scaliness, pain, and nipple tenderness, discharge, or inversion (ACS, 1995). Breast health programs should instruct women how to assess for these signs and symptoms and to report any changes to a health care provider. A health care provider may suggest a waiting period because many breast conditions are caused by normal hormonal changes. However, if a woman chooses this option, she must be committed to regular follow-up. It is extremely important that if a woman does not agree with this waiting period that she voice her concern. A second opinion from a breast specialist or surgeon may be required. Women on a fixed income or in rural areas should call the local ACS office or health department for names of providers who provide this service at no cost or at a reduced cost.

Treatment

Although a diagnosis of breast cancer is frightening, it is a survivable disease that can be cured with early diagnosis and treatment. The 5-year survival rate for localized breast cancer is 94%. If detected in the early stages when most often curable, breast cancer is highly treatable by surgery, radiotherapy, chemotherapy, and hormonal therapy. Fortunately, the methods for treating breast cancer have changed over the years. Newer approaches, considering the medical situation and the woman's preferences, include breast conservation and breast reconstruction and are becoming an important part of treatment and rehabilitation. In addition, recent innovations tailor adjuvant therapy to the woman's risk for recurrence (Pressman & Hirshaut, 1994). However, these new less "damaging" approaches may not be available to women without insurance or who are underinsured or live in medically underserved areas. Physician preference can also play a role in the treatment decision (Edward E. Partridge, MD, personal communication, September, 1995).

Implications

There is no empiric evidence for primary prevention strategies for breast cancer. However, there are encouraging prospects in this area. A possible link of dietary fat with breast cancer has prompted the National Cancer Institute (NCI) and the ACS to recommend that women reduce fat intake to 30% or less of daily calories. Others have questioned studies that link dietary fat to cancer. In Italy, dietary chemoprevention in a synthetic form of vitamin A is being tested in women who have already had breast cancer. These scientists are hoping to prevent cancer from developing in the opposite breast. Others are investigating the protective potential of other vitamins, such as C and E. Researchers are examining naturally occurring chemicals, called phytochemicals, found in common edible plants. If these chemicals are cancer-fighting substances, they can be extracted, purified, and added to women's diets.

The known breast cancer risk factors are not easily changed through a woman's health habits. Thus, the focus for breast cancer management has been on secondary prevention (early detection) through recommended screening. The ACS (1995) and the American College of Obstetricians and Gynecologists (ACOG, 1991a) make the following recommendations for asymptomatic women:

Mammograms

- by age 40: screening mammogram
- aged 40 to 49: mammogram every 1 to 2 years
- aged 50 and over: mammogram every year

Breast Examination

- CBE: every 3 years for women 20 to 40
- CBE: every year for women over 40
- BSE: monthly for women beginning at age 20

Not all cancer agencies support the ACS recommendations. A recent report has created much confusion over the efficacy of mammography in women aged 40 to 49 (Fletcher, Black, & Harris, 1993). Based on these findings, the NCI has revised its recommendations to include routine screening every 1 to 2 years with mammography and CBE for women 50 years of age and over (NCI, 1993). Most authorities, including the American Academy of Family Physicians, ACS, ACOG, American College of Physicians, Canadian Task Force on the Periodic Health Examination, and U.S. Preventive Services Task Force, recommend yearly screening for women 50 years of age and older (U.S. Department of Health and Human Services [DHHS], 1994a).

The professional organization of oncology nurses, Oncology Nurses Society (ONS), addressed the screening controversy in the following statement:

> ONS supports the right of each woman to make an informed decision about her need, regardless of age, for screening mammogram. It is the position of the ONS that the nurse's role is to promote public understanding of the issues and controversies relating to screening guidelines, and secondly, to advocate an informed decision-making process for individual consumers. The ONS calls for research that will provide a scientific basis for breast cancer screening guidelines for all women. In addition, the ONS supports legislation which insures access to insurance coverage for women ages 40-49 who desire screening mammography (*ONS News*, 1994, p. 3).

Mammography is the most effective screening modality for the early detection of breast cancer. However, mammography is not 100% accurate with sensitivity estimates of 70% to 90% and specificity estimates of 90% to 95% (Eddy, 1991). A woman needs to verify that her mammography facility uses only dedicated mammography equipment that meets minimum safety and image quality standards. Fortunately, as of October 1, 1994, all U.S. mammography facilities must be certified by the Food and Drug Administration as providing quality mammography.

If a mammogram looks suspicious, ultrasound and focal spot magnification may be needed to decide if biopsy is necessary (Rebecca Bryant, MSN, OCN, personal communication, October, 1994). In addition, breast magnetic resonance imaging is under study as a diagnostic tool (Orel et al., 1994).

The Breast Cancer Prevention Trial (BCPT) is a randomized study of the drug tamoxifen in women who are at increased risk for breast cancer. Tamoxifen reduces the occurrence of new cancers in the opposite breast of women who already had breast cancer and is being used in the BCPT. The BCPT is a study within the National Surgical Adjuvant Breast and Bowel Project (NSABP). Recent revelations about the inclusion of faulty data in the NCI's NSABP study B-06 (lumpectomy trials) have shaken the confidence of many health care providers and the public. A second credibility gap for NCI relates to the NSABP study B-14, which tests tamoxifen's ability to prevent a second occurrence of breast cancer in women with ER positive, node-negative cancer. A breast cancer is estrogen receptor positive if the tumor cells contain a receptor that attracts estrogen. When estrogen attaches to the tumor cell, it affects the metabolism of the tumor. Hormonal therapy, such as with tamoxifen, is used to block estrogen from those receptors. (John T. Carpenter, Jr, MD, personal communication, March 25, 1996). These concerns about clinical trials and scientific misconduct have led women to question studies related to breast cancer and the value of screenings. However, breast cancer experts, such as Dr. Susan Love, have been outspoken about the questionable studies and have continued to support the study results. For more information related to this issue contact NCI's PDQ system (1-800-4-CANCER), or Internet via computer, and CancerFAX, reached by fax machine (*ONS News*, 1994).

Lung Cancer

Epidemiology

In 1986, lung cancer surpassed breast cancer as the leading cause of cancer deaths in women. Lung cancer continues to be the leading cancer killer among Americans, killing an estimated 64,300 women and 94,400 men in 1996. In this same year, an estimated 78,100 women and 98,900 men developed lung cancer. Although the rate of lung cancer is dropping among Caucasian men, it is increasing among African American men and among women of both races.

Each year about 3000 nonsmoking adults die of lung cancer as a result of sidestream cigarette smoke. According to the ACS (1995), the risk of dying of lung cancer is 30% higher for a nonsmoker living with a smoker than that for a nonsmoker living with another nonsmoker. There is some discussion that women may be more vulnerable to lung cancer than men (Keller & Howe, 1993; McGinn & Haylock, 1993). Stockwell et al. (1992) found an elevated risk for nonsmoking women with at least a 22 smoke-year exposure and that risk was higher for women with non-adenocarcinoma of the lung. These researchers found that the overall risk was increased threefold when lifetime exposure was at least 40 years whether the exposure occurred during childhood/adolescence or adulthood. Yet, others have found that studies are skewed toward higher risks of mortality and that the research does not support heart and cancer deaths in nonsmokers (Mantel, 1992).

Etiology, Antecedents, and Risk Factors

The increased incidence of lung cancer–related deaths in men in the 1930s and in women in the 1960s followed the pattern of increased acceptance of smoking behavior, first in men and then in women. In fact, smoking among female adolescents is higher than among male adolescents (DHHS, 1994c). It is estimated that 79% of lung cancer deaths among women are related to smoking (ACS, 1995). In addition, tobacco has been linked to cancers of the mouth, pharynx, larynx, esophagus, pancreas, uterine cervix, kidney, and bladder (McGinn & Haylock, 1993). Tobacco, the real culprit, is a major source of carcinogens in industrialized nations. Lung cancer risk is related to cumulative dose, which for cigarettes is measured in pack-years. The latency period between initiation of smoking and the development of lung cancer is 15 to 20 years (DHHS, 1986). Additional risk factors include exposure to certain substances, such as arsenic and asbestos, particularly in people who smoke. Radiation exposure and radon exposure may also increase risk, especially in cigarette smokers. Sidestream cigarette smoke increases the risk of lung cancer for nonsmokers (ACS, 1995). Thirty percent of lung cancers are adenocarcinoma and large cell carcinoma and are less frequently associated with smoking than squamous and small cell types. In fact, adenocarcinoma is the most common cell type occurring in nonsmokers, especially young women (NCI PDQ system, 1994).

Symptoms, Disease Patterns, and Responses to Disease

Lung cancer has no early symptoms. When symptoms do appear they include persistent cough, chest pain, wheezing breath sounds, shortness of breath, coughing up blood, and recurring pneumonia or bronchitis. Without early symptoms, early detection is almost impossible; thus, the 5-year relative survival rate is only 13% (ACS, 1995). Chest radiography, analysis of the types of cells in a sputum specimen, and fiberoptic examination of the bronchial passages assist diagnosis.

Treatment

There are two kinds of lung cancer based on cell type: small cell and non-small cell. Small cell lung cancer, sometimes called oat cell lung cancer, is usually found in individuals who smoke or who were former smokers. Treatments for small cell lung cancer are surgery, radiation therapy, and chemotherapy. Chemotherapy is the most common treatment for all stages of small cell lung cancer. Non-small cell lung cancer is usually associated with prior smoking, passive smoking, or radon exposure. Surgery and radiation therapy are used to treat non-small cell lung cancer. However, these treatments often do not cure the disease.

Implications

Primary lung cancer prevention focuses on decreasing the number of new smokers and helping present smokers to quit. Deciding not to smoke cigarettes is the most important thing a woman can do to decrease her chance of developing cancer. For individuals who have smoked less than 20 years, who stop smoking, their lung cancer risk steadily declines, and approaches, but does not quite reach, that of nonsmokers after 15 years of abstinence (Tabbarah, Lowitz, & Casciato, 1988, p. 115).

The tobacco industry advertising is alluring to young persons, portraying models who smoke as being provocative, seductive, and thin. Cigarette smoking does decrease appetite and increase metabolism and appeals to a woman's need to control her weight. Smoking cessation programs must address these concerns of women to be effective. Over half of female smokers begin smoking before age 13; thus, prevention efforts must be begin at the junior high age group or younger (Penny & Shell, 1991).

Some researchers are more optimistic about the treatment for lung cancer. According to Bunn (1993), progress has been made in the treatment of non-small cell lung cancer. Although continued research is needed, long-term survival has improved. New approaches to lung cancer include the creation of agents that inhibit lung cancer growth factors, monoclonal antibodies that react with lung cancer cell surface antigens, and gene therapy.

Colorectal Cancer

Epidemiology

In the United States, colorectal cancer in both men and women is the second most common cause of death after lung cancer, accounting for approximately 55,300 deaths annually (ACS, 1995). In 1995, about 100,000 Americans were diagnosed with colon cancer and about 38,200 with rectal cancer. In this same year, women's deaths from colorectal cancer were third (28,100), and the incidence of 65,900 is a distant third after breast and lung cancer. Men have a higher incidence of colon cancer, 40.6/100,000, compared to women, 29.6/100,000. Rectal cancer is also higher in men, 18.1/100,000, than in women, 10.6/100,000 (Miller et al., 1992). The risk of developing colorectal cancer increases with age. Among those over 65 years of age, the incidence is an alarming 337.1/100,000.

There is good news for the Caucasian population as both incidence and mortality rates of colorectal cancer have begun to decline (Hoel et al., 1992). From 1985 to 1988, the incidence rates had fallen slightly more for women, 11% as compared to 8% for men. The decline in incidence may be explained by an increased awareness for primary prevention by some groups and by the professional community's approach to early treatment of colorectal polyps (DeCosse, Tsioulias, & Jacobson, 1994). Mortality rates remain unchanged in African American women and are actually increasing in African American men (Miller et al., 1992). Hispanics and African Americans are also more likely to have a more advanced stage of colorectal cancer at the time of presentation than their Caucasian counterparts (Steele, Winchester, Menck, & Murphy, 1993).

Etiology, Antecedents, and Risk Factors

The most significant risk factor for colorectal cancer, besides age (40 years) is diet. According to Greenwald, Lanza, and Eddy (1987), a diet high in fat, particularly animal fat, is associated with high risk, and a diet high in fiber is associated with low risk. Diets high in fat have been linked with persons with sedentary lifestyles and obesity, which can be additional risk factors for the development of this type of cancer. Diets that include fruits and vegetables, vitamin D, and calcium are protective against colorectal cancer. The role of diet, alcohol, and sex hormones in the development of colorectal cancer is complex and cannot be described fully here (For more information on this subject read Ingram, Bennett, Wilcox, & deKlerk, 1987, and Rose, Goldman, Connolly, & Strong, 1991). A personal or family history of colon or rectal polyps or a history of chronic or inflammatory bowel disease such as ulcerative colitis or Crohn's disease increases the risk of colorectal cancer. An additional risk factor for women developing colorectal cancer is a family or personal history of breast, ovarian, or endometrial cancer.

Antecedents

Adenomatous polyps of the large bowel are considered precursors of colorectal cancer. About 15% of all patients with colorectal cancer have a family history of adenomatous polyps. Possible explanations include a genetic abnormality or an environmental exposure. Only 1% of colorectal cancer patients have familial adenomatous polyposis, an autosomal dominant condition, which if untreated, develops into colorectal cancer.

Symptoms, Disease Patterns, and Responses to Disease

Symptoms vary based on the location of the cancer but may include obstructive symptoms, abdominal pain, rectal bleeding, blood in the stool, and change in bowel habits. Based on the reduction of Caucasian women developing colorectal cancer, it appears that these women are getting the message that dietary changes and early detection are key to avoiding this cancer. Poor women are less likely to participate in screening (Weinrich, Weinrich, Boyd, Johnson, & Frank-Stromborg, 1992), and their cancers are found in later stages.

Gender differences are apparent in the development of colorectal cancers. The hormonal effects of nutrition may help explain these differences in incidence and site distribution. In developed countries, the sigmoid is the most common primary site of colon cancer in both men and women. However, as age of onset increases, right-sided tumors become more common, especially in older women (Alley & McNee, 1986; Butcher et al., 1985). In addition, cholecystectomy may be associated with a small increase in risk of right-sided colon cancer in women (Llamas, Torlach, Ward, & Bain, 1986).

Treatment

Fortunately, about 85% of individuals diagnosed with colorectal cancer can have surgery intended for cure. For postmenopausal women with curable colon cancer removal of the ovaries is also recommended to prevent subsequent primary ovarian cancer and to remove any possibility of occult metastasis from the colon (Brief, Brener & Goldenkranz, 1991). The ACS (1995) states that surgery or surgery with radiation is the most effective method of treating this cancer. Combining chemotherapy and immunologic agents is showing promise for individuals with a more advanced stage of colorectal cancer. According to the National Cancer Data Base, treatment trends are beginning to show the influence of recent data showing benefit for multimodality therapy, and this treatment pattern was consistent regardless of race or socioeconomic strata (Steele et al., 1993). Persons with ulcerative colitis or familial adenomatous polyposis need to be educated about their risk of developing colorectal cancer and the surgical procedures available (Wilson, 1993).

Implications

Primary colorectal cancer prevention includes making dietary changes because a high-fat or low-fiber diet may be associated with increased risk. Other primary prevention strategies may soon include taking aspirin or NSAIDS. Risk of colorectal cancer declined with long-term use of aspirin among women in the Nurse's Health Study (Giovanucci et al., 1995).

Studies indicate that more colorectal cancers are diagnosed at a localized stage among Caucasians than among African Americans (Miller et al., 1992). This is also true of the cancer in women of lower socioeconomic status who present late in the disease. In contrast, women of higher socioeconomic status are more likely to have regular examinations and screening that includes an annual stool specimen for guaiac and a sigmoidoscopy every 3 to 5 years after the age of 50. In a study of 211 persons (mean age 72), mostly women (77.1%), only 5% reported that they had received information about colorectal cancer from their physician although nearly all had seen a doctor within the preceding year (Weinrich et al., 1992). Information and screening are important; for example, with an annual fecal occult blood testing (with rehydration of the sample, which increases significantly the sensitivity of the test), there is a significant reduction in mortality from colorectal cancer (Mandel et al., 1993).

Cervical Cancer

Epidemiology

An increasing number of women are at risk for cancer of the cervix. Although the incidence of invasive cervical cancer has been reduced, the number of women with cervical intraepithelial neoplasia (CIN) has increased at alarming rates (DiSaia & Creasman, 1994). Cervical carcinoma in situ, a precancerous condition, is now more frequent than invasive cancer, especially in women under age 50 (ACS, 1996). Invasive cancer of the cervix will occur in 15,700 women in 1996 and 4900 will die of the disease. In addition there will be 65,000 who are diagnosed with carcinoma in situ. Fortunately, over the past 50 years the incidence of invasive cervical cancer has decreased 50% for most American women and the relative survival rates have increased.

If the diagnosis is invasive cervical cancer, it is most often squamous cell carcinoma although some are adenocarcinomas (Gusberg & Runowicz, 1991). Cervical cancer is associated with young women, but older women even into their eighties have been diagnosed with the disease (Chapman, 1992). This is a significant but often neglected population of elderly women diagnosed with cervical cancer. Among certain ethnic groups cervical cancer continues to be a major killer. In fact, the mortality rate is more than twice as high for African American women as for Caucasian women (ACS, 1995). In 1991, cervical cancer claimed the lives of 1344 minority women as follows: African American, 983; Hispanic, 292; Native American, 42; Chinese, 17; and Japanese, 10 (ACS, 1995).

Etiology, Antecedents, and Risk Factors

Studies report that cervical cancer can be considered a sexually transmitted disease (ACS, 1995; Nelson, Averette, & Richart, 1984), due to the following risk factors; first intercourse at an early age, multiple sexual partners, and a nonmonogamous male partner. Viral agents, including herpes simplex virus, human papillomavirus (HPV), human immunodeficiency virus, are likely cofactors in the development of cervical cancer. Certain forms of HPV are known to cause cervical cancer. Although tobacco abuse is a major risk factor for cancer of the esophagus, larynx, and oral cavity, it has also been associated with both cervical cancer and stomach cancer (Cresanta, 1992).

Symptoms, Disease Patterns, and Responses to Disease

No symptoms are associated with the preinvasive stage of this cancer. The most common symptoms of invasive cervical carcinoma are abnormal bleeding and vaginal discharge (ACS, 1995). Pain and systemic symptoms are late manifestations of the disease. According to Gusberg and Runowicz (1991), persistent aching pain in the lower quadrant or low back pain occurs when a tumor reaches the pelvic side wall pressing against nerve trunks.

Treatment

Fortunately, most of the women with an abnormal Pap smear have a treatable precancerous condition called cervical dysplasia or CIN. The ability to locate and precisely define the size and distribution of CIN by colposcopy has allowed a more conservative approach to the disease. A magnified view of the cervix via colposcopy enhances these abnormalities to determine if cervical changes are benign or cancerous. Colposcopy allows clinicians to closely follow patients with abnormal Pap smears (Yaeger, 1994). The conservative approaches include local excision, cryotherapy (destruction of cells by extreme cold), electrocoagulation (destruction of cells through intense heat by electric current), by carbon dioxide laser, and by a loop electrodiathermy excision procedure. Treatment for invasive cervical cancer is generally by surgery or radiation or both. The survival rate for women with localized disease is 91% (ACS, 1996). If cervical cancer is allowed to progress, more aggressive treatment is needed.

Implications

As a sexually transmissible disease cervical cancer could be controlled with barrier methods of contraception. However, if it occurs deaths should be few because it has a lengthy preinvasive state, an effective screening test (Pap test), and various treatment options (Yoder & Rubin, 1992). The reasons women give for not having a Pap test are fear, embarrassment, and no need if symptoms are not present. All women need to be educated about the importance of regular cancer examinations. According to the ACS (1996), the Pap test should be performed annually with a pelvic examination in women who are sexually active, regardless of age, or who have reached age 18 years. Annual testing is important because of the incidence of abnormal Pap smear increasing, due to the rising incidence of cervicitis, HPV, inflammation, dysplasia, carcinoma in situ, and microinvasive carcinoma. Other women, such as those whose mothers took diethylstilbestrol, must be followed more closely.

Unfortunately, many women who have cervical cancer have never had a Pap smear and many die from this disease (McKie, 1993). In some areas, 75% of elderly women have not had a Pap smear within the previous 5 years (Mandelblatt & Fahs, 1988; Mandelblatt, Gogaul, & Wistreich, 1986). These data together with the fact that over 25% of invasive cervical cancers occur in women older than 65 and that 40% to 50% of all women who die from cervical cancer are over 65 years of age (DHHS, 1994b) makes one wonder if there should be an upper limit to Pap test screening as proposed by some groups. This implies that older women are not sexual beings, or if they are sexually active, they must only be in a mutually monogamous relationship, or that they are expendable. A better approach in deciding when to discontinue Pap testing would be to assess each woman, regardless of age, as an individual. The clinician should complete a thorough health history that includes a sexual history. This would allow the clinician and woman to make an informed decision about the frequency of Pap testing.

Uterine Cancer

Epidemiology

Gynecologic cancers can affect any organ of a woman's reproductive system, but the most common type is cancer of the uterus. The uterus is composed of two layers of tissue, the endometrium or inner layer and the muscular outer layer known as the myometrium. Cancer may occur in either layer but develops more often in the endometrium. An entirely different form of this cancer, uterine sarcoma, arises from connective tissue, such as smooth muscle (Disaia & Creasman, 1994). Among all Americans, cancer of the uterus is fourth in incidence. It affects approximately 31,000 women annually and kills 5900. This disease occurs most often in women between the ages of 60 and 74. Seventy-five percent of endometrial cancer is diagnosed in women over age 50. Gusberg and Runowicz (1991) explain that the rise in the relative prevalence of endometrial tumors is probably related to an aging population, high-fat diets, and estrogen replacement therapy without the protective benefit of progesterone.

Etiology, Antecedents, and Risk Factors

According to the ACOG (1991b), the principal factor that predisposes women to the development of endometrial cancer is chronic, unopposed exposure to estrogen. This exposure may be related to endogenous factors, such as early menarche, late menopause, history of infertility, failure to ovulate, and obesity, or exogenous factors, such as the ingestion of unopposed estrogen. Other risk factors include pelvic radiation therapy, hypertension, and diabetes mellitus. However, the latter two are more likely related to obesity (ACOG, 1991a).

Endometrial hyperplasia, a precursor to the development of endometrial cancer, is an abnormal increase in the number of endometrial cells and stromal cells, which support endometrial tissue. If this condition is not treated, it can progress to invasive cancer in 25% of cases. Endometrial cancer has a long preclinical stage, suggested by its development late in life and the recognition of its precursor lesions. The development of this tumor is highly preventable (Gusberg & Runowicz, 1991).

Although there is no genetic marker for this cancer, in 12% to 28% of cases the tumor has occurred in families (Gusberg & Runowicz, 1991). In addition, women who have had breast or ovarian cancer are at higher than average risk for developing endometrial cancer.

Symptoms, Disease Patterns, and Responses to Disease

The one and only significant sign of endometrial cancer is abnormal uterine staining or bleeding. One-third of women with postmenopausal bleeding have a malignancy. Bleeding in pre- and perimenopausal women is associated with endometrial cancer only in a small number of cases (Gusberg & Runowicz, 1991). As with other cancers, pain and weight loss occur late in the disease (ACS, 1995).

Treatment

The uterine lesions resulting from hormonal imbalance are often reversible with adequate progestin therapy (ACOG, 1991b). If uterine cancer is detected, the treatment depends on the stage of the tumor, the size of the uterus, the degree of cancer cell differentiation, and the woman's age and medical condition. The mainstay of treatment is hysterectomy, with or without radiation therapy. Other treatments include hormones or chemotherapy. The cure rate for endometrial cancer is very high because these tumors tend to be well differentiated and localized. However, about 15% of tumors develop quickly and are deadly. Early detection of this cancer, before it has extended beyond the uterus, boasts a 94% 5-year survival rate. When diagnosed in a regional stage, the survival rate drops to 67% (ACS, 1995).

Implications

There is no effective screening method to detect endometrial cancer. The ACS (1995) suggests that women at high risk of developing endometrial cancer have an endometrial biopsy evaluated at menopause and that women on hormone replacement therapy or tamoxifen get regular examinations. ACOG's (1991b) outpatient evaluation of a woman suspected of having endometrial cancer consists of a careful inspection of the cervix, vulva, vagina, and anus; Pap smear; test for occult blood in the stool; and a thorough pelvic examination. In addition, biopsy should be performed on any suspicious genital lesion, and an endometrial biopsy and endocervical curettage done in postmenopausal women with vaginal bleeding or perimenopausal women with a menstrual abnormality.

Ovarian Cancer

Epidemiology

The grim statistics are that ovarian cancer ranks second in incidence among women's gynecologic cancers, but ranks first in the cause of death compared with other cancers of the female reproductive system (ACS, 1996). In 1996, the ACS estimates that 14,800 women with ovarian cancer will die of this disease, and approximately 26,700 women will learn that they have the disease. More specifically 1 in every 70 women, without a family history of the disease, will develop ovarian cancer (Teneriello & Park, 1995). Most of these cancers occur in women over age 40. The high mortality rate is related to the absence of symptoms in the early stages of the disease. Screening for early stage ovarian cancer has proven to be a challenge.

Three-fourths of all malignant ovarian tumors derive from different types of epithelial cells. Epithelial tumors of the ovary are the most common type in adults and have a peak incidence in the 40- to 70-year-old age group. Although children and adolescents are not invulnerable to the disease, ovarian cancer in this population is rare and more often associated with germ cell tumors. Tumors arising from the coelomic epithelium covering the ovary account for approximately 85% to 90% of all malignancies. These epithelial ovarian cancers are far more common in Western industrialized nations than anywhere else in the world. In the United States, the disease occurs more often in older women of Northern European descent (Daly, 1992; Deppe & Lawrence, 1988).

Etiology, Antecedents, and Risk Factors

The cause of ovarian cancer is unknown; however, current evidence suggests that altered endocrine function may contribute to its development. It is a common occurrence for women with breast, colon, or endometrial cancer to develop ovarian cancer at about the same time; therefore, these cancers may have a common etiology. The number of years a woman ovulates is a factor in the development of this disease because protection is provided through reducing the number of ovulations through events such as pregnancy before age 25, early menopause, and 10 or more years of oral contraceptive use (WHO Collaborative Study, 1991). Conversely, women with more than 40 ovulation years belong to the high-risk group: women with late menopause or those of few births, decreased fertility, and delayed childbearing.

Ovarian cancer has a tendency to run in families. Women who have a mother or sister with this disease have as much as a 50% risk of developing ovarian cancer. Although this is an important finding, it represents only 1% to 3% percent of women with ovarian cancer (Creasman & DiSaia, 1991). It is not clear whether familial clustering represents a genetic susceptibility or a shared environmental exposure. Because the disease is more common in highly industrialized countries, environmental factors may be involved. Exposure to talc and asbestos is associated with an increased risk of ovarian cancer. Women report exposure to talc from barrier contraceptives and feminine hygiene products. Some women use talc on the perineum as part of personal hygiene practice (J. Holcombe, personal communication, December, 1994).

Symptoms, Disease Patterns, and Responses to Disease

The major obstacle in fighting ovarian cancer is its remarkable lack of symptoms. For most women, at the time of diagnosis, it has spread to organs of the pelvis and abdomen. Unlike other gynecologic cancers, women with this cancer rarely have vaginal bleeding. According to the ACS (1996), the most common sign of ovarian cancer is enlargement of the abdomen. With this increase in girth, women may complain of an inability to fasten skirts and pants. They may experience vague gastrointestinal symptoms including abdominal discomfort, upper abdominal fullness, and early satiety. For this reason, the ACS (1996) recommends that women over 40 with vague digestive disturbances, not explained by any other cause, need a thorough evaluation for ovarian cancer. According to clinicians, the most frequently noted physical symptom of ovarian cancer is pelvic pain and ascites associated with a pelvic mass (ACOG, 1991c).

Treatment

Surgery, radiation, and chemotherapy are all treatment options for ovarian cancer. The choice of treatment is determined by several things including the properties of the tumor and age and reproduction status of the woman. Surgery is aimed at resection of as much tumor as is safely possible (ACOG, 1991c). Since the early 1980s platinum-based combination chemotherapy has been the standard treatment for advanced epithelial ovarian cancer (Qazi & McGuire, 1995; Thigpen, Vance, & Lambuth, 1988). There is also a "second look" operation after a prescribed course of chemotherapy to determine the usefulness of additional chemotherapy. An alternative to chemotherapy is external radiotherapy (Gusberg & Runowicz, 1991). For a woman with ovarian cancer that is no longer responding to the standard chemotherapy there is new hope. Paclitaxel (Taxol) is a relatively new anticancer drug that has been particularly useful in ovarian cancer. This drug, derived from the bark of the yew tree, is costly to produce, and its use is limited to only women who have demonstrated progressive or persistent disease (Runowicz, 1992). Synthetic forms of the drug are being tested. Oncology nurses and other providers are becoming knowledgeable about the guidelines for Taxol administration and the management of toxicities. Women with ovarian cancer need good information on the available therapies to make informed decisions about their treatment (Hillig-Noone & Fioravanati, 1994).

Implications

Unfortunately, there are no effective methods of mass screening to detect ovarian cancer. According to the NCI and ACOG, women who have become sexually active or are 18 years of age and older should have an annual pelvic examination as part of a periodic health examination. For women at high risk of developing ovarian cancer, new screening technologies show promise in uncovering the disease earlier. Transvaginal ultrasonography can detect ovarian enlargement and color Doppler ultrasonography helps to distinguish malignant from benign growth. A tumor marker such as CA 125 is useful for the detection of advanced ovarian cancer, but its sensitivity is reduced in early stage disease and is even less reliable for early diagnosis. These new methods are complex and costly and are not useful for mass screening; yet, they do provide a basis for the creation of clinical trials, according to Gusberg (1992).

Methods of prevention include prophylactic removal of the ovaries for women aged 45 and older who are undergoing hysterectomy. For women with a strong family history of ovarian cancer, it is recommended that they undergo surgery at age 40.

The current challenge to gynecologic oncologists and other health care providers is to care for the women with advanced disease. Improved surgeries and knowledge of the therapies that are most successful have increased the number of survivors of ovarian cancer.

Cancer's Relevance for Women Across the Lifespan

Cancer is not just another chronic disease; it evokes many of the deepest fears of mankind (Weisman, 1979). Many men and women identify cancer as the most feared disease (Murray & McMillan, 1993). However, women are more frightened of cancer than men, who describe more fear of heart disease. Women also report anxiety and fear after having gone through tests to rule out cancer. Benedict, Williams, and Baron (1994) found that women reported an increased frequency of thinking about breast cancer and fear of breast cancer after a benign breast biopsy.

Others have found that women awaiting the results of a biopsy for cancer are more vulnerable to psychological morbidity than women having gallbladder surgery (Hughson, Cooper, McArdales, & Smith, 1988). Holcombe's (1985) work with women with gynecologic cancer found that the uncertainty that accompanies the diagnosis of cancer combined with the potential threat to the feminine identity can create adjustment problems. In addition, the relevance that cancer has for a woman changes throughout the life cycle, from youth, midlife, and into old age.

Young Women

From her first menstruation, around the age of 13, a young woman begins to learn about her body and the intricate changes that are occurring. These changes are usually benign because youth is considered a time of low cancer risk. As the young woman matures she may question bodily changes as potential signs of disease, including cancer, but her time is usually spent in other pursuits. For example, learning about her fertility/fecundity is an important part of a young woman's development. Decisions about family planning methods start early for many women, and these choices have implications in terms of cancer risk. Choosing a barrier method of contraception, such as condoms, offers some protection from cervical cancer (Rosenberg, Davidson, Chen, Judson, & Douglas, 1992); however, if the choice is an oral contraceptive she must ask the most controversial question surrounding pill use, "Do oral contraceptives cause cancer?" (Coker, Harlap, & Fortney, 1993; Coker, McCann, Hulka, & Walton, 1992). Women must weigh the pill's risk versus its benefits. For example, the benefit could outweigh the risk for a woman with a strong family history of ovarian cancer because long-term pill use offers protection against the number one gynecologic killer (Lynch, Albano, Lynch, Lynch, & Campbell, 1982).

In the United States, the average woman will become pregnant and bear just under two children in her lifetime. Cancer during pregnancy, once rare, is now becoming more common as women choose childbearing into their forties. Malignant disease complicates 1 in 1000 pregnancies, with breast cancer diagnosed in 1 in 3500 (Titcomb, 1990). Women who become pregnant are also at risk for gestational trophoblastic neoplasia (GTN), which represents a unique array of diseases originating from the placenta (ACOG, 1993). The benign form of GTN is called hydatidiform mole and represents 80% of cases. However, approximately 20% of women with primary hydatidiform mole will develop malignant sequelae. The malignant forms of GTN are the invasive mole (chorioadenoma destruens) and the frankly malignant form (choriocarcinoma). Molar pregnancy occurs in about 1 in every 1500 to 2000 pregnancies among Caucasians in the United States; the incidence is much higher among Asian women (1/800). In the Far East the incidence is even higher for Asian women, accounting for 1 in every 125 to 200 pregnancies.

Cancer is generally believed to carry a worse prognosis during pregnancy because of the potential adverse effects of anticancer treatments on the fetus and of pregnancy-related hormonal and immunologic modifications on the disease (*Lancet,* June 24, 1994). In breast cancer, however, several studies suggest that prognosis depends more on the woman's age than on gestational age at diagnosis

(Baron, 1994a, 1994b; Barron, 1984; Dansforth, 1991) or on a delay in diagnosis (Saunders & Baum, 1993). More common are women who must decide about child-bearing after cancer. In one study approximately 18,000 of the 180,000 women who were diagnosed with breast cancer were under age 40, and of those diagnosed with cancer, an estimated 7% went on to have children. Oncology professionals do not agree on the safety of pregnancy after breast cancer.

A woman's decisions about various treatments for cancer, particularly during her young adult years, have lifelong implications. Fortunately, with improved survival rates there is an increased emphasis on quality of life issues. Ferrell, Grant, and Padilla (1991) studied the experience of chronic pain and perceptions of quality of life and developed a quality of life model. The model consists of four dimensions: physical well-being, psychological well-being, social concerns, and spiritual well-being. The investigators' report that there were gender differences in the four dimensions; for example, women described more social concerns with child care. Another important quality of life issue, for a woman and her partner, from both a physiologic and psychological perspective, is the impact that cancer and its treatment have on fertility and sexual functioning (Holcombe, 1985; Smith, 1994). Fertility can be adversely affected by chemotherapy and radiation therapy. Women who desire children are often devastated by the loss of fertility. In fact, for some individuals certain aspects of their lives are so vital to self-concept that without it they feel less alive or less like living.

Common cancers, such as breast, cervical, and uterine, have a profound affect on a woman's sexuality. A common way that cancer treatment affects a woman's sexuality is by causing premature menopause. Menopausal symptoms may cause a woman to experience hot flashes and vaginal atrophy (vagina becomes tight and dry). Hormone replacement therapy may relieve these problems, but women with cancer of the breast or uterus usually cannot take estrogen. Even so-called minor treatments for preinvasive cervical cancer destroy special mucous-producing cells (cervical crypts) and reduce vaginal lubrication, which is important to a woman's sexual functioning. Others have found that women treated for cervical cancer with radiation experienced more painful intercourse and decreased sexual desire than women treated with hysterectomy only (Schover, Fife, & Gershenson, 1989).

Women who lose a part of their body to cancer, especially if it is a breast or an area of the genitals, may miss the pleasure they felt from these areas being touched during lovemaking or self-pleasuring (Lidster & Horsburgh, 1994). Because breast cancer is the most common cancer in women, sexual problems have been linked to mastectomy (the most common treatment) more often than to any other cancer treatment. Fortunately, more health care providers and patients are discussing the subject of sexuality at all stages of therapy, but especially in the beginning, when the treatment for cancer is being planned (Burke, 1994).

Midlife Women

The majority of women in midlife have good health, yet chronic illnesses such as cancer become increasingly prevalent. According to Mitchell and Helson (1990), the "prime of life" is a useful concept in this stage of a woman's development. At the same time, midlife women use health services at relatively high rates. Many women appear more sensitive to symptoms of illness and are more active in their orientation toward the detection and treatment of disease than are men (Dennerstein, 1995). This, of course, is not true for all women in midlife. One subset of women who neglect cancer screening as well as other health care encounters are lesbian women (Bradford, Ryan, & Rothblum, 1994; Buenting, 1992). The attitude of health care providers toward lesbians is a factor in this self-neglect (Stevens, 1992). Lesbian women describe health care providers' behaviors as hostile and rejecting. Because of their negative experiences, lesbian women may delay seeking health care services until signs or symptoms of cancer persist.

Postmenopausal women are another group who have unique needs. No longer concerned about the risk of pregnancy, these women must now decide whether they should take hormone replacement therapy, which has a known beneficial effect on the cardiovascular and skeletal systems. Much attention has been focused on the use of this therapy on women at risk for or with breast cancer. However, any cancer that thrives in an estrogen-rich environment is cause for concern. Clinicians who work in women's health or with women cancer survivors must be thoroughly informed to answer questions objectively and to assist women in making decisions about hormone replacement therapy (Vassilopoulou-Sellin, 1993).

Midlife is also a time when women play multiple roles in daily management of family life. Women, more often than men, nurture children and provide the care and support of extended family members. When a woman is diagnosed with cancer, her ability to perform these important roles can be severely limited and have a negative impact on the entire family system (Northouse, 1991, 1993). Many researchers have described cancer as a family disease (Germino, 1987; Lewis, Woods, & Hough, 1989). Women and their families have benefited from the earlier diagnosis of cancer and improved treatments that allow many women to return to work or remain working throughout the course of the disease. Work here includes family responsibilities, domestic duties, and the workforce (Bonam-Crawford & Orlick, 1994). For many midlife women return to work is essential for their economic and emotional well-being; however, there are many barriers to employment for cancer patients. The financial cost of cancer for the family can be devastating (Hartung, 1996). Less is known about the informal costs of cancer care. Given, Given, and Stommel (1994) studied family and out-of-pocket costs for women with breast cancer. This study is important in describing the informal costs of breast cancer. Additional studies are needed that will examine the family care costs together with the formal and direct reimbursable medical costs of all cancer affecting women and their families.

Older Women

As a group, older women look forward to the so-called golden years. However, more and more older adults are raising grandchildren or caring for an ill spouse or sibling. Over half of the 31 million people 65 years of age and older coexist with a disability that limits their daily activities, and the percentage climbs to 60% for minority groups (U.S. Bureau of the Census, 1992). It is little wonder that older women do not notice subtle changes in their own bodies, or if noticed, they consider the change a normal part of aging or an aspect of a chronic condition. Yet, cancer should be considered a possible explanation because the incidence of cancer increases with age and a disproportionate number of elders die of the disease (ACS, 1995; Frank-Stromborg, 1986).

As a woman ages she and her health care provider must take physical changes seriously. Gender disparities in clinical decision-making have been noted (American Medical Association, 1994). Older women must be encouraged to report changes and concerns to their health care providers, and these must *be taken as seriously as* those of their male counterparts.

Older women, who are more often the nation's socioeconomically disadvantaged, are not benefiting from early detection provided through cancer screening. In addition to cost, other factors that prevent this population from using cancer screening include accessibility, availability, lack of knowledge, health care provider variables, and lack of community involvement (Brown & Williams, 1994).

By using resources in the community older women may be able to obtain low cost cancer screening. Through the efforts of organizations such as the ACS and the NCI research and education projects are ongoing. Included in this are over 100 community demonstration projects that provide cancer education messages and programs to the poor and underserved in the United States (ACS, 1995).

Health care providers must incorporate cancer control and early detection methods into their practice with older women. Older women have shown that they will adhere to suggestions for screening if given the same opportunity as younger women. In addition to encouraging women to seek screening, if a diagnosis of cancer is made, the health care provider must be ready to support the older woman in her informed decisions about treatment. The ACS and NCI also provide educational materials, such as films and pamphlets to health professionals. The toll-free number, 1-800-4-CANCER, connects calls with the office that serves their area. People who have cancer, their families, and health care professionals who care for persons with cancer need up-to-date, accurate information about cancer and its treatment. To help meet these needs, NCI developed the Physicians Data Query Base (PDQ). This computer data base provides quick and easy access to state-of-the-art treatment information for patients and doctors, screening guidelines, information about clinical trials, and names of organizations and physicians involved in the care of people with cancer (NCI, 1993).

As women age, the incidence of cancer increases; yet, older women are often excluded from clinical trails and are often denied standard cancer treatments based solely on age and not on scientific data (Derby, 1991; Yellen, Cellen, & Leslie, 1994). Ensuring that the older woman has the same opportunity for the state-of-the-art treatment or is enrolled in clinical trails is of utmost importance.

Summary

This chapter described the cancers that are unique to or that are increasing in women. In addition, the relevance that cancer has for women across the life cycle was addressed. To achieve the NCI's cancer control objectives for the nation, women, as well as men, must work together with their communities and their health care providers to reduce cancer mortality. It is important that women—young, middle aged, and older—learn the good news about early screening for some cancers. Should cancer be detected, every woman needs up-to-date information about new treatments and available clinical trials. There is good news in the fight against certain women's cancer and women need to be informed in a way that takes into perspective their uniqueness as women in addition to their diversity.

Acknowledgments

The author acknowledges the assistance of Ms. Rebecca Bryant, MSN, OCN, UAB Comprehensive Cancer Center Director of the Alabama Black Belt Cancer Linkage Initiative in her careful review of the chapter.

The author wishes to express her appreciation to Dr. Judy Holcombe, Associate Professor at the University of Alabama School of Nursing, University of Alabama at Birmingham, for her review of the section on gynecologic cancer.

References

Alley, P. G., & McNee, R. K., (1986). Age and sex differences in right colon cancer. *Diseases of the Colon and Rectum, 29,* 227-229.

American Cancer Society. (1994). *Cancer facts and figures.* Atlanta, GA: Author.

American Cancer Society. (1995). *Cancer facts and figures.* Atlanta, GA: Author.

American Cancer Society. (1996). *Cancer facts and figures.* Atlanta, GA: Author.

American College of Obstetricians and Gynecologists. (1991a). *Carcinoma of the breast* (Technical Bulletin No. 142, pp. 1-7).

American College of Obstetricians and Gynecologists. (1991a). *Carcinoma of the endometrium* (Technical Bulletin No. 162, pp. 1-6).

American College of Obstetricians and Gynecologists. (1991b). *Cancer of the ovary* (Technical Bulletin No. 141, pp. 1-7).

American College of Obstetricians and Gynecologists. (1993). *Management of gestational trophoblastic disease* (Technical Bulletin No. 178, pp. 1-7).

American Medical Association, Council on Ethical and Judicial Affairs. (1994). Gender disparities in clinical decision making. *Journal of the American Medical Association, 266*(4), 559-562.

Baron, R. H. (1994a). Dispelling the myths of pregnancy-associated breast cancer. *Oncology Nursing Forum, 21*(7), 507-512.

Baron, R. H. (1994b). Treatment options for patients with pregnancy-associated breast cancer [Letter to the editor]. (A correction in Table 2 describing the treatment options for pregnant patients by stage and trimester of this article appears in the *Oncology Nursing Forum, 21*(7), 1135.

Barron, W. M. (1984). The pregnant surgical patient: Medical evaluation and management. *Annals of Internal Medicine, 101,* 683-691.

Benedict, S., Williams, R., & Baron, P. (1994). The effect of benign breast biopsy on subsequent breast cancer detection practices. *Oncology Nursing Forum, 21*(9), 1467-1475.

Bonam-Crawford, D., & Orlick, M. (1994). Helping patients with cancer achieve their work potential. *Clinical Perspectives in Oncology Nursing, 1*(1), 3.

Bradford, J., Ryan, C., & Rothblum, E. D. (1994). National lesbian health care survey: Implications for mental health care. *Journal of Consulting and Clinical Psychology, 62*(2), 228-242.

Breen, N., & Kessler, L. (1994). Changes in use of screening mammography: Evidence from the 1987 and 1990 National Health Interview surveys. *American Journal of Public Health, 84*(1), 62-67.

Brief, D. K., Brener, B. J., & Goldenkranz, R., et al. (1991). Defining the role of subtotal colectomy in the treatment of carcinoma of the colon. *Annals of Surgery, 213,* 248-252.

Brown, L. W., & Williams, R. D. (1994). Culturally sensitive breast cancer screening programs for older black women. *Nurse Practitioner, 19*(3), 21, 25-26, 31-32.

Buenting, J. A. (1992). Health life-styles of lesbian and heterosexual women. *Health Care for Women International, 13*(2), 165-171.

Bunn, P. (1993). Future directions in the management of non-small cell lung cancer. *Lung Cancer,* 9(Suppl. 2), S91-S107.

Burke, M. B. (Ed.). (1994). Face to face. *Oncology Patient Care, Practical Guidelines for the Specialized Nurse, 4*(1), 4.

Butcher, D, Hassanein, K., Dudgeon, M., et al. (1985). Female gender is a major determinant of changing subsite distribution of colorectal cancer with age. *Cancer, 56,* 714-716.

Calle, E. E., Flanders, D., & Thun, M. J. (1993). Demographic predictors of mammography and Pap smear screening in U.S. women. *American Journal of Public Health, 83*(1), 53-60.

Chapman, G. (1992). Survival of advanced age females with cervical carcinoma, *Gynecologic Oncology, 46*(3), 287-291.

Coker, A. L., Harlap, S., & Fortney, J. A. (1993). Oral contraceptives and reproductive cancers: Weighing the risks and benefits. *Family Planning Perspective, 25* (1), 17-23, 36.

Coker, A., McCann, M., Hulka, B., & Walton, L. (1992). Oral contraceptive use and cervical intraepithelial neoplasia. *Journal of Clinical Epidemiology, 45*(10), 1111-1118.

Cresanta, J. L. (1992). Epidemiology of cancer in the United States. *Primary Care, 19* (3), 419-441.

Creasman, W. T., & DiSaia, P. J. (1991). Screening in ovarian cancer. *American Journal Obstetrics and Gynecology, 165,* 7-10.

Dansforth, D. N. (1991). How subsequent pregnancy affects outcome in women with a prior breast cancer. *Oncology, 5* (11), 23–31, 35.

Daly, M. B. (1992). The epidemiology of ovarian cancer. *Hematological/Oncology Clinics of North America, 6*(4), 729-738.

Deckers, P. J., & Ricci, A., Jr. (1992). Pain and lumps in the female breast. *Hospital Practice, 27*(2A), 67-73, 77-78, 87-94.

DeCosse, J. J., Tsioulias, G. J., & Jacobson, J. S. (1994). Colorectal cancer: Detection, treatment, and rehabilitation. *CA: A Cancer Journal for Clinicians, 44*(1), 27-42.

Dennerstein, L. (1995). Gender, health, and ill-health. *Women's Health Issues, 5* (2), 53–59.

Deppe, G., & G. Lawrence, W. D. (1988). Cancer of the ovary. In S. Gusberg, H. Shingleton, & G. Deppe (Eds.), *Female genital cancer* (pp. 379-425). New York: Churchill Livingstone.

Derby, S. E. (1991). Ageism in cancer care of the elderly. *Oncology Nursing Forum. 18* (15) 921–926.

DiSaia, P. J. & Creasman, W. T. (1992). *Clinical gynecologic oncology* (4th ed). St. Louis: Mosby Year Book.

Eddy, D. M. (1991). Screening for breast cancer. In D. M. Eddy (Ed.), *Common screening tests* (Chap. 9). Philadelphia: American College of Physicians.

Ferguson, M. K., Skosey, C., Hoffman, P. C., & Golomb, H. M. (1990). Sex-associated differences in presentation and survival in patients with lung cancer. *Journal of Clinical Oncology, 8*(8), 1402–7.

Ferrell, B. R., Grant, M., & Padilla, G. (1991). The experience of pain and perceptions of quality of life: Validation of a conceptual model. *Hospice Journal, 7*(3), 9-22.

Feuer, E. J., Wun, L. M., Boring, C. C., Lap-Ming, W., Flanders, W., Timmel, M., & Tong, T. (1993). The lifetime risk of developing breast cancer. *Journal of the National Cancer Institute, 85*(11), 892-897.

Fletcher, S. W., Black, W., Harris, R., Rimer, B. K., & Shapiro, S. (1993). Report of the International Workshop on screening for breast cancer. *Journal of the National Cancer Institute, 85*(20), 1644–1656.

Frank-Stromborg, M. (1986). The role of the nurse in early detection of cancer: Population sixty-six years of age and older. *Oncology Nursing Forum, 13*(3), 66-73.

Germino, B. (1987). *The impact of cancer on the patient, the family and the nurse.* Living with cancer: The Fifth National Conference on Cancer Nursing. Arlington, VA: American Cancer Society.

Giovannucci, E., Egan, K. M., Hunter, D. J., Stampfer, M. J., Colditz, G. A., Willett, W.C., Speitzer, F. E. (1995). Aspirin and the risk of colorectal cancer in women. *New England Journal of Medicine, 333*(10), 609-614.

Given, B. A., Given, C. W., & Stommel, M. (1994). Family and out-of-pocket costs for women with breast cancer. *Cancer Practice, 2*(3), 187-193.

Greenwald, P., Lanza, E., & Eddy, G. A. (1987). Dietary fiber in the reduction of colon cancer risk. *Journal of the American Dietetic Association, 87,* 1178-1188.

Gusberg, S. B. (1992). The challenge of ovarian cancer. *CA: A Cancer Journal for Clinicians, 42*(6), 325-326.

Gusberg, S. B., & Runowicz, C. D. (1991). Gynecologic cancers. In A. I. Holleb, D. J. Fink, & G. P. Murphy (Eds.), *American Cancer Society textbook of clinical oncology*. Atlanta, GA: American Cancer Society.

Hartung, P. (1996). Financial resources for adults with cancer. *Cancer Practice, 4* (2), 105–108.

Hillig-Noone, M., & Fioravanti, S. G. (1994). Taxol: Past, present, and future. In S. Molloy-Hubbard, P. E. Green, & M. T. Knobf (Eds.), *Oncology nursing patient treatment and support, 1*(4), 1-8, 12.

Hoel, D. G., Davis, D. I., Miller, A. B., et al. (1992). Trends in cancer mortality in 15 industrialized countries, 1969-1986. *Journal of the National Cancer Institute, 84,* 313-320.

Holcombe, J. (1985). *Social support, perception of illness, and self-esteem of women with gyneco-logical cancer.* Dissertation, University of Alabama-Birmingham, p. 152.

Hughson, A., Cooper, A., McArdales, C., & Smith, D. (1988). Psychosocial morbidity in patients awaiting breast biopsy. *Journal of Psychosomatic Research, 32*(2), 173-180.

Ingram, D. M., Bennett, F. C., Wilcox, D., & deKlerk, N. (1987). Effect of low-fat diet on female sex hormone levels. *Journal of the National Cancer Institute, 79,* 1225-1229.

Isaacs, J. H. (1992). History and physical examination and breast self-examination. In J. H. Isaacs (Ed.), *Textbook of breast disease.* St. Louis: Mosby-Year Book.

Keller, J. E., & Howe, H. L. (1993). Risk factors for lung cancer among nonsmoking Illinois residents. *Environmental Research, 60*(1), 1-11.

Lewis, F. M., Woods, N. F., & Hough, E. E. (1989). The family's functioning with chronic illness in the mother: The spouse's perspective. *Social Science and Medicine, 20,* 1261-1269.

Lidster, C. A., & Horsburgh, M. E. (1994). Masturbation—Beyond myth and taboo. *Nursing Forum, 29*(3), 18-27.

Llamas, K. J., Torlach, L. G., Ward, M., & Bain, C., (1986). Cholecystectomy and adenomatous polyps of the large bowel. *Gut, 27,* 1181-1185.

Lynch, H. T., Albano, W. A., Lynch, J. F., Lynch, P. M., & Campbell, A. (1982). Surveillance and management of patients at high genetic risk for ovarian carcinoma. *Obstetrics and Gynecology, 59*(5), 589-596.

Mack, E., McGrath, T., Pendleton, D., & Zieber, N. A. (1993). Reaching poor populations with cancer prevention and early detection programs. *Cancer Practice, 1*(1), 35-39.

Makuc, D. M., Freid, V. M., & Parsons, P. E. (1994, August 3). Health insurance and cancer screening among women. *Advance data from vital and health statistics* (No. 254). Hyattsville, MD: National Center for Health Statistics.

Mandel, J., Bond, J., Church, T., Snover, D., Bradley, G., Schuman, L. M., & Ederer, F. (1993). Reducing mortality from colorectal cancer by screening for fecal occult blood. *New England Journal of Medicine, 328*(19), 1365-1371.

Mandelblatt, J. S., & Fahs, M.C. (1988). The cost-effectiveness of cervical cancer screening for low-income elderly women. *Journal of the American Medical Association, 259*(16), 2409-2413.

Mandelblatt, J. S., Gogaul, I., & Wistreich, M. (1986). Gynecological care of elderly women: Another look at Papanicolaou testing. *Journal of the American Medical Association, 256*(3), 367-371.

Mantel, N. (1992). Dubious evidence of heart and cancer deaths due to passive smoking. *Journal of Clinical Epidemiology, 45* (8), 809-813.

McGinn, K. A., & Haylock, P. J. (1993). *Women's cancers.* Alameda, CA: Hunter House.

McKie, L. (1993). Women's views of the cervical smear test: Implications for nursing practice— Women who have not had a smear test. *Journal of Advanced Nursing, 18*(6), 972-979.

Miller, B. A., Ries, L. A. G., & Hankey, B. F., et al. (1992). *Cancer statistics review 1973-89* (NIH Publication No. 92-2789). Bethesda, MD: National Cancer Institute.

Mitchell, V., & Helson, R. (1990). Women's prime of life: Is it in the 50's? *Psychology of Women Quarterly, 14*(4), 451–470.

Murray, M., & McMillan, C. L. (1993). Gender differences in perceptions of cancer. *Journal of Cancer Education, 8*(1), 53-62.

National Cancer Institute. (1993). *Understanding breast changes: A health guide for all women* (NIH Publication No. 93-3536). Bethesda, MD: Author.

Nelson, J., Averette, H., & Richart, R. (1984). Dysplasia, carcinoma in situ, and early invasive cervical carcinoma. *CA: A Cancer Journal for Clinicians, 4,* 306-325.

Northouse, L. (1991). Psychologic consequences of breast cancer on partner and family. *Seminars in Oncology Nursing, 7*(3), 216-223.

Northouse, L. (1993). Cancer and the family: Strategies to assist spouses. *Seminars in Oncology Nursing, 9*(2), 74-82.

ONS News. (1994). Board reacts to BCPT concerns. *9*(7), 1, 3, 13.

Orel, S. G., Schnall, M. D., LiVolsi, V. A., et al. (1994). Suspicious breast lesions: MR imaging with radiologic-pathologic correlation. *Radiology, 190*(2), 485-493.

Penny, S. L., & Shell, J. A. (1991). Lung cancer. In S.E. Otto (Ed.). *Oncology nursing* (p. 52). St. Louis: Mosby-Year Book.

Pisani, P. (1992). Breast cancer: Geographic variation and risk factors. *Journal of Environmental Pathology, Toxicology and Oncology, 11*(5/6), 313-316.

Powell, D. E., & Stelling, C. B. (1994). *The Diagnosis and Detection of Breast Disease.* St Louis, Mosby.

Pressman, P., & Hirshaut, Y. (1994, September/October). Breast cancer: Past, present and progress. *Coping: Living with cancer,* 34-35.

Qazi, F., & McGuire, W. P. (1995). The treatment of epithelial ovarian cancer. *CA: A Cancer Journal for Clinicians, 45*(2), 88-101.

Robischon, T. (1988). New screening guidelines for breast cancer sought. *Oncology & Biotechnology News,* 23.

Rose, D. P., Goldman, M., Connolly, J. M., & Strong, L. E. (1991). High-fiber diet reduces serum estrogen concentrations in premenopausal women. *American Journal Clinical Nutrition, 54,* 520-525.

Rosenberg, M. J. Davidson, A. J., Chen, J. H., Judson, F. N., & Douglas, J. M. (1992). Barrier contraceptives and sexually transmitted diseases in women: A comparison of female dependent methods and condoms. *American Journal of Public Health, 82*(5), 669-674.

Runowicz, C. D. (1992). Advances in the screening and treatment of ovarian cancer. *CA: A Cancer Journal for Clinicians, 42*(6), 327-349.

Saunders, C. M., & Baum, M. (1993). Breast cancer and pregnancy: A review. *Journal of the Royal Society of Medicine, 86,* 162-165.

Schover, L. R., Fife, M. B., & Gershenson, D. M. (1989). Sexual dysfunction and treatment for early stage cervical cancer. *Cancer, 63*(1), 204-212.

Smith, D. B. (1994). Sexuality and the patient with cancer: What nurses need to know. *Oncology Patient Care, Practical Guidelines for the Specialized Nurse, 4*(1), 1-3, 15.

Steele, G. D., Winchester, D. P., Menck, H. R., & Murphy, G. P. (1993). Clinical highlights from the National Cancer Data Base: 1993. *CA: A Cancer Journal for Clinicians, 43*(2), 71-82.

Stevens, P. E., (1992, April-June). Lesbian health care research: A review of the literature from 1970-1990. *Health Care for Women International, 13*(2), 91-120.

Stockwell, J., Goldman, A., Lyman, G., Noss, C., Armstrong, A., Pinkham, P., Candelora, E., & Brusa, M. (1992). Environmental tobacco smoke and lung cancer risk in nonsmoking women. *Journal of the National Cancer Institute, 84*(18), 1417-1422.

Strax, P. (1990). Detection of breast cancer. *Cancer, 66,* 1336-1340.

Tabbarah, H. J., Lowitz, B. B., & Casciato, D. A. (1988). Lung cancer. In D. A. Casciato & B. B. Lowitz (Eds.), *Manual of clinical oncology* (2nd ed.). Boston: Little, Brown.

Teneriello, M. G., & Park, R. C. (1995). Early detection of ovarian cancer. *CA: A Cancer Journal for Clinicians, 45*(2), 71-87.

Thigpen, J. T., Vance, R. B., & Lambuth, B. W. (1988). Ovarian carcinoma: The role of chemotherapy. *Seminars in Oncology, 15,* 16-23.

Titcomb, C. L. (1990). Breast cancer and pregnancy. *Hawaii Medical Journal 49* (1),18, 20–22,24.

U.S. Bureau of the Census. (1992). *Statistical abstract of the United States: 1992* (112th ed.). Washington, DC: Author.

U.S. Department of Health and Human Services. (1986). *The health consequences of using smoke-less tobacco: A report of the Advisory Committee to the Surgeon General* (NIH Publication No. 86-2874). Washington D.C.: U.S. Government Printing Office.

U.S. Department of Health and Human Services. (1994a). Mammography. In *Clinician's handbook of preventive services* (pp. 191-194). Washington, DC: U.S. Government Printing Office.

U.S. Department of Health and Human Services. (1994b). Papanicolaou smear. In *Clinician's handbook of preventive services* (pp. 195-200). Washington, DC: U.S. Government Printing Office.

U.S. Department of Health and Human Services. (1994c). Tobacco. In *Clinician's handbook of preventive services* (pp. 115-118). Washington, DC: U.S. Government Printing Office.

Varricchio, C. G. (1995). Issues to consider when planning cancer control interventions for women. *Women's Health Issues, 5* (2), 64–72.

Vassilopoulou-Sellin, R., (1993). Estrogen replacement therapy in women at increased risk for breast cancer. *Breast Cancer Research and Treatment, 28*(2), 167-177.

Weinrich, S., Weinrich, M., Boyd, M., Johnson, E., & Frank-Stromborg, M. (1992). Knowledge of colorectal cancer among older persons. *Cancer Nursing, 15* (5), 322-330.

Weisman, A. D. (1979). *Coping with cancer.* New York: McGraw-Hill.

WHO Collaborative Study of Neoplasia and Steroid Contraceptives. (1991). Breast cancer and depot medroxyprogesterone actate: A multinational study. *Lancet, 338,* 834-838.

Wilson, R. (1993). Patient teaching for an ileoanal reservoir. *Journal of ET Nursing, 20*(5), 199-203.

Yaeger, K. (1994, July). Colposcopy: A valuable tool, an opportunity for nurses. *Advances for Nurse Practitioners,* 21-24.

Yellen, S. B., Cella, D. F., Leslie, W. T. (1994). Age and clinical decision making in oncology patients. *Journal of the National Cancer Institute, 86* (23), 1766–1770.

Yoder, L., & Rubin, M. (1992). The epidemiology of cervical cancer and its precursors. *Oncology Nursing Forum, 19*(3), 485-493 (reprinted in ACS Professional Education Publication).

Young, J. L., Percy, C., & Asire, A. J. (Eds.). (1981). *Incidence and mortality data: 1973-77* (National Cancer Institute Monograph 57, DHHS Publication No. NIH 81-2330). Washington, DC: U.S. Government Printing Office.

CHAPTER 12

Infectious Diseases

Consuelo M. Beck-Sague
Suzanne Vernon
Trent MacKay

Introduction

Although great strides have been made in the control of infectious diseases in the last 50 years, their overall impact remains considerable. In the United States, according to the National Health Interview Survey of 1991, 46,104,000 cases of acute infective and parasitic diseases per year (18/100 persons) occurred (Hoeprich, Jordan, & Ronald, 1994). These yielded 154,768,000 days of restricted activity, 68,703,000 bed-bound days, 18,727,000 days lost from work in persons over 17 years of age, and 72,000,000 days lost from school among children under 18 years of age. Some infectious diseases, notably human immunodeficiency virus (HIV) infection and related diseases, are common causes of death among young adults (Centers for Disease Control and Prevention [CDC], 1994).

Some infections are specific to the female reproductive system or breast. Others, such as tuberculosis (TB), appear to have a somewhat more virulent course or a different presentation in women. Because of the unique anatomic and physiologic processes related to menarche, reproduction, and contraception, sexually transmitted diseases (STDs) are of particular importance among women of reproductive age.

Sexually Transmitted Diseases

In many STDs, the sequelae are much more severe among women than among men and frequently include infertility and sometimes death (Grimes, 1986; Shepard & Jones, 1989; Westrom, 1980). STDs affect women across the lifespan: in childhood, due to sexual abuse; in adolescence and adulthood, due to sexual behavior, pregnancy, and childbearing; and in later life, due to complications such as cervical cancer. The impact encompasses adverse reproductive outcomes, including low birthweight, fetal wastage, and vertical transmission; infertility; ectopic pregnancy; and chronic pelvic pain. The most important STDs in women are syphilis, gonorrhea, *Chlamydia trachomatis* genital infections, genital herpes, human papillomavirus (HPV) infections, including genital warts and cervical dysplasia, and HIV infection. A detailed discussion of each follows.

Syphilis

Epidemiology

Congenital syphilis was recognized even in the 1600s as a distinct syndrome related to adult infection, thought to be inherited by infants from fathers, or acquired from wet-nurses and other caretakers (Chiu & Radolf, 1994; Murphy & Patamasucon, 1985). Transplacental transmission from infected asymptomatic mothers was appreciated only in the early 1900s, when reactive serologic tests for syphilis in asymptomatic mothers confirmed them as the source of infections.

The rate of primary and secondary syphilis among women peaked in 1945 (121/100,000, Caucasian women; 970/100,000, women of other races) and then declined until the 1960s, because of penicillin treatment and screening and identification of sexual partners through contact tracing (Brown et al., 1970).

The increase in rate of infection in the 1960s, although often attributed to the "sexual revolution," coincided with sweeping cuts in funding of programs to reduce transmission of STDs (Chiu & Radolf, 1994). After declines in the 1970s, a dramatic upsurge in cases of primary and secondary syphilis was first recognized in large cities in 1985 and 1986 (CDC, 1987) (Fig. 12–1). In all cases, outbreaks were among disadvantaged racial minority populations, and male/female ratios approached 1:1 (Finelli, Budd, & Spitalny, 1993). During the epidemic, women were at higher risk of syphilis than men who engaged in the same high-risk activities. Prostitution and drug use, particularly noninjectable, smoked cocaine ("crack"), appeared to play a role in outbreaks (Siegal et al., 1993).

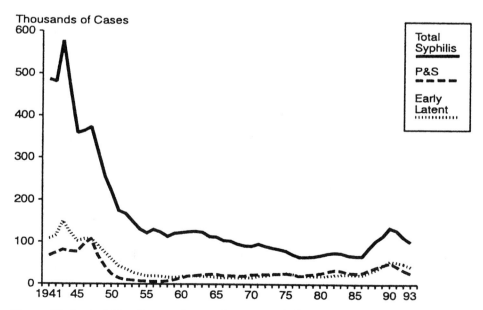

Figure 12-1. Syphilis—Reported cases by stage of illness: United States, 1941-1993. (Source:Centers for Disease Control and Prevention.)

Primary and secondary syphilis rates among women peaked in 1990 at 17.6/100,000 (122 and 10/100,000 among African American and Hispanic women, respectively). Incidence of congenital syphilis tends to closely reflect incidence of primary and secondary syphilis among women (Dunn, Webster, Nakashima, & Sylvester, 1993). The number of congenital syphilis cases rose dramatically from a low of 104 in 1978 to 4406 in 1991 (Fig. 12–2). Although a change in surveillance definition of congenital syphilis was in part responsible for this increase, even before the change, 558 cases were reported, the highest number in over 30 years. Since 1990, a decline observed in syphilis has been attributed to control programs begun during the epidemic.

The rate of primary and secondary syphilis was higher among females than males in the 10- to 24-year age groups; women 20 to 24 years of age had the highest rate of any U.S. age group in 1993, 30.6/100,000.

Etiology

Syphilis is caused by *Treponema pallidum* subspecies *pallidum*. Women with untreated syphilis are most infectious to both their sexual partners and fetuses, during primary and secondary (lesion) stages of syphilis. About 30% of sexual partners of a person with lesion syphilis become infected. Over 90% of pregnancy outcomes to women with lesion syphilis are stillbirths, premature infants, or infants with congenital syphilis (Chiu & Radolf, 1994).

During latent syphilis, when there are no symptoms or signs, microscopic abrasions occurring during intercourse can result in a sexual partner being exposed to

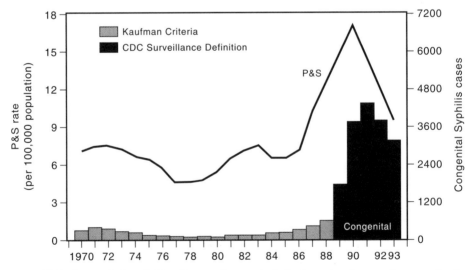

Figure 12-2. Congenital syphilis—Reported cases in infants under 1 year of age and rates of primary and secondary syphilis among women: United States, 1970–1993. (Source: Centers for Disease Control and Prevention.)

blood during spirochetemia, and transplacental transmission of *T. pallidum* from the maternal bloodstream readily occurs in the second and third trimester of pregnancy. Therefore, both vertical and sexual transmission can occur during latency. The risk of transmission gradually falls with increasing duration of latency.

Clinical Symptoms

The primary lesion, or chancre, is usually a painless genital ulcer. The chancre may be intravaginal, cervical, or vulvar and often is unnoticed. This lesion resolves without treatment, and, although often accompanied by lymphadenopathy, is rarely associated with systemic symptoms.

The secondary stage, which occurs within 6 weeks of healing of the primary lesion, is characterized by a generalized rash with palmar and plantar predilection. Except for vesicular rashes, any type of rash is seen in secondary syphilis.

The latency period after lesion syphilis and before symptoms of late syphilis occur is divided into early latency (< 1 year) and late latency (≥ 1 year). During this period, the only evidence of infection is a reactive serologic test. Women are more likely to present during latency because lesions or their significance are often not recognized by the patient.

Occasionally, women with HIV infection may have unusual clinical manifestations or an atypical course of early syphilis, with more frequent presentation, and persistence of chancres, in the secondary stage (Hutchinson, Hook, Shepherd, Verley, & Rompalo, 1994). Titers may be higher in HIV-infected patients, and biologic false-positive results have been described. HIV-infected persons with syphilis should be evaluated with lumbar puncture and should be treated with regimens effective in eradicating central nervous system infection (CDC, 1993b).

Therapeutic and Behavioral Interventions

Injectable penicillin is the optimal therapy. Nonpenicillin regimens are less effective and subject to noncompliance. Oral desensitization should be used for penicillin-allergic pregnant or HIV-infected women and for neurosyphilis.

Primary prevention of syphilis and other STDs includes deferring initiation of sexual activity, reducing the number of sexual partners, and using effective barrier methods of contraception. Additionally, the epidemiology of syphilis in the late 1980s and 1990s suggests that focusing prevention strategies on prostitutes and their partners, drug users, and pregnant women would greatly reduce the incidence of syphilis among women (Ernst, Romolo, & Nick, 1993). Standard interventions in secondary prevention, including identification of sexual partners of heterosexual men with early syphilis, have contributed to the decline of syphilis in the 1990s; these efforts merit continuing support.

Implications

The most important implication of the syphilis diagnosis in a female patient is that this is among the most prominent risk factors for HIV infection, presumably because of high-risk behaviors and because genital ulcers may increase transmission of HIV (Otten, Zaidi, Peterman, Rolfs, & Witte, 1994). Women with syphilis are candidates for HIV screening and intervention to reduce risk of HIV transmission. Syphilis may also increase heterosexual transmission of hepatitis B (Bratos et al., 1993). Women diagnosed with syphilis should be questioned regarding their last menstrual period, and pregnancy tests should be offered to determine the need for measures to prevent congenital syphilis (CDC, 1993b).

Gonorrhea

Epidemiology

The incidence of gonorrhea, like the incidence of primary and secondary syphilis, rose during the late 1960s. The rate for gonorrhea peaked in 1976, then declined, diverging from trends in primary and secondary syphilis in 1985 (Fig. 12–3). However, gonorrhea continues to be the most common reportable infectious disease in the United States (CDC, Division of STD/HIV Prevention, 1994). Rates of gonorrhea are much higher than rates of primary and secondary syphilis and are high or rising among female African American children (10–14 years of age) and adolescents (15–19 years of age). Incidence of gonorrhea among female children and adolescents is higher than among male children and peaks in adolescence.

The epidemiology of gonorrhea has changed since 1981, with increasing concentration of cases in "core" groups, consisting of highly sexually active individu-

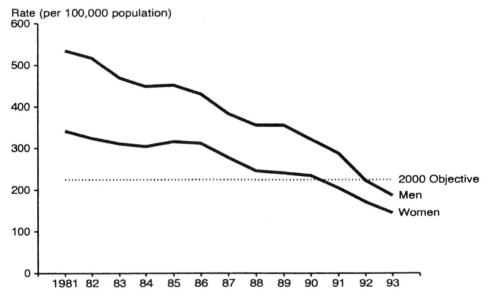

Figure 12-3. Gonorrhea—Rates by gender: United States, 1981-1993 and the year 2000 objective. (Source: Centers for Disease Control and Prevention, Division of STD/HIV Prevention.)

als, often disadvantaged members of racial minorities. The strongest risk factors for gonorrhea among women is young age at first intercourse. In some core groups, drug use and prostitution are also risk factors (Phillips, Hanff, Wertheimer, & Aronson, 1988).

Among women, lower genital tract gonorrhea is often asymptomatic (Morse & Holmes, 1994). The risk of acquiring gonorrhea is approximately 35% among men after one exposure to an infected woman, but rises to 75% with reexposures. Risk of gonorrhea transmission from the male to female partner is higher. Pharyngeal infection is more common among women because fellatio is more likely than cunnilingus to result in pharyngeal infection.

As many as 50% of women who become infected develop pelvic inflammatory disease (PID) (see below) (Morse & Holmes, 1994). Women account for most cases of disseminated gonococcal infection (DGI) because they are less likely to be recognized as being infected early in the course of infection and because menstruation, pregnancy, and pharyngeal gonorrhea are all risk factors for dissemination (Holmes, Counts, & Beaty, 1971).

Etiology

The etiologic agent of gonorrhea is a gram-negative diplococcus, *Neisseria gonorrhoeae*. The site of infection is the columnar epithelium of the endocervix.

Clinical Symptoms

Genital Infection. The true rate of symptoms among women with gonorrhea is uncertain and varies considerably with the clinical setting. Most women with gonorrhea who experience symptoms complain of vaginal discharge due to cervicitis, unilateral labial swelling and pain (bartholinitis), abnormal menstrual bleeding, Bartholin abscess, or lower abdominal pain with tenderness on adnexal palpation. Rate of *N. gonorrhoeae* recovery varies from 6% among some asymptomatic populations to 30% to 82% of women with PID (Morse & Holmes, 1994).

Anorectal Infection. The primary site of infection is usually the endocervix, with secondary contamination of the anorectal area due to vaginal discharge. Direct infection also probably occurs during anal intercourse. Anorectal infection is more common in women than in heterosexual men and may be asymptomatic or present with tenesmus, constipation, mucopurulent rectal discharge, and bleeding (Morse & Holmes, 1994).

Disseminated Gonococcal Infection. Since the introduction of antimicrobials, women have tended to predominate among DGI cases because they are more likely to be asymptomatic and less likely to receive early treatment (Holmes et al., 1971).

Arthritis is the most common manifestation of DGI (Holmes et al., 1971). Two clinical forms exist. The first, or bacteremic form, presents with fever, chills, gonococcemia, and polyarticular arthritis or tenosynovitis. This polyarthritis generally presents with scant effusion and affects knees, wrists, ankles, elbows, and the small joints of the hands. Typical skin lesions are generally seen with this form of gono-coccal arthritis, beginning as small red papules or petechiae that may either resolve or evolve through vesicular then pustular stages to form a necrotic center on a he-morrhagic base.

The second, or monarticular form, presents with joint effusion, absence of bac-teremia and skin lesions, and positive cultures for *N. gonorrhoeae* from the synovial fluid. The bacteremic form may precede the septic joint stage.

Pregnancy has been recognized as a precipitating factor to dissemination in 28% to 40% of women reported with gonococcal arthritis; pregnancy or menstruation pre-cipitate dissemination in over 70% of women (Graber, Sanford, & Ziff, 1968). Gonococcal arthritis is diagnosed primarily in the last trimester but can occur earlier.

Subacute gonococcal endocarditis, most frequently involving the aortic valve, has been reported in women with DGI, generally preceded by polyarthritis (Holmes et al., 1971). Myocarditis, pericarditis, or rarely, meningitis is sometimes seen in gonococcemic patients.

Gonococcal Pelvic Inflammatory Disease. PID or acute salpingitis, is prob-ably the most common severe complication of gonorrhea (Westrom, 1980). Among the sequelae of PID are infertility due to tubal occlusion, chronic abdominal pain, and occasionally death, generally caused by rupture of tubo-ovarian abscesses (TOA), resulting in generalized peritonitis. Ectopic pregnancy also is strongly asso-ciated with past PID (Chow, Daling, Cates, & Greenberg, 1987).

Therapeutic and Behavioral Interventions

Therapy for gonorrhea and the decision to admit depend primarily on whether dissemination has occurred, the severity of symptoms, and lifespan issues, such as whether the patient is a child (CDC, 1993b). Intramuscular treatment with ceftriax-one is recommended for uncomplicated anal or genital gonorrhea. The diagnosis of gonorrhea in a child warrants admission and should prompt evaluation for sexual abuse. Adult PID patients should be managed as inpatients if the diagnosis is un-certain and emergencies such as ectopic pregnancy cannot be excluded; if pelvic abscess is suspected; if the patient is pregnant, is an adolescent, has HIV infection, or is unable to tolerate or follow outpatient management; or if clinical follow-up cannot be ensured (CDC, 1993b). Patients with DGI should always be admitted.

Gonorrhea and *C. trachomatis* infection tend to coexist, so patients treated for gonorrhea should also be treated for *C. trachomatis* (CDC, 1993b). In general, one-dose treatments are preferred.

Implications

Suppurative STDs, including gonorrhea and chlamydia infections, facilitate HIV heterosexual transmission, so the diagnosis of these common infections in popula-tions with high HIV infection prevalence suggests the possible need for screening and counseling for risk reduction (Laga et al., 1993). The link between these infec-tions and PID requires that management include measures to rule out or detect PID.

Chlamydia trachomatis

Epidemiology

Infection with *C. trachomatis* is the most common bacterial STD diagnosed in U.S. women. The prevalence has been estimated to be as high as 8% to 40% among sexually active women (Cates & Wasserheit, 1991). The incidence of *C. trachomatis* infection among U.S. women has risen considerably in the last 10 years; part of this apparent increase is due to increased availability of funding for testing in family planning clinics (Division of STD/HIV Prevention, CDC, 1994) (Fig. 12–4). Core groups, such as have been described for gonorrhea, have not been described for chlamydia infections (Zimmerman et al., 1990). Adolescents and young adults tend to have the highest prevalence. Risk factors for *C. trachomatis* infection among women include oral contraceptive use, cervical ectopy (endocervical tissue ectopically found in the exocervix), and sexual partners with nongonococcal urethritis (Harrison et al, 1985). Because cervical ectopy is commonly seen in adolescence and oral contraceptive use tends to induce ectopy, these risk factors may be linked. Endocervical cells are the targets of *C. trachomatis*, so ectopy may not only increase the risk of infection, but also the likelihood of recovering the organism during routine studies.

Etiology

Chlamydia trachomatis is one of two species in the genus *Chlamydia* (Arno & Jones, 1994). Serovars D, E, F, G, H, I, J, and K cause conjunctivitis, cervicitis, PID,

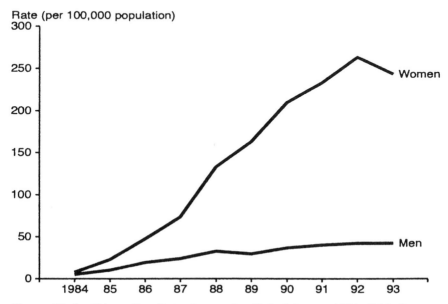

Figure 12-4. Chlamydia—Rates by gender: United States, 1984-1993. (Source: Centers for Disease Control and Prevention, Division of STD/HIV Prevention.)

and infant pneumonia. Several diagnostic tests exist, including culture, nucleic acid probes, enzyme-linked immunoassays, and polymerase chain reaction tests.

Clinical Manifestations

Manifestations of *C. trachomatis* infection in women include cervicitis, with scant cervical discharge, contact bleeding, and friability; dysuria and urgency; PID, which is often silent; and, less commonly, perihepatitis and pelvic abscess. Mucopurulent cervicitis, often with friability, is often seen, but the majority of women with infections are asymptomatic.

Therapeutic Interventions

Azithromycin 1 g orally allows treatment in one dose with efficacy similar to doxycycline (CDC, 1993b). Treatment of infected pregnant women with erythromycin may prevent infant infection (CDC, 1993b). Patients should be instructed to refer sexual partners for treatment.

Implications

Among the important implications are the possibilities of infertility and ectopic pregnancy. Reinfection is extremely common, so past *C. trachomatis* infection is an indication for frequent reexamination (CDC, 1993b). Research on the safety of one-dose regimens in adolescents aged less than 15 years is vital because they are at high risk of infection, recurrence, and noncompliance.

Pelvic Inflammatory Disease

Epidemiology

The number of hospitalizations for PID in the United States has decreased during the 1980s, whereas the number of patients seen in physicians' offices did not vary significantly, suggesting a decrease in incidence of the more severe manifestations or changes in patterns of hospitalization (Rolfs, Galaid, & Zaidi, 1992). The proportion of cases of PID caused by *N. gonorrhoeae* varies considerably by population. *N. gonorrhoeae* and *C. trachomatis* cause about 50% of PID; other organisms, including *Mycoplasma* species and anaerobic organisms, cause the rest.

Etiology

See Gonorrhea and *C. trachomatis* infections.

Clinical Manifestations

PID tends to present with lower abdominal pain and adnexal tenderness. Spread of infection into the abdomen may cause perihepatitis with adhesions. Fitz-

Hugh–Curtis syndrome is typified by right upper quadrant pain, a friction rub, and "violin string" adhesions between the liver capsule and the pelvic organs. Women with PID may have higher rate of HIV seropositivity (Hoegsberg et al., 1990).

Therapeutic Considerations

Cefoxitin 2g every 6 hours and Doxycycline 100 mg every 12 hours is usually effective (CDC, 1993).

Implications

PID may be more severe in women with HIV infection and with more surgical interventions and pelvic abscesses (Hoegsberg et al., 1990). *N. gonorrhoeae* tends to cause a more severe clinical picture, but PID due to *C. trachomatis* is more likely to result in tubal occlusion; ectopic pregnancy and infertility may result.

Vaginitis and Vaginosis

Epidemiology

Vaginal discharge is the common presenting complaint of inflammatory processes causing vaginitis and bacterial vaginosis, which result from replacement of the normal H_2O_2-producing *Lactobacillus* species with anaerobic bacteria. The number of visits to physicians for trichomoniasis has remained stable for over 30

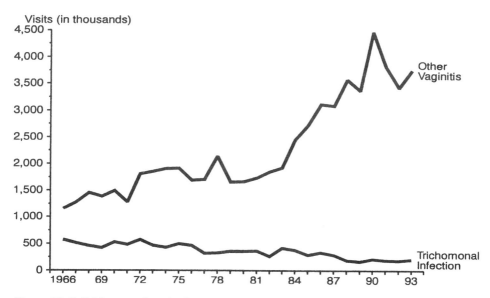

Figure 12-5. Trichomonal and other vaginal infections—Initial visits to physicians' offices: United States, 1966-1993. (Source:National Disease and Therapeutic Index [IMS America, Ltd].)

years, but the number of visits for other types of vaginitis has increased considerably (Fig. 12–5).

Etiology

The three common diseases characterized by vaginal discharge include trichomoniasis (caused by *Trichomonas vaginalis*), bacterial vaginosis (caused by replacement of the normal vaginal flora by overgrowth of anaerobes, including *Bacteroides* species and *Mobiluncus* species, *Gardnerella vaginalis*, and *Mycoplasma hominis*) (CDC, 1993b), and candidiasis due to *Candida albicans*. Candidiasis is not usually transmitted sexually and is frequently seen in women during pregnancy, with use of antimicrobials that allow overgrowth of *C. albicans*, and in hyperglycemic women. Cervicitis due to *C. trachomatis* and *N. gonorrhoeae* sometimes presents with discharge.

Forgotten tampons, pessaries, diaphragms, and other foreign bodies in the vagina often present with vaginal discharge, usually foul smelling. Douching and deodorants may result in vaginitis.

Clinical Manifestations

Vaginal discharge is the most common presenting complaint, along with local irritation, itching, burning, and odor. Although laboratory diagnosis is needed to confirm the etiologic agent, hyperemic appearance of the vaginal mucosa, with hemorrhagic petechiae in the posterior fornix and cervix ("strawberry vagina") suggests trichomoniasis. Thick, white curdlike discharge suggests candidiasis. A white, homogeneous, noninflammatory discharge suggests bacterial vaginosis.

Narrow-range pH paper can confirm pH of vaginal discharge greater than 4.5, which suggests bacterial vaginosis or trichomoniasis (CDC, 1993b). Preparations of discharge specimens diluted in 0.9% normal saline solution examined under low and high dry power can show motile *T. vaginalis* or clue cells, which suggest bacterial vaginosis. Preparations diluted in 10% potassium hydroxide can show pseudohyphae and yeast of *Candida* species.

Therapeutic Considerations

Only women with symptomatic vaginal disease require treatment for bacterial vaginosis, candidiasis, or trichomoniasis; screening for asymptomatic disease in healthy women is not needed. However, metronidazole treatment of bacterial vaginosis in asymptomatic women may reduce postabortion PID, and in pregnant women, may reduce risk of premature labor.

Women with bacterial vaginosis may be treated with one dose of 2 g metronidazole (CDC, 1993b). For vulvovaginal candidiasis, topical azole drugs are more effective than nystatin. Trichomoniasis is treated with metronidazole for 7 days.

Implications

Speculum examination in postpubertal women with vaginal discharge can rule out such causes as foreign bodies. Laboratory diagnosis is essential to diagnose coinfections and confirm etiology. Systemic illnesses, such as diabetes or HIV, should be considered in women with severe, recurrent candidal vulvovaginitis in the absence of obvious risk factors, such as pregnancy, particularly if associated with unexplained weight loss and other suggestive symptoms. Bacterial vaginosis, or the altered vaginal microflora characteristic of bacterial vaginosis, is associated with *Escherichia coli* introital colonization and acute cystitis in women who use diaphragms and may cause premature labor (Hooton, Fihn, Johnson, Roberts & Stamm, 1989) (see section on urinary tract infections).

Herpes Simplex Virus

Epidemiology

Approximately 30 million U.S. persons have had herpes simplex virus-2 (HSV-2) infection (Johnson et al., 1989). The number of initial visits to physicians for genital herpes may be increasing (Division of STD/HIV Prevention, CDC, 1994).

Etiology

Genital herpes is caused by infection with HSV-1 or HSV-2, with most cases caused by serotype HSV-2. Most women infected with HSV never recognize the infection and in only a minority are the symptoms recurrent.

Genital ulcer disease may be nonspecific and more than one pathogen may coexist in a genital lesion, so diagnosis by tissue culture may aid clinical decision-making (see section on lifespan of STDs). Viral isolation in tissue culture is the most sensitive and specific method of confirming a diagnosis of genital herpes.

Clinical Manifestations

Most women with primary genital HSV-2 infection report a prolonged duration of systemic and local symptoms, including fever, headache, myalgia, and malaise (Kinghorn, 1993), which appear early in the course of the disease, peak within the first 4 days after onset of lesions, and gradually recede. Painful lesions in the vulva, vagina, and cervix; itching; severe dysuria, both internal and external, due to urine touching the lesions; vaginal discharge; and tender inguinal adenopathy are reported by most women. Widely spaced bilateral ulcerative or pustular lesions on the external genitals are common. Some women's lesions start as vesicles or papules, but often, only local pain is reported. The lesions generally coalesce into large areas of ulceration (Fig. 12–6). The mean time from onset of lesions to last positive culture and to complete reepithelialization is longer in women than in men.

Therapeutic Considerations

Systemic acyclovir provides partial relief from symptoms and signs of genital herpes when used to treat the first clinical episode or when used as suppressive therapy (CDC, 1993b).

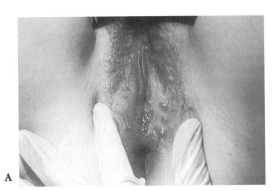
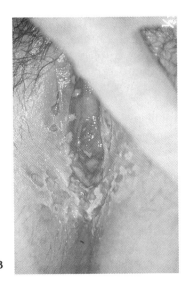

A   B

*Figure 12-6. Initial vesicular appearance of vaginal herpetic lesions (**A**) and coalescence into large ulcerations with inflammatory cells (**B**) typical of vulvovaginal herpes simplex infection. (Source: CDC Still Pictures Archive.)*

Implications

Patients should be advised to abstain from sexual activity while lesions are present and about the natural history of the disease, with emphasis on possible recurrences, asymptomatic viral shedding, and sexual transmission even without symptoms (Merz, Bendetti, Ashley, Selke, & Corey, 1992). Both male and female patients should be advised of the need for condom use, the risk of neonatal infection, and the fact that genital herpes appears to promote HIV transmission (Hook et al., 1992; Maccato, 1993).

Condylomata Acuminata, Cervical Cancer, and Other Human Papillomavirus Infections

Epidemiology

In 1842, Rigoni-Stern hypothesized that cervical cancer had an infectious sexually transmitted etiology. Since that time, numerous studies have confirmed the association between sexual risk factors and cervical cancer (Reeves, Rawls, & Brinton, 1989). The association between the putative etiologic agent, HPV, and cervical cancer was formally proposed in 1974 (zur Hausen, Meinhof, Schreiber, & Bornkamm, 1974). The first reports demonstrating HPV DNA in cervical cancer biopsies appeared in 1983, and the first case-control study associating HPV types 16/18 with cervical cancer was published in 1989 (Dürst, Gissman, Ikenberg, & zur Hausen, 1983; Reeves et al., 1994).

Cervical cancer exhibits many epidemiologic features of an STD. A woman's risk of cervical cancer increases significantly with increased number of sexual partners and younger age of sexual debut, with these two factors apparently function-ing independently. Male sexual behavior is also important. Spouses of women with cervical cancer have had more sex partners, earlier age at first intercourse, more ex-tramarital affairs, and are more likely to have used prostitutes than spouses of healthy women (Reeves et al., 1994). Factors including race, socioeconomic status, and obstetric history affect risk of cervical cancer. Other risk factors including diet, smoking, and host genetics have emerged in some studies.

Cervical cancer progresses from mild dysplastic lesions to cancer over a pro-longed period of at least 10 years, so early detection by Pap smear has significantly reduced the incidence of cervical cancer. But cervical cancer is the fourth most common cancer in African Americans, Hispanics, and Native Americans where less screening or other factors may play a role.

Etiology

Over 70 different HPV types infect human beings, and at least 25 of these in-fect the genital epithelium. These 25 types have been categorized as low risk (iden-tified in benign genital warts) or high risk (identified in genital cancers). HPVs initiate infection and replicate only in squamous epithelial cells.

Clinical Manifestations

Infection with HPV types 6 and 11 results in genital warts or condyloma acumi-nata. These warts most frequently form on the exposed vagina, vulva, or perineal area. Genital warts seldom progress to more than a benign warty lesion. Infection with high-risk HPV types, such as 16 and 18, can cause precancerous dysplastic le-sions of the squamous epithelium, variously termed cervical intraepithelial neopla-sia (CIN) or squamous intraepithelial lesions (SIL) (Lundberg, 1989). Nearly all women with cervical cytologic findings of SIL have cervical HPV infection, and at least 25% to 50% of these are infected with HPV types 16 and 18 (Koutsky et al., 1992; Schiffman et al., 1993). Precancerous dysplastic lesions left untreated may progress to high-grade or invasive disease. As many as 40% of women with low-grade lesions may develop moderate to severe CIN lesions within 24 months of first detection of HPV 16 or 18 (Lundberg, 1989).

Therapeutic and Screening Considerations

Cervical cancer control programs use Papanicolaou (Pap) smears for the detec-tion of precancerous lesions. Early and aggressive treatment of cervical dysplasia has resulted in significant decreases in morbidity and mortality due to cervical can-cer while preserving fertility in many women. Sexually active women should have cervical Pap smears every 1 to 3 years as part of their initial and routine gyneco-logic care. The current practices are that if a Pap smear shows low-grade SIL, care-givers refer the woman for colposcopic evaluation and biopsy, if indicated (Cole, 1993). Some others follow this woman with repeat Pap smears at frequent intervals (eg, every 3–6 months). If a Pap smear indicates high-grade SIL or squamous cell carcinoma, the woman should be referred for colposcopic examination, and possibly, colposcopically directed biopsy for histologic confirmation. Standard treatment of CIN is to ablate dysplastic lesions. Currently, cervical cancer control programs do not include routine HPV testing (Lundberg, 1989). Prospective randomized trials are necessary to determine the efficacy of HPV testing as part of screening or in treatment selection.

Implications

As with any viral infection, the majority of cervical HPV infections are subclinical; a high proportion of low-grade lesions will spontaneously regress. Cervical HPV infection is more common among women infected with HIV, and prevalence of infection and cervical disease increase with immunosuppression (Vernon et al., 1994).

Human Immunodeficiency Virus

Epidemiology

Acquired immunodeficiency syndrome (AIDS) is being increasingly diagnosed in women; in 1990, only 10% of cases were reported in women, whereas in 1993, 16% were reported in women (Wortley, Chu, & Berkelman, 1995). HIV infection was now the leading cause of death among women 25 to 44 years of age in 15 East Coast U.S. cities with populations of more than 100,000 in 1992 (Selik & Chu, 1994). African American and Hispanic women are disproportionately affected, accounting for 76% of cases in 1993 (Chu & Wortley, 1995). Incidence rates for African American and Hispanic women were 77 and 41/100,000, respectively, in 1992, compared with 8, 5, and 3/100,000 for Native American, Caucasian, and Asian women, respectively.

The geographic distribution of the HIV epidemic among women is different from that among men; among women, it is concentrated in inner city areas of the Northeast and Southeast; rural areas in Southeast have also been affected.

The median age of patients at the time of AIDS diagnosis was 34 years in 1993, and more than 90% were reported in women aged 20 to 50 (Chu & Wortley, 1995); 28% of women were diagnosed under 30 years of age, indicating that many were infected during adolescence or early adulthood.

Most cases of AIDS among women are related to injection drug use, either because the women acquire HIV infection through injection drug use or through heterosexual transmission from injection drug users; the geographic distribution of AIDS is similar to that of drug use among women (Chu & Wortley, 1995) (Fig. 12–7). Injectable cocaine, because it is administered more frequently than heroin, appears to be associated with increased needle sharing. Crack cocaine, though not injectable, is associated with increased tendency to engage in unsafe sexual activity with multiple partners, especially exchanging sex for money or drugs, which greatly increases the likelihood for HIV transmission.

The proportion of AIDS cases attributed to heterosexual transmission more than doubled from 15% in 1983 to 39% in 1992 and exceeds the proportion infected through injection drug use in the South and in Puerto Rico (Chu & Wortley, 1995). Female-to-female transmission has been reported but is rare.

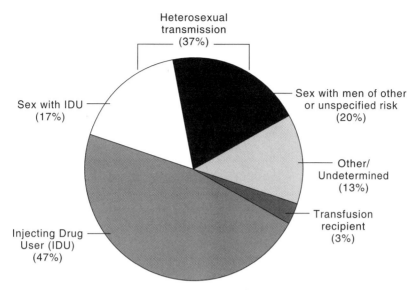

Figure 12-7. Women with AIDS, by mode of HIV transmission, United States, 1993. (Source: Centers for Disease Control and Prevention, Division of HIV/AIDS.)

In 1993, the case definition of AIDS was expanded to include all persons with HIV infection who had a CD4 cell count less than 200 microliters (CDC, 1993a). Three AIDS-defining illnesses were also added: TB, recurrent pneumonia, and invasive cervical carcinoma. A 126% increase in reported cases over 1992 was attributed to earlier reporting in the course of HIV disease, with the effect of increasing the number of persons living with AIDS. Even before the change in surveillance, the percentage increase for AIDS cases among women was greater (167%) than that for men (120%) (Chu & Wortley, 1995).

The increased incidence of HIV infection among young African American women tested through Job Corps applications and increased rates of STDs suggests that AIDS cases resulting from heterosexual transmission among disadvantaged women may continue to rise.

Etiology

Most AIDS cases and related illnesses are caused by HIV-1, a retrovirus, although most complications are due to opportunistic infections and malignancies (Abimuku & Gallo, 1995). Another retrovirus, HIV-2, also causes AIDS, mostly in West Africa.

Symptoms and Natural History

The extremely varied presentation of HIV infection is based on the fundamental abnormality, the progressive decrease in the number CD4+ lymphocytes

(DeHovitz, 1995). The decline in CD4 lymphocyte count is one of the most important predictors of disease progression and development of opportunistic infections.

Natural History. The natural history of HIV infection follows a series of stages usually defined by clinical disease and CD4 count (DeHovitz, 1995). Although some of the early clinical manifestations of symptomatic HIV disease are similar in men and women, some important differences are apparent. The most common gender-related clinical findings due to HIV infection in women are vulvovaginal candidiasis, cervical dysplasia, and carcinoma in situ (DeHovitz, 1995). Although some of these conditions do not meet the surveillance definition of AIDS, they have a clinical course or require management that is complicated by HIV infection.

In late HIV disease, patients generally have CD4 counts that range from 0 to 200, consistent with the case definition of AIDS. They are at high risk for developing a wide range of opportunistic infections, including *Pneumocystis carinii* pneumonia, toxoplasmosis, lymphoma, and cryptococcal meningitis (DeHovitz, 1995). Women with late HIV disease have a different distribution of opportunistic infection compared with men; *Candida* esophagitis and HSV and cytomegalovirus (CMV) infections are more common in women.

Genital Ulcers and Vaginal Candidiasis. Vaginal candidiasis is extremely common in women, and chronic vulvovaginal candidiasis is seen frequently in women with HIV infection. It is associated with development of severe opportunistic infections within a short period of time (DeHovitz, 1995; Fleming, Ciesielski, Byers, Castro, & Berkelman, 1991). Some studies suggest that candidiasis in women with HIV infection is more severe, has a higher tendency to recur, and may be more likely to be caused by non-*Albicans* species. The initial therapeutic approach should be with standard topical antifungal medication (Currier, 1995). Should that fail, or if candida vulvovaginitis recurs in the absence of such causes as oral contraceptives or antimicrobials, oral therapy with fluconazole may be used with careful monitoring of liver function tests.

Herpetic ulcers may take longer to resolve, warranting long-term use of suppressive doses of acyclovir (Currier, 1995). Dark-field negative genital ulcers have been described with negative HSV and chancroid cultures, which failed to respond to empirical syphilis treatment and resolved with zidovudine.

Cervical Human Papillomavirus Infection. Among patients with cervical cancer, women with HIV infection appear to have more rapid progression to advanced disease and more prompt recurrence (DeHovitz, 1995). Some HIV-infected women have died of cervical cancer, so that it is essential to screen HIV-infected women. Guidelines for the use of Pap tests recommend screening at intake, 6-month follow-up, and yearly, as long as the specimens were adequate for interpretation and were normal (CDC, 1993b).

Therapy

Primary care for HIV-infected women includes antiretroviral therapy, prevention and management of opportunistic infections, and the specific management of gynecologic manifestations of HIV disease (Currier, 1995). Too few women have been included in clinical trials to date to have interpretable data regarding gender-specific toxicities. Screening for TB (including tuberculin skin tests) and cervical disease are vital aspects of management.

Implications

The diagnosis of HIV infection in women has obvious implications for the long-term plans, contraception, prenatal care, and medical and psychosocial care of the patient, covered in different sections of this book (Dehovitz, 1995).

Sexually Transmitted Diseases Across the Lifespan

Sexual Abuse in Childhood

About 25% of the more than 2 million cases of suspected abuse or neglect reported each year in the United States are sexual abuse (Finkelhor, Hotaling, Lewis, & Smith, 1990; U.S. Department of Health and Human Services, 1988). Most victims are girls, possibly because of reporting bias.

In children in whom sexual abuse has occurred or is suspected, several studies should be routinely performed, even in asymptomatic children. Examination of the genitalia and the perianal area for warts, vaginitis, and evidence of trauma or other lesions should be performed (CDC, 1993b). Speculum examination should not be performed on prepubertal girls. The decision to evaluate children by collecting specimens for STDs when they are asymptomatic and have no physical findings suggestive of STDs should be made on an individual basis. If specimens are collected because of the suspicion of sexual abuse, collection should be according to a protocol designed to maximize the predictive positive and negative powers of such tests. Genital examination under anesthesia may be desirable for specimen collection.

The most frequently diagnosed STD in sexually abused children is gonorrhea, although *C. trachomatis* is often isolated from sexually abused children as well (Hammerschlag, 1994; Ingram, 1994). In children with evidence of one STD, it is essential to test for others.

Vulvovaginitis

Vulvovaginitis is a common complaint in prepubertal girls. Only rarely is an STD implicated. Other frequent causes include streptococcus or enteric organisms and infestations and rarely candidiasis. However, vaginitis is the most common presentation of gonococcal infection in children (Ingram, 1994). The neutral to alkaline pH and thin, atrophic nature of the prepubertal vagina predisposes to diffuse vaginitis and dysuria. The incubation period is brief, and although some children are asymptomatic, the child usually develops a purulent, sometimes foul-smelling discharge accompanied by labial erythema. PID presenting as lower abdominal pain and tenderness, rebound, decreased bowel sounds, and vaginal discharge occur in about 6% of prepubertal children with gonococcal vaginitis. All children with purulent vaginitis should have specimens for Gram stain and culture obtained from the hymen, outer first millimeters of the vagina, or from the discharge.

Chlamydia infection is generally asymptomatic but may present with vaginitis in children (Hammerschlag, 1994). Bacterial vaginosis and trichomoniasis can cause discharge in sexually abused girls but have been described without evidence of sexual activity (Jones, Yamauchi, & Lambert, 1985; Rudloff, 1991).

Anogenital Lesions

Anogenital lesions are less common in prepubertal children and may be more likely to be sexually acquired than vaginitis (Frasier, 1994). Warts, chancres, ulcers, and vesicles or pustules should be evaluated for HPV and HSV infection and syphilis.

Syphilis is relatively rare in sexually abused children. However, when it is diagnosed during the primary and secondary stages, it generally presents as anogenital condylomata lata. If a child has evidence of other STDs, is in a high syphilis prevalence population, or if the assailant is not available for testing but is suspected to belong to a high-risk group (eg, drug abuser), serologic screening for syphilis may be needed but will not be reactive during incubation.

Typically, HPV anogenital infection in prepubertal girls presents as verrucous, flesh-colored or reddish papules; the most common location is perianal in both boys and girls. The lesions may extend into the anal canal, the urethra, or hymen. The lesions are often asymptomatic or may become infected, causing pain, bleeding, dysuria, pruritus, or vaginitis. Other conditions, such as molluscum contagiosum, and skin tags should be considered in the differential diagnosis (Frasier, 1994).

It may be useful in determining the mode of transmission of anogenital warts in children to perform HPV DNA typing of anogenital warts (Frasier, 1994). Warts due to HPV types common in genital infection are more likely to be due to sexual transmission than those due to types seen in common skin warts, but sexual abuse should be considered in all children with genital warts.

Genital HSV infection presents in children as painful perineal lesions, dysuria, or vulvovaginitis. A history of sexual contact is common among children with genital herpes. Autoinoculation from oral lesions may result in genital herpes in children who have not been abused; this is particularly likely in children where eruption of genital tract vesicles was immediately preceded by oral lesions. But even in genital herpes due to HSV-1, evidence of sexual abuse should be sought in all cases.

Adolescence

Infection with *C. trachomatis* is the most frequently diagnosed STD in female adolescents, but gonorrhea is extremely common as well. PID is one of the most serious outcomes of STDs in adolescents. It is estimated that 16% to 20% of the women hospitalized with PID yearly are adolescents and that sexually active 15-year-old girls have 10 times the risk of PID that a 24-year-old has (Golden, Neuhoff, &

Cohen, 1989). HSV infection appears to be common among adolescents, and HPV and HIV infection and cervical dysplasia are increasingly common among adolescents (Gayle & d'Angelo, 1991).

The rate of primary and secondary syphilis among adolescent women (aged 15–19) increased by 112% in the years from 1985 through 1991; by 1991, their rate was almost twice that of adolescent men (CDC, Division of STD/HIV Prevention, 1994) (Fig. 12–8). During the syphilis epidemic, substance abuse, incarceration, prostitution, other STDs, and history of past sexual abuse were identified as risk factors for syphilis.

The STDs in adolescent women are generally detected by screening. Screening for STDs that are common and often asymptomatic should be part of routine care for sexually active adolescents. Urine-based screening strategies should be considered in populations with a high prevalence. Pap smears (and serologic tests for syphilis in high prevalence areas) should be performed on sexually active adolescents at least at intake.

Childbearing Years

Pregnancy

Prenatal care tends to be underused in precisely the populations where it is most urgently needed for the diagnosis and treatment of STDs: disadvantaged populations, adolescents, and drug users. This is due in large part to unavailability of services, long waits, overcrowding, and unacceptable service delivery, all of which reduce the possibility of early enrollment and screening. Treatment of STDs in preg-

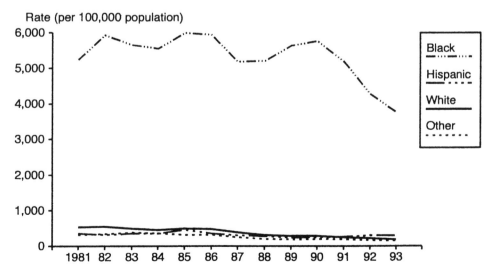

Figure 12-8. Gonorrhea—Reported rates for 15- to 19-year-old females by race and ethnicity: United States, 1981–1993. (Source: Centers for Disease Control and Prevention, Division of STD/HIV Prevention.)

nant women is limited by lack of research on use of several effective drugs during pregnancy, as well as the need to ensure safe treatment for the fetus.

Syphilis. Even in very low prevalence populations, routine syphilis screening during pregnancy with nontreponemal serologic tests is cost effective (Frau & Alexander, 1985). Untreated syphilis may cause fetal wastage, spontaneous abortion, prematurity, and congenital syphilis.

Gonorrhea and C. Trachomatis Infections. The incidence of gonorrhea among screened U.S. pregnant women has ranged from less than 1% to 7.5%; in 1983, positive cervical cultures for *N. gonorrhoeae* from prenatal and obstetric clinics and hospital inpatient obstetrics services ranged from 2.2% to 2.9% (Frau & Alexander, 1985).

Gonorrhea and *C. trachomatis* infections are associated with vertical transmission and adverse pregnancy outcomes, infant conjunctivitis, and other evidence of perinatal infection (Christmas et al., 1989). Coinfection may increase the likelihood of vertical transmission. Gonorrhea is also associated with postabortion endometritis.

Pharyngeal infection appears to be somewhat higher in antenatal populations than in similar nonpregnant populations; in two studies, the throat was the only infected site in 15% and 36% of pregnant women screened, respectively (Stutz, Spence, & Duangmani, 1976). This finding may be associated with behavior changes during pregnancy, such as an increase in fellatio (Solberg, Butler, & Wagner, 1973).

Gonococcal PID rarely occurs during pregnancy because it is difficult for the gonococci to traverse the barrier of the intact cervix and uterus during pregnancy. Nevertheless, some possible mechanisms of infection include infection at the time of fertilization or soon after, before uterine cavity closure, instrumentation, or ascending infection with threatened abortion and intrauterine bleeding (Acosta, Mabray, & Kaufman, 1970). Pelvic abscess can occur at any time of gestation, but acute PID in pregnancy, consistent with the mechanisms proposed, typically occurs in the first trimester (Blanchard, Pastorek, & Weeks, 1987). Pelvic abscesses and acute PID can generally be managed medically, so awareness of these entities may spare pregnant women abdominal surgery. Even with prompt medical treatment, fetal loss is common in pregnancies complicated by PID, approaching 50% (Acosta et al., 1970).

Screening with culture at the first prenatal visit is the ideal method of prevention, particularly in high prevalence populations. Probe-based assays are about as sensitive as culture. All patients with evidence of gonococcal infection early in pregnancy should have repeat testing during the last weeks of gestation. Testing for *C. trachomatis* should be performed late in the pregnancy.

Herpes Simplex Virus. From 1500 to 2000 cases of neonatal herpes (200–500/100,000 live births) occur yearly in the United States (Arvin & Prover, 1990). Approximately 67% to 80% are caused by HSV-2, generally because of contact with the birth canal, although some are due to postnatal or intrauterine HSV infection (Arvin & Prover, 1990). Primary maternal infection before 20 weeks of gestation is associated with abortion, stillbirth, hydrocephaly, and chorioretinitis. Cesarean section within 24 hours of rupture of membranes reduces the transmission rate to high-risk infants. Examination at onset of labor, with cesarean section in women who have genital herpes lesions at that time, is the most cost-effective strategy (Libman, Dascal, Kramer, & Mendelson, 1991).

Human Papillomavirus. Genital warts in women tend to become larger during pregnancy or cell-mediated immunosuppression and may complicate vaginal delivery. Podophyllin and podofilox for the treatment of condylomata acuminata are contraindicated during pregnancy (CDC, 1993b). Lesions tend to proliferate and become friable during pregnancy, so some experts advocate removal. Cesarean delivery should only be performed if the pelvic outlet is obstructed by genital warts or if vaginal delivery would result in excessive bleeding.

Human Immunodeficiency Virus. Yearly, approximately 1000 cases of HIV infection are reported among infants and children; over 90% are vertically acquired (CDC, 1994).

Prevalence of HIV infection among infants born to infected mothers generally ranges from 13% to 40%. Several maternal factors are associated with increased risk of HIV transmission to the infant (St. Louis et al., 1993). The highest transmission risk appears to be associated with maternal p24 antigenemia, low CD4+ lymphocyte counts, maternal CD8+ counts greater than 1.80×10^9/L, and placental membrane inflammation in women without the other risk factors. Infants delivered without complications and those delivered by uncomplicated cesarean section are less likely to be infected.

Zidovudine use during the pregnancy and delivery, with treatment of the infant during the neonatal period, reduces the risk of vertical transmission by over 60% (CDC, 1994), so pregnant women should be encouraged to receive pretest counseling, HIV testing, and information on zidovudine use. Breast-feeding should be discouraged.

Hepatitis B Immunization. Universal hepatitis B immunization at birth is currently recommended to prevent perinatal transmission.

Midlife and Beyond

The greatest impact of STDs after the childbearing years is from cervical cancer and HIV infection. Increasingly, women aged 50 and over are being diagnosed with AIDS; these women accounted for 8% of reported cases in 1993 (DeHovitz, 1995). Because of a failure to appreciate the role of these diseases in the care of perimenopausal women, and the fact that most women receive screening for cervical cancer in the context of contraception and may be less likely to be screened once contraception is no longer sought, HIV and STD screening for older women may be suboptimal. Although changes in sexual activity generally do result in decreased risk of STDs in the woman over age 35, the long-term consequences of such infections persist through life.

Other Gynecologic and Obstetric Infections

There is no routine surveillance of most gynecologic and obstetric infections. Most information about them is derived from series and studies. Because these infections are often related to reproductive activities (contraception, childbearing), they are seen most commonly in women of childbearing age. These are caused by a wide variety of organisms, among them anaerobic or sexually transmitted organisms, mycoplasmas, *Gardnerella* species, *Haemophilus influenzae*, and group B streptococcus.

The most common serious gynecologic infections are TOAs and postoperative, postpartum, and pregnancy-related infections.

Tubo-ovarian Abscess

Pelvic inflammatory disease, postoperative infections, and pelvic infections associated with an intrauterine device can result in a TOA. TOAs occur in approximately 10% to 15% of women with clinically recognized PID (Sweet & Gibbs, 1990). However, in several series, less than 50% of the women who developed TOAs had a history of PID. A TOA forms when purulent material collects in the area of the fallopian tube and ovary and encapsulation occurs, often with involvement of surrounding structures such as bowel, omentum, and bladder. It may be difficult to distinguish between a true abscess and a tubo-ovarian complex consisting of adherent tube, ovary, and adjacent structures without an actual abscess cavity. The microbiology of TOAs is poorly defined although anaerobic organisms such as *Bacteroides* are the most common isolates. TOA rupture is a surgical emergency and may result in overwhelming sepsis and death if not managed aggressively. Symptoms of a TOA are similar to those of PID, although if the abscess is unilateral, the pain may be localized on one side; they are most common in the third and fourth decades of life.

The diagnosis of TOA is by clinical examination, supplemented by ultrasonography, computed tomography (CT) scanning, or magnetic resonance imaging (MRI). Ultrasonography is adequate for diagnosis in most cases and is less expensive than CT or MRI. Most women with TOA will respond to intravenous antibiotic therapy using one of the regimens recommended for PID. Antibiotic regimens should include medications effective against anaerobes such as clindamycin, metronidazole or second- or third-generation cephalosporins; 60% to 70% of women with a TOA will respond to intravenous antibiotic with improvement in symptoms and reduction in fever, white blood cell count, or erythrocyte sedimentation rate. If improvement does not occur, surgical intervention must be considered. Alternatives include total abdominal hysterectomy and bilateral salpingo-oophorectomy, posterior colpotomy, unilateral adnexectomy, percutaneous ultrasound or CT-guided drainage, or laparoscopic drainage. All of the procedures, except hysterectomy/salpingo-oophorectomy, may allow future fertility.

Postoperative Pelvic Infections

Because gynecologic surgical procedures frequently involve exposure to vaginal organisms, postoperative infections caused by these organisms are common. Many of the organisms found in the normal vaginal flora have the potential to produce postoperative pelvic infection, particularly in women with predisposing factors including pelvic malignancy, obesity, immunosuppression, and medical problems such as diabetes or collagen vascular or cardiovascular disease. Patients undergoing emergency, prolonged, or extensive surgery may also be at increased risk.

Pelvic cellulitis or a pelvic abscess after an abdominal or vaginal hysterectomy typically presents with fever, leukocytosis, and lower abdominal pain within the first 72 hours postoperatively (Darney, 1987). Physical examination reveals tenderness in the lower abdomen and in the vaginal cuff and parametrial areas. If an abscess or infected hematoma is present, a mass may be present adjacent to the vaginal cuff. Because postoperative infections are typically polymicrobial and include gram-negative and gram-positive aerobes and anaerobes, broad-spectrum antibiotic coverage is indicated. A variety of antibiotic regimens have proven successful in eradicating postoperative infections including combinations of an aminoglycoside with second- or third-generation cephalosporins or with clindamycin or metronidazole. If a cuff abscess or infected hematoma is identified, vaginal drainage is indicated.

Postoperative endometritis may occur after an induced abortion or, infrequently, after diagnostic dilatation and curettage. The incidence of postabortal endometritis is approximately 1% and is frequently associated with retained tissue. On pelvic examination, the uterus is tender and, if tissue is present, the uterus is softened and enlarged beyond the expected size. Ultrasound will verify the presence of tissue. Treatment includes antibiotics and vacuum aspiration of tissue, if necessary. If the symptoms are mild and tenderness is confined to the uterus, outpatient antibiotic therapy with doxycycline or amoxicillin-clavulanate should be given for 7 to 10 days. If the patient is febrile or has evidence of peritonitis, she should receive intravenous antibiotics (Darney, 1987).

Antibiotic prophylaxis reduces the risk of postoperative infections in all women undergoing vaginal hysterectomy and in women at high risk undergoing abdominal hysterectomy. A single dose of a first-generation cephalosporin such as cefazolin or cephalothin should be given at least 30 minutes before surgery. Women at increased risk for postabortal infection may benefit from preoperative prophylaxis with doxycycline.

Postpartum Infection

Postpartum endometritis occurs in only 1% to 2% of women who give birth vaginally, but in women undergoing cesarean delivery the rate may be as high as 50%. Risk factors include prolonged labor, prolonged rupture of membranes, chorioamnionitis, use of internal fetal monitoring, and multiple cervical examinations. Infection rates are also higher among women of lower socioeconomic status. Postpartum and postcesarean endometritis are polymicrobial infections, and the vaginal flora is the usual source of organisms. Other implicated organisms include group A β-hemolytic streptococci, sexually transmitted organisms, and mycoplasmas. However, the role of sexually transmitted organisms as primary pathogens is unclear (Gibbs & Sweet, 1994).

Signs and symptoms of postpartum infection include fever, lower abdominal pain, uterine tenderness, and foul-smelling and purulent lochia. Blood and uterine cultures should be obtained, but antibiotic choice is usually empirical. Postpartum endometritis often responds rapidly to a combination of a penicillin and an aminoglycoside. Postcesarean endometritis may require more aggressive therapy, and appropriate antibiotic regimens include second- and third-generation cephalosporins, clindamycin-gentamicin, penicillin-β-lactamase inhibitors, and extended-spectrum penicillins. In patients with risk factors for infection, antibiotic prophylaxis reduces the risk of postcesarean endometritis and wound infection by approximately 50%. A single- or three-dose regimen of a first-generation cephalosporin should be started immediately after the cord is clamped.

Infections During Pregnancy

Many nonsexually transmitted infections may occur during pregnancy, but few (including toxoplasmosis, rubella, group B streptococcus, and CMV) affect the fetus severely.

Toxoplasmosis is caused by the intracellular protozoan, *Toxoplasma gondii*, that is contracted from ingesting infected raw or undercooked meat or from contact with the feces of infected domestic cats (American College of Obstetricians and Gynecologists [ACOG], 1994; Gibbs & Sweet, 1994). Approximately one-third of pregnant women in the United States have acquired immunity. Seroconversion during pregnancy is uncommon, with approximately 1 to 3 newborns per 1000 showing evidence of congenital infection. The rate of fetal infection increases with gestational age from about 20% in the first trimester to 60% in the third trimester. The severity of fetal infection decreases with advancing gestational age. Maternal infection is often subclinical but may be associated with headache, fatigue, myalgia, and cervical lymphadenopathy. Congenital infection is also frequently subclinical but may be associated with the triad of chorioretinitis, microcephaly or hydrocephalus, and intracerebral calcifications. When infection is suspected during pregnancy, serologic testing through a recognized reference laboratory may provide confirmation. With severe fetal infection, ultrasound may reveal microcephaly or hydrocephaly, growth retardation, or hepatosplenomegaly. Infection early in pregnancy is associated with approximately a 15% risk of severe congenital infection, and, particularly if there is ultrasound evidence of infection, pregnancy termination may be considered. Antibiotic treatment with sulfadiazine, pyrimethamine, and spiramycin appears to decrease the risk of congenital infection in the face of documented maternal infection. However, prevention is the cornerstone of management in the United States. Pregnant women should avoid eating undercooked meat and should wash their hands and kitchen surfaces after handling raw meat. Domestic cats should be kept indoors; maternal contact with the litter should be avoided (ACOG, 1994; Gibbs & Sweet, 1994).

Group B streptococcus may be found in the vaginal flora of 5% to 40% of women and may associated with severe neonatal illness. The rate of colonization appears to be highest among women under age 20. Preterm and low-birthweight infants are at greatest risk for infection. Prolonged rupture of the membranes and maternal fever are also risk factors for infection. Transmission may occur with ascent of the organisms from the vagina after membrane rupture or in the birth canal at the time of delivery. The transmission rate is approximately 60%, but the attack rate for serious infection is much lower, approximating 0.1% to 0.3% for early onset and 0.05% for late onset infection. Early onset disease usually occurs within 24 hours of birth and is associated with fulminant sepsis and pneumonia. The case fatality rate is approximately 10% to 20%, with the higher rates among premature and low-birthweight infants. Late onset disease occurs more than 7 days after birth, is typically manifested by meningitis, and may be associated with subsequent neurologic sequelae in up to 50% of infected infants. The management of group B streptococcus colonization during pregnancy and the prevention of neonatal infection remain controversial. Universal screening at 26 to 28 weeks and treatment of colonized women intrapartum if risk factors, such as prolonged membrane rupture, are present, and universal antimicrobial treatment of unscreened women who present in labor with a risk factor have been recommended. The most commonly used drug is ampicillin during labor (ACOG, 1994).

Cytomegalovirus is the most common cause of congenital infection, affecting approximately 1% of all live births (Cederqvist, 1994). Ten percent of infected newborns will have symptomatic disease with serious neurologic sequelae including mental retardation and sensorineural hearing loss. Approximately 4000 symptomatic infants are born annually in the United States. An additional 6000 infected, asymptomatic infants will develop milder late sequelae such as hearing loss and learning disabilities. Primary maternal infection during early pregnancy is most likely to result in severe congenital infection. However, recurrent maternal infections may also result in congenital infection although the risk of serious neurologic sequelae is small. Maternal seroprevalence is lowest in higher socioeconomic groups, and approximately 50% of higher-income women are susceptible to primary infection during pregnancy. Maternal infection is invariably asymptomatic, and the majority of newborns born with congenital infection are also asymptomatic. Management of CMV during pregnancy is complicated by the high rate of asymptomatic maternal virus excretion (about 10%) and the lack of symptoms with primary infection. Routine serologic screening is not indicated because there is no vaccine, and detection of the virus provides little prognostic information. No treatment is available (Cederqvist, 1994).

Although immunization has markedly reduced the incidence of rubella in the United States, approximately 10% of pregnant women are susceptible. Seronegative women of reproductive age should be identified and immunized before pregnancy. Up to 50% of rubella infections in the first trimester will result in the congenital rubella syndrome including cataracts, mental retardation, deafness, or congenital heart defects. Maternal infection is characterized by a macular rash, malaise, arthralgia, and postauricular adenopathy. Acute and convalescent serologic tests will document infection. Because of the high risk of fetal damage, women with documented first trimester rubella infection may consider abortion.

Because these infections are generally related to reproduction and contraception, they are a concern for women largely from adolescence through late thirties. Women receiving family planning and prenatal services, and during labor and delivery, particularly cesarean delivery, are the focus of preventive efforts to reduce the incidence and complications of gynecologic infections.

Therapeutic Interventions

Aside from specific antimicrobial and surgical procedures to treat these infections, guidelines that are highly effective in reducing the risk of these infections and early detection and effective treatment should be incorporated in surgical, delivery and intrauterine device management procedures. For example, careful preoperative management of women with diabetes before surgical procedures, avoidance of retention of fetal parts after abortion, reduction of unnecessary examinations and instrumentation during labor and delivery, and preconceptional counseling and prenatal care in high-risk women may greatly reduce the risk and severity of these infections.

Implications

Aside from the short-term real risk, though small, of death, TOA and other gynecologic infections are associated with increased risk of infertility, chronic pelvic pain, adhesions, and other problems, particularly when complicated by peritonitis.

Tuberculosis

Epidemiology

The number of cases of TB in the United States has increased considerably in the late 1980s and early 1990s, primarily because of increases among immigrant and underserved minority populations and the effect of HIV infection on the risk of activation (Cantwell, Snider, Cauthen, & Onorato, 1994; Selwyn et al., 1989). The clinical course of TB, with infection, latency, and reactivation, is well described. Reactivation of infections during adolescence is somewhat more common in females. Active TB is primarily pulmonary, even in persons with HIV infection. Pelvic TB is is very rare among U.S. women but is occasionally seen in immigrants, and in some areas of the developing world. One case was described after occupational infection (Shireman, 1992). Rarely, cases of vulvar primary lesions have occurred, but most cases of pelvic TB are secondary to an extragenital source, usually pulmonary (Anonymous, 1978).

Etiology

Mycobacterium tuberculosis is the most common cause of granulomatous pelvic infections, the typical presentation of pelvic TB (Anonymous, 1978). Pelvic TB almost always primarily involves the fallopian tubes.

Clinical Manifestations

The most common symptom of genital TB in women is infertility although dysmenorrhea and dyspareunia are also frequently reported (Margolis, Wranz, Kruber, Joubert, & Odendal, 1992). Most women with pelvic TB have no specific symptoms suggestive of TB, and pelvic TB is most often diagnosed by culture of menstrual fluid (De Vynck et al., 1990; Oosthuizen, Wessels, & Hefer, 1990). Tuberculous salpingitis generally presents in a similar fashion as PID caused by other etiologies. Ascites in a younger woman with adnexal masses and a fixed uterus suggests the possibility of pelvic TB with secondary peritonitis.

Risk Factors

The most important risk factor for reactivation from infection to active TB among women, as among men, is HIV infection (Cantwell et al., 1994). Pregnancy can also cause reactivation although some studies suggest that the risk associated with pregnancy is overstated (Margono, Mrouech, Garely, White, & Minkoff, 1994). Diabetes, particularly insulin-dependent diabetes, is an important risk factor for reactivation as well. Women who are being treated for autoimmune and other disease with immunosuppressive doses of corticosteroids and malnourished and homeless women are also at high risk of progression.

Complications, including preterm labor and intrauterine growth retardation, have been reported in women with TB (Margono et al., 1994). Pregnant women with drug-susceptible strains can be treated safely with isoniazid, rifampin, and ethambutol. The safety of pyrazinamide to the fetus is uncertain.

In general, infertility among women in very high TB prevalence populations should prompt inclusion of pelvic TB in the differential. PID in women with a history of TB, refractory to effective antimicrobial therapy, or occurring in young virginal or in elderly, postmenopausal patients suggests tuberculous etiology (De Vynck, 1990; Oosthuizen et al., 1990; Margolis et al., 1992). PPD skin testing, with allergy testing, should be performed in persons with HIV infections and HIV testing should be offered to women with TB.

Therapeutic Considerations

The cornerstone of TB treatment is chemotherapy with three or more antituberculous drugs, including isoniazid and rifampin. Intrauterine pregnancy is rare after genital TB, occurring when genital TB is diagnosed and treated early with both chemotherapy and surgical reconstruction; ectopic pregnancy can occur after therapy and may be catastrophic (Durukan, Urman, Yrali, Arikan, & Beykal, 1990).

Urinary Tract Infections

Epidemiology

Approximately one-third of women have a urinary tract infection (UTI) during their lives (Stamm, McKevitt, Roberts, & White, 1991). Uncomplicated UTI in women of reproductive age prompt 6 to 7 million office visits a year, making this the most common problem seen by physicians in primary care in this population. Many women suffer multiple recurrences of UTI in their lifetime. After menopause, the frequency of UTIs and recurrences increases considerably (Privette, Cade, Peterson, & Mars, 1988). UTIs are an important cause of hospitalization and are the most common hospital- and nursing home-acquired infection among women (Gleckman, 1992). UTIs are particularly common among catheterized women in nursing homes and are the most common cause of community-acquired bacteremia.

Etiology

Escherichia coli is the most common cause of acute bacterial cystitis, acute symptomatic pyelonephritis, and asymptomatic bacteriuria among patients at home, hospitals, and nursing homes (Gleckman, 1992). *E. coli* causes over 85% to 90% of these infections in young women and slightly fewer in elderly women. The distal urethra normally is colonized by enteric and perineal bacteria, particularly fecal *E. coli*, which enter the bladder through urethral trauma, retrograde movement during intercourse or masturbation, and turbulent flow in the short female urethra.

Staphylococcus saprophyticus is the second most common uropathogen in young women with acute symptomatic bacterial cystitis but is a very unusual pathogen in elderly women with symptomatic UTI. Other pathogens, such as enterococci and *Candida* species, are seen in hospitalized, institutionalized, and older women. *C. trachomatis* can cause urethritis in young, sexually active women. Group B streptococcus can cause UTI in nonpregnant women, and in pregnant women, group B streptococcus bacteriuria is associated with spontaneous abortion, premature rupture of membranes, endometritis, and neonatal infection. In recurrent UTIs and those associated with catheterization, other, more resistant gram-negative organisms may be seen.

Clinical Manifestations

Throughout their lifespan, women are more likely to develop UTIs than men, for anatomic, physiologic, and hormonal reasons, which play different roles during their lifetimes. However, among newborns, UTIs are more common in boys and generally present as nonspecific signs of sepsis, decreased activity, and feeding. In young girls, cystitis may present as daytime dribbling, nocturnal enuresis, dysuria, frequency, urgency, abdominal and suprapubic pain, low-grade fever, or hematuria or pyuria (Marks, 1987). Foul-smelling urine may be the only complaint in girls who have otherwise asymptomatic bacteriuria and normal genitourinary tracts. Dysuria and frequency are also common among reproductive age women with cystitis.

In elderly persons, UTIs may present with nonspecific symptoms and signs of lowered mental status, confusion, lethargy, and loss of interest in eating, drinking, socialization, and self-care. Elderly women with central nervous system disorders who have unexplained changes in mental status, such as stupor, anorexia, or aggressiveness, should be evaluated for UTI because these are frequently associated with bacteriuria and pyuria. Frequency, incontinence, nocturia, and abdominal pain are often seen in noncatheterized women with UTI. Fever is a common sign in elderly women, but hypothermia is also seen.

The classic symptoms and signs of pyelonephritis (chills, fever, flank pain, and costovertebral angle tenderness) are unusual in young children, somewhat more common in older children and young women, and not a constant finding at any age. Renal parenchymal infection can often be demonstrated in asymptomatic UTI. Recurrence is common after pyelonephritis.

Lifespan Issues

Urinary tract infection in young girls after infancy should prompt obtaining of a careful history with particular attention to previous UTIs, trauma, foreign bodies, sexual activity, and neuropsychiatric conditions (Marks, 1987). Specimen collection for urinalysis and urine culture and sensitivity should be done with a midstream clean-catch technique if therapy can be temporarily withheld and the child can cooperate.

Sexual intercourse, obesity, and diaphragm or contraceptive jelly use for contraception are associated with increased incidence of bacteriuria and UTI (Forland, 1993). Bacterial vaginosis, or the altered microflora associated with the high vaginal pH seen in bacterial vaginosis, is also associated with *E. coli* vaginal colonization and UTI among women who use diaphragms (Hooton et al., 1989). The incidence of bacteriuria appears to increase during pregnancy. Bacteriuria and UTI during pregnancy have been implicated in premature labor, low birthweight, other adverse outcomes, and neonatal UTI and sepsis. Prompt diagnosis and treatment of UTI during pregnancy may result in reduction in risk of prematurity.

In premenopausal women, circulating estrogens encourage colonization of the vagina by lactobacilli. These organisms produce lactic acid from glycogen, which inhibits the growth of uropathogens. Menopause is associated with reduction of lactobacilli, increase in vaginal pH, and vaginal colonization with uropathogens, particularly *E. coli*. Other factors associated with aging, including incomplete bladder emptying, incontinence, and poor perineal hygiene, also play a role in the increased risk of UTI. Many elderly institutionalized women with asymptomatic bacteriuria have upper UTI (Gleckman, 1992).

Therapeutic Considerations

Prevention. Considerable research has been undertaken to reduce UTI recurrence. In children, when an underlying cause of obstruction or infection can be defined, such as fecal contamination, foreign body, pinworms, or detergent irritation, removal or avoidance of these factors will reduce recurrences (Marks, 1987). No evidence of renal damage or other adverse outcomes has been identified in children with recurrent UTIs if not due to underlying etiologies. Once these are ruled out, with careful clinical and bacteriologic surveillance and antimicrobials when indicated, the prognosis for girls with recurrent UTIs is good (Marks, 1987).

In sexually active women whose UTIs are temporally related to diaphragm use, diaphragm and spermicide use should be discontinued (Forland, 1993). In other sexually active women with recurrent UTIs, postcoital quinolone prophylaxis may be effective (Pfau & Sacks, 1994). A variety of antimicrobial regimens have documented prophylactic efficacy for prevention of acute UTI, including trimethoprim-sulfamethoxazole 40/200 mg/d two or three times weekly (Nicolle, 1992). Antimicrobial prophylaxis is highly effective in preventing cystitis, bacteriuria, and pyelonephritis; resistance to trimethoprim-sulfamethoxazole was observed to increase in the last 5 years, but the proportion of *E. coli* strains resistant to ampicillin and nitrofurantoin did not increase (Durukan et al., 1990).

Among menopausal women, decreasing vaginal pH by topical application of intravaginal estriol cream has reduced UTI recurrence (Raz & Stamm, 1993). Systemic estrogen use, with antimicrobials, has also been effective (Privette et al., 1988). The use of cranberry beverages among elderly women to acidify urine reduces the frequency of bacteriuria (Avorn et al., 1994).

In hospitals and nursing homes, reduction of catheterization and mobilization reduce UTI incidence (Wong & Hooton, 1983). Intermittent and closed system catheterization greatly reduce UTI risk.

Antimicrobial Therapy. Commonly, antimicrobial therapy is initiated before isolation of the pathogen on the basis of the most likely organism. In many outpatient settings, it is appropriate, when the patient has no evidence of systemic disease, to use one-dose or short-term regimens without culture confirmation (Forland, 1993; Hooton & Stamm, 1991).

Summary

Although great strides have been made in the control of infectious diseases in the last 50 years, the overall impact of infectious diseases remains considerable. In the United States, according to the National Health Interview Survey of 1991, 46,104,000 cases of acute infective and parasitic diseases per year (18/100 persons) occurred. These yielded 154,768,000 days of restricted activity, 68,703,000 bed-bound days, 18,727,000 days lost from work in persons over 17 years of age and 72,000,000 days lost from school among children under 18 years of age. Some infectious diseases, notably HIV infection and related diseases, are common causes of death among young adults.

Some infections are specific to the female reproductive system or breast. Others, such as TB, appear to have a somewhat more virulent course or a different presentation in women. Because of the unique anatomic and physiologic processes related to menarche, reproduction, and contraception, STDs are of particular importance among women of reproductive age.

References

Abimuku, A. G., & Gallo, R. C. (1995). HIV: Basic virology and pathophysiology. In H. L. Minkoff, J. A. Dehovitz, & A. Duerr (Eds.), *HIV infection in women* (pp. 13-31). New York: Raven Press.

Acosta, A. A., Mabray, C. R., & Kaufman, R. H. (1970). Intrauterine pregnancy and coexistent pelvic inflammatory disease. *Obstetrics and Gynecology, 37,* 282-285.

American College of Obstetricians and Gynecologists. (1994). *Precis V.* Washington, DC: Author.

Anonymous. (1978). Tuberculosis of the female genital tract [Editorial]. *British Medical Journal, 1,* 1286.

Arno, J. N., & Jones, R. B. (1994). Venereal chlamydial infections. In P. D. Hoeprich, M. C. Jordan, & A. R. Ronald (Eds.), *Infectious diseases: A treatise of infectious processes* (5th ed.). Philadelphia: Lippincott.

Arvin, A. M., & Prober, C. G. (1990). Herpes simplex virus infections. *Pediatric Infectious Disease Journal, 9,* 765-778.

Avorn, J., Monane, M., Gurwitz, J. H., Glynn, R. J., Choodnovskiy, I., Lipsitz, L. A. (1994). Reduction of bacteriuria and pyuria after ingestion of cranberry juice. *Journal of the American Medical Association, 271,* 751-754.

Blanchard, A. C., Pastorek, J. G., & Weeks, T. (1987) Pelvic inflammatory disease during pregnancy. *Southern Medical Journal, 80,* 1363-1365.

Bratos, M. A., Eiros, J. M., Orduna, A., et al. (1993). Influence of syphilis in hepatitis B transmission in a cohort of female prostitutes. *Sexually Transmitted Diseases, 20,* 257-261.

Brown, W. J., Donohue, J. F., Axnick, N. W., Blount, J. H., Jones, O. G., & Ewen, N. H. (1970). *Syphilis and other venereal diseases* (Vital and Health Statistics Monographs, American Public Health Association, pp. 152-182). Cambridge, MA: Harvard University Press.

Cates, W., & Wasserheit, J. N. (1991). Genital chlamydial infections: Epidemiology and reproductive sequelae. *American Journal of Obstetrics and Gynecology, 164,* 1771-1781.

Cantwell, M. F., Snider, D. E., Jr., Cauthen, G. M., & Onorato, I. M. (1994). Epidemiology of tuberculosis in the United States, 1985-1992. *Journal of the American Medical Association, 272,* 535-539.

Cederqvist, L. L. (1994). Cytomegalovirus infection. In J. G. Pastorek (Ed.), *Obstetric and gynecologic infectious disease*. New York: Raven Press.

Centers for Disease Control. (1987). Increases in primary and secondary syphilis—United States. *Morbidity and Mortality Weekly Report, 36,* 393-396.

Centers for Disease Control and Prevention. (1992). 1993 Revised classification system for HIV infection and expanded surveillance case definition for AIDS among adolescents and adults. *Morbidity and Mortality Weekly Report, 41,* 1-19.

Centers for Disease Control and Prevention. (1993). 1993 Sexually transmitted diseases treatment guidelines. *Morbidity and Mortality Weekly Report, 42,* 1-102.

Centers for Disease Control and Prevention. (1994). Recommendations of the U.S. Public Health Service Task Force on the use of zidovudine to reduce perinatal transmission of human immunodeficiency virus. *Morbidity and Mortality Weekly Report, 43,* 1-20.

Centers for Disease Control and Prevention, Division of STD/HIV Prevention. (1994). *Sexually transmitted disease surveillance, 1993*. Atlanta, GA: Author.

Chiu, M. J., & Radolf, J. D. (1994). Syphilis. In P. D. Hoeprich, M. C. Jordan, & A. R. Ronald, (Eds.), *Infectious diseases: A treatise of infectious processes* (5th ed., pp. 694-714). Philadelphia: Lippincott.

Chow, W. H., Daling, J. R., Cates, W., Jr., & Greenberg, R. S. (1987). Epidemiology of ectopic pregnancy. *Epidemiologic Reviews, 9,* 70-93.

Christmas, J. T., Wendel, G. D., Bawdon, R. E., Farris, R., Cartwright, G., & Little, B. B. (1989). Concomitant infection with *Neisseria gonorrhoeae* and *Chlamydia trachomatis* in pregnancy. *Obstetrics and Gynecology, 74,* 295-298.

Chu, S. Y., & Wortley, P. M. (1995). Epidemiology of HIV/AIDS in women. In H. L. Minkoff, J. A. Dehovitz, & A. Duerr (Eds.), *HIV infection in women* (pp. 1-12). New York: Raven Press.

Cole, H. M. (1993). Diagnostic and therapeutic technology assessment (DATTA). *Journal of the American Medical Association, 270,* 2975-2981.

Currier, J. S. (1995). Medical management of HIV disease in women. In H. L. Minkoff, J. A. Dehovitz, & A. Duerr (Eds.), *HIV infection in women* (pp. 125-155). New York: Raven Press.

Darney, P. D. (1987). *Handbook of ambulatory and gynecologic surgery.* Oradell, NJ: Medical Economics Company.

Dehovitz, J. A. (1995). Natural history of HIV infection in women. In H. L. Minkoff, J. A. Dehovitz, & A. Duerr, (Eds.), *HIV infection in women* (pp. 57-71). New York: Raven Press.

De Vynck, W. E., Kruger, T. F., Joubert, J. J., Scott, F., Van Der Merwe, J.P., Hulme, V. A., & Swart, Y. (1990). Genital tuberculosis associated with female infertility in the western Cape. *South African Medical Journal, 77,* 630-631.

Dunn, R. A., Webster, L. A., Nakashima, A. K., & Sylvester, G. C. (1993). Surveillance for geographic and secular trends in congenital syphilis—United States, 1983-1991. *Morbidity and Mortality Weekly Report, 42*(SS-6), 59-71.

Durst, M., Gissman, L., Ikenberg, H., & zur Hausen, H. (1983). A new papillomavirus DNA from a cervical carcinoma and its prevalence in cancer biopsy samples from different geographic regions. *Proceedings of the National Academy of Sciences of the United States of America, 80,* 3812-3815.

Durukan, T., Urman, B., Yrali, H., Arikan, U., & Beykal, O. (1990). An abdominal pregnancy 10 years after treatment for pelvic tuberculosis. *American Journal of Obstetrics and Gynecology, 163,* 594-595.

Ernst, A. A., Romolo, R., & Nick, T. (1993). Emergency department screening for syphilis in pregnant women without prenatal care. *Annals of Internal Medicine, 22,* 781-785.

Finelli, L., Budd, J., & Spitalny, K. C. (1993). Early syphilis. Relationship to sex, drugs, and changes in high-risk behavior from 1987-1990. *Sexually Transmitted Diseases, 20,* 89-95.

Finkelhor, D., Hotaling, G., Lewis, I. A., & Smith, C. Sexual abuse in a national survey of adult men and women: Prevalence, characteristics and risk factors. *Child Abuse and Neglect, 14,* 19-28.

Fleming, P. L., Ciesielski, C., Byers, R. H., Castro, K. G., & Berkelman, R. L. (1991). Gender differences in reported AIDS indicative diagnoses. *Journal of Infectious Diseases, 168,* 61-67.

Forland, M. (1993). Urinary tract infection: How has its management changed? *Postgraduate Medicine, 93,* 371-86.

Frasier, L. D. (1994). Human papillomavirus infections in children. *Pediatric Annals, 23,* 354-360.

Frau, L. M., & Alexander, E. R. (1985). Public health implications of sexually transmitted diseases in pediatric practice. *Pediatric Infectious Disease Journal, 4,* 453-467.

Gayle, H. D., & D'Angelo, L. J. (1991). Epidemiology of acquired immunodeficiency syndrome and human immunodeficiency virus infection in adolescents. *Pediatric Infectious Disease Journal, 10,* 322-328.

Gibbs, R. S., & Sweet, R. L. (1994). Maternal and fetal infections, clinical disorders. In Creasy, R. K., & Resnik, R. *Maternal-fetal medicine principles and practice.* Philadelphia: Saunders.

Gleckman, R. A. (1992). Urinary tract infection. *Clinics in Geriatric Medicine, 8,* 793-803.

Golden, N., Neuhoff, S., & Cohen, H. (1989). Pelvic inflammatory disease in adolescents. *Journal of Pediatrics, 114,* 138-143.

Graber, W. J., III, Sanford, J. P., & Ziff, M. (1968). Sex incidence of gonococcal arthritis. *Arthritis and Rheumatism, 11,* 569-578.

Grimes, D. A. (1986). Deaths due to sexually transmitted diseases: The forgotten component of reproductive mortality. *Journal of the American Medical Association, 255,* 1727-1729.

Hammerschlag, M. R. (1994). *Chlamydia trachomatis* in children. *Pediatric Annals, 23,* 349-353.

Harrison, H. R., Costin, M., Meder, J. B., et al. (1985). Cervical *Chlamydia trachomatis* infection in university women, relationship to history, contraception, ectopy, and cervicitis. *American Journal of Obstetrics and Gynecology, 153,* 244-249.

Hoegsberg, B., Abulafia, O., Sedlis, A., et al. (1990). Sexually transmitted diseases and human immunodeficiency virus infection among women with pelvic inflammatory disease. *American Journal of Obstetrics and Gynecology, 165,* 1135-1139.

Hoeprich, P. D., Jordan, M. C., & Ronald, A. R. (1994). Preface. In P. D. Hoeprich, M. C. Jordan, & A. R. Ronald (Eds.), *Infectious diseases: A treatise of infectious processes* (5th ed., pp. xvii-xviii). Philadelphia: Lippincott.

Holmes, K. K., Counts, G. W., & Beaty, H. N. (1971). Disseminated gonococcal infection. *Annals of Internal Medicine, 74,* 979-993.

Hook, E. W., Cannon, R. O., Nahmias, A. J., Lee, F. F., Campbell, C. H., Glasser, D., & Quinn, T. C. (1992). Herpes simplex virus infection as a risk factor for human immunodeficiency virus infection in heterosexuals. *Journal of Infectious Diseases, 165,* 251-255.

Hooton, T. M., Fihn, S. D., Johnson, C., Roberts, P. L., & Stamm, W. E. (1989). Association between bacterial vaginosis and acute cystitis in women using diaphragms. *Archives of Internal Medicine, 149,* 1932-1936.

Hooton, T. M., & Stamm, W. E. (1991). Management of acute complicated urinary tract infections in adults. *Medical Clinics of North America, 75,* 339-357.

Hutchinson, C. M., Hook, E. W., Shepherd, M., Verley, J., & Rompalo, A. M. (1994). Altered clinical presentation of early syphilis in patients with human immunodeficiency virus infection. *Annals of Internal Medicine, 121,* 94-100.

Ingram, D. L. (1994). *Neisseria gonorrhoeae* in children. *Pediatric Annals, 23,* 341-348.

Johnson, R. E., Nahmias, A. J., Madger, L. S., Lee, F. K., Brooks, C. A., & Snowden, C. B. (1989). A seroepidemiologic survey of the prevalence of herpes simplex virus type 2 infection in the United States. *New England Journal of Medicine, 321,* 7-12.

Jones, J. G., Yamauchi, T., & Lambert, B. (1985). *Trichomonas vaginalis* infestation in sexually abused girls. *American Journal of Diseases of Children, 139,* 846-847.

Kinghorn, G. R. (1993). Genital herpes: Natural history and treatment of acute episodes. *Journal of Virology, 1* (Suppl.), 33-38.

Koutsky, L. A., Holmes, K. K., Critchlow, C. W., et al. (1992). A cohort study of the risk of cervical intraepithelial neoplasia grade 2 or 3 in relation to papillomavirus infection. *New England Journal of Medicine, 327,* 1272-1278.

Laga, M., Manoka, A., Kivuvu, M., Malele, B., Tuliza, M., Nzila, N., Goeman, J., et al. (1993). Non-ulcerative sexually transmitted diseases as risk factors for HIV-1 transmission in women: Results from a cohort study. *AIDS, 7,* 95-102.

Libman, M. D., Dascal, A., Kramer, M. S., & Mendelson, J. (1991). Strategies for the prevention of neonatal infection with herpes simplex virus: A decision analysis. *Review of Infectious Diseases, 13,* 1093-1104.

Lundberg, G. D. (1989). The 1988 Bethesda system for reporting cervical/vaginal cytological diagnoses. *Journal of the American Medical Association, 262,* 931-934.

Maccato, M. (1993). Herpes in pregnancy. *Clinical Obstetrics and Gynecology, 36,* 369-377.

Margolis, K., Wranz, P. A. B., Kruger, T. G., Joubert, J. J., & Odendal, H. J. (1992). Genital tuberculosis at Tyberberg Hospital—Prevalence, clinical presentation and diagnosis. *South African Medical Journal, 81,* 12-15.

Margono, F., Mrouech, J., Garely, A., White, D., & Minkoff, H. L. (1994). Resurgence of active tuberculosis among pregnant women. *Obstetrics and Gynecology, 83,* 911-914.

Marks, M. (1987). Cystitis. In R. F. Feigin & J. C. Cherry, (Eds.), *Textbook of pediatric infectious diseases* (2nd ed., pp. 521-529). Philadelphia: Saunders.

Merz, G. J., Bendetti, J., Ashley, R., Selke, S. A., & Corey, L. G. (1992). Risk factors for the sexual transmission of genital herpes. *Annals of Internal Medicine, 116,* 197-202.

Morse, S. A., & Holmes, K. K. (1994). Gonococcal infections. In P. D. Hoeprich, M. C. Jordan, & A. R. Ronald (Eds.), *Infectious diseases: A treatise of infectious processes* (5th ed., pp. 670-684). Philadelphia: Lippincott.

Murphy, F. K., Patamasucon, . (1985). Congenital syphilis. In K. K. Holmes, P. A. Mardh, P. F. Sparling, & P. J. Wiesner (Eds.), *Sexually transmitted diseases* (pp. 352-374).

Nicolle, L. E. (1992). Prophylaxis: Recurrent urinary tract infection in women. *Infection, 20,* S203-S207.

Nicolle, L. E., Muir, P., Harding, G. K. M., & Norris M. (1987). Localization of urinary tract infection in elderly institutionalized women with asymptomatic bacteriuria. *Journal of Infectious Diseases, 157,* 65-69.

Oosthuizen, A. P., Wessels, P. H., & Hefer, J. N. (1990). Tuberculosis of the female genital tract in patients attending an infertility clinic. *South African Medical Journal, 77,* 562-564.

Otten, M. W., Zaidi, A. A., Peterman, T. A., Rolfs, R. T., & Witte, J. J. (1994). High rate of HIV seroconversion among patients attending urban sexually transmitted diseases clinics. *AIDS, 8,* 549-53.

Pfau, A., & Sacks, T. G. (1994). Effective postcoital quinolone prophylaxis of recurrent urinary tract infections in women. *Journal of Urology, 152,* 136-138.

Phillips, R. S., Hanff, P. A., Wertheimer, A., & Aronson, A. D. (1988). Gonorrhea in women seen for routine gynecologic care: Criteria for testing. *American Journal of Medicine, 85,* 177-182.

Privette, M., Cade, R., Peterson, J., & Mars, D. (1988). Prevention of recurrent urinary tract infections in postmenopausal women. *Nephron, 50,* 24-27.

Raz, R. M., & Stamm, W. E. (1993). A controlled trial of intravaginal estriol in postmenopausal women with recurrent urinary tract infections. *New England Journal of Medicine, 329,* 753-756.

Reeves, W. C., Gary, H. E., Johnson, P. R., Icenogle, J. P., Brenes, M. M., de Britton, R. M., Dobbins, J. G., & Schmid, D. S. (1994). Risk factors for genital papillomavirus infection in populations at high and low risk for cervical cancer. *Journal of Infectious Diseases, 170,* 753-758.

Reeves, W. C., Rawls, W. E., & Brinton, L. A. (1989). Epidemiology of genital papillomaviruses and cervical cancer. *Review of Infectious Diseases, 11,* 426-439.

Rolfs, R. T., Galaid, E. I., & Zaidi, A. A. (1992). Pelvic inflammatory disease: Trends in hospitalizations and office visits, 1979 through 1988. *American Journal of Obstetrics and Gynecology, 156,* 983-90.50.49.

Rudloff, M. D. (1991). Significance of *Garnerella vaginalis* in a prepubertal female. *Pediatric Infectious Disease Journal, 10,* 709-710.

Schiffman, M. H., Bauer, H. M., Hoover, R. N., et al. (1993). Epidemiologic evidence showing that human papillomavirus infection causes most cervical intraepithelial neoplasia. *Journal of the National Cancer Institute, 85,* 958-964.

Selik, R., & Chu, S. Y. (1994). HIV infection as leading cause of death among young adults in U.S. cities and states. *Journal of the American Medical Association, 271,* 903.

Selwyn, P. A., Hartel, D., Lewis, V. A., et al. (1989). A prospective study of the risk of tuberculosis among intravenous drug users with human immunodeficiency virus infection. *New England Journal of Medicine, 320,* 545-550.

Shepard, M. K., & Jones, R. B. (1989). Recovery of *Chlamydia trachomatis* from endometrial and fallopian tube biopsies in women with infertility of tubal origin. *Fertility and Sterility, 52,* 232-238.

Shireman, P. K. (1992). Endometrial tuberculosis acquired by a health care worker in clinical laboratory. *Archives of Pathology and Laboratory Medicine, 116,* 521-523.

Siegal, H. A., Carlson, R. G., Falck, R., Forney, M. A., Wang J., & Li, L. (1992). High-risk behaviors for transmission of syphilis and human immunodeficiency virus among crack cocaine-using women. A case study from the Midwest. *Sexually Transmitted Diseases, 19,* 266-271.

Solberg, D. A., Butler, J., & Wagner, N. N. (1973). Sexual behavior in pregnancy. *New England Journal of Medicine, 238,* 1098-1108.

Stamm, W. E., McKevitt, M., Roberts, P. L., & White, N. J. (1991). Natural history of recurrent urinary tract infections in women. *RID, 13,* 77-84.

St. Louis, M. E., Kamenga, M., Brown, C., et al. (1993). Risk for perinatal HIV-1 transmission according to maternal immunologic, virologic, and placental factors. *Journal of the American Medical Association, 269,* 2853-2859.

Stutz, D. R., Spence, M. R., & Duangmani, C. (1976). Oropharyngeal gonorrhea during pregnancy. *Journal of the American Venereal Disease Association, 3,* 65-67.

Sweet, R. L., & Gibbs, R. S. (1990). *Infectious diseases of the female genital tract.* Baltimore: Williams & Wilkins.

U.S. Department of Health and Human Services. (1988). *Study of national incidence and prevalence of child abuse and neglect* (Office of Human Development Services contract 105-85-1702). Washington, DC: Author.

Vernon, S. C., Reeves, W. C., Clancey, K. A., Laga, M., StLouis, M., Gary, H. E., Ryder, R. W., Manoka, A. T., & Icenogle, J. P. (1994). A longitudinal study of human papillomavirus DNA detection in HIV-1 seropositive and seronegative women. *Journal of Infectious Diseases, 169,* 1108-1112.

Westrom, L. (1980). Incidence, prevalence, and trends of acute pelvic inflammatory disease and its consequences in industrialized countries. *American Journal of Obstetrics and Gynecology, 138,* 880-892.

Wong, E. S., & Hooton, T. M. (1983). *Guidelines for prevention of catheter-associated urinary tract infections. Guidelines for prevention and control of nosocomial infections* (pp. 1-5). Atlanta, GA: Centers for Disease Control and Prevention.

Wortley, P. M., Chu, S. Y., & Berkelman, R. L. The epidemiology of HIV/AIDS in women and the impact of the expanded 1993 CDC surveillance definition of AIDS. In D. Cotton, H. Watts (Eds.), *Medical management of AIDS in women.* New York: John Wiley & Sons, Inc.

Zimmerman, H. L., Potterat, B. A., Dukes, R. L., et al. (1990). Epidemiologic differences between chlamydia and gonorrhea. *American Journal of Public Health, 80,* 1338-1342.

zur Hausen, H., Meinhof, W., Schreiber, W., & Bornkamm, G. W. (1974). Attempts to detect virus-specific DNA sequences in human tumors: Nucleic acid hybridization with complementary RNA of human wart virus. *International Journal of Cancer, 13,* 650-656.

Bibliography

Blythe, M. J., Katz, B. P., Batteiger, B. E., Ganser, J. A., & Jones, R. B. (1992). Recurrent genitourinary chlamydial infections in sexually active female adolescents. *Journal of Pediatrics, 121,* 487-493.

Centers for Disease Control and Prevention. (1992). Projections of the number of persons diagnosed with AIDs and the number of immunosuppressed HIV-infected persons, United States, 1992-1994. *Morbidity and Mortality Weekly Report, 41*(RR18), 1-29.

Reeves, W. C., Brinton, L. A., Garcia, M., et al. (1989). Human papillomavirus infection and cervical cancer in Latin America. *New England Journal of Medicine, 320,* 1437-1441.

CHAPTER 13

Alcohol and Other Drug Use, Abuse, and Dependence

Karen Moses Allen
Elaine Feeney

Introduction

When discussing alcohol and other drug (AOD) use, abuse, and dependence, various terms are applied interchangeably. Some use the term *substance* use, abuse, and dependence, whereas others prefer the term *chemical* use, abuse, and dependence. Still others use the word *addiction* when addressing the problem of AOD dependence. The Center for Substance Abuse Prevention would prefer to include tobacco in discussions of AOD dependence, but political pressures related to categorizing tobacco usage as an addiction have influenced them to stick to the phrase "alcohol and other drugs."

With so much variation, those who are not in the field have difficulty grasping the concepts, which are confusing even to experts, practitioners, and researchers who are in the field. In this chapter, the term used will be AOD use, abuse, and dependence, based on the *Alcohol and Other Drug Thesaurus* (National Institute on Alcohol Abuse and Alcoholism [NIAAA] and Center for Substance Abuse Prevention, 1993). The "other drug" category includes nicotine, caffeine, marijuana, cocaine, central nervous system depressants and stimulants, hallucinogens, opiates, over-the-counter (OTC) drugs, prescription drugs, and inhalants.

Alcohol or other drug *use* is defined as self-administration of a psychoactive substance. Alcohol or other drug *abuse* is defined as the use of a psychoactive substance for a purpose not consistent with legal or medical guidelines, as in the non-medical use of prescription medications. Alcohol or other drug *dependence* is defined as the need for repeated doses of alcohol or other drugs to feel good or to avoid feeling bad. *Dependence* is a "cluster of cognitive, behavioral, and physiologic symptoms that indicate a person has impaired control of psychoactive substance use and continues use of the substance despite adverse consequences." (NIAAA and Center for Substance Abuse Prevention, 1993). Dependence refers to both physical and psychological elements. Psychological or psychic dependence refers to the experience of impaired control over drinking or drug use, whereas physiologic or physical dependence refers to tolerance and withdrawal symptoms (NIAAA and Center for Substance Abuse Prevention, 1993).

Epidemiology

Historical Use

The overall picture of AOD use, abuse, and dependence among women has varied over time. Changes have occurred in patterns of use, drugs of choice, combinations of drugs, methods of administration, prevalence of use, reasons for use, impact of use, and treatment related to use.

Worth (1991) cited a number of sources in providing an historical look at AOD use, abuse, and dependence among women. Alcohol was the drug used most often by American women before the 18th century. However, during the 18th century, both alcohol and other drugs were consumed, mostly in the form of patent medicines. Women consumed alcohol-based elixirs containing opiates for dental problems, painful menstruation and "female organ" problems, and coughs. These remedies and elixirs were often manufactured and promoted by unregulated medical practitioners.

During the 19th century, use of opium derivatives increased among women in the United States, with the highest rate of opiate addiction being among women from the South where it was prescribed to ease pain and treat gastrointestinal illnesses and infectious diseases. From 1850 to 1880, the number of American women addicted to legal remedies, alcohol, opiates, and analgesic and coca products outnumbered men by 2:1 (Worth, 1991).

Worth (1991) noted that a number of the women received the drugs from their physicians. However, Witters, Venturelli, and Hanson (1992) pointed out that during the 19th century the average opiate addict—who was white, middle-aged, living at a middle to upper socioeconomic level, married, a housewife, and from the south—obtained her opium or morphine legally by mail order from Sears, Roebuck or the local store. In addition to taking drugs, these women continued to drink alcohol (mostly whiskey), whereas women from the lower socioeconomic levels drank gin (Worth, 1991).

Incidence and prevalence of AOD use, abuse, and dependence among minority women during the 19th century has not been well documented. Women in general were barely given social recognition during that time period— minority women were given none. Far from being viewed as a distinct group worthy of study, they were virtually considered nonexistent.

Current Use

Alcohol

Mercer and Khaveri (1990) conducted a study in 1977 to determine frequency of drinking, amount per occasion, maximum amount per occasion, and frequent maximum amount consumed among women and men. They repeated the study in 1985 and found that, although in both studies men reported drinking more alcohol than women, when the results were examined based on differences in body weight and adjustments were made, the amount of alcohol consumed per pound of body weight was the same for both men and women. Other findings from the Mercer and

Khaveri study showed a significant increase in the maximum amount of beer that women drank from 1977 to 1985. The women tended to drink liquor in such quantities that their blood alcohol concentrations equaled those reported for men. Based on the above data, the researchers concluded that the disparate drinking between men and women in 1977 converged in 1985, indicating a greater risk for women who drink.

Grant et al. (1991) used data from the 1988 National Health Interview Survey (NHIS) to document that 4.36% of women met criteria for the 1-year combined alcohol abuse and dependence prevalence rate based on *DSM-III-R* criteria. Data collected 2 years after the 1988 NHIS revealed an increase in that prevalence rate.

Dawson (1993) examined three components of alcohol intake—number of drinking occasions, number of drinks per occasion, and ethanol content per drink—and found that the male/female ratio of drinks per occasion was almost identical to the ratio of the number of drinks per year. In addition, women's average alcohol content per drink was higher than that of men because they were more likely to consume spirits and wine.

Kessler (1994) examined data from the 1990–1992 National Comorbidity Study and estimated a combined alcohol abuse and dependence prevalence rate of 5.3% for women.

A 1994 report revealed that of 26,615 women (aged 18–44) surveyed by the 1991 Behavioral Risk Factor Surveillance System on alcohol consumption among women of childbearing age, 50% were nondrinkers, 45% light drinkers, 3% moderate drinkers, and 2% heavy drinkers (Centers for Disease Control and Prevention [CDC], 1994a). Among all drinkers, 21% reported binge drinking, and a total of 4% drank while being pregnant.

A 1994 Gallup poll showed that 70% of men and 61% of women drink alcohol, that is, 7 in 10 men and 6 in 10 women currently identify themselves as drinkers. The overall trends of the poll showed that for the first time since 1985, the percentage of women drinkers now exceeds 60% (Hanson & Venturelli, 1995).

Other Drugs

A major survey used to depict incidence and prevalence of AOD use among women is the National Household Survey on Drug Abuse, which provides information specific to licit and illicit drug use.

National surveys strive to provide a picture representative of the entire United States population of women. Therefore, attempts have been made to determine the incidence and prevalence of AOD use, abuse, and dependence of *some* women using this methodology. Although the U.S. General Accounting Office (1993) found these surveys to be fraught with weaknesses, such as methodologic problems leading to overestimates and underestimates, findings exclusive of large segments of the population (homeless, incarcerated, institutionalized, certain minority groups, and so on), reliance on self-reports, language difficulties, lack of privacy during interviews, and statistical problems, results viewed with caution can provide some idea of current AOD use among women.

The 1993 National Household Survey on Drug Abuse revealed that alcohol was still the most widely used drug, with 84% lifetime use. The next highest used drug was tobacco, with 71% lifetime use. Marijuana was the most commonly used illicit drug (34% of the population) followed by 11% lifetime use for nonmedical use of psychotherapeutic drugs and 11% lifetime use of cocaine. Heroin, hallucinogens, and inhalants were used by fewer than 9% of the population in their lifetimes (Substance Abuse and Mental Health Services Administration [SAMHSA], 1994a).

Licit Drugs

Based on population estimates from the 1993 Household Survey on Drug Abuse (SAMHSA, 1994a), the alcohol use rate among women was 10% less than among men in the past year and 14.9% less among women than men in the past month. These rates show a fair amount of difference between women and men in the rates of use for alcohol and illicit drugs.

Unfortunately, however, the drug that kills nearly 500,000 people a year shows close rates of use among women and men. According to data from the CDC (1994b), smoking prevalence was the same in 1991 and 1992 for both adult men and women, all racial/ethnic groups, individuals representative of all educational levels, and persons with incomes above poverty level. There was a substantial increase in the prevalence of smoking among women who live below the poverty level. In addition, the 1993 population estimates reported by the Household Survey on Drug Abuse (SAMHSA, 1994a) show that only a 5.8% difference existed between women and men (26.6 to 32.4, respectively) in cigarette use rates during the past year and just a 3.9% difference existed in cigarette use rates during the past month (22.3 for women and 26.2 for men).

An estimated 70% of all psychoactive prescription drugs used by people under age 30 are obtained without the user having a prescription. Pharmacist's records show that about $60.7 billion is spent on psychoactive drug prescriptions each year (U.S. Bureau of the Census, 1993). Such figures show that it may be more difficult to find people who do not use prescription drugs than people who do (Hanson & Venturelli, 1995).

Illicit Drugs

Results of the 1993 Household Survey on Drug Abuse showed a 4.6% difference between women and men (9.6 to 14.2, respectively) in the rates of illicit drugs use in the past year, and a 3.3% difference between women and men (4.1 to 7.4, respectively) in the rates of illicit drug use in the past month (SAMHSA, 1994a). According to the National Institute on Drug Abuse (NIDA), 5.5% of women completing a pregnancy and health survey used some illicit drug during pregnancy.

Contextual Use

Alcohol

Much of the diversity in drinking habits between the genders can be linked to the frequency and nature of social situations. Although men drink more than women, a great deal of similarity exists in the patterns of the sexes within situations in that, for both sexes, average consumption increases on weekends in bars, with friends, at parties, and as a function of duration (Harford, 1994).

Thomas C. Harford of the Division of Biometry and Epidemiology of the National Institute on Alcohol Abuse and Alcoholism has been an advocate of looking at the context of AOD use when examining epidemiology. In 1978, he suggested that rates of alcohol consumption be viewed as products of the numerous interactional and situational contexts in which drinking occurs. Certain drinking contexts are associated with heavier drinking because of interactional dynamics present, such as treating to and sharing rounds or toasting at weddings (Clark, 1985).

Shore and Batt (1991) examined contextual factors associated with the drinking behaviors of business and professional women. Results suggested that social context may be important in understanding women's drinking. Variables directly related to drinking, such as time spent in drinking situations or settings and drinking habits of spouses and best friends, correlated with increased drinking. Other contextual variables played a preventive role; for example, increased numbers of memberships in professional organizations were predictive of decreased alcohol consumption.

Herd and Grube (1993) found that 80% of Caucasian women and 46% of African American women drank while having dinner in a restaurant. Caucasian women were also more likely to drink in the context of eating lunch at a restaurant; going to a bar, tavern, or cocktail lounge; and entertaining friends. African American women reported drinking during a quiet evening at home or while at a club or organizational meeting. Although both groups of women drank in equal proportions in the context of associating with friends in a public place such as a park, street, or parking lot, African American women had more average number of drinks per month in this context than Caucasian women. However, a larger proportion of African American women's alcohol use occurred at home.

Emotional state is another contextual situation that has an impact on the incidence and prevalence of alcohol use, abuse, and dependence among women. According to Klein and Pittman (1993) a definite relationship exists between emotional state and alcohol consumption. Using a national probability sample they found that:

1) Men drank significantly more beer in response to negative emotional states (particularly loneliness) as opposed to women.
2) Women drank beer more heavily when experiencing positive emotions such as stimulation, festiveness, and romance.
3) Women consumed more wine when experiencing positive affect; men did not.

Raskin and Miller (1993) studied the prevalence of comorbidity of psychiatric and addiction disorders in the general (nonclinical) population. With the exception of antisocial personality, women had comorbidity disorders at approximately three times the rate of men.

Other Drugs

Prevalence of other drug use among women is related to context and situation as well. According to Allen (1992), the majority of subjects in her study stated that they began use of cocaine (which was their drug of choice) for social reasons. Using drugs in contextual situations—such as getting high with spouses or lovers, partying, passing the joint around when sitting with a group of female friends talking, using cocaine because it allows completion of prostitution jobs, and so on—mirrors the contextual influences described for drinking.

Henderson, Boyd, and Mieczkowski (1994) found that women were more likely to begin drug use or maintain their drug use in the context of more intimate relationships with the opposite sex.

Use Among Ethnic Groups

African American Women

Available data suggest that although alcohol use begins later among African American women than among Caucasian women, the onset of alcohol-related problems appears earlier among African Americans (SAMHSA, 1994b). Patterns of drug use among African American women, as reflected in studies of women in treatment, indicate that they are more likely than other women in treatment to use opiates. In the past they were found to be less likely to use psychotherapeutic drugs for nonmedical uses; however, the 1992 Household Survey on Drug Abuse revealed that they were likely to do so. Between 1988 and 1992, the use of cocaine among African American women rose slightly, whereas it decreased among Hispanic and Caucasian women.

Among African American women, marital status was an important determinant of heavier drinking, with effects being moderated by age and employment status. Unmarried middle-aged women (40–59 years) and unmarried women who were homemakers were among the African American women at greatest risk for heavy drinking (Herd, 1988). According to Darrow, Russell, Cooper, Mudar, and Frone (1992), heavier drinking among African American women was associated with higher parity, and church attendance was a protective factor against heavier drinking for this group.

American Indian Women

American Indians are a large segment of the population that is left out of the annual Household Survey on Drug Abuse. Although American Indian women drink less than men, they are particularly susceptible to alcohol-related health problems. According to LaDue (1990), alcoholism is the predominant health problem for American Indian women in what has been described as a triad that includes violence and depression. The rates of these problems have increased significantly since 1970.

American Indian women who use drugs began doing so at a young age (often 10 or 11); marijuana, stimulants, and inhalants are popular (Leland, 1984). However, because prevalence rates among American Indians are not a part of the national surveys it is hard to say exactly what specific AOD use, abuse, and dependence looks like among women from this ethnic group. Hence, what remains is to present the devastating effects of AOD use and abuse on this population of women.

In all age groups, the alcohol-related mortality rates were significantly higher for American Indian women than for other women (LaDue, 1990). In fact, American Indian women aged 15 to 24 show an age-specific alcoholism death rate that exceeds the American Indian male rate by 40% (Indian Women's Health Care Round Table Final Report, 1991). Further, when compared across the lifespan, the mortality rate from alcoholism of American Indian women exceeds that of Caucasian women by 3% to 19%.

The fetal alcohol syndrome rate among American Indian populations is reportedly as high as 1/50, significantly higher than that of the general population of women (LaDue, 1990).

Asian American and Pacific Island Women

Asian American and Pacific Islanders are *not* a homogeneous ethnic group. This label represents more than 60 different Asian and Pacific Islander groups, each with a distinct cultural, language, and ethnic identity. They have emigrated from countries and cultures as diverse as Japan, China, Vietnam, Cambodia, Thailand, Korea, India, and the Philippines. To date, there are no incidence- and prevalence-of-use data collected at the national level pertaining to this vast Asian/Pacific Islander population. The three major annual national surveys—the National Household Survey on Drug Abuse, the NIDA National Adolescent School Health Survey, and the High School Senior Survey—do not report results pertaining to Asian/Pacific Islanders (Kim, McLeod, & Shantzis, 1992).

It is believed that Asians have the lowest alcohol prevalence rate of any major ethnic group in the United States, regardless of gender, and therefore Asian women are thought to have a lower alcohol consumption rate than African American, Caucasian, and Hispanic women. Kitano & Chi (1989) reported that Asian female heavy drinkers were more likely to be between 26 and 35 years of age. Further, among Asian women, the highest percentage of heavy drinking occurs as follows: Japanese, 12%; Filipinos, 4%; Koreans, 0.8%; and Chinese, 0%.

The Institute of Medicine (1990) reported that acculturation over the generations leads to an increase in prevalence rates of AOD use among these women. Sun (1991) noted that the low prevalence rates could be due to low reporting of AOD use or low use of professional mental health and social services among this group of women. If these things changed, it is more than likely that the prevalence rates among Asian women would increase. Orlandi, Weston, and Epstein (1992) noted that the rate of cigarette, alcohol, and tranquilizer abuse among Asian women already seems to be increasing.

Hispanic Women

Epidemiologic data specific to ethnicity indicate that Caucasian women have higher lifetime AOD use rates than Hispanic women, 83% versus 69%, respectively (NIDA, 1992). However, Hispanic women were more likely to report use of illicit drugs in the month before the survey than were Caucasian women.

Although the National Household Survey on Drug Abuse reports information on Hispanics, developers of the survey do not break down Hispanic women into their specific subgroups. This is important because the rates of use and abuse vary with place of origin.

According to Caetano (1988), Hispanic women from South and Central America have the highest rates of abstention (74%), followed by Mexican women (71%), Cuban women (48%), and Puerto Rican women (45%). In addition, for United States-born Hispanic women, there is a smaller percentage reported for abstention, particularly among second-generation women.

Amaro et al. (1990) stated that increased drug use occurs with increased acculturation. Levels of drinking in Hispanic women are associated with increased income, education, and increased drinking by the woman's husband (Corbett, Mora, & Ames, 1991).

Use Among Older Women

To date, the household surveys have grouped women aged 35 and older together, making it difficult to determine the extent of AOD use, abuse, and dependence among elderly women. Alcohol or other drug abuse is the second most common disorder affecting the elderly; it has an impact on an estimated 30% of elderly suicides and is seen in high rates among the institutionalized elderly (Solomon, Cutler, & Pierce, 1990). According to Dawson et al. (1992), the majority of persons in nursing homes are women, and two-thirds of persons in nursing homes receive psychotropic drugs. Adams, Yuan, Barboriak, and Rimm (1993) reported a prevalence rate of 14.8/10,000 women aged 65 and older for alcohol-related diagnoses in hospital admissions.

Epidemiologic researchers Robins and Regier (1991) reported that the lifetime prevalence rates of alcohol abuse or dependence in women aged 65 and over in the general population range from 0.36% to 1.14%. Even with these numbers it is believed that the rate of alcohol and drug abuse in the elderly is underestimated by researchers and underdiagnosed by health care providers (Szwabo, 1993).

A task force on the elderly with alcohol and drug problems validated this when they found that alcoholism among the elderly is largely overlooked or dismissed, up to 70% of elderly hospitalizations are alcohol related, and the average number of prescriptions for the elderly is 15 per year (SASSI Institute, 1994).

Drugs are disproportionately prescribed for older women, who are also more likely to use multiple drugs such as sedatives, antihypertensives, cardiac medications, vitamins, analgesics, laxatives, and hormones. They use prescribed drugs at rates 2.5 times higher than men. Although they only constitute 7% of the population, they receive 17% of psychoactive drugs and 20% of sedative hypnotics prescribed (Szwabo, 1993).

Another factor that contributes to the incidence and prevalence of AOD use and abuse among elderly women is their tendency to use OTC drugs to treat their own illnesses. This practice is more common among minority and low-income elderly women because they cannot afford the expense of seeing a physician (Kail, 1989).

Caetano (1994) recently summarized findings concerning alcohol use among African American, Hispanic, and Caucasian women (Display 13–1). Caetano also noted that in 1995 the Alcohol Research Group would begin a survey updating epidemiologic data about women's drinking. American Indian and Asian American women are not to be included, however. These ethnic groups are lamentably ignored even in the simple task of counting, so it comes as no surprise that they are neglected in the effort to understand the causes and antecedents for alcohol use and determine the most effective treatment.

Epidemiologic data provide a picture of the magnitude of AOD use, abuse, and dependence among women, and inspire a search for the causes, contributing factors, or antecedents of this problem. The urgency of the task is heightened by the devastating consequences and effects on women of AOD use, abuse, and dependence (discussed later).

Etiology

Etiologic research related to AOD use among women continues to be a top priority because much of what is known is based on data obtained from men. However, theories, models, and antecedents of alcohol, tobacco, and other drug use, abuse,

DISPLAY 13-1

Alcohol Use Among African American, Hispanic, and Caucasian Women

1. Drinking deceases with age among women in all three groups, and the variation is such that rates of abstention are two times higher among women who are 60 years of age and older than among women 18 to 29 years of age.

2. African American and Hispanic women have higher rates of abstention than do Caucasian women in almost all age groups.

3. Factors such as having an annual family income higher than $30,000 and being single increase the likelihood of Hispanic women drinking frequently.

4. A direct relationship exists between drinking, income, and education for women in all three groups. African American women are more likely to be drinkers if employed, whereas Caucasian women are more likely to be drinkers if they are single, have a high income, and are employed. Hispanic women are more likely to be drinkers if they are employed, educated, and acculturated (having adopted the norms, social values, and overall culture of the host country).

5. In general, the proportion of Caucasian women who reported alcohol-related problems was higher than the proportions of African American and Hispanic women.

Adapted from Caetano, R. (1994). Drinking and alcohol-related problems among minority women. *Alcohol Health and Research World,* 18(3), 233–241.

and dependence specific to women, or based on data gathered from women, are being developed.

Biologic Causes

Genetics has long been viewed as a key factor in the etiology of AOD use, abuse, or dependence. Research conducted to obtain empirical data in support of this theory usually includes examining aspects of twins or adoptees to promote heredity as a significant factor.

Bohman, Sigvardsson, and Cloninger (1981) found that alcohol problems among adopted daughters were linked to alcoholism in the biologic mother. The development of alcohol problems, however, was variable when the biologic father was the alcohol abuser. Although mild alcohol abuse by the biologic father was associated with significantly more alcohol abuse in the adopted daughter, severe alcohol abuse was not.

Genetic factors are expressed differently in women with a family history of alcoholism than in men of a similar background. For example, Cloninger, Bohman, Sigvardsson, and Von Korring (1985) examined familial and genetic factors in inheritance of alcoholism and established the existence of two clinically identifiable alcohol dependence syndromes. Type I is "milieu limited" because it points to environmental causative factors and is characterized by having a later onset. Type II is "male limited" and is characterized by early onset of alcohol-related problems, impulsivity, risk taking, belligerence, and criminal activity. Alcoholism in women with "milieu-limited" alcoholic fathers is shaped by the environment. Female type II alcoholism is expressed primarily as somatization (head, neck, and abdominal pain), whereas in men it is expressed by criminality.

According to Kendler, Heath, Neale, Kessler, and Eaves (1992), genetics plays a major role in the etiology of alcoholism in women. Their results showed that estimates for the heritability of liability to alcoholism in women in the sample ranged from 53% to 61%, depending on the definition of the illness. These authors further stated that "the findings suggest that the role of genetic factors in the etiology of alcoholism among women is substantial; and that at least half of the total liability to alcoholism is a result of genetic factors" (p.88).

In addition, Kendler et al. (1992) found that environmental factors also play a major role in etiology of alcoholism among women, particularly individual-specific environmental risk factors. However, childhood family-environmental factors, such as social class, parental disciplinary practices, or parental drinking behavior had only a minor role etiologically for women.

It is important to note that all of the subjects in the Kendler et al. study were Caucasian. There is a need for studies of other racial and ethnic groups, following the same techniques, in order to validate these findings. However, NIDA (1994) has confirmed that genetic factors contribute substantially to individual differences in vulnerability to AOD addiction.

Biochemical Causes

Another etiologic perspective of AOD abuse has come from the biochemical arena. According to Uhl, Blum, Noble, and Smith (1993), dopamine systems are intimately involved with the actions of addictive substances. Addicting drugs such as amphetamine and cocaine act on the dopamine transporter. Even drugs such as alcohol and nicotine, which do not directly alter dopamine function, can indirectly activate the mesolimbic-mesocortical dopamine system (the biochemical reward system that causes intense sense of well-being and pleasurable feelings), reinforcing more drug use.

Uhl et al. (1993) posited that although other genetic and environmental influences remain likely to determine the majority of variance in individual vulnerability to substance abuse, interindividual differences in gene-encoding proteins involved in dopaminergic neurotransmission could explain some of the genetic bases for interindividual differences in vulnerability to substance abuse. Their recent work outlined some differences in gene-based vulnerability among ethnic groups. In the future, gender differences may be identified as well.

NIDA (1994) reported that clear biochemical and functional changes occur in the brains of cocaine addicts that may account for the compulsive, nonvolitional drug taking of addiction. Decreases in dopamine D2 receptors are associated with reduced brain activity in areas of the brain that control repetitive and impulsive behaviors related to all AOD addiction. NIDA also validated that the limbic system (the brain's reward system) does reinforce AOD use, abuse, and addiction.

Psychological and Emotional Causes

Psychological or emotional issues as antecedents to AOD use, abuse, and dependence among women have also been documented. Among the women in their study, Korolenko and Donskih (1990) found that the desire to drink alcohol was correlated with current troubles, unpleasant situations, and emotional trauma. In addition, the women exhibited a sense of helplessness and had problems controlling negative feelings and coping with anxiety. From a theoretical perspective, Korolenko and Donskih (1990) viewed alcoholism, drug abuse, and other self-destructive behaviors as symptoms of an addictive disorder. They concluded that addicted women use alcohol and other substances to alter their consciousness and expand their awareness. They also stated that life stressors such as divorce, loneliness, and dissatisfaction with a career may exacerbate tendencies to abuse alcohol or other drugs.

According to Grover and Thomas (1993), unhealthy anger management, as evidenced in physiologic symptoms, may be viewed as an antecedent in self-medication through either alcohol or OTC medications. In their study, 61% of persons designated as being "high anger" drank alcoholic beverages, compared with 36% of those designated as "low-anger." The profile of the high-anger OTC user was an older woman having less education, experiencing somatic anger, and using more prescription medications.

High rates of childhood victimization for women with alcohol problems suggest the presence of a link between victimization and the development of alcohol problems among women aged 18 to 45 (Miller, Downs, & Testa, 1993).

Stress as a cause of AOD use, abuse, and dependence among women was supported by Lindenberg, Gendrop, and Reiskin (1993). They developed the Social

Stress Model of Substance Abuse, which builds on and integrates knowledge from various psychosocial theories and models. This model posits that "the likelihood of someone engaging in drug abuse is a function of the stress level and the extent to which it is offset by stress modifiers such as social networks, social competence, and resources" (p. 351). They identified the following as major stressors:

- catastrophic life events
- life transitions
- daily hassles
- enduring life strains
- developmental stresses

Lindenberg et al. (1993) pointed out that the ways in which one interprets and copes with stress may influence the ability to access resources and select appropriate models of success. When individuals have social networks, social competence, and resources available, they are able to cope better. If these are absent, however, then they turn to substance abuse. In addition, drugs may be used as a temporary method to relieve stress, giving the individual a false sense of coping.

According to Wilsnack, Klassen, Schur, and Wilsnack (1991), women who are already predisposed to alcoholism may begin to drink in response to crises or stressful experiences of life such as divorce, separation, or loss of a loved one due to death. Being divorced or separated seems to contribute to the highest percentage of heavy drinking among women. They concluded that social factors also predict the onset of women's problem drinking.

Social Causes

Social issues that contribute to AOD use and abuse among women include, but are not limited to, family violence, community violence, homelessness, societal intolerance of differences such as race, sexual preference, or religion (discrimination), or societal norms and expectations. According to Worth (1991), "critical changes in drug abuse patterns and their intensity among women are linked to major upheavals in their lives. Their polydrug use has a long history linked to social, economic and political oppression" (p. 7).

Theories of AOD use, abuse, and dependence are a way of understanding the problem as it exists in individuals, families, and communities. Because a number of theories and models are used to interpret or describe AOD use, abuse, and dependence, special attention must be paid to those that are specific to women or have had women as subjects for validity testing. The best approach to understanding the cause of this problem among women is to accept that multiple and dynamic factors influence a woman's decision to drink or use drugs in a manner that leads to abuse or dependence.

Social causes play a large role in the use of alcohol and other drugs among African American, American Indian, Asian American, and Hispanic women. Caetano (1994) stated that more recently explanations of these women's drinking have placed considerable emphasis on use of alcohol to minimize stress related to immigration, acculturation, poverty, racial discrimination, and powerlessness. In addition, drinking occurs because of ordinary adaptations to changes in norms, attitudes toward drinking, and an increase in disposable income. He posited that to understand drinking by African American and Hispanic women (probably Asian and American Indian women as well) one must consider the interplay of cultural, historical, and socioeconomic factors just beginning to emerge from ethnic studies.

Symptoms, Disease Patterns, and Responses to Disease

Experts have concluded that problems associated with alcohol and other drugs stem from a biopsychosocial cause. No one reason can be used to explain them. As shown thus far in this chapter, biologic, psychological, and social forces join together to promote the problem of AOD use, abuse, and dependence among women. The following sections outline the physical or biologic effects and discuss interventions that address the need to treat the biologic, psychological, and social aspects of AOD abuse and/or addiction in a woman's life.

Symptoms, Course of Illness, and Disease Patterns

The most common description of the symptoms and course of illness for AOD use, abuse, and dependence follows a model for alcohol addiction developed by E. M. Jellinek in 1952—the disease model (medical model). The disease model is viewed as a cornerstone in describing addictions. Jellinek (1960) posited that alcoholism is a primary disease with 43 specific symptoms that progress through three phases: early, middle, and late stages. The early stage is characterized by having blackouts; the middle stage is differentiated by experiencing a loss of control in attempting to modify the use of the drug; and the third stage is identified by the development of physical dependence and tolerance with subsequent withdrawal if use of the drug is discontinued.

Although Jellinek collected data from female alcohol addicts, he did not use it in developing his model because the disease seemed to develop more rapidly in women, and their phases of progression were not as clear-cut as the phases of progression for men. The existence of this rapid development phenomenon is evidenced by the fact that women become intoxicated after drinking smaller quantities of alcohol than are needed to produce intoxication in men, and women begin to experience alcohol-related problems after having drunk for a shorter period of time than men.

Based on interviews with subjects from Alcoholics Anonymous, Elder (1973) reported that onset of the problem drinking period averaged 2.8 years for men, but only 1.1 years for women. Later, Orford and Keddie (1985) found that the median number of years since problem onset was 11 for men as opposed to 3.6 for women. Furthermore, studies show that the interval between onset of drinking-related problems and entry into treatment is shorter for women than for men (Hasin, Grant, & Weinflash, 1988; Piazza, Vrbka, & Yeager, 1989). This could be because women progress more rapidly than men from onset of drinking through later stages of alcoholism. This is indicated by the acceleration or rapid development of cardiovascular, gastrointestinal, and liver diseases, otherwise known as telescoping (NIAAA, 1990;

Orford & Keddie, 1985; Piazza et al., 1989; Van Thiel & Gavaler, 1988). Several physiologic factors are believed to contribute to telescoping of alcoholism in women.

Whether you are providing care, conducting research, educating students, or writing and deciding policy that relates to addicted women, it is important to be aware of the above information because it describes the expected progression of the problem among women.

Response Effects of Alcohol

Metabolism

Women have lower total body water content (lower mean body water volume) than men of comparable size, 51% versus 65%, respectively (Lex, 1991). After alcohol is consumed, it diffuses uniformly into all body water, both inside and outside of cells. Because of their smaller quantity of body water, women achieve higher concentrations of alcohol in their blood than do men after drinking equivalent amounts of alcohol (NIAAA, 1990).

Another physiologic difference in women is diminished activity of alcohol dehydrogenase (the primary enzyme involved in the metabolism of alcohol) in the stomach. This may contribute to the gender-related differences in blood alcohol concentrations and a woman's heightened vulnerability to the physiologic consequences of drinking (NIAAA, 1990).

Julkunen, Tannenbaum, Baraona, and Lieber (1985) demonstrated that a certain amount of alcohol is metabolized by gastric alcohol dehydrogenase in the stomach before it enters the systemic circulation. This first-pass metabolism decreases the availability of a certain amount of alcohol to the system. Frezza et al. (1990) studied blood alcohol levels in women and found them high because of diminished activity of gastric alcohol dehydrogenase. As a result of this diminished activity, first-pass metabolism was decreased in women compared to men and virtually nonexistent in alcoholic women.

In other words, the amount of alcohol available to the system is much higher in women than in men. Specifically, these researchers found that women get about 30% more alcohol into the bloodstream than do men who are of a similar weight and drink the same amount. In addition, women's absorption rates and blood alcohol levels are more variable and are affected by progesterone levels that fluctuate across the menstrual cycle (rising after ovulation and before onset of menses) or during pregnancy (Lex, 1991).

Hormonal Effects

Johnson and Williams (1985) suggested that the combined effect of estrogens and alcohol may augment liver damage. Other research indicated that chronic alcohol abuse has been associated with menstrual cycle-related problems such as amenorrhea and anovulation (Seki, Yoshida, & Okamura, 1991). Gaveler (1988) found that alcoholic women had a higher rate of early menopause than nonalcoholic women. Becker, Tonnesen, Kaas-Claesson, and Gluud (1989) documented that alcoholic women had a higher frequency of irregularity in menstrual duration or flow or both.

In contrast, Gavaler et al. (1991) reported that the increase in estrogen levels associated with moderate alcohol drinking in postmenopausal women may explain the apparent protective effects of alcohol against coronary disease.

In a recent review of research related to alcohol and the menstrual cycle, Lammers, Mainzer, and Breteler (1995) found no evidence that menstrual cycles cause significant instability in the absorption, metabolism, and action of alcohol.

Neurophysiologic Effects

Long-term alcohol abuse is associated with alterations in electrical and structural properties of the brain (for reviews see Hunt & Nixon, 1993; Nixon, 1993).

Hill and Steinhauser (1993) found that alcoholic women had significantly smaller P300s (brain waves that occur in response to external stimuli) than nonalcoholic women. Based on this and other data, they concluded that low P300 intensity (as measured by an electroencephalogram) may be a marker for assessing the risk for developing alcoholism in young women.

Using computed tomography, Jacobson (1986) examined alcoholic women and found enlarged brain ventricles and widened sulci. According to Nixon (1994) because the brain occupies a closed space within the skull, these findings indicate shrinkage of the brain tissue. Further, the degree of brain shrinkage detected in women was similar to that reported in the literature for alcoholic men, despite women having reported lower peak alcohol consumption. Earlier, Mann, Batra, Gunther, and Schroth (1992) also found similar levels of brain shrinkage in alcoholic men and women, even though the women had shorter drinking histories. Suspected neurophysiologic changes and differences in the brains of alcoholic men and women lead to the expectation of change in neuropsychological aspects among these persons as well.

Neuropsychological Effects

According to Nixon (1994), most research suggests that female alcoholics share the same pattern of neuropsychological dysfunction as men, despite typically reported shorter or less severe alcoholic drinking patterns than the men. Based on a review of Parsons' (1993) study, neurophysiologic function tends to recover progressively in alcoholic men and women over approximately a 2- to 5-year period of abstinence. Verbal skills appear to recover earliest, but subtle deficits, particularly in abstraction and problem solving, may persist.

According to Nixon (1994) in tests of speed and accuracy, although both alcoholic men and women took longer to complete tests than nonalcoholics, only the alcoholic women were less accurate than their matched controls. When efficiency ratios were considered, alcoholic men and women were equally impaired despite a shorter drinking history.

This information provides support for the telescoping of disease discussed earlier that occurs physiologically in women. This is important to remember when treating alcoholic women because client responses to assignments and in therapy sessions will be influenced by these neurophysiologic and neuropsychological cognitive deficits. The comprehension of the women as a whole might be decreased, so unreasonable expectations related to interventions and treatment should be avoided. As noted by Nixon (1994), continued abstinence is necessary for sustained recovery of neurophysiologic function. Alcoholic men and women who resume drinking, even at a greatly reduced rate, remain cognitively impaired when retested.

Morbidity and Mortality

Chronic AOD abuse exacts a greater physical toll on women than on men. Female alcoholics have death rates 50% to 100% higher than male alcoholics. A greater percentage of women die from suicides, alcoholic-related accidents, circulatory disorders, and cirrhosis of the liver (NIAAA, 1990). In addition to vulnerability to liver disease, duration of alcohol use was found to be shorter in women with pancreatitis than in men although no differences in daily alcohol consumption were detected (NIAAA, 1994).

Witteman et al. (1990) conducted a follow-up study of women who had normal blood pressure at baseline and found that two to three drinks per day were associated with a 40% greater risk for hypertension, a leading cause of cardiovascular and cerebrovascular disease.

Findings from the CDC (1990) revealed that the estimated alcohol-related mortality rate of cardiovascular disease among women was almost three times the rate for men (17.6:6.6). Alcohol-related years of potential life lost to life expectancy for women was more than for men with cardiovascular disease, respiratory diseases, digestive diseases, and other alcohol-related diagnoses.

Stroke in the United States accounts for a higher percentage of deaths in women than in men, in all stages of life. Data consistently indicate that young women have about a 50% excess of subarachnoid hemorrhage, the least common form of stroke (Office of Research on Women's Health, 1992). Heavy drinking is associated with a fourfold increase in the risk of hemorrhagic stroke (NIAAA, 1994).

Response Effects of Other Drugs

Physiologic differences are evident between men and women in the effects of marijuana and barbiturates. According to Babor, Lex, Mendelson, and Mello (1984), the patterns of marijuana consumption for men and women are distinct, which could be related to the fact that there is a greater amount of lipid or fat tissue in women that can store and gradually release tetrahydrocannabinol, the main mood-altering chemical in marijuana. Witters et al. (1992) state that "[i]n general, the more lipid soluble the barbiturate is, the more easily it enters the brain, the faster it will act, and the more potent it will be as a depressant" (p. 163).

Metabolism

Fat solubility of barbiturates influences the duration of the drugs effects. Fat-soluble barbiturates are stored in fatty tissue; consequently, the fat content of the body can influence the effects the user experiences. Women have a higher body fat ratio than men; therefore, the effect of the barbiturate is more potent and lasts longer. Hence, their reaction to the drug is different (Witters et al., 1992).

Hormonal Effects

According to Mello, Mendelson, and Teoh (1989) in addition to alcohol use, cocaine, marijuana, and opiates also adversely affect the female reproductive system. Cocaine, marijuana, and opiates have been implicated in amenorrhea, anovulation, and spontaneous abortion. Marijuana and opiates have been implicated in luteal phase dysfunction; cocaine and opiates have also been implicated in hyperprolactinemia.

Human Immunodeficiency Virus/Acquired Immunodeficiency Syndrome

In 1994, of the 79,674 persons aged 13 or older reported to have acquired immunodeficiency syndrome (AIDS), 18% were women. This is nearly three times the number 10 years ago. The median age of women with AIDS was 35 and women aged 15 to 44 accounted for 84% of cases. More than 75% of the cases were African American and Hispanic women with rates being 16 and 17 times higher, respectively, than in Caucasian women. The most important thing to note here is that 41% of women with AIDS reported drug use; and of all women with AIDS who were initially reported as being without risk but were reclassified later, 27% had a history of intravenous drug use (CDC, 1995).

Fetal Effects

During 1993, approximately 1000 to 2000 infants were perinatally infected with human immunodeficiency virus (HIV), which assumes a transmission rate of 15% to 30% (CDC, 1995).

Although alcohol use is the drug with the most documented negative effects on fetuses based on use during pregnancy, crack cocaine is also frequently associated with adverse pregnancy outcomes. The most common obstetric complications of cocaine abuse include abruptio placentae, preterm labor, fetal distress, and stillbirth (Acker et al., 1983; Chasnoff et al., 1985; Oro & Dixon, 1987). Cocaine use contributes to optic nerve malformation or atrophy, delayed visual maturation, and eyelid edema (Good, Ferriero, Golabi, & Kobori, 1992).

In addition, the babies of mothers using drugs are frequently born in withdrawal. Gerada, Dawe, and Farrell (1990) found that women opiate users often give birth to small-for-date, sometimes premature babies who have to be treated for drug withdrawal symptoms.

Response Effects on Older Women

Although evidence shows the devastating physiologic response to and impact of AOD use on fetuses and babies (the very young), it is even more of a danger for older women. According to Glantz and Backenheimer (1988), women aged 60 and older accounted for twice as many drug-related emergency room visits as men.

Although moderate drinking in the postmenopausal years appears protective to some degree, in reality older women are faced with even greater susceptibility than younger women, or than men, to physical damage from substance abuse. According to Szwabo (1993), aging physiologically affects absorption, distribution, metabolism, and excretion of drugs. Renal function decreases, with a diminished creatinine clearance, altering filtration and excretion of toxic substances. Decreased liver function contributes to slower drug metabolism. Increased body fat increases the half-life of fat-soluble drugs. Older women face increased time that alcohol is in the blood and therefore sustained effects of the drugs used. The symptoms, course of illness, physiologic response, and consequences of AOD use, abuse, and dependence among women are clearly different in women than in men. Women who use, abuse, or are dependent on alcohol or other drugs experience devastating consequences, which makes treatment a necessity for them.

Clinical, Therapeutic, and Behavioral Interventions

Treatment

The early treatment of AOD use, abuse, and dependence was mainly directed toward men. The number of treatment programs increased in the 1970s, and although many women were admitted to them, it quickly became evident that these programs were geared toward treating male alcoholics who were predominantly Caucasian. In 1976, a special hearing on alcohol abuse among women was held by the Congressional Subcommittee on Alcoholism and Narcotics. As a result, an initiative from the NIAAA established funding for 40 treatment programs specifically for women.

This seems to be the trend for addressing AOD issues among women. First, political action is taken, then federal service and research agencies provide funding to meet identified needs. In 1986, the Office for Substance Abuse Prevention was formed as legislated by the federal government, and 2 years later began to fund demonstration projects to address AOD abuse in women, with a goal of reducing their AOD use during pregnancy.

With the Reorganization Act of 1992 (P.L. 102-321) mandated by federal legislation, the Substance Abuse and Mental Health Services Administration (SAMHSA) was established. Within the office of the SAMHSA administrator, several offices were given designated responsibilities. One such office is the Office of Women's Services (OWS).

The OWS provides leadership and guidance in creating and maintaining an agency-wide focus for addressing the AOD and mental health needs of women. This office performs the following functions (SAMHSA, 1992):

1) coordinates SAMHSA activities for women
2) is an advocate for comprehensive service provision for AOD abusing and mentally ill women among professional and constituency groups and within the Public Health Service, other federal agencies, and state and local governments
3) uses research-based literature as one of many major sources for obtaining necessary information to use in coordinating and advocating prevention and treatment needs of AOD abusing and dependent women

Within SAMHSA are a number of branches, including one for women and children. Using experts in addiction among women, along with current research specific to addicted women and their needs, this branch developed and published recommendations for comprehensive treatment for addicted women.

These recommendations were based on research from NIDA (1994), which shows that women drug abusers get better when treatment takes care of all their basic needs. Their needs were identified as food, shelter, clothing, transportation, child care, parenting training, medical care, mental health therapy, and legal assistance. NIDA stated that good treatment also needs to provide reading, basic education, and job-finding skills. They also felt that treatment was more effective when the women could be with their children (p. 9).

As shown in Figure 13–1, SAMHSA (1994b) posits that a comprehensive treatment model must make clear that caring for women with AOD problems must be part of a broad public health and social services response. The figure depicts the interrelationships between the community as a whole and a treatment program offering comprehensive services for women. It shows the various aspects of the community that influence the client and with which she may interact in the process of initiating AOD use, continuing its use, and engaging in and continuing the recovery process (SAMHSA, 1994b).

Critical components of a *Comprehensive Treatment Model of Addicted Women* recommended by SAMHSA (1994b) include the following:

Medical Interventions

- testing and treatment for infectious diseases, including hepatitis, tuberculosis, HIV, and sexually transmitted diseases
- screening and treatment of general health problems, including anemia and poor nutrition, hypertension, diabetes, cancer, liver disorders, eating disorders, dental and vision problems, and poor hygiene
- obstetric and gynecologic services, including family planning, breast cancer screening, periodic gynecologic screening (eg, Pap smears), and general gynecologic services
- infant and child health services, including primary and acute health care for infants and children, immunizations, nutrition services (including assessment for Women, Infants, and Children [WIC] program eligibility), and developmental assessments performed by qualified personnel

Substance Abuse Counseling and Psychological Counseling

- counseling regarding the use and abuse of substances directly, as well as other issues, which may include low self-esteem; race and ethnicity issues; gender-specific issues; disability-related issues; family relationships; unhealthy interpersonal relationships; violence (including incest, rape, and other abuse); eating disorders; sexuality; grief related to loss of children, family, or partners; sexual orientation; and responsibility for one's feelings including shame, guilt, and anger
- parenting counseling, including information on child development, child safety, and injury prevention
- treatment for the presence of dual diagnoses and relapse prevention

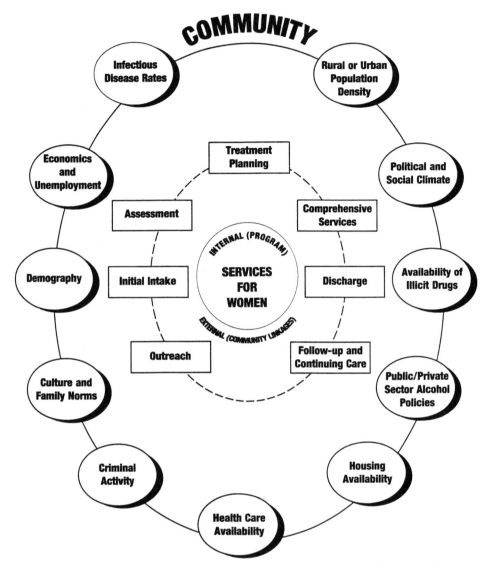

Figure 13-1. SAMSHA (1994b). Practical approaches in the treatment of women who abuse alcohol and other drugs. (DHHS publication no. SMA 94-3006.) Washington, DC: U.S. Government Printing Office.

Health Education and Prevention Activities

- health education and prevention activities covering: HIV/AIDS, the physiology and transmission of sexually transmitted diseases, reproductive health, preconception care, prenatal care, childbirth, female sexuality, childhood safety and injury prevention, physical and sexual abuse prevention, nutrition, smoking cessation, and general health

Life Skills

- education regarding practical life skills, vocational evaluation, financial management, negotiating access to services, stress, management and coping skills, and personal image building
- parenting, including infant/child nutrition, child development, and child/parent relationships
- educational training and remedial services with access to local education/general equivalency degree programs and other educational services as identified at intake
- literacy assessment and English language competency programs
- job counseling, training and referral, if possible, via case managed/coordinated referrals to community programs

Other Social Services

- transportation for clients to gain access to substance abuse treatment services and related community services
- child care
- legal services
- housing

Comprehensive treatment validates the understanding that forces from the biologic, psychological, and social realms that cause the problem need to be addressed for true recovery to begin.

When addressing the care needs of pregnant addicted women, it is important to note that they enter the health care system by way of routine prenatal care and through drug abuse treatment. It is recommended by SAMHSA (1993) that pregnant addicted women entering the system by way of prenatal care should receive the care outlined in Figure 13–2 (pp.278-279) and Display 13-2 (p.282), regardless of how far along the pregnancy has advanced. Actually, it would be good to apply the initial screening and assessment steps to all pregnant women to ascertain if a problem exists. A pregnant addicted woman entering the health care system by way of drug abuse treatment should receive the care outlined in Figure 13–3 (pp.280-281) and Display 13-3 (p.283).

In general, neither the early nor the late onset of AOD abuse among older people comes to the attention of the substance abuse/addictions treatment professional through the usual referral networks (courts, employers, spouses, families). Older women may be isolated from their community and family because they may no longer drive, may have retired from their jobs, and may be living alone because of separation or death. Widows may be a particularly vulnerable population for alcohol and prescription drug abuse (SAMHSA, 1994b).

The primary route of intervention and treatment for this group of women may be through the health care system, including the health care provider(s) and the acute care setting where older women seek treatment for age-related health problems. Specific programming for older women has not, for the most part, become standard in substance abuse/addictions treatment programs. This is true partly because the proportion of substance abusing women in older age groups is significantly lower than that of younger age groups (SAMHSA, 1994b).

Currently, there is a rush at the federal level to develop, open, and evaluate programs for pregnant and postpartum women. In doing so, however, we are neglecting a whole other population that needs intervention of a different kind. Aging causes unique issues that compound AOD use, abuse, and dependence among women; therefore, detoxification procedures, lecture sessions, group therapy programs, exercise activities, family sessions, and even recovery plans for older women must be different from those for teenage girls or younger women.

Barriers to Treatment

With all the progress made in tailoring AOD treatment to women's needs, they are still underrepresented in treatment. In a survey conducted by the National Association of State Alcohol and Drug Abuse Directors (NASADAD), it was found that within the 31 responding states, 4,004,803 women needed AOD abuse treatment. However, only 548,326 (13.69%) were receiving it. Further, of the 250,362 pregnant women who needed AOD abuse treatment, only 29,842 (11.9%) were receiving it (NASADAD, 1990). It is clear that women of all ethnic groups are facing barriers to treatment for their AOD abuse problem.

Researchers have been investigating just what these barriers are. Allen (1994) reviewed the literature and posited a theoretical definition of barriers as being subjective phenomena—beliefs or perceptions arising from within the person; or external phenomena—health care system, structural characteristics of programs, sociocultural-environmental factors; or anything that constructs, restrains, or serves as an obstacle to the person receiving care or treatment for a particular problem. Allen's review also led to conceptualizing barriers to treatment for AOD abusing women as coming from three domains: treatment program, individual characteristics, and socioenvironmental issues.

Allen (1994) developed the barriers to treatment instrument based on these three domains, which allows addicted women to identify what their perceptions are of the barriers that keep them from receiving help for their problem. This instrument is currently being used in research to alter the underrepresentation of women in treatment.

Summary and Implications

Although women use, abuse, and become dependent on alcohol and other drugs at a rate less than that of men, it is quickly becoming similar to that of men. And they experience more devastating physical, emotional, psychological, and social responses and consequences than do men. Therefore, the following implications for research, practice, and policy will hopefully inspire experts in women's health to lobby politically, inquire scientifically, and institute clinically the necessary factors to prevent and treat AOD use, abuse, and dependence among women.

Research

There are numerous implications for research in the area of AOD use, abuse, and dependence among women. However, space limitations allow only a few to be mentioned. Research designed to demonstrate the rates of use among all women needs to change the title "Household Survey" to incorporate runaway teen-age girls, homeless women, incarcerated women, older women in nursing homes, and women living on reservations. In addition, it needs to delineate the varying types of Hispanic, American Indian, Asian American, and African American groups. Therefore, it might be time to begin to document incidence and prevalence of AOD use, abuse, and dependence in a book for women only.

Research needs to expand in the area of etiology to become empirically based using women as subjects, as well as women from a variety of culturally different backgrounds. Questions such as "How much is genetics a factor among African American women or American Indian women from a particular tribe?" "Is there a specific biochemical D2 response in the addiction process that is relevant only to women?" are the types of questions that begin to address gender-specific, culturally relevant, and age-related etiology.

Research is needed for delineating what the stages and symptoms of AOD use, abuse, and dependence are in women. Maybe a model such as Jellinek proposed will never work for women, but large-scale inquiry related to this needs to be implemented.

Currently, work is being done on physiologically different responses of women to AOD use. This work will continue to be significant to how we approach detoxifying, treating, and supporting sobriety for these women.

Although attempts are being made to establish gender-specific treatment programs, more large-scale research into the degree of effectiveness over traditional programs is needed. In addition, research related to effectiveness of specific components within gender-specific treatment programs is needed.

Practice

Although AOD use, abuse, and dependence are not listed among the leading causes of death for women, the top two causes (cardiovascular disease and lung cancer) are overwhelmingly influenced by alcohol and tobacco usage. This is a powerful argument for including primary and secondary preventive measures for AOD use, abuse, and dependence in practice.

Implications for treatment include providing components of care that are supported by research rather than opinion. Research of all kinds is acceptable. It can be based on hard numbers or women's experiences, but treatment needs to be based on what has been researched and proven to be appropriate and effective.

Treatment needs to be accessible, available, and affordable (in some cases free) for all women. After this has been put into place, a mechanism for determining what sociocultural barriers are keeping these women out of treatment should be established.

To really design relevant and effective treatment programs, recovering women from all socioeconomic strata need to have input at the federal level in the OWS of SAMHSA.

Policy

Implications for policy are most urgent. Legislators, lobbyists, and policymakers are in a position to insist that more direction be provided for establishing a data base

(text continues on page 284)

All Pregnant, Substance-Using Women

Prenatal Intake →	Prenatal Followup →	Labor/Delivery with Prenatal Care →	Labor/Delivery with No Prenatal Care →
• Complete detailed health history	• Identify medical and psychosocial problems	• Complete detailed health history	• Follow all guidelines in previous column, if possible, plus perform:
• Perform physical exam	• Provide health education opportunities	• Perform physical exam	−Sonogrom
• Complete family history	• Obtain random urine and/or blood toxicologies	• Query for *recent* AOD use	−Complete baseline laboratory tests
• Complete health history of baby's father, if possible	• Reinforce importance of AOD treatment	• Repeat hepatitis B and HIV screens and syphilis test, if previously negative	
• Complete routine prenatal panel	• Reinforce importance of other service providers	• Complete urine and/or blood toxicologies	
• Complete other tests, including tuberculin test with antigen panel, urine toxicology/blood screening, and baseline sonogram	• Discuss reproductive options	☑ Follow universal precautions and OSHA standards	
• Optional tests as needed	• Manage common complications	☑ Notify pediatric, nursing, and social services	
☑ Check for tracks, abscesses, poor general hygiene, poor dental hygiene, infections	• Encourage involvement of father of baby or significant other	• Monitor fetus	
• Refer for AOD treatment, social services, nutrition counseling, parenting education, employ- ment couseling, others as needed		• Provide pain management	
• Review sexual practices and provide education on safer sexual practices		• Select delivery method	
• Obtain written release		• Insert central line if needed	

☑ **Additions for HIV-Positive Women**

• Refer for specific HIV medical treatment	• Reinforce importance of HIV medical treatment	• Provide special handling of cord, placenta, and neonate	• Follow guidelines in previous column
• Conduct extensive review of symptoms	• Repeat CD4 count every trimester		
• Obtain T4 of CD4 count	• Ensure special pediatric followup		

Figure 13–2. Pregnant, substance-using women. Point of entry: Prenatal care.

All Pregnant, Substance-Using Women

→ Postpartum →	Neonatal →	Nutrition →	Refer for
• Encourage continued participation in AOD treatment • Encourage and educate about family planning • Permit breastfeeding in methadone-maintained mothers • Initiate preventive health maintenance program • Provide for child care and parenting education • Conduct post-partum followup	• Obtain urine and/or blood toxicologies • Monitor for effects of drugs on the infant • Treat appropriately, depending on drug • Review case with mother and educate her regarding special care of infant • Encourage involvement of father of baby or significant other, and family members	• Provide for nutrition assessment • Develop special care plans according to specific effects of each drug: –Alcohol –Cigarettes –Marijuana –Heroin –Cocaine –Other • Provide for: –Prevention and intervention –Nutrition counseling –Multivitamin and mineral supplements –Special concerns	Alcohol and Other Drug Treatment (See Display 13-2)

LEGEND

☑	Medical caution
AOD	Alcohol and other drugs
Substance-Using:	Women at risk for problems resulting from their use/abuse of alcohol and other drugs

☑ Additions for HIV-Positive Women

• Conduct postpartum followup • Breastfeeding contraindicated • Encourage continued participation with HIV specialist for medical followup for mother and infant • Educate mother regarding special needs of infant • Encourage and educate about family planning	• Ensure special pediatric followup

All Pregnant, Substance-Using Women

Assessment ——————➤ Medical Withdrawal and Treatment ———————————➤

Drug Use/Abuse	Alcohol	Cocaine

• History
  –Duration of use
  –Frequency, type, amount
  –Routes of administration
  –Social context of use
  –Past treatment
  –Support group involvement
• Consequences
• Relapse factors
• Motivation for treatment/ continued use
• Refer for prenatal care
	• Setting
	  –Inpatient
	  –Under medical supervision
	• Follow admission procedures
	☑ Monitor for S/S of AWS
	☑ Antabuse: contraindicated
	• Inpatient AOD treatment whenever possible
	• Outpatient AOD treatment with special focus on pregnancy issues and drug use
	• Encourage and monitor continued prenatal care
		• Setting
		  –Inpatient most effective
		• Follow admission procedures
		☑ Medication contraindicated, except in cases of extreme agitation
		• Inpatient AOD treatment whenever possible
		• Outpatient AOD treatment if necessary, with special focus on pregnancy issues and drug use
		• Encourage and monitor continued prenatal care

Psychosocial • Family history • Support system • Attitudes about pregnancy • Education • Employment • Abuse: physical, emotional, sexual • Legal • Current crises • Relationship to other children		
Mental Health • Mental status • Psychiatric symptoms • History of mental Illness • Suicide risk • Family history of mental illness • DSM-III-R diagnosis • Treatment recommendations		

FIGURE 13-3. *Pregnant, substance-using women. Point of entry: Alcohol and other drug treatment.*

All Pregnant, Substance-Using Women

→ **Refer for**

Opiates	Methadone	Sedative-Hypnotics	Prenatal care (see Display 13-3)
• Setting −Outpatient or Inpatient • Follow admission procedures • Methadone maintenance recommended with psychosocial counseling • Medical withdrawal not recommended • Encourage and monitor continued prenatal care	• Medical withdrawal from methadone not recommended • Encourage and monitor continued prenatal care	• Setting −Inpatient −Under medical supervision • Follow admission procedures ☑ Monitor for severe symptoms: seizures, delirium ☑ Determine risk/benefit ratio when considering use of medications • Encourage and monitor continued prenatal care	

LEGEND

☑	Medical caution
AWS	Alcohol withdrawal syndrome
AOD	Alcohol and other drugs
Substance-Using:	Women at risk for problems resulting from their use/abuse of alcohol and other drugs
S/S	Signs and symptoms

DISPLAY 13-2
Referral for Alcohol and Other Drug Treatment

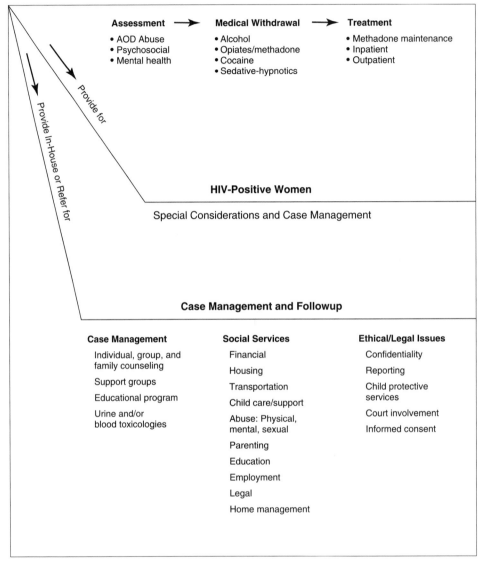

Alcohol and Other Drug Treatment

Assessment → **Medical Withdrawal** → **Treatment**

- AOD Abuse
- Psychosocial
- Mental health

- Alcohol
- Opiates/methadone
- Cocaine
- Sedative-hypnotics

- Methadone maintenance
- Inpatient
- Outpatient

Provide for

Provide In-House or Refer for

HIV-Positive Women

Special Considerations and Case Management

Case Management and Followup

Case Management

Individual, group, and family counseling

Support groups

Educational program

Urine and/or blood toxicologies

Social Services

Financial

Housing

Transportation

Child care/support

Abuse: Physical, mental, sexual

Parenting

Education

Employment

Legal

Home management

Ethical/Legal Issues

Confidentiality

Reporting

Child protective services

Court involvement

Informed consent

DISPLAY 13-3
Referral for Prenatal Care

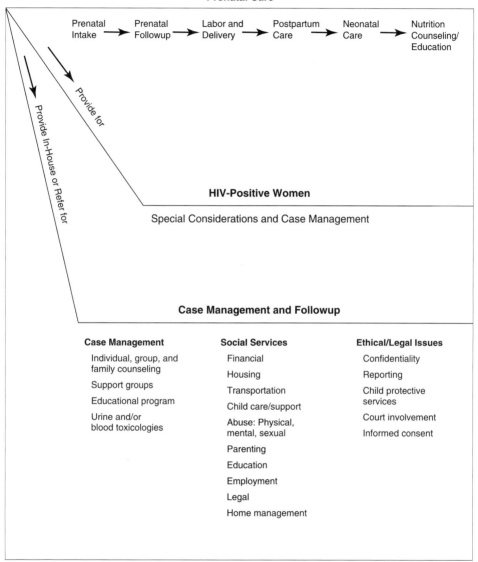

Prenatal Care

Prenatal Intake → Prenatal Followup → Labor and Delivery → Postpartum Care → Neonatal Care → Nutrition Counseling/Education

Provide for

Provide In-House or Refer for

HIV-Positive Women

Special Considerations and Case Management

Case Management and Followup

Case Management	Social Services	Ethical/Legal Issues
Individual, group, and family counseling	Financial	Confidentiality
Support groups	Housing	Reporting
Educational program	Transportation	Child protective services
Urine and/or blood toxicologies	Child care/support	Court involvement
	Abuse: Physical, mental, sexual	Informed consent
	Parenting	
	Education	
	Employment	
	Legal	
	Home management	

specific to detailing incidence and prevalence of AOD use, abuse, and dependence among all ethnic and cultural groups of women (whether in households, incarcerated, homeless, or on reservations). Policymakers must also increase research funding to promote national studies on the barriers to treatment from the perspective of the AOD abusing or dependent woman.

Other implications for policy include having recovering women representative of all communities on the SAMHSA OWS advisory council. They could share their treatment and recovery experiences so that their recommendations can be implemented and tested for effectiveness on a national level.

Alcohol and other drug use, abuse, and dependence is a major issue in women's health. The incidence and prevalence is higher than previously flawed methodology led us to believe, and the impact is as devastating, as has been documented. Future plans for addressing women's health must allow the true picture of this problem to be seen, understood, and addressed.

References

Acker, D., Sachs, B., Tracey, K., et al. (1983). Abruptio placentae associated with cocaine use. *American Journal of Obstetrics and Gynecology, 146,* 220-221.

Adams, W., Yuan, Z., Barboriak, J., & Rimm, A. (1993). Alcohol-related hospitalizations of elderly people. *Journal of the American Medical Association, 270*(10), 1222-1225.

Allen, K. (1992). Establishing reliability of the Community Oriented Program Evaluation Scale on chemically-dependent black females. *International Journal of the Addictions, 27*(1), 93-106.

Allen, K. (1994). Development of an instrument to identify barriers to treatment for addicted women, from their perspective. *International Journal of the Addictions, 29*(4), 429-444.

Allen, K., & Dixon, M. (1994). Psychometric assessment of the Allen barriers to treatment instrument. *International Journal of the Addictions, 29*(5), 545-563.

Amaro, H., Whitaker, R., & Coffman, G., et al. (1990). Acculturation and marijuana and cocaine use: Findings from HHANES 1982–84. *American Journal of Public Health, 80*(Suppl.), 54-60.

Babor, T., Lex, B., Mendelson, J., & Mello, N. (1984). Marijuana effect and tolerance: A study of subchronic self-administration in women. In L. Harris (Ed.), *Problems of drug dependence.* (NIDA Research Monograph No. 49). Washington, DC: U.S. Government Printing Office.

Becker, U., Tonnesen, H., Kaas-Claesson, N., & Gluud, C. (1989). Menstrual disturbances and fertility in chronic alcoholic women. *Drug and Alcohol Dependence, 24*(1), 75-82.

Bohman, M., Sigvardsson, S., & Cloninger, C. (1981). Maternal inheritance of alcohol abuse crossfostering analysis of adopted women. *Archives of General Psychiatry, 38,* 965-969.

Caetano, R. (1988). Alcohol use among Hispanic groups in the United States. *American Journal of Drug and Alcohol Abuse, 14,* 293-308.

Caetano, R. (1994). Drinking and alcohol-related problems among minority women. *Alcohol Health and Research World, 18*(3), 233-241.

Centers for Disease Control. (1990). Alcohol-related mortality and years of potential life lost—United States 1987. *Morbidity and Mortality Weekly Report, 39*(11), 173-190.

Centers for Disease Control and Prevention. (1994a). Frequent alcohol consumption among women of childbearing age—Behavioral risk factor surveillance system, 1991. *Morbidity and Mortality Weekly Report, 43*(18), 328-329.

Centers for Disease Control and Prevention. (1994b). Cigarette smoking among adults—United States, 1992, and changes in the definition of current cigarette smoking. *Morbidity and Mortality Weekly Report, 43*(19), 342-346.

Centers for Disease Control and Prevention. (1995). Update: AIDS among women—United States, 1994. *Morbidity and Mortality Weekly Report, 44*(5), 81-84.

Chasnoff, I., Burns, W., Schnoll, S., et al. (1985). Cocaine use in pregnancy. *New England Journal of Medicine, 313,* 666-669.

Clark, W. (1985). Alcohol use in various settings. In E. Single (Ed.), *Public drinking and public policy.* Toronto: Addiction Research Foundation.

Cloninger, C., Bohman, M., Sigvardsson, S., & Von Korring, A. (1985). Psychopathology in adopted-out children of alcoholics: The Stockholm adoption study. In M. Galanter (Ed.), *Recent developments in alcoholism* (Vol. 3). New York: Plenum Press.

Corbett, K., Mora, J., & Ames, G. (1991). Drinking patterns and drinking-related problems of Mexican-American husbands and wives. *Journal of Studies on Alcohol, 52*(3), 215-223.

Darrow, S., Russell, M., Cooper, M., Mudar, P., & Frone, M. (1992). Sociodemographic correlates of alcohol consumption among African-American and white women. *Women's Health, 18*(4), 35-51.

Dawson, N., Dadheech, G., Speroff, T., et al. (1992). The effect of patient gender on the prevalence and recognition of alcoholism on a general medicine inpatients service. *Journal of Internal Medicine, 7,* 38.

Dawson, D. (1993). Patterns of alcohol consumption: Beverage effects on gender differences. *Addiction, 88,* 133-138.

Elder, T. (1973). Alcoholism and its onset in a population of admitted alcoholics: An A.A. study. *British Journal of Addiction, 68,* 291.

Frezza, M., DiPadova, C., Pozzato, G., Terpin, M., Baraona, E., & Lieber, C. (1990). High blood alcohol levels in women: The role of decreased gastric alcohol dehydrogenase and first-pass metabolism. *New England Journal of Medicine, 322*(2), 95-99.

Gavaler, J. (1988). Effects of moderate consumption of alcoholic beverages on endocrine function in post-menopausal women: Bases for hypotheses. In M. Galanter (Ed.), *Recent developments in alcoholism* (Vol. 6). New York: Plenum Press.

Gavaler, J., Love, K., Van Thiel, D., Farholt, S., et al. (1991). An international study of the relationship between alcohol consumption and postmenopausal estradiol levels. *Alcohol Abuse and Alcoholism, Suppl. 1,* 327-330.

Gerada, C., Dawe, S., & Farrell, M. (1990). Management of the pregnant opiate user. *British Journal of Hospital Medicine, 43,* 138-141.

Glantz, M., & Backenheimer, M. (1988). Substance abuse among elderly women. *Clinical Gerontology, 8,* 3.

Good, W., Ferriero, D., Golabi, M., & Kobori, J. (1992). Abnormalities of the visual system in infants exposed to cocaine. *Ophthalmology, 99*(3), 341-346.

Grant, B., Harford, T., Chou, P., Pickering, R., Dawson, D., Stinson, F., & Noble, J. (1991). Epidemiologic Bulletin No. 27. Prevalence of DSM-III-R alcohol abuse and dependence: United States, 1988. *Alcohol Health and Research World, 15*(1), 91-96.

Grover, S., & Thomas, S. (1993). Substance use and anger in mid-life women. *Issues in Mental Health Nursing, 14,* 19-29.

Hanson, G., & Venturelli, P. (1995). *Drugs and society* (4th ed.). Boston: Jones and Bartlett.

Harford, T. (1994). *Alcohol consumption patterns among women.* Paper presented at the American Psychological Association Conference. Psychosocial and behavioral factors in women's health: Creating an agenda for the 21st century. Washington, DC.

Hasin, D., Grant, B., & Weinflash, J. (1988). Male/female differences in alcohol-related problems: Alcohol rehabilitation patients. *International Journal of the Addictions, 23*(5), 437-448.

Henderson, D., Boyd, C., & Mieczkowski, T. (1994). Gender, relationships and crack cocaine. *Research in Nursing and Health, 17*(4), 265-272.

Herd, D. (1988). Drinking by black and white women: Results from a national survey. *Social Problems, 35*(5), 493-505.

Herd, D., & Grube, J. (1993). Drinking contexts and drinking problems among black and white women. *Addiction, 88,* 1101-1110.

Hill, S., & Steinhauser, S. (1993). Event-related potentials in women at risk for alcoholism. *Alcohol, 10*(5), 349-354.

Hunt, W., & Nixon, S. (1993). *Alcohol-induced brain damage.* National Institute on Alcohol Abuse and Alcoholism Research Monograph No. 22. (NIH Publication No. 93-3549). Washington, DC: U.S. Government Printing Office.

Indian Women's Health Care Round Table Final Report. (1991). *Indian women's health care consensus statement*. Indian Health Service, Office of Planning, Evaluation and Legislation. Rockville, MD: Author.

Institute of Medicine. (1990). Populations defined by functional characteristics. In *Broadening the base of treatment for alcohol problems*. Washington, DC: Author.

Jacobson, R. (1986). Female alcoholics: A controlled CT brain scan and clinical study. *British Journal of Addiction, 81*(5), 661-669.

Jellinek, E. (1960). *The disease concept of alcoholism*. New Haven, CT: College and University Press.

Johnson, R., & Williams, R. (1985). Genetic and environmental factors in the individual susceptibility to the development of alcoholic liver disease. *Alcohol Abuse and Alcoholism, 20* (2), 137-160.

Julkunen, R., Tannenbaum, L, Baraona, E., & Lieber, C. (1985). First pass metabolism of ethanol: An important determinant of blood levels after alcohol consumption. *Alcohol, 2*(3), 437-441.

Kail, B. (1989). Drugs, gender and ethnicity: Is the older minority woman at risk? Introduction to drug use and minority older women. *Journal of Drug Issues, 29,* 171.

Kendler, K., Heath, A., Neale, M., Kessler, R., & Eaves, L. (1992). A population-based twin study of alcoholism in women. *Journal of the American Medical Association, 268*(14), 1877-1882.

Kessler, R. (1994). Lifetime and 12-month prevalence of DSM-III-R psychiatric disorders in the United States. *Archives of General Psychiatry, 51,* 8-19.

Kim, S., McLeod, J., & Shantzis, C. (1992). Cultural competence for evaluators working with Asian-American communities: Some practical considerations. In M. Orlandi, R. Weston, & L. Epstein (Eds.), *Cultural competence for evaluators, a guide for alcohol and other drug abuse prevention practitioners working with ethnic/racial communities*. (DHHS Publication No. ADM 92-1884). Rockville, MD: Office for Substance Abuse Prevention.

Kitano, H., & Chi, I. (1989). Asian Americans and alcohol: The Chinese, Japanese, Koreans, and Filipinos in Los Angeles. In: D. Spiegler, D. Tate, S. Aiken, & C. Christian (Eds.), *Alcohol use among ethnic minorities: Proceedings of a conference on the epidemiology of alcohol use and abuse among ethnic minority groups*. NIAAA Research Monograph No. 18. (DHHS Publication No. ADM 89-1435). Washington, DC: U.S. Government Printing Office.

Klein, H., & Pittman, D. (1993). The relationship between emotional state and alcohol consumption. *International Journal of the Addictions, 28*(1), 47-61.

Korolenko, C., & Donskih, T. (1990). Addictive behavior in women: A theoretical perspective. *Drugs and Society, 4*(3/4), 39-65.

LaDue, R. (1990). Coyote returns: Survival for Native American women. In P. Roth (Ed.), *Alcohol and drugs are women's issues, Vol. 1: A review of the issues*. Metuchen, NJ: Women's Action Alliance and Scarecrow Press.

Lammers, S., Mainzer, D., & Breteler, M. (1995). Do alcohol pharmacokinetics in women vary due to the menstrual cycle? *Addiction, 90,* 23-30.

Leland, J. (1984). Alcohol use and abuse in ethnic minority women. In S. Wilsnack & L. Beckman (Eds.), *Alcohol problems in women: Antecedents, consequences, and intervention*. New York: Guilford Press.

Lex, B. (1991). Some gender differences in alcohol and polysubstance users. *Health Psychology, 10*(2), 121-132.

Lindenberg, C., Gendrop, S., & Reiskin, H. (1993). Empirical evidence for the social stress model of substance abuse. *Research in Nursing and Health, 16,* 351-362.

Mann, K., Batra, A., Gunther, A., & Schroth, G. (1992). Do women develop alcoholic brain damage more readily than men? *Alcoholism: Clinical and Experimental Research, 16,* 1052-1056.

Mello, N., Mendelson, J., Teoh, S. (1989). Neuroendocrine consequences of alcohol abuse in women. *Annals of the New York Academy of Sciences, 562,* 211-240.

Mercer, P., & Khavari, K. (1990). Are women drinking more like men? An empirical examination of the convergence hypothesis. *Alcoholism: Clinical and Experimental Research, 14*(3), 461-166.

Miller, B., Downs, W., & Testa, M. (1993). Interrelationships between victimization experiences and women's alcohol use. *Journal of Studies on Alcohol, Suppl. 11,* 109-117.

National Association of State Alcohol and Drug Abuse Directors. (1990). Survey finds 250,000 pregnant women need treatment. *Alcohol and Drug Abuse Week*.

National Institute on Alcohol Abuse and Alcoholism. (1990, October). *Alcohol and women.* Alcohol Alert, No. 10. Rockville, MD: Author.

National Institute on Alcohol Abuse and Alcoholism. (1994). *Eighth special report to the U.S. Congress on alcohol and health.* (NIH Publication No. 94-3699). Alexandria, VA: EEI.

National Institute on Alcohol Abuse and Alcoholism and Center for Substance Abuse Prevention. (1993). *The alcohol and other drug thesaurus: A guide to concepts and terminology in substance abuse and addiction.* Washington, DC: Author.

National Institute on Drug Abuse. (1992). *National household survey of drug abuse: Population estimates 1991.* (DHHS Publication No. ADM 92-1887). Washington, DC: U.S. Government Printing Office.

National Institute on Drug Abuse. (1994, September/October). *NIDA reflects on 20 years of neuroscience research.* NIDA Notes, special section. Washington, DC: U.S. Government Printing Office.

Nixon, S. (1993). Application of theoretical models to the study of alcohol-induced brain damage. In W. A. Hunt & S. J. Nixon (Eds.), *Alcohol-induced brain damage.* National Institute on Alcohol Abuse and Alcoholism Research Monograph No. 22. (NIH Publication No. 93-3549). Washington, DC: U.S. Government Printing Office.

Nixon, S. (1994). Cognitive deficits in alcoholic women. *Alcohol Health and Research World, 18* (3), 228-231.

Office for Research on Women's Health. (1992). *Report of the National Institutes of Health: Opportunities for research on women's health.* (NIH Publication No. 92-3457). Washington, DC: U.S. Government Printing Office.

Orford, J., & Keddie, A. (1985). Gender differences in the functions and effects of moderate and excessive drinking. *British Journal of Clinical Psychology, 24,* 265-279.

Orlandi, M., Weston, R., & Epstein, L. (1992). *Cultural competence for evaluators, a guide for alcohol and other drug abuse preventioners working with ethnic/racial communities.* (DHHS Publication No. ADM 92-1884). Rockville, MD: Office for Substance Abuse Prevention.

Oro, A., & Dixon, S. (1987). Perinatal cocaine and methamphetamine exposure: Maternal and neonatal correlates. *Journal of Pediatrics, 111,* 571-578.

Parsons, O. (1993). Impaired neuropsychological cognitive functioning in sober alcoholics. In W. A. Hunt & S. J. Nixon (Eds.), *Alcohol-induced brain damage.* National Institute on Alcohol Abuse and Alcoholism Research Monograph No. 22. (NIH Publication No. 93-3549). Washington, DC: U.S. Government Printing Office.

Piazza, N., Vrbka, J., & Yeager, R. (1989). Telescoping of alcoholism in women alcoholics. *International Journal of the Addictions, 24*(1), 19-28.

Raskin, V., & Miller, N. (1993). The epidemiology of the comorbidity of psychiatric and addictive disorders: A critical review. *Journal of Addictive Diseases, 12*(3), 45-57.

Robins, L., & Regier, D. (1991). *Psychiatric Disorders in America.* New York: The Free Press.

SASSI Institute. (1994, May). *News & Reports.* Vol. 4.

Seki, M., Yoshida, K., & Okamura, Y. (1991). A study on hyperprolactinemia in female patients with alcoholism. *Arukoru Kenkyo-to Yakubutsu Ison, 26*(1), 49-59.

Shore, E., & Batt, S. (1991). Contextual factors related to the drinking patterns of American business and professional women. *British Journal of Addiction, 86,* 171-176.

Solomon, K., Cutler, L., Pierce, E. (1990). Alcoholism and drug abuse in the elderly. In R. Corman, D. Rogers, & D. Williams (Eds.), *Proceedings of the Seventh Annual Conference of the Maryland Gerontological Association.* Baltimore: Maryland Gerontological Association.

Substance Abuse and Mental Health Services Administration. (1992, December). *SAMHSA Mission.* Paper presentation at the SAMHSA New Directions Conference, Baltimore, Maryland.

Substance Abuse and Mental Health Services Administration, Center for Substance Abuse Treatment. (1993). *Pregnant substance abusing women: Treatment improvement protocol series.* (DHHS Publication No. SMA 93-1998). Rockville, MD: Author.

Substance Abuse and Mental Health Services Administration. (1994a). *National household survey on drug abuse: Population estimates, 1993.* (DHHS Publication No. SMA 94-3017). Washington, DC: U.S. Government Printing Office.

Substance Abuse and Mental Health Services Administration, Center for Substance Abuse Treatment. (1994b). *Practical approaches in the treatment of women who abuse alcohol and other drugs*. (DHHS Publication No. SMA 94-3006). Washington, DC: U.S. Government Printing Office.

Sun, A. (1991). Issues for Asian American women. In P. Roth (Ed.), *Alcohol and other drugs are women's issues, Vol. 1: A review of the issues*. Metuchen, NJ: Women's Action Alliance and Scarecrow Press.

Szwabo, P. (1993). Substance abuse in older women. *Clinics in Geriatric Medicine, 9* (1), 197-208.

Uhl, G., Blum, K., Noble, E., & Smith, S. (1993). Substance abuse vulnerability and D2 receptor genes. *Trends in Neurosciences, 16* (3), 83-87.

U.S. Bureau of the Census. (1993). *Statistical abstract of the United States, 1993, 113th ed.* Washington, DC: U.S. Government Printing Office.

U.S. General Accounting Office. (1993). *Drug use measurement. Strengths, limitations, and recommendations for improvement*. Washington, DC: Author.

Van Thiel, D., & Gaveler, J. (1988). Ethanol metabolism and hepatotoxicity: Does sex make a difference? In M. Galanter (Ed.), *Recent developments in alcoholism* (Vol. 6). New York: Plenum Press.

Wilsnack, S., Klassen, A., Schur, B., & Wilsnack, R. (1991). Predicting onset and chronicity of women's problem drinking: A five-year longitudinal analysis. *American Journal of Public Health, 81* (3), 305-318.

Witteman, J., Willett, W., Stampfer, M., Colditz, G., et al. (1990). Relation of moderate alcohol consumption and risk of systemic hypertension in women. *American Journal of Cardiology, 65* (9), 633-637.

Witters, W., Venturelli, P., & Hanson, G. (1992). *Drugs and society* (3rd ed.). Boston: Jones and Bartlett.

Worth, D. (1991). American women and polydrug abuse. In P. Roth (Ed.), *Alcohol and drugs are women's issues, Vol. 1: A review of the issues*. Metuchen, NJ: Women's Action Alliance and Scarecrow Press.

CHAPTER 14

Eating Disorders

Jenny H. Conviser
Marian L. Fitzgibbon

Over the last 20 years, the United States has witnessed a rise in the incidence of eating disorders; current estimates indicate that seven million women in this country suffer from eating disorders (National Association of Anorexia Nervosa and Associated Disorders [ANAD], 1995). Many other women struggle with less serious forms of disordered eating that do not meet all diagnostic criteria for eating disorders. On average, women who fulfill diagnostic criteria for eating disorders outnumber men by a ratio of 10:1 (Lucas, Beard, O'Fallon, & Kurland, 1991). Eating disorders may be more prevalent among women than men, in part, because women tend more often to diet to lose or control body weight. This assumption is supported by data that show the highest incidence of eating disorders in populations most concerned about dieting. In 1989, Americans spent approximately $30 billion on weight loss products and programs (Goode, 1990), which suggests that our society is preoccupied with body weight and therefore at risk for eating disorders.

This chapter addresses three categories of disordered eating: anorexia nervosa (anorexia), bulimia nervosa (bulimia), and binge eating. Factors related to symptoms, etiology, illness patterns, and treatment are discussed. Finally, the implications and recommendations for women are summarized.

Anorexia

Anorexia nervosa is characterized by a preoccupation with dieting, body shape, and weight. Those diagnosed with anorexia nervosa have a body weight of 15% or more below ideal weight. Anorectic individuals harbor intense fear of weight gain and attempt to assuage these fears with increased caloric restriction and exercise. The refusal to maintain a minimally normal body weight can result in amenorrhea or the absence of normal menstrual cycle function. Despite the critically low body weight that threatens health and well-being, the anorectic individual is often unaware of being "too thin" and is actually tormented by persistent feelings of being overly fat. Distorted perception of shape and weight, refusal to maintain minimally normal body weight, amenorrhea, and intense fear of gaining weight are diagnostic features of anorexia nervosa (American Psychiatric Association [APA], 1994).

Anorexia tends to be more prevalent among women than men, with prevalence rates of 269.9 for women and 22.5 for men per 100,000 population (Lucas et al.,

1991). Anorexia is more prevalent in middle and upper socioeconomic classes, industrialized and developed countries, and among individuals exposed to social pressures to maintain a thin body (Vandereycken & Hoek, 1992). The age of onset is most often during early adolescence and is common among 15- to 19-year-old girls. Current theory points to the combination of psychological, social, familial, environmental, and biologic factors that predispose an individual to this illness. Maturational problems and sociocultural factors are believed to precede the precipitation of anorectic symptoms in psychologically vulnerable women. Anorexia is complex in characteristics and variable in severity of symptoms. Women with weight and body concerns comprise a heterogeneous population; therefore, it is important to note that *not* all women with weight and body preoccupation meet the criteria for anorexia.

Many psychological factors are implicated in the predisposition to anorexia. Hilde Bruch (1973) was one of the earliest researchers to formally describe the psychological components of anorexia. She believed that failed early parent–child interactions, faulty perception of body boundaries, profound sense of ineffectiveness, and lack of autonomy characterized individuals with this illness. Other emotional traits commonly observed among anorectics include extreme compliancy, emotional reserve, compulsivity, lack of independence, avoidance of such maturational problems as individuation from family, poor self-esteem, and depression. Dysfunctional family dynamics can predispose and maintain disordered eating patterns such as anorexia. Dysfunctional patterns in families of anorectics often include conflict avoidance, extreme emotional constraint, affective lability, child involvement in marital conflict, overly intrusive parent–child interactions, poor boundaries among family members, and intolerance of change (Strober, 1992).

The results of summary data from 68 outcome studies estimate that 60% of anorectics achieve normal weight and normal menstruation and 49% achieve normalized eating patterns (Steinhausen, 1995). On average, about 40% of anorectics recover, 33% improve, and 20% endure chronic symptoms (Steinhausen, 1995). Unfavorable prognostic factors include history of vomiting, bulimia, extreme weight loss, and chronicity. A short interval between onset of symptoms and beginning of treatment is associated with a more favorable outcome. Conclusions based on outcome studies of anorexia nervosa are limited because of the numerous methodologic problems associated with such studies. The methodologic problems include overreliance on data from clinical centers, overreliance on telephone interview data, poor psychiatric assessment methods, and heterogeneous samples with regard to onset of the disease and length of follow-up.

Tracey Gold, star of the popular ABC television show, "Growing Pains," recently described her struggle with anorexia nervosa (Levitt, 1994). Diagnosed at the age of 12, Tracey reported calorie restriction, frequent weighing, and abstention from fatty foods, as well as the use of diuretics and laxatives to purge. Her highest body weight reached 133 lb at age 19 and her lowest weight was 80 lb. Tracey described herself as being fearful of uncontrollable weight gain should she allow herself even a small weight gain: "I was always saying, well, I don't want to eat this now because there might be something I'd rather eat later. Of course, that time never came." Tracey became increasingly controlled by her patterns of starvation and denial. Now at age 24, Tracey's weight continues to hover around 92 lb, 17 lb below a recommended body weight. Although Tracey feels that she is well along a positive course of recovery, her mother disagrees: "She sees a lump of butter and shudders."

In addition to Tracy's personal frustrations with anorexia, those nearest to Tracey who witnessed her struggle were also traumatized. Like so many other family members and friends who witness the effects of this disease, Tracey's boyfriend and parents wanted desperately to help her recover from anorexia, but they felt unable to intervene in beneficial ways. "Tracey went through hell," says her boyfriend, "and I had to sit there helplessly watching it." Tracey and her parents (Levitt, 1994) grew familiar with the relatively long and variable course of recovery that can often occur with eating disorders, even with the best professional treatment and family support.

Bulimia

Bulimia is characterized by episodes of rapid consumption of large amounts of food followed by uncomfortable feelings such as loss of control, guilt, depression, or fear of gaining weight (APA, 1994). The bulimic's view of self is powerfully influenced by body shape and weight, and therefore the fear of gaining weight is particularly distressful. In an effort to cope with these feelings, compensatory behaviors such as self-induced vomiting, laxative or diuretic use, enemas, excessive exercise, severely restrictive eating (low calorie intake), or periods of fasting follow. Bulimics of the "purging type," regularly engage in self-induced vomiting, laxative, diuretic, or enema use. Bulimics of the "nonpurging type" engage in compensatory behaviors such as fasting or excessive exercise, but do not regularly engage in self-induced vomiting, laxative, diuretic, or enema use. The diagnostic criteria for bulimia nervosa describe the frequency of the binge episodes and inappropriate compensatory behaviors as occurring on average of at least twice a week for 3 months (APA, 1994). The individual struggling with bulimic symptoms is usually aware of the disordered nature of these behaviors but is unable to refrain from such behavior.

The prevalence of bulimia among adolescent and young adult women is approximately 1% to 3% (APA, 1994). As many as 19% of female students responding to questionnaires report bulimic symptoms (Lucas et al., 1991). The average age of onset for bulimia is 18 years, with a range of 9 to 45 years (Johnson & Connors, 1987). Bulimic symptoms often begin after a period of restrictive eating or prolonged dieting. Other common precipitants include family problems, being teased about appearance, problems in romantic relationships, leaving home, or failures in school or work (Johnson & Connors, 1987). Emotional upset such as depression, loneliness, boredom, and anger may also occur at the time of onset of bulimic symptoms.

The degree of psychological difficulties present in bulimic individuals varies although some psychological features are common among bulimics:

- Bulimics often suffer from poor self-esteem, impulsivity, excitability, affective lability, and dysphoria.

- Bulimics may feel persistently ineffective, sensitive to rejection or nonreward, out of control, and helpless.
- Social role expectations may be confusing or overwhelming.
- Family chaos or conflict, high achievement expectations, and the pursuit of thinness are frequent sources of great stress.
- Bulimics have difficulty identifying, articulating, and controlling their various mood and bodily states.
- Regulating affective states and behavior is sometimes perceived by the individual as frightening and impossible.
- Binging and purging behaviors can serve as the bulimic's efforts to use external behaviors to gain control over internal difficulties.
- Binging can also serve as an opportunity for the overly controlled or obsessive individual to be out of control.

Outcome studies of bulimia are primarily retrospective and predominantly short- and intermediate-term studies. Few prognostic studies of bulimia exist, and therefore outcome data are currently far from conclusive. However, it is estimated that 50% of bulimia nervosa patients are asymptomatic 2 to 10 years after beginning cognitive/behavior therapy and participating in some follow-up treatment (Hsu, 1995). Approximately 20% of treated patients remain symptomatic despite treatment, and about 30% of patients treated experience periods of remission and relapse (Hsu, 1995). Left untreated, bulimia has a poor short-term prognosis. Additional data on bulimic individuals who are left untreated are needed.

Catherine is a 29-year-old, single, bulimic, woman who is currently employed as an attorney. Although repeatedly called "scrawny" as a child, she felt fat. Catherine may have had a biologic propensity for weight gain given that her parents and grandparents have histories of obesity. Catherine's father is a successful businessman and has high expectations for his children. Catherine's mother tries to be her daughter's best friend. Despite well meaning intentions, her mother is overly intrusive and controlling. Both parents have histories of problem eating. Catherine's father engages in obsessive exercise behavior and has anorectic symptoms. Catherine's mother is repulsed by obesity and sometimes binge eats but is also known for preparing and serving large portions of high-fat and high-calorie foods at frequent family functions. Catherine's mother is easily angered and offended if others decline her invitations to dine.

Catherine gained weight during high school to 130 lb and then during her freshman year at college to 165 lb. She reduced her weight to 110 lb through restrictive eating and purging. When "in control," Catherine runs 5 miles daily, eats only vegetarian foods, eats three meals a day and never snacks between meals, eats low-fat or nonfat foods, eats the same foods each day, and counts the number of bites of food she eats and the calories per bite consumed. She has observed that binging occurs more often when she feels stressed. Binging can occur as often as five times daily and 7 days a week. A single binge can include one-half of a cake, a pint of ice cream, up to 10 donuts, one-half a pizza, a bag of potato chips, and 8 to 10 ounces of cheese. She self-induces vomiting several times during and after the binge. After purging she feels weak and light-headed. Her eyes tear and her throat is sore. Her voice has a raspy quality caused by the irritation associated with the purging. After purging, Catherine initially feels some sense of "relief" or calm, and she feels "good" about "it" being over. Later she feels more depressed and angry with herself about the loss of control. After binging and purging, Catherine refuses invitations to see friends and family, cancels plans, goes to work late, or misses days of work. She hates that she is unable to "kick this thing" on her own.

Binge Eating

The diagnosis, binge eating disorder (BED), used in the *Diagnostic and Statistical Manual of Mental Disorders* (*DSM IV*) (APA, 1994) as a research diagnosis, has been conceptualized as an eating disorder characterized by binge eating without the compensatory behavior to avoid weight gain as seen in bulimia nervosa (Spitzer et al., 1991, 1992, 1993). Criteria include:

- recurrent binge eating (characterized by a larger amount of food than most people would eat under similar circumstances, plus a perceived loss of control over eating)
- associated behavioral features such as rapid or solitary eating
- marked distress
- minimum average occurrence of binge eating 2 days a week for at least 6 months
- binge eating that does not occur during the course of bulimia or anorexia nervosa (Spitzer et al., 1993)

Although binge eating in the obese population has been recognized for many years (Gormally, Black, Daston, & Rardin, 1982; Loro & Orleans, 1981; Marcus, Wing, & Lamparski, 1985; Stunkard, 1959), research has only recently focused on the prevalence and significance of binge eating as it relates to obesity treatment outcome (Marcus, Wing, & Hopkins, 1988). Binge eating is an important clinical feature among some obese individuals and has been associated with a range of characteristics. It is estimated that 20% to 50% of those individuals seeking weight management treatment have significant binge eating problems (Marcus & Wing, 1987).

Compared to individuals who do not binge, obese binge eaters show higher levels of psychopathology (Fitzgibbon & Kirschenbaum, 1991), more dietary restraint, preoccupation with eating, and unhealthy diet behavior (Goldfein, Walsh, La Chaussee, Kissileff, & Devlin, 1993); experience more weight fluctuations and increased fat body weight (Goldfein et al., 1993; Telch, Agras, & Rossiter, 1988); express more concern with body shape and weight (Marcus, Smith, Santelli, & Kaye, 1992); and appear to respond less well to traditional behavioral interventions (Marcus, Wing, & Hopkins, 1988). The mounting evidence to suggest that binge eaters are a distinct subgroup among the obese population has led to the inclusion of binge eating as a separate eating disorder diagnosis in *DSM IV*.

Data from multisite studies (Spitzer et al., 1991, 1993) suggest an overall prevalence of approximately 30% of BED in weight control samples. Associated findings in these studies indicate that compared to obese nonbingers, individuals with BED have histories of more severe obesity, extreme weight fluctuations, an earlier onset of obesity, significant dieting behavior, and more general psychopathology. Although the 1991 study indicated a higher prevalence of BED in women, this was not replicated in the 1993 study.

Susan is a 22-year-old, single, woman diagnosed with BED. She is of average weight at 5 feet 3 inches and 126 lb. She works part-time as a receptionist and attends college. Susan complains of a 4-year history of eating problems including constant worry about her weight and appearance, preoccupation with calorie and fat intake, and low-calorie eating. She feels these eating-related problems are increasingly out of control and troubling. She has no prior history of anorexia or bulimia. She describes the food intake during daily binges as increasingly large and more debilitating: "I stuff myself until I am paralyzed," she says. Susan binges once daily, usually when her time is unscheduled in the afternoon and she is alone. She notices that she is particularly prone to binging when she is avoiding a necessary task in which she has little interest. Before the binge she is aware of feeling anxious, restless, and unable to sit still or concentrate on other activities such as television or reading. During one binge episode lasting 45 minutes, she may consume one-half a pizza, a large box of breakfast cereal with milk, one-half jar of peanut butter, and a box of cookies. After binging Susan feels painfully full, has difficulty breathing, and feels that she cannot stand, sit, or move for 1 to 2 hours. Later, she feels extreme guilt, self-hate, and anger. Susan's binges are followed by more restrictive eating and promises to herself to refrain from binging the next day, but these promises are increasingly hard to keep. She worries that the binges will affect her weight, appearance, mood, and the ability to focus on other activities or important relationships. Susan believes that except for her eating problems, her life is "perfect."

Etiology and Risk Factors

At present, there is no single cause of eating disorders. Experts agree that psychological, biologic, sociocultural, environmental, and familial factors often converge to cause disordered eating. Some factors related to the risk of eating disorders in women are discussed below.

Cultural Emphasis on Thinness

The belief that fat is synonymous with ugly, bad, weak, or failure is pervasive in the United States. However, this notion is certainly not universal. Although obesity has been associated with the increased risk of such health problems as high blood pressure, diabetes, and premature death, it may represent the ability to afford food, medical care, and increased survival rates in periods of famine for people living in poor countries. Obesity in some countries is admired and is symbolic of success and economic security. In some cultures, particularly in less affluent and developing areas such as Latin America, Puerto Rico (Dolan, 1991), and the Philippines (Stunkard, 1977), a positive correlation exists between body weight and socioeconomic status.

There appears to be greater societal pressure to maintain a thin shape among individuals in Western countries (Bordo, 1993). Over the past 20 years, the standard for women's body weight and shape in the United States has become increasingly thin. The average weight of Playboy centerfold models declined between 1959 and 1979 with models in 1979 weighing only 84% of the average woman (Garner & Garfinkel, 1980). During this same time period, Miss America Pageant winners had a 0.37-lb weight decline per year (Garner & Garfinkel, 1980). This downward weight trend generally continued in the next 10-year period (1979–1988) with 69% of the Playboy centerfold women and 60% of Miss America contestants having weights of 15% or more below the expected weight for their age and height (Wiseman, Gray, Mosimann, & Ahrens, 1992). Being thin is equated with attractiveness, desirability, sex appeal (Fallon & Rozin, 1988), accomplishment, success, and control (Barsky, 1988; Glassner, 1988). The current "thin ideal" (McCarthy, 1990) ranks far below the actual *average* weight of women in this country (Garner, 1985). One theory maintains that women who develop eating disorders have internalized this unrealistic thin ideal to a greater extent than others.

Women in the United States generally express greater dissatisfaction with their body weight than do men. In a survey of Americans, 96% of the respondents indicated that they would like to change something about their bodies; 78% of women, as opposed to 58% of men, wanted to change their body weight (Harris, 1987). In a study of newspaper personal ads for dating, 70% of the ads specified weight, shape, or height characteristics, and women described themselves as 89.4% less than the ideal body weight (Anderson, Woodward, Spalder & Koss, 1993). Women's magazines are estimated to contain 10.5 times as many advertisements and articles promoting weight loss as compared to men's magazines (Anderson & DiDomenico, 1992). It is hypothesized that a relationship exists between sociocultural reinforcements that advocate thinness (such as magazine advertisements) and the incidence of eating disorders.

Family History

Children who come from families in which one or more individuals suffer from eating disorders are at increased risk for also developing eating disturbances (Strober, 1995).

Research has shown that eating disorders are more prevalent among biologic relatives of patients than in the population at large in which the lifetime expectancy for anorexia nervosa is 0.5% to 1.5% (Strober & Humphrey, 1987). Interestingly, the siblings of patients with eating disorders seem to have a greater likelihood of developing eating problems, weight-related problems, and mood and substance abuse disorders (Vandereycken, 1995). Parental traits and child management styles have also been studied with varying results. One common observation is that parents of patients with eating disorders tend to disagree about childrearing issues and have difficulty finding age-appropriate balance between control and autonomy for their children (Vandereycken, 1995). Parents of bulimic patients are often remembered as uncaring—mothers as neglectful and fathers as controlling and unaffectionate.

Initial presentation with the family of an eating-disorder patient may reveal an idealized family unit complaining only of the eating disorder problem and denying other family conflict or limitation with regard to stability, nurturance, or caring

(Vandereycken, 1995). However, observational studies show that families of anorectic children have greater family discord, extreme alienation of affection, rigid family organization, poor interpersonal boundaries, and extreme restriction of autonomy. Mothers of anorectics are described as intrusive, overprotective, anxious, perfectionistic, and fearful of separation; fathers of anorectics are described as emotionally constricted, obsessional, moody, withdrawn, passive, and ineffectual (Strober & Humphrey, 1987). A full range of psychological disturbances from mild to severe appear to be present in some parents of those with anorexia nervosa.

Bulimics perceive their families to be more disturbed in their relationships than do normal weight controls (Humphrey, 1989; Wonderlich, 1992). In particular, they observed greater conflict, isolation, less cohesion, less involvement, less nurturing, and less expressiveness among family members than do the normal controls. Families of bulimics also use complex and contradictory interpersonal messages. They sometimes communicate opposite messages to their daughters such as appearing to offer them freedom and understanding while at the same time controlling their daughters' behavior and feelings (Humphrey, 1989).

Little research on adults with eating disorders and their marital relationships exists. Empirical data is scarce. One common clinical observation of couples in marriage is the presence of marital dissatisfaction. Patients sometimes attribute marital discord to the eating disorder. Other clinical observations of marital couples include evidence of lack of intimacy, communication difficulties, conflict avoidance, and power struggles in the relationship (Woodside, Shekter-Wolfson, Brandes, & Lackstrom, 1993).

Although various disturbed family interaction patterns have been observed and descriptions of family members have been collected, specific causal relationships related to eating disorders have not yet been demonstrated.

History of Abuse

Sexual abuse among individuals with eating disorders has been a difficult topic to study accurately. However, it is estimated that approximately 30% of patients with eating disorders have had a history of sexual abuse during childhood (Connors & Morse, 1992). This rate of abuse approximates rates found in non–eating-disorder populations. Child abuse (physical or sexual) does not appear to increase the likelihood of developing a specific disorder such as bulimia nervosa, but it may increase the diversity of psychopathology if any pathology exists (Rorty, Yager, & Rossotto, 1994). No causal relationship between childhood sexual experiences and later eating disorders has been evidenced (Palmer, 1995).

History of Psychiatric Illness

Women with greater body dissatisfaction, thinner body ideal, and more depression tend to have an earlier onset of eating disorders. The biologic relatives of bulimics may have an increased tendency for mood disorders. Individuals with bulimia tend to have poor treatment outcomes when they have had previous psychiatric hospitalizations (Fahy & Russell, 1993). Additionally, poor prognosis has been associated with bulimic individuals who have been diagnosed with a personality disorder (Fahy & Russell, 1993).

Substance Abuse

Higher than expected rates of current and past substance abuse are found among individuals with either anorexia or bulimia (Wilson, 1995). As many as 3% to 49% of bulimic women experience alcohol abuse, dependence, or treatment during their lifetime (Mitchell, Hatsukami, Ekert, & Pyle, 1985). In addition, bulimic women are more likely to have alcoholism in a first-degree relative than are nonbulimic women (Bulik, 1987). Studies of the relationship between substance abuse and binge eaters have produced mixed results (Wilson, 1995).

Explanations for the relationship between eating disorders and the higher incidence of substance abuse may be found in the examination of personality disorders. Recent research indicates that a higher incidence of both alcohol and tranquilizer abuse, as well as laxative and diuretic abuse, may occur only among those eating-disorder patients with psychiatric disorders or those specifically diagnosed with borderline personality disorder (Koepp, Schildbach, Schmager & Rohner, 1993). It is argued that substance abuse is correlated positively with the diagnosis of a personality disorder and not with eating disorders. Therefore, when the diagnosis of borderline personality disorder is statistically controlled for, women with eating disorders do not appear to differ from non–eating-disorder women with respect to alcohol abuse.

Other explanations for the comorbidity of eating disorders and substance abuse may be found in further research concerning personality traits, personality disorders, and genetic factors. Personality traits such as poor impulse control, chronic depression, and low frustration tolerance have been documented and may be traits expressed as disordered eating and substance abuse (Krahn, 1991). Genetic factors may also play a role in the development of both eating disorders and substance abuse (Holderness, Brooks-Gunn, & Warren, 1994; Kendler et al., 1991) although the specifics of such factors have not yet been delineated.

Sexual Orientation

The issue of sexual orientation as a mediator for risk for eating problems was explored by some researchers with mixed results. Herzog, Newman, and Warshaw (1991) noted that membership in a male homosexual culture is associated with greater interest in an underweight ideal than measured among heterosexual men, therefore leaving homosexual men at increased risk for developing eating disorders. The emphasis on attractiveness in the homosexual male subculture has also been associated with increased body dissatisfaction and disregulated eating (Mishkind, Rodin, Silberstein, & Striegel-Moore, 1986). Conversely, some lesbian women may have a different relationship to social norms than do homosexual men or heterosexual women. Therefore, they may be somewhat protected from the effects of stereotypical thinking related to physical attractiveness. Some researchers have found that lesbians are less invested in the "thin ideal" and the associated cultural norms for attractiveness, which may possibly lessen their less risk for disordered eating (Brown, 1987; Mayer, 1983; Stein, 1989). One study showed that whereas 67% of cohabiting men rated attractiveness of their partner as important, only 35% of lesbians rated physical attractiveness as important (Blumstein & Schwartz, 1983).

Findings concerning lesbians' risk for eating disorders relative to heterosexual women are mixed. Methodologic problems in this research (such as small sample size and unreliable assessment tools) have resulted in inconclusive data.

Athletics or Dance

Eating disorders may more prevalent in environments that are particularly stressful and competitive. Individuals and groups in which ideal body weight and appearance are greatly emphasized, such as entertainers, models, dancers, and some athletes are also at risk (Crago, Yates, Beutler, & Arizmendi, 1985; Druss & Silverman, 1979; Yates, Leehey, & Shisslak, 1983). Although precise prevalence rates have yet to be confirmed, eating disorders are a significant problem among some college athletic teams (Garner & Rosen, 1991). As many as 62% of team members suffer from eating disorders when under the combined pressures to excel and to maintain specific weight and appearance requirements (Rosen & Hough, 1988). Eating disorders and related problems frequent women's sports where special emphasis is placed on appearance and weight (Lopiano & Zotos, 1992). Such sports typically include figure skating, diving, ballet, distance running, and gymnastics. In some sport environments, well meaning but poorly informed coaches and teachers encourage calorie counting, restrictive eating, and dieting to promote optimal performance and appearance. For unmet weight requirements, they might institute punishments such as public ridicule, excessive exercise requirements, or elimination from traveling teams or competition. In other cases, it is not the coaches, but parents, friends, fellow athletes, and fans who impose punishment for weight gain or body imperfection. Even officials and judges have been accused of placing greater importance on appearance rather than skills and assigning lower scores accordingly. Because athletic officials hold much power in determining medal winners, title winners, qualifiers for special teams or final competitions, college scholarship awards, and endorsement contracts, the consequences of weight prejudice can be dire.

College gymnasts may be especially susceptible to eating disorders given the pressure to maintain a very low body weight at an age when the body's natural tendency may be to gain weight and develop rounder hips and breasts. Moreover, the revealing clothing worn in competition, the fact that the gymnasts are scored not only on skill, but also on appearance, and the popular belief that thinner is somehow better, impose additional pressures. Thinner, however, is *not* always better. Dieting and weight loss can result in both less fat and muscle mass, which can hamper athletic performance (Yeager, Agostini, Nattiv, & Drinkwater, 1993). In addition, poor nutrition can result in increased fatigue, anemia, electrolyte imbalance, and depression, all of which alone or in combination threaten health and well-being and disrupt athletic performance (Yeager et al., 1993). Christy Henrich, an accomplished world class gymnast, was a recent casualty of anorexia nervosa at age 22. She was described as having been a "straight A student" and a "perfectionistic" in all endeavors. She not only struggled with disordered eating but reportedly (Noden, 1994) abused laxatives and exercised compulsively. Christy described her life as an anorectic as "a horrifying nightmare. It feels like there is a beast inside me, like a monster. It feels evil" (Noden, 1994). Christy lapsed into a coma and died on July 26, 1994, of organ failure secondary to starvation. At 4 feet 10 inches tall, Christy had weighed as little as 47 lb. She was 61 lb when she died.

Ethnicity

Early research has suggested a lower prevalence of eating disorders among non-Caucasian than Caucasian individuals. However, such data may have been compromised by research biases. Non-Caucasian individuals may have been referred less frequently for treatment and therefore have been underrepresented in the data. Recent studies suggest that minorities are similar to Caucasian individuals with regard to prevalence of disturbed eating behaviors.

Obesity

A familial tendency toward obesity may exist in families of those with eating disorders, but this has not been conclusively documented. A recent study by Telch and Agras (1994) support the relevance of the BED diagnosis and the importance of assessing BED in research with obese populations. Findings from this study of 107 obese women diagnosed with BED indicated a significant positive relationship between binge eating severity and degree of psychiatric symptomatology; degree of obesity and psychopathology were unrelated. The authors suggest that binge eating may account for the observed relationship between obesity and psychopathology reported in previous studies (Telch & Agras, 1994) and may clarify some inconsistencies in the research.

A number of researchers and clinicians have suggested that to effectively treat the psychological and behavioral disturbances associated with obesity, competently designed treatment approaches tailored to individual needs must be implemented (Brownell, 1993). Fitzgibbon, Stolley, and Kirschenbaum (1993) underscored the important differences in the obese population by comparing three matched groups: obese individuals seeking treatment, obese persons not seeking treatment, and normal weight controls. They were measured on the level of psychopathology, binge eating, and negative emotional eating. Results indicated that obese people seeking treatment reported significantly greater psychopathology and binge eating than either those who had not sought treatment or normal weight controls. The authors stressed the importance of evaluating such variables because these individuals may not do well in standard behavior programs (Fitzgibbon et al., 1993).

Symptoms and Illness Patterns

Symptoms that are often associated with increased risk for an eating disorder are listed in Display 14-1. Individuals experiencing any one or more of those behaviors need comprehensive and professional evaluation for eating disorders.

Those suffering from eating disorders are also beset with considerable somatic or medical complications, emotional distress, disrupted interpersonal functioning, and in many cases, financial burden.

DISPLAY 14-1
Symptoms Indicating an Increased Risk for an Eating Disorder

1. Inability to maintain a minimum recommended body weight
2. Engaging in secretive eating
3. Self-induced or spontaneous vomiting after eating
4. Use of medications, laxatives, or diet pills to control weight
5. Chewing and spitting out food or drink
6. Amenorrhea not explained by other medical conditions
7. Frequent weighing of oneself
8. Mood change after eating
9. Mood change after weighing
10. Persistent feelings of dissatisfaction with body weight or shape
11. Persistently feeling fat despite others telling you that you are thin
12. Feeling a loss of control when eating
13. Feeling fearful of uncontrollable weight gain
14. Discomfort or embarrassment experienced when eating in front of other people
15. Receiving comments from other people regarding weight, eating, or exercise behavior
16. Mood change or increased worry about shape or weight when abstaining from exercise

Medical complications secondary to eating disorders (ANAD, 1994; APA, 1994) are many and can range from mild to severe. The most apparent physical feature of anorexia is emaciation. Primary or secondary amenorrhea is common. Abdominal pain, cold intolerance, lethargy, and potassium deficiency are also common. Excess energy, hypotension, constipation, and lanugo or fine body hair growth are often seen in individuals who are starving. Abnormal heart rate or bradycardia is common in anorectic individuals. Dry or yellowing skin is also common. Peripheral edema or water retention in the body's extremities can accompany refeeding and can be especially distressing for the anorectic individual.

The physical signs and symptoms associated with purging-type bulimia are often related to the body's fluid and electrolyte balance (ANAD, 1994; APA, 1994). Fluid imbalance resulting in irregular heart activity, called cardiac arrhythmia, poses the most serious threat to health and requires close medical monitoring and intervention. Edema, sometimes observed in feet and ankles, can indicate electrolyte imbalance caused by long periods of starvation, excessive vomiting, or use of laxatives or diuretics. Insufficient fluid intake or excessive fluid elimination can result in dry skin. Rashes and blemishes may be related to vomiting and laxative abuse. Inadequate nutrition or vomiting can result in erosion of tooth enamel, teeth that are increasingly sensitive to hot and cold, and tooth decay. Cuts or scarring from teeth can result from self-induced vomiting and may be visible on the back of the hands. Swelling, pain, and tenderness of the salivary glands, and especially the parotid gland, can result from frequent vomiting. Feelings of fullness with accompanying abdominal distention may persist after the person eats. Feelings of fullness may be caused by slow intestinal activity resulting from chronic laxative use or poor nutrition or emotional factors such as worry or anxiety regarding ingested food. Insufficient body fat, excessive exercise, and binge–purge cycles can disrupt normal hormonal function and trigger irregular menstrual cycles or amenorrhea. The symptoms associated with purging-type bulimia nervosa are likely to be more severe than those with nonpurging type.

Individuals with eating disorders frequently complain of persistent and at times severe emotional distress. Depressed mood often occurs with eating disorders. Other related complaints from those with eating disorders often include poor concentration, preoccupation with food and eating, irritability, frustration, sleep disruption, fatigue, and poor self-esteem. Anxiety related to fears of uncontrollable eating, weight gain, or body shape may persist. Such emotional difficulties can disrupt occupational and educational pursuits, or interpersonal relationships. Individuals with eating disorders can feel at odds with others, misunderstood, unsupported, isolated, and alone. Intervention or help from others can be perceived by the patient with an eating disorder as bothersome, interfering, unnecessary, or provocative. Secretive eating, binging, or behaviors such as medication use and abuse can also lead to avoidant and isolating behaviors that separate the individual from others. Depression, anxiety, occupational stressors, conflictual relationships, and social isolation can further exacerbate the cycle of binging, purging, and disordered eating.

Financial problems related to eating disorders can be burdensome, an issue not often acknowledged. Medical, psychological, and psychiatric treatment can be costly in terms of both time and dollars. Health insurance policies vary widely in their coverage of eating disorders and eating-related issues. Some policies are profoundly limited in the amount of coverage or the number of sessions covered for treatment of eating disorders. Patients and their families must carefully plan to manage their financial resources to accommodate what can sometimes be long-term and multicomponent treatment.

Food expenses for those with bulimia can be costly as well. Multiple daily grocery store and restaurant stops can result in costs as high as $100 a day. Depression and illnesses relating to eating disorders can also result in missed work or job loss and corresponding loss of income.

Relevance Across the Lifespan

A serious potential consequence of insufficient body weight is amenorrhea, which is usually associated with a reduction in estrogen levels. Because estrogen protects the skeletal structure, amenorrheic women may experience bone loss and therefore be at greater risk for bone fractures. In fact, amenorrheic athletes have higher rates of fractures than do female athletes with normal menstrual cycles (Rankin, 1993). Poor nutrition and low body weight are two factors related to eating disorders that can increase the risk for premature osteoporosis. Interestingly, even such factors as bed rest and traveling in outer space increase bone mass loss. Conversely, physical activity is associated with bone health in premenopausal and postmenopausal women. Athletes have a higher bone density than inactive individuals. One 3-year study of women nursing home residents with an average age of 81 examined the effects of exercise while the women were seated in a chair. Women who participated in this exercise regimen had a 2.3% increase in radial bone mineral density. Nonparticipants had a 3.3% decline in this same measurement (Rankin, 1993).

Maintenance of adequate body weight to sustain normal menstrual function, good nutrition with adequate consumption of calcium especially during childhood and adolescence, and adequate amounts of weight-bearing exercise can reduce the risk of osteoporosis. Without sufficient nutrition and adequate body weight, anorectic individuals are at increased risk for premature osteoporosis.

Treatment

Without treatment, the prognosis for women with eating disorders can be poor. With professional help, most women with eating disorders will have a promising recovery. If symptoms occur, women should seek treatment as soon as possible. Delaying treatment may exacerbate symptoms, which can lead to the need for more intensive and longer treatment. When seeking diagnostic information and treatment advice, patients should consult more than one professional for opinions and recommendations. Multicomponent treatment is not necessary for all eating-disorder patients but should be available to patients if it is needed. For treatment of most serious symptoms or for those symptoms that endure over time, multicomponent treatment is recommended. This treatment includes medical management, pharmacotherapy, nutrition education, behavioral management, psychodynamic psychotherapy, cognitive therapy, family therapy, and group therapy.

Pharmacotherapy is sometimes beneficial for these patients. In the past, eating-disorder patients, especially bulimics, were treated successfully with antidepressant medication (Kennedy & Goldbloom, 1991; Walsh, 1991). Use of antidepressant medications such as tricyclic antidepressants, monoamine oxidase inhibitors, serotonin reuptake inhibitors, and atypical antidepressants like bupropion and trazodone are most importantly associated with improved mood, as well as improved body image, less obsessive focus on food and dieting, and reduced binge frequency (Walsh, 1992). However, other medications, such as antianxiety agents and more rarely, antipsychotic agents, are useful as well. Serotonergic agents are used to treat obsessive–compulsive symptoms. Cyproheptadine, an antihistamine, is associated with weight gain and relief of depressive symptoms in some patients with anorexia nervosa (Walsh, 1995).

Individual evaluation will determine if a medication trial is indicated. This evaluation is best conducted by a psychiatrist or health care practitioner with specialized training and experience in treating eating disorders. Any medication regimen should be carefully monitored by the prescribing health care practitioner. Medication used to treat eating disorders is most often prescribed in combination with psychotherapy.

Most individuals with eating disorders can be treated successfully without inpatient hospitalization. However, a small number of individuals with the most serious and immediate life-threatening symptoms, such as threatened self-harm, severe depression, or substance abuse, may require one or more medical or psychiatric hospitalizations. Hospitalization may also be indicated if the patient fails to respond adequately to outpatient treatment. Professionals formally trained in treating eating disorders are best able to determine whether inpatient treatment is necessary. Inpatient hospitalization can be most beneficial when it offers a protective environment; empathic and available health care practitioners with specialized training in the treatment of eating disorders; support for individual expression, growth, and change; reliable organization and structure; and the capacity to manage problematic behavior or health problems that may arise during the hospitalization.

Failure to respond to treatment is associated with factors such as older age of onset, longer duration of problem symptoms left untreated, lower body weight, poor childhood adjustment, the presence of other substance dependence or abuse, poor family relationships, and previous psychiatric history.

Implications

A unified and collective effort on the part of Americans is needed to reduce the prevalence of eating disorders. It is essential that men and women continue to become informed regarding the 1) sociocultural pressures to achieve and maintain thin ideals, 2) hazards of dieting and weight loss, and 3) consequences of eating disorders. Parents, teachers, coaches, health care practitioners, as well as the weight loss and beauty industries, can all influence beliefs and attitudes regarding body weight, shape, appearance, and beauty.

The beauty industry promotes the image of thinness as superior, which infers that weight loss and dieting are necessary to achieve this standard. Clothes are designed and marketed for the subnormal weight female body, and hair and makeup products are modeled by thin and waiflike models. Weight loss products are linked to other promises such as becoming more attractive, more desirable, and somehow more able to achieve a better life or personality. Susan Faludi, author of (1992) *Backlash, War Against Women*, argues that the feminine traits celebrated by the beauty industry in the 1980s were unnatural and that such traits could only be achieved with "harsh, unhealthy, and punitive measures" (p. 201). Faludi also maintains that

> ...the beauty industry seems the most superficial of the cultural institutions..., but its impact on women was, in many respects, the most intimately destructive to both female bodies and minds. Following the orders of the '80's beauty doctors made many women literally ill..., silicone injections left painful deformities. Cosmetic liposuction caused severe complications, infections, and even death. Internalized, the decade's beauty dictates played a role in exacerbating an epidemic of eating disorders (p. 203).

Individuals can reduce their own risk of eating disorders and support healthy eating behaviors by following the recommendations outlined in Display 14-2. Display 14-3 suggests some ways that parents can reduce the risk of eating disorders and support healthy eating behaviors in their children. Hopefully, parents can model positive self-evaluation, reduce their own emphasis on appearance, avoid instituting a "diet mentality" in the home, and provide experiences that build a sense of self in their children that is not contingent alone on weight and appearance.

Teachers can also assist their students in learning about the importance of proper nutrition and the hazards of dieting by creating learning environments that promote acceptance and respect for all body types and minimize competition around appearance, weight, and body shape. Educational opportunities should be provided for women to learn to critically evaluate advertisements, sales pitches, and marketing strategies for weight loss and beauty products. Teachers can help women learn to make informed choices about products and behaviors that may have short- and long-term health consequences. Everyone should learn the importance of early recognition of the signs and symptoms of disordered eating. This may be difficult given the private nature of many aspects of this type of illness. Individuals suffering with disordered eating and related problems may prefer to work on the problem themselves, or they may feel embarrassed or ashamed to discuss their problems with others. However, when such symptoms are observed or reported, early assessment and intervention are vital. Individuals with disordered eating can be reminded that:

DISPLAY 14-2
Recommendations for Reducing the Risk of Eating Disorders

1. Eat a variety of nutritious meals and snacks periodically throughout the day.
2. Do not deny yourself or abstain from eating your favorite foods, rather eat such foods in moderation.
3. Avoid skipping meals or becoming overly hungry.
4. Keep healthy foods available.
5. Avoid storing large quantities of foods with which you feel you have little control.
6. Eat in an eating place such as a kitchen or dining room.
7. Avoid eating in environments where you feel less control, such as in front of the television, buffet dining, or in the company of certain people.
8. Find alternatives for managing uncomfortable feelings such as sadness, anger, anxiety, or fear.
9. Avoid overly restrictive dieting.
10. Avoid frequent weighing.
11. Problem solve or seek advice regarding decisions to enter environments that leave you feeling pressured about your body weight, shape, and appearance.

DISPLAY 14-3
Guidelines for Parents to Reduce the Risk of Eating Disorders in Children

---

1. Model healthy eating and exercise behavior.
2. Encourage eating a variety of nutritious meals and snacks periodically throughout the day.
3. Avoid use of food as a punishment or a reward.
4. Seek professional treatment for eating difficulties, psychiatric disturbance, substance abuse, family conflict, or marital difficulties.
5. Offer plentiful praise for accomplishments and attributes that are not weight or appearance related.
6. Discourage dieting.
7. Model acceptance and respect for all body types, shapes, and weights.
8. Consult a professional or arrange for an assessment if eating or weight-related problems arise.

---

1. An assessment is an opportunity to gather information and does not mean that treatment is necessary.
2. Assessment does not necessarily lead to a diagnoses of an eating disorder.
3. Early assessment can prevent additional and more complex eating-related problems.
4. Eating disorder assessments for adults are confidential.
5. An assessment can help an individual feel less alone and more understood in terms of his or her eating disorders.

Health care practitioners are in a powerful position to intervene. They can help reduce the risk of eating disorders in several ways:

1. Become well informed regarding the prevalence and risks of eating disorders.
2. Become well informed regarding the hazards of restrictive dieting.
3. Become familiar with the symptoms and medical complications associated with eating disorders.
4. Ask patients directly and specifically about problematic behaviors such as self-induced vomiting, binging, starvation diets, low body weight, use of laxatives, diuretics, and weight loss medications.
5. Provide patients with accurate information regarding healthy eating and realistic weight management strategies.
6. Refer patients for eating disorders treatment when appropriate.

It is important for health care practitioners to know that symptoms of eating disorders usually do not spontaneously remit; early assessment and intervention are most helpful in preventing further complications.

Finally, it is an individual responsibility to challenge one's own thinking and judgment in response to people of high or low body weight. Stereotypical reactions, labels, and verbal comments should be avoided. The challenge is to look beyond physical appearance when evaluating oneself or others.

References

American Psychiatric Association. (1994). *Diagnostic and statistical manual of mental disorders* (4th ed.). Washington, DC: Author.

Anderson, A. E., & DiDomenico, L. D. (1992). Diet vs. content of popular male and female magazines: A dose-response relationship to the incidence of eating disorders? *International Journal of Eating Disorders, 11,* 283-287.

Anderson, A. E., Woodward, P. J., Spalder, A., & Koss, M. (1993). Body size and shape characteristics of personal (in search of) ads. *International Journal of Eating Disorders, 14,* 111-116.

Barsky, A. J. (1988). *Worried sick: Our troubled quest for wellness.* Boston: Little Books.

Blumstein, P., & Schwarz, P. (1983). *American couples: Money, work and sex.* New York: William Morrow.

Bordo, S. (1993). *Unbearable weight: Feminism, Western culture, and the body.* Berkeley, CA: University of California Press.

Brown, L. (1987). Lesbians, weight and eating: New analyses and perspectives. In Boston Lesbian Psychologies Collective (Eds.), *Lesbian psychologies: Explorations and challenges* (pp. 294-309). Chicago: University of Illinois Press.

Brownell, K. (1993). Whether obesity should be treated. *Health Psychology, 12,* 339-341.

Brownell, K. D. (1991). Dieting and the search for the perfect body: Where physiology and culture collide. *Behavior Therapy, 22,* 1991.

Bruch, H. (1973). *Eating disorders: Obesity, anorexia nervosa, and the person within.* New York: Basic Books.

Bulik, C. M. (1987). Alcohol use and depression in women with bulimia. *American Journal of Drug and Alcohol Abuse, 13,* 343-355.

Connors, M. E., & Morse, W. (1992). Sexual abuse and eating disorders: A review. *International Journal of Eating Disorders, 13,* 1-11.

Crago, M., Yates, A., Beutler, L. E., & Arizmendi, T. G. (1985). Height-weight ratios among female athletes: Are collegiate athletics the precursors to an anorexic syndrome? *International Journal of Eating Disorders, 4,* 79-87.

Dolan, B. (1990). Cross-cultural aspects of anorexia nervosa and bulimia. *International Journal of Eating Disorders, 10,* 67-78.

Druss, R. G., & Silverman, J. A. (1979). Body image and perfectionism of ballerinas: Comparison and contrast with anorexia nervosa. *General Hospital Psychiatry, 1,* 115-121.

Fahy, T. A., & Russell, G. F. M. (1993). Outcome and prognostic variables in bulimia nervosa. *International Journal of Eating Disorders, 14,* 135-145.

Fallon, A. E., & Rozin, P. (1985). Sex differences in perceptions of desirable body shape. *Journal of Abnormal Psychology, 94,* 102-105.

Faludi, S. (1991). *Backlash: The undeclared war against American women.* New York: Crown.

Fitzgibbon, M. L., & Kirschenbaum, D. S. (1991). Distressed binge eaters as a distinct subgroup among obese individuals seeking treatment. *Addictive Behaviors, 16,* 441-451.

Fitzgibbon, M. L., Stolley, M. R., & Kirschenbaum, D. S. (1993). Obese people who seek treatment have different characteristics than those who do not seek treatment. *Health Psychology, 12,* 342-345.

Garner, D. M., & Garfinkel, P. E. (1980). Socio-cultural factors in the development of anorexia nervosa. *Psychological Medicine, 10,* 647-657.

Garner, D. M., & Rosen, L. W. (1991). Eating disorders among athletes: Research and recommendations. *Journal of Applied Sport Science Research, 5,* 100-117.

Glassner, B. (1988). *Bodies: Why we look the way we do and how we feel about it.* New York: Putnam.

Goode, E. E. (1990, May). Getting slim. *U.S. News and World Report, 108,* 56-65.

Goldfein, J. A., Walsh, B. T., LaChaussee, J. L., Kissileff, H. R., & Devlin, M. J. (1993). Eating behavior in binge eating disorder. *International Journal of Eating Disorders, 14*(4), 427–431.

Gormally, J., Black, S., Daston, S., & Rardin, D. (1982). The assessment of binge eating severity among obese persons. *Addictive Behaviors, 7,* 47-55.

Harris, L. (1987). *Inside America*. New York: Vintage Books.

Herzog, D. B., Newman, K. L., & Warshaw, M. (1991). Body image dissatisfaction in homosexual and heterosexual males. *Journal of Nervous and Mental Disease, 179* (6), 356-359.

Holderness, C. C., Brooks-Gunn, J., & Warren, M. P. (1994). Co-morbidity of eating disorders and substance abuse review of the literature. *International Journal of Eating Disorders, 16*, 1-34.

HSU, L. K. G. (1995). Outcome of bulimia nervosa. In K. D. Brownell & C. G. Fairburn (Eds.). *Eating disorders and obesity* (pp. 165-170). New York: Guilford Press.

Humphrey, L. (1989). Is there a causal link between disturbed family processes and eating disorders? In W. G. Johnson (Ed.), *Advances in eating disorders* (pp. 119-136). Greenwich, CT: JAI Press.

Johnson, C., & Connors, M. E. (1987). Demographic and clinical characteristics. In *The etiology and treatment of bulimia nervosa* (pp. 32). New York: Basic Books.

Kendler, K. S., MacLean, C., Neale, M., Kessler, R., Heath, A., & Eaves, L. (1991). The genetic epidemiology of bulimia nervosa. *American Journal of Psychiatry, 148*, 1627-1637.

Kennedy, S. H., & Goldbloom, D. S. (1991). Current perspectives on drug therapies for anorexia nervosa and bulimia nervosa. *Drugs, 41*, 367-377.

Koepp, W., Schildbach, S., Schmager, C., & Rohner, R. (1993). Borderline diagnosis and substance abuse in female patients with eating disorders. *International Journal of Eating Disorders, 14*(1), 107-110.

Krahn, D. D. (1991). The relationship of eating disorders and substance abuse. *Journal of Substance Abuse, 3*, 239-254.

Levitt, (1994, January 31). Weight and see. *People Magazine*, 50-54.

Lopiano, D. A., & Zotos, C. (1992). Modern athletics: The pressure to perform. In K. D. Brownell, J. Rodin, & J. H. Wilmore (Eds.), *Eating, body weight, and performance in athletes: Disorders of modern society* (pp. 275-292). Philadelphia: Lea & Febiger.

Loro, S. D., & Orleans, C. S. (1981). Binge eating in obesity: Preliminary findings and guidelines for behavioral analysis and treatment. *Addictive Behaviors, 6*, 155-166.

Lucas, A. R., Beard C. M., O'Fallon, W. M., & Kurland, L. T. (1991). Fifty year trends in the incidence of anorexia nervosa in Rochester, Minnesota: A population-based study. *American Journal of Psychiatry, 148*(7), 917-922.

Marcus, M. D., Smith, D., Santelli, R., & Kaye, W. (1992). Characterization of eating disorder behavior in obese binge eaters. *International Journal of Eating Disorders, 12*(3), 249-255.

Marcus, M. D., & Wing, R. R. (1987). Binge eating among the obese. *Annals of Behavioral Medicine, 9*, 23-27.

Marcus, M. D., Wing, R. R., & Hopkins, J. (1988). Obese binge eaters: Affect, cognitions and response to behavioral weight control. *Journal of Consulting and Clinical Psychology, 56*, 433-439.

Marcus, M. D., Wing, R. R., & Lamparski, D. M. (1985). Binge eating and dietary restraint in obese patients. *Addictive Behaviors, 10*, 163-168.

Mayer, V. F. (1983). The forward. In L. Schoenfielder & B. Wieser (Eds.), *Shadow on a tightrope: Writings by women on fat oppression* (pp. ix-xvii). Iowa City, IA: Aunt Lute Book Co.

McCarthy, M. (1990). The thin ideal, depression and eating disorders in women. *Behavior Research Therapy, 28*, 205-215.

Mishkind, M. E., Rodin, J., Silberstein, L. R., & Striegel-Moore, R. H. (1986). The embodiment of masculinity. *American Behavioral Scientist, 29*, 545-562.

Mitchell, J. E., Hatsukami, D., Ekert, E. C., & Pyle, R. L. (1985). Characteristics of 275 patients with bulimia. *American Journal of Psychiatry, 142*, 482-485.

National Association of Anorexia Nervosa and Associated Disorders. (1995). *Brief description of therapies used in anorexia nervosa and bulimia*. Highland Park, IL: Author.

Noden, M. (1994, August 8). For many women athletes, the toughest foe is anorexia. Gymnast Christy Henrich lost her battle. *Sports Illustrated*, 52.

Palmer, R. L. (1995). In K. D. Brownell & C. G. Fairburn (Eds.), *Sexual Abuse and Eating Disorders* (pp. 230-237). New York: Guilford Press.

Rankin, J. W. (1993). Diet, exercise, and osteoporosis. *American College of Sports Medicine News, 3*, 1-4.

Rorty, M., Yager, J., & Rossotto, E. (1994). Childhood sexual, physical, and psychological abuse and their relationship to comorbid psychopathology in bulimia nervosa. *International Journal of Eating Disorders, 16*(4), 317-334.

Rosen, L. W., & Hough, D. O. (1988). Pathogenic weight control behaviors of female college gymnasts. *Physician and Sportsmedicine, 16,* 141-146.

Spitzer, R. O., Devlin, M., Walsh, B. T., Hasin, D., Wing, R., Marcus, M., Stunkard, A., Wadden, T., Yanovski, S., Agras, S., Mitchell, J., & Nonas, C. (1992). Binge eating disorder: A multisite field trial of the diagnostic criteria. *International Journal of Eating Disorders, 11*(3), 191-203.

Spitzer, R. O., Yanovski, S., Wadden, T. A., Wing R. R., Marcus, M. D., Stunkard, A. J., Mitchell, J., Hasin, D., Horne, R. (1993). Its further validation in a multisite study. *International Journal of Eating Disorders, 13,* 137-153.

Stein, A. (1989). All dressed up, but no place to go? Style wars and the new lesbianism. *Out/Look: National Lesbian and Gay Quarterly,* 34-42.

Steinhausen, H. C. (1995). The course and outcome of anorexia nervosa. In K. D. Brownell & C. G. Fairburn (Eds.), *Eating disorders and obesity* (pp. 234-237). New York: Guilford Press.

Strober, M. (1992). Family-genetic studies. In K. Halmi (Ed.), *Psychobiology and treatment of anorexia nervosa and bulimia nervosa* (pp. 61-76). Washington, DC: American Psychiatric Press.

Strober, M. (1995). Family-genetic perspectives on anorexia nervosa and bulimia nervosa. In K. D. Brownell & C. G. Fairburn (Eds.), *Eating disorders and obesity* (pp. 165-170). New York: Guilford Press.

Strober, M., & Humphrey, L. L. (1987). Familial contributions to the etiology and course of anorexia nervosa and bulimia. *Journal of Consulting and Clinical Psychology, 55*(5), 654-659.

Stunkard, A. J. (1959). Eating patterns and obesity. *Psychiatric Quarterly, 33,* 284-292.

Stunkard, A. J. (1977). Obesity and social environment: Current status, future prospects. *Proceeding of the New York Academy of Sciences, 300,* 298-320.

Telch, C. F., & Agras, W. S. (1994). Obesity, binge eating, and psychopathology: Are they related. *International Journal of Eating Disorders, 15,* 53-61.

Telch, C. F., Agras, W. S., & Rossiter, E. M. (1988). Binge eating increases with increasing adiposity. *International Journal of Eating Disorders, 7,* 115-119.

Vandereycken, W. (1995). The families of patients with an eating disorder. In K. D. Brownell & C. G. Fairburn (Eds.), *Eating disorders and obesity* (pp. 165-170). New York: Guilford Press.

Vandereycken, W., & Hoek, H. W. (1992). Are eating disorders culture-bound syndromes? In K. A. Halmi (Ed.), *Psychobiology and treatment of anorexia nervosa and bulimia nervosa* (pp. 19-36). Washington, DC: American Psychiatric Press.

Walsh, B. T. (1991). Psychopharmacologic treatment of bulimia nervosa. *Journal of Clinical Psychiatry, 52,* 34-38.

Walsh, B. T. (1992). Pharmacological treatment of eating disorders. In K. Halmi (Ed.), *Psychobiology and treatment of anorexia nervosa and bulimia nervosa* (pp. 329-340). Washington, DC: American Psychiatric Press.

Walsh, B. T. (1995). Pharmacotherapy of eating disorders. In C. G. Fairburn & G. T. Wilson (Eds.), *Eating disorders and obesity* (pp. 313-317). New York: Guilford Press.

Wilson, G. T. (1995). Eating disorders and addictive disorders. In K. D. Brownell & C. G. Fairburn (Eds.), *Eating disorders and obesity* (pp. 165-170). New York: Guilford Press.

Wiseman, C. V., Gray, J. J., Mosimann, J. E., & Ahrens, A. H. (1992). Cultural expectations of thinness in women: An update. *International Journal of Eating Disorders, 11,* 85-89.

Wonderlich, S. (1992). Relationship of family and personality factors in bulimia. In J. H. Crowther, D. L. Tennenbaum, S. E. Hobfoll, & M. A. Parris Stephens (Eds.), *The etiology of bulimia nervosa: The individual and familial context* (pp. 103-126). Washington and Philadelphia: Hemisphere Publishing.

Woodside, D. B., Shekter-Wolfson, L. F., Brandes, J. S., & Lackstrom, J. B. (1993). *Eating disorders and marriage: The couple in focus.* New York: Brunner/Mazel.

Yates, A., Leehey, K., & Shisslak, C. M. (1983). Running—An analogue of anorexia? *New England Journal of Medicine, 308,* 251-255.

Yeager, K. K., Agostini, R., Nattiv, A., & Drinkwater, B. (1993). The female athlete triad: Disordered eating, amenorrhea, osteoporosis. *Medicine and Science in Sports and Exercise,* 775-777.

CHAPTER 15

Obesity

Jacqueline A. Walcott-McQuigg

Introduction

Obesity is prevalent in all affluent populations and the prevalence is increasingly becoming a major public health problem. About 35% of women and 31% of men between 20 and 74 years of age are obese. Obesity is complex and multifactorial. A disease of appetite regulation and energy metabolism, it involves genetics, physiology, biochemistry, the neurosciences, and environmental, psychosocial, and cultural factors (Thomas, 1995). Obesity is an excessive accumulation of body fat greater than or equal to 30% in women or 25% in men. Severe obesity is defined as 40% body fat in women or 35% in men (Bray, 1989). Although technically incorrect, the terms overweight and obesity are used interchangeably (Wilmore, 1993).

Measurement of Obesity

Measurement of obesity is complex and may be controversial because there are no direct measures of body fat (Perri, Nezu, & Viegener, 1992). Underwater weighing is the gold standard for measuring body fat. An individual is weighed under water and out of the water to determine the density of body fat. Unfortunately, this method is cumbersome and not practical for use in large population studies or with individuals who are unwilling to be submerged in water. Other measures such as skinfold thickness and relative weight may not be accurate. Skinfold thickness data may present problems related to the reliability of the measurement (Perri et al., 1992). Relative weight, calculated by dividing a person's actual weight by the "ideal" weight produces a ratio that is calculated into a percentage (ie, 1.30 = 30% overweight). Limitations to using relative weight as an indicator of obesity include use of weight tables, such as the Metropolitan Life tables, that were developed with a sample in which women, ethnic and racial minorities, and people in lower socioeconomic groups were not well represented (Harrison, 1985). Tables also do not provide information on fat distribution or degree of obesity, and age-specific weights are inaccurate (Perri, et al., 1992).

Body fat measurement can also be determined by using a tetrapolar bioelectrical impedance plethysmograph. This method, based on the principal that an applied electrical current is conducted by the body fluids and electrolytes, assesses total body fat, lean body mass, and total body water and their compartments. This method of assessing body composition has been validated with several populations (Lukaski & Bolonchuk, 1988). Bioelectrical impedance analysis (BIA) is useful for estimating change in total body water and fat-free mass during weight loss by obese populations. Individual assessments are subject to large errors (±1.4 kg). Some of these errors may be caused by variable hydration fraction of fat tissue in obesity and the specificity of equations developed in one population (Lukaski & Bolonchuk, 1988). However, BIA was more accurate than skinfold analysis for measuring change in body composition in obese populations (Kushner et al., 1990). Plethysmography machines are portable and easy to use. Future investigations with varied populations may validate the BIA as a useful measure of body fat in population studies. Results of studies testing other new technologic developments to measure body fat, such as x-ray densitometry, infrared interactance, and computed tomography, are not generalizable to obese populations (Perri et al., 1992).

Body mass index (BMI) is the most widely used descriptor of obesity. It is an alternative weight/height ratio that is used to classify individuals into obesity categories and estimate the degree of obesity in large populations (Olson, 1993). BMI is calculated by dividing weight in kilograms by the square of height in meters. BMI calculations have higher correlations with hydrostatic weighing (rs = .70–.80) than other height/weight ratios (Perri et al., 1992).

For people aged 20 years and older, overweight is defined as body mass index (BMI) equal to or greater than 27.8 in men and 27.3 in women (U.S. Department of Health and Human Services [DHHS], 1991). BMI values correspond to 20% above ideal weight (27.2% men, 26.9% women) using the 1983 Metropolitan Life tables. Several classification systems for types of obesity have been developed for studying and treating obese individuals (Bray, 1989, 1992; Garrow, 1988; Perri et al., 1992). The classification systems are based on the known cause of the obesity, probability of improvement, associated health risks, and type of treatment required (Perri et al., 1992).

Prevalence of Obesity

In both adults and children the prevalence of obesity has escalated rapidly since World War II (Berg, 1993). Ten-year follow-up data from the first National Health and Nutrition Examination Survey (NHANES I) revealed that major weight gain was two times higher for women than men, was greatest in persons aged 25 to 35, peaked in both sexes between the ages of 35 to 44 years, and continued to increase in women until age 55, while it declined in men (Williamson, 1993).

Data from the second National Health and Nutrition Examination Survey (NHANES II) showed that women (27.1%) are more overweight than men (24.2%), are more severely overweight (10.85% versus 8.0%), (Kuczmarski, 1992), and between the ages of 25 to 74 years, had greater amounts of cumulative weight gain (7.3 kg) than men (4.5 kg) and more fluctuations (Williamson, 1993; Williamson, Kahn, & Byers, 1991). Among women aged 35 to 55, 30% of European American and 60% of African American women were overweight (VanItallie, 1985).

Obesity is a problem for all women especially as they grow older (Wing, 1992). Ethnic and income differences exist in the prevalence of overweight: 48.5% in African American, 47.25% in Mexican (Kuczmarski, Flegal, Campbell, & Johnson, 1994), 39.8% in Puerto Rican, 31.9% in Cuban (Williamson, Kahn, Remington, & Anda, 1990), and 40% in Native American Indian/Alaska Native women (Young, 1993), compared with 32.1% in European American women (Kuczmarski et al., 1994). Data are scarce on rates of obesity in other ethnic minority groups. Berg (1993) reported that Native Hawaiians have among the highest rates of obesity and related chronic disease. Women on the island of Molokai have an average BMI of 31 between the ages of 20 to 59. Two-thirds of women and men have BMIs over 27.3, and 42% of the women are severely overweight with a BMI over 31. Additionally, 5-year longitudinal data show that America Samoan women have an average BMI range between 32 and 34. However, disease rates are not as great among Samoans given the rates of obesity. Additionally, recent evidence indicates a rise in obesity in Asian American populations (Kumanyika, 1994a).

In the past, across all age groups, the prevalence of overweight was significantly higher for women below the poverty line than for those above it (Kumanyika, 1987; Sobol & Stunkard, 1989). For men the overweight prevalence was slightly higher for those above the poverty line than for those below it (VanItallie, 1985). However, recent data using educational attainment as a measure of socioeconomic status revealed 39% of men and women with less than a high school education were overweight compared to 36% with a high school education and 29% with some college education (Thomas, 1995).

Analysis of gender data from NHANES III shows the highest rates of overweight for women occur at age 50 to 59, whereas the lowest rates are at age 20 to 29, when only 20% are overweight (Berg, 1994). Racial and ethnic differences show that Mexican American women have highest rates of weight gain at age 40 to 49 and African American women at age 60 to 69.

A national health objective for the year 2000 is to reduce overweight to a prevalence of no more than 20% among people aged 20 and older and no more than 15% among adolescents aged 12 to 19 (DHHS, 1991). Table 15-1 lists the 1976–1980 baseline data used to establish year 2000 target percent reductions in weight for low-income and ethnic minority women. However, the increasing prevalence of obesity presents a dismal probability of reaching the year 2000 target goals for reduction of obesity.

Health Risks of Obesity

An increase in body weight of 20% or more constitutes a serious health hazard (National Center for Health Statistics, 1988). The risks of obesity depend on total body fat as well as distribution of body fat. When the fat is distributed in the chest and abdominal region it is called the android pattern (apple shape). Far more common in men, it is associated with greater risk for diabetes, cardiovascular disease, hypertension, and mortality (Bjorntorp, 1986). The gynoid pattern, in which fat is distributed in the hips and thighs (pear shape), is more common in women

Table 15-1.   Prevalence of Obesity Among Special Population Targets

Target Groups	1976–1980 Baseline	Year 2000 Target
Low-income women	37%	25%
African American women	44%	30%
Hispanic women	—	25%
Mexican American women	39%+	
Puerto Rican women	37%+	
Cuban women	34%+	
American Indian/Alaska Natives	29–75%	30%

Source: Adapted from U.S. Department of Health and Human Services. (1991). *Healthy people 2000: National health promotion disease prevention objectives* (p. 114). Washington, DC: U.S. Government Printing Office.

(Markham, 1987). Women with the gynoid pattern have a lower resting metabolic rate, greater tendency to gain weight, and more difficulty trying to lose weight (Westrate et al., 1990).

The waist/hip ratio (WHR) measures body fat distribution. This measurement involves comparing the circumference of the waist to the circumference of the hips. WHRs that exceed 0.8 for women and 1.0 for men suggest a significantly increased health risk (Bjorntorp, 1986). In both men and women higher WHRs are associated with increased risk of diabetes, hypertension, stroke, and death (Lapidus & Bengtsson, 1988). In a study of 41,837 women aged 55 to 69, Folsom et al. (1993) found WHR, more so than BMI, was strongly and positively associated with mortality in a dose-response manner in older women. Excess weight gained during adulthood is usually distributed in the trunk and correlates with a greater health risk of cardiovascular disease than a history of childhood obesity (Olson, 1993). Several studies revealed a greater tendency for upper body obesity in minority populations (Curb et al., 1991; Folsom et al., 1991; Keenan, Strogatz, James, Ammerman, & Rice, 1992), especially in Mexican Americans of both sexes (Haffner, 1986). However, in a study of 42 African American women, Dowling and Pi-Sunyer (1993) found that upper body obesity was less detrimental in the risk of developing diabetes and cardiovascular disease than it was for European American women.

Obesity is associated with more advanced breast cancer, especially post-menopausally (Verreault, Brisson, Deschenes, & Naud, 1989), coronary artery disease, and cancer of the colon, rectum, and prostate in men; cancer of the gallbladder, biliary passages, uterus, and ovaries (National Institutes of Health [NIH], 1995); functional limitations (Kral, 1985); digestive diseases, pulmonary problems, endocrine disorders, sleep apnea, orthopedic and dermal difficulties, and hematologic and immunologic differences (Berg, 1993; Bray, 1985, Sjostrom, 1992). Significant health risks at lower levels of overweight can present hazards, especially in the presence of diabetes, hypertension, heart disease, and cerebrovascular or associated risks factors (Pi-Sunyer, 1993).

Health risks depend on the number of years the individual has been obese and whether the person is gaining or maintaining weight (Olson, 1993). Most studies on body weight are with predominantly Caucasian, middle-income, and middle-aged men (Olson, 1993), yet women are 90% of participants in surgical (Brolin, 1992) and other types of weight control programs (Brownell & Wadden, 1992; Hyman, Sempos, Saltsman, & Glinsmann, 1993). In gender-only studies, European American women are usually the subjects (Kumanyika, 1994a), which may account for the lack of consistent evidence for a significant association between obesity and mortality in ethnic minority populations (Kumanyika, 1993).

Many health risks are associated with obesity. An examination of the literature reveals that some health risks occur with small increases in weight, whereas others are more likely to occur with major weight gain. Ethnic minority women are more obese than European American women. Despite the high rates of obesity among all ethnic minority women, African American women suffer a disproportionate number and severity of health risks (Kumanyika, 1994a).

The next sections address obesity and selected disease processes as they relate to women.

Obesity and Cardiovascular Disease

Obesity is a major risk factor in cardiovascular disease. One in nine women have heart disease between the ages of 45 to 54 with an increase of one in three over the age of 65. In a 28-year follow-up of 5209 men and women in the Framingham study, rates of heart disease were significantly associated with higher increments of weight (Higgens, Kannel, Garrison, Pinsky, & Stokes, 1988). Additionally, higher BMIs affected the risk of coronary disease, myocardial infarction, congestive heart failure, and sudden death (Hubert, Feinleib, McNamara, & Castelli, 1983).

In an 8-year study of 115,888 nurses aged 30 to 55 years, free of coronary disease, stroke, and cancer, a significant association was found between obesity and nonfatal myocardial infarction and fatal coronary heart disease (Manson et al., 1990). Even women as little as 5% overweight had an increased risk of complications and women of average weight had coronary risks 30% higher than the lean women. Controlling for the independent contribution of obesity, the researchers demonstrated that across all weight categories, obesity accounted for 40% of coronary events and 70% for women within the heaviest category (BMI > 29) (Perri et al., 1992). More than 25% of American women aged 35 to 64 have a BMI greater than 29 (Kuczmarski et al., 1994); for African American women within this age group, the BMI is as high as 58.7 (Croft et al., 1992).

Although the death rate from heart disease has declined steadily over the past years, the decline has slowed substantially for African American men, African American women, and European American women (DHHS, 1993). The 1987 age-adjusted death rate was 55% higher among African American women than European American women (Saunders, 1991). Death rates are higher among African American women; however, when heart disease rates are compared within income levels, the rates are lower than those of European American women (DHHS, 1991). Although Hispanic and Native American women have high rates of obesity, heart disease mortality rates are lower than those for European American women (Berg, 1993; Heckler, 1985).

Obesity contributes to heart disease through its strong risk factor association with hypertension, high blood cholesterol, and diabetes (DHHS, 1991). Obesity is the next best predictor of cardiovascular disease risk after age and blood pressure (Garrow, 1988). Most population studies show a rise in blood pressure with an increase in body weight or other indicators of body fatness (Bray, 1984; Schotte & Stunkard, 1990). Persons with high blood pressure are defined as those with a systolic and diastolic pressure of greater than or equal to 140/90 mm Hg or those on antihypertensive medications. Fifty-two percent of overweight women have hypertension compared to 19% non-overweight women (National Heart, Lung and Blood Institute [NHLBI], 1993). Nearly 50% of African American women over age 60 have hypertension (Heckler, 1985; Nickens, 1991). African American women may have a shorter life expectancy than European American women because of hypertension and its complications, cerebrovascular accident (stroke), and hypertensive heart disease (DHHS, 1993). Although the proportion of hypertension attributable to obesity is higher for European American women, the prevalence of obesity and hypertension is higher in African American women (Kumanyika, 1989).

High blood cholesterol is defined as cholesterol levels greater than 240 mg/dL. The condition most closely associated with coronary heart disease, elevated plasma lipids, especially cholesterol is known as hyperlipidemia or hyperlipoproteinemia (Winston, 1988). Among overweight women, 38% have high blood cholesterol levels as compared to 25% of non-overweight women. In the study on nurses (Manson et al., 1990) hypertension, serum cholesterol levels, and diabetes were two to five times more prevalent among women with BMIs greater than 29.

Obesity and Diabetes

Approximately 13 million persons in the United States have diabetes (Douglas & Milligan, 1994). Of these aged 20 and older, 90% to 95% have type II or non–insulin-dependent diabetes mellitus (NIDDM). Obesity is the major risk factor for NIDDM. Estimates of the prevalence of obesity among individuals with NIDDM range from 60% to 90% (American Diabetes Association [ADA], 1993). Excess abdominal fat increases the potential for NIDDM (Bjorntorp, 1993) and the risk of developing NIDDM increases twofold for the mildly obese, to fivefold for moderately obese, and exceeds tenfold for the severely obese (U.S. National Commission on Diabetes, 1975).

The prevalence of diabetes is highest in the ethnic minority populations of the United States. About 25% of African Americans, 33% of Hispanics, and 17% of European Americans have diabetes by ages 65 to 74 (ADA, 1993). One in 3 Native Americans are at risk for developing NIDDM as compared to 1 in 20 in the general population (Young, 1993).

Diabetes incidence in minority women tends to be higher than in European American women (Harris, 1990). Rates of diabetes between the ages of 20 and 74 are 30% higher in European American women as compared to 100% higher in African American women (Harris, 1990; Pi-Sunyer, 1990). Mexican American women are two times as likely to develop diabetes as non-Hispanic Americans living in the same area. The higher incidence rate in Mexican women probably results from genetic factors and a higher prevalence of risk factors, such as obesity (ADA, 1993); for African American women, obesity alone does not explain the differential prevalence (Harris, 1990). Puerto Rican women are two times as likely to develop diabetes as non-Hispanic Americans. Data on Native American women reveal an incidence rate of 40% for women aged 45 to 64 (Young, 1993); the rate increases to over 65% for women over age 65.

Complications of diabetes are more prevalent and associated with higher morbidity and mortality (Summerson, Konen, & Dignan, 1989). Women with diabetes have at least twice the risk of developing heart disease as nondiabetic women. More than 80% of people with diabetes die with some form of heart disease (NIH, 1992).

Obesity and Cancer

Numerous epidemiologic studies examine obesity and site-specific cancer (Miller, 1988); the largest is the American Cancer Society (ACS) study involving more than one million men and women. In the 12-year prospective study the mortality ratio between obesity and cancer was 1.55 for women compared to 1.33 for men (Pi-Sunyer, 1993). Rates of endometrial (5.42), gallbladder (3.58), cervical (2.39), ovarian (1.63), and breast cancer (1.53) were significantly associated with obesity (Garfinkel, 1985; Pi-Sunyer, 1993; St. Joer, 1993). European American women have the highest incidence of breast cancer, and African American women have the highest mortality rates (ACS, 1995). Obesity has been consistently associated with advanced breast cancer at diagnosis and obese cancer patients are generally found to have higher rates of recurrence and shorter survival times than lean patients (Greenberg, Vessey, & McPherson, 1985). Two explanations were given for these findings. First, the association of body weight with breast cancer prognosis could result from delayed diagnosis among overweight women. The presence of marked obesity may interfere with the physician's examination, causing a delayed or missed diagnosis (VanItallie & Lew, 1992). Second, the growth and spread of breast cancer may be enhanced in obese women. In a study of 656 women, Verreault et al. (1989) found that body weight may influence the course of hormone-responsive breast cancer. Production of nonovarian estrogens were significantly increased in obese women before and after menopause during the preclinical phase of the disease. Postmenopausal women (Pi-Sunyer, 1993) and women with android obesity (Schapira, Kumar, Lyman & Cox, 1990) and premenopausal African American women (Schatzkin et al., 1987) may be at greater risk.

The site-specific cancers in women are related to nutritional intake. However, the intake of dietary fat may confound the relationship between obesity and cancer. Kumanyika (1994b) suggests that racial and ethnic issues in diet and cancer epidemiology would be better delineated by appropriately designed racial and ethnic comparison studies.

Other Obesity-Related Physical Health Problems

Osteoarthritis has a dose-response rate by weight, race, and gender with obese African Americans experiencing a higher incidence (Anderson & Felson, 1988).

Sleep apnea, a compromise in the performance of the respiratory control system during sleep, occurs in many severely obese individuals. Unfortunately, weight loss may not alleviate the condition (Kales, Vela-Bueno, & Kales, 1987). Women may have menstrual irregularities, reduced fertility, and high-risk pregnancies (Berg, 1993) that end in stillbirth (VanItallie & Lew, 1992). Body weight before pregnancy and weight gain during pregnancy influence the progression and outcome of labor (Bray, 1985).

Gallbladder disease is more common in women, especially in European American women (Sichieri, Everhart, & Roth, 1990). The prevalence of gallstones increases with age, parity, and obesity. By age 60, nearly one-third of obese women will develop gallbladder disease (Bray, 1985). Blood cholesterol influences the development of gallbladder disease. Gallstones are primarily composed of cholesterol, bile is more saturated with cholesterol in obese individuals, and hepatic secretion of bile is high (Bray, 1985).

Obesity and Psychological Risks

Many people, women more so than men, experience social discrimination and psychological distress as a consequence of their weight (Wadden & Stunkard, 1985, 1992). Depression, anxiety, stress, low self-esteem, and psychological well-being are also linked to obesity.

Determinants of Obesity

Obesity is multifactorial in origin. Determinants of obesity may operate as singular causes or in concert as complex interrelationships. Complex interactions of genetic, physiologic, behavioral, cultural, and psychological variables produce and maintain obesity.

Genetics

Data from twin studies, adoption studies, and family studies show that genetic influences largely determine whether a person can become obese, but the environment determines whether a person does become obese and the extent of that obesity (Meyer & Stunkard, 1992).

Bouchard (1991, 1994) proposes a genetic link to obesity that may interact with nongenetic influences, such as interactions between genes and environment, different and interactive genetic and environmental influences on eating, food preferences, physical activity, and metabolism. His genetic research focuses on distinguishing between necessary and susceptibility genes. Necessary genes permit excess body mass to develop and are important in body fat distribution; susceptibility genes lower the threshold for a person to develop obesity. The susceptibility gene is not necessary for the development of obesity, but it may make the individual more sensitive to environmental or lifestyle factors, such as dietary fat, energy intake, and level of activity. Future research may reveal the presence of both genes in ethnic and racial minority groups, providing explanations for their greater propensity for the development of obesity.

A recent breakthrough in gene research by geneticist Jeffrey Friedman at the Howard Hughes Medical Institute at Rockefeller University is the discovery of an obesity gene in mice (Marx, 1994). The gene, similar to one found in human beings, when mutated causes a severe hereditary obesity in mice. This discovery gives obesity researchers the opportunity to study an aspect of obesity that has not been available in the past.

Energy Expenditure

Daily energy expenditure can be divided into three components: resting metabolic rate (RMR), the thermic effect of food (TEF), and the thermic effect of exercise (TEE). RMR is the energy expended by resting in bed in the fasting state under comfortable conditions (Ravussin & Swinburn, 1992). This energy maintains the systems of the body and the body temperature at rest. It accounts for 60% to 70% of daily energy expenditure. It is proportional to the amount of lean or muscle tissue that an individual has (Perri et al., 1992). In obese individuals who have more muscle than lean tissue, differences in TEF and TEE may offset a higher RMR. Women have less lean tissue than men; therefore, their RMR is lower (Perri et al., 1992). The aging process results in loss of lean tissue and a decline in RMR and caloric expenditure. If caloric intake is not decreased, an individual will gain weight. Results from prospective and longitudinal studies suggest lowered RMR may influence the development and maintenance of obesity (Perri et al., 1992).

Liebel, Rosenbaum, and Hirsch (1995) repeatedly measured 24-hour total energy expenditure, resting and nonresting, and the TEF in 18 obese subjects and 23 subjects who had never been obese. Usual body weight, 10% to 20% of weight loss due to underfeeding, or 10% weight gain due to overfeeding were studied. Findings revealed that when a subject's weight dropped 10% the body's metabolic rate fell 15% to compensate, burning fewer calories. When subjects increased their weight by 10% the amount of energy burned was 16%. Thus, maintenance of reduced or elevated body weight was associated with compensatory changes in energy expenditure, which opposed the maintenance of body weight that is different from usual weight. The findings mean that women who lose 10 lb will burn 10% to 15% fewer calories on exercising than women who effortlessly maintain that weight. Women who gain 10 lb, will burn about 10% to 15% more calories while exercising.

Thermogenesis is an increase in RMR in response to stimuli, such as food, psychological influences, drugs, or hormones. TEF, the major form of thermogenesis accounts, for 10% of daily energy expenditure. TEE accounts for 20% to 30% of energy expenditure in sedentary individuals or a significant amount of calories in active individuals (Ravussin & Swinburn, 1992). Decreased thermogenesis is not as likely an explanation for significant degrees of obesity (Ravussin & Swinburn, 1992) as low levels of physical activity (Perri et al., 1992).

Other Physiologic Determinants

The set-point theory proposed by Keesey (1989) suggests that at any particular point in time there is but one body weight for each individual. Physiologic mechanisms operate to maintain body weight at a constant level or set point. Evidence for the set-point theory has been supported by research (Perri et al., 1992; Liebel et al., 1995).

Obesity involves the storage of excessive amounts of fat. In humans fat cell development occurs mainly in infancy and puberty. Although most obesity is adult onset, obese children and adolescents are 50% more likely to become obese adults (Castiglia, 1989). In a study of Pima Indians, maternal diabetes is a determinant of obesity in their children. Children of women who were diabetic during pregnancy were more likely to develop obesity during childhood and young adulthood than those who were nondiabetic (Young, 1993).

Physiologic factors are likely to play a significant role in the struggle to maintain weight. Lipoprotein lipase (LPL) is an enzyme that mobilizes fatty acids for lipid storage (Young, 1992). Increased levels of LPL are associated with increased adipose storage (Wadden & Letizia, 1992). In animals and in human beings, higher levels of LPL have been found after weight loss. These higher levels may indicate a greater propensity for weight gain, even in the presence of diet control and increased exercise activity.

Behavioral or Lifestyle Factors

Dietary intake and activity levels are associated with rates of obesity (U.S. Public Health Service, 1988). Americans eat more meals out of the home and have questionable dietary knowledge, attitudes, and practices (Berg, 1994). American adults consume 36% of their total calories from fat, with 13% of calories from saturated fat. Women between the ages of 19 to 50 consume only 12 g fiber, half the recommended amount (DHHS, 1991). Alcohol is an important determinant of weight gain. Consumption of alcohol accounts for about 6% of caloric intake and may promote fat storage in much the same way as fat (Flatt, 1993).

Twenty-two percent of adults perform light to moderate physical activity for 30 minutes five or more times a week (DHHS, 1991); 33% of people participate in strenuous activity three times a week (*The Nation's Health*, 1993), and 25% of adults are sedentary. Although women report lower activity than men (White et al., 1987), child care and other role responsibilities interfere with women's ability to engage in leisure activity (Henderson, 1990; King et al., 1993; SeChrist, Walker, & Pender, 1987; Walcott-McQuigg, 1992, 1994). Women, especially European American women, are more likely than men to consider themselves overweight (Horm & Anderson, 1993), are more likely to attempt to lose weight (Levy & Heaton, 1993), and are seven times more likely to be involved in formal weight loss programs (Wing, 1993). African American women's lifestyle factors are studied more often than other ethnic minority women. Even when Hispanic, Native Americans, and Asian/Pacific Islanders are subjects, data on African Americans are more often analyzed and discussed (Horm & Anderson, 1993). Examination of minority population obesity data may show that they eat more, eat more regularly, and have decreased opportunities for physical activities (Kumanyika, 1994a).

Research on African American women and weight supports this proposition. In a 10-year study of weight change among women, African American women were less likely to lose weight (Kahn & Williamson, 1991), less likely to exercise (Burke, et al., 1992; Folsom et al., 1991; Kumanyika, 1987; Kumanyika & Adams-Campbell, 1991), and less likely to diet to lose and maintain weight (Kumanyika, Obarzanek, Stevens, Hebert, & Whelton, 1991; Williamson, Serdula, Anda, Levy, & Byers, 1992). Studies on Latino populations show lower rates of participation in physical activity than for European Americans (Bernal & Perez-Stable, 1994).

Culturally patterned behaviors and beliefs also contribute to the development and maintenance of obesity (Brown, 1992). Minority cultures may be more sensitive to larger body size than European American cultures (Brown, 1992; Kumanyika, 1994a; Walcott-McQuigg, 1992). Attitudes toward body size and value revealed that fewer African American women perceived themselves as overweight (Allan, Mayo, & Michel, 1993; Dawson, 1988; Rand & Kuldau, 1990), did not define being overweight as unhealthy (Allan et al., 1993; Walcott-McQuigg et al., 1995) or unattractive (Kumanyika, Wilson, & Guilford-Davenport, 1993), and were primarily bothered by their inability to wear and "look good" in certain fashions (Walcott-McQuigg et al, 1995). African American women were less likely to feel it was necessary to be slim to be attractive or that weight affected desire to participate in sex, sports, and other exercise activities (Thomas & James, 1988; Walcott-McQuigg et al., 1995).

Massara (1980) found that Puerto Rican female migrant workers did not think obese figures were "too heavy." Within the Puerto Rican culture a traditional fear of "thinness" due to fatal complications is related to acceptance of a larger body size (Massara, 1989). In a Mexican American mother and daughter study, daughters were more likely than their mothers to identify a slim body size as more attractive (Hall, Cousins, & Power, 1990). A study of 21 Mexican/Mexican American and 16 Puerto Rican women (Walcott-McQuigg, 1994) revealed that women did not feel it was necessary to be slim to be attractive and did not define overweight as being unhealthy.

In a study of Native Americans, over 70% of Eastern Cherokee women perceived themselves as overweight and were satisfied with their current weight. Seventy-five percent of the women had engaged in weight reduction such as self- and medically prescribed diets, use of drugs, and participation in exercise (Terry & Bass, 1984).

Emotions such as stress, anger, and depression are associated with eating behavior, weight gain, and obesity (Dipietro, Anda, Williamson, & Stunkard, 1992; Foreyt, Brunner, Goodrick, Cuter, Brownell, & St. Joer, 1995; Ganley, 1989; Istvan Zavela, & Weidner, 1992; Thomas & Donnellan, 1991; Walcott-McQuigg, 1993). Binge eating, snacking, and eating large meals are food patterns associated with weight gain in obese individuals. Binge eating is the most clearly defined pattern of food intake with obese individuals (Stunkard, 1992). Binge eating disorder is the same as bulimia nervosa except that the person does not vomit. Binges make a substantial contribution to the excess calories that contribute to weight gain in obese individuals. Adverse emotional reactions such as depression, nervousness, weakness, and irritability are consequences of dieting (Wadden & Stunkard, 1985, 1992).

In addition to emotional reactions, physical risks also occur with dieting behavior, such as the formation of gallstones (Berg, 1993).

The effect of "weight cycling," more common in women, has generated controversy regarding its role in weight fluctuations and variability in disease risks. Several studies found an increase in coronary heart disease, increase in WHR in premenopausal women, and decrease in weight loss ability (Berg, 1993; St. Joer, 1994). However, other studies have not revealed similar relationships between disease risks and body fat distribution (Berg, 1993). The controversy exists because of lack of standardization in weight cycling measurement (Berg, 1993; Wing, 1993).

Weight Loss Therapy

Many programs and services exist to help individuals lose and maintain weight. Studies show that individuals who complete weight loss programs lose approximately 10% of their body weight, only to regain most of it within 1 year and for some all of it in 5 years (Thomas, 1995). Although the success of weight loss programs is controversial, evidence shows that positive benefits come from weight loss efforts.

Reduction in body weight can lower blood pressure (Trials of Hypertension Prevention Group, 1992) and improve blood cholesterol levels in overweight individuals (Wood, Stefanick, Williams, & Haskell, 1991). Goldstein (1992) reviewed the medical effects of modest weight reduction (10% or less) in patients with obesity-associated medical complications. For obese patients with NIDDM, hypertension, or hyperlipidemia, weight reduction improved glycemic control and reduced blood pressure and cholesterol levels.

In a study to assess the effects of physical fitness, 3120 women were given a baseline treadmill test to assess fitness and followed for 8 years. Women in the least fit quintile had a significantly higher age-adjusted all-cause mortality rate than women in the most fit quintile (Blair, Kohl, & Paffenbarger, 1989).

Types of programs can be classified into self-initiated or do-it-yourself programs, nonclinical programs, and clinical programs (Thomas, 1995). Do-it-yourself programs may include self-imposed diets, joining a community group for social support, such as Overeaters Anonymous or Take Off Pounds Sensibly. Nonclinical programs are the commercial programs such as Weight Watchers, Jennie Craig, or Nutrisystem. Commercial programs rely on trained counselors to provide services to clients. Clinical programs staffed by licensed professionals may provide various services such as nutrition, medical, behavior therapy, exercise, and psychological counseling. They may use very low-calorie diets, medications, and surgery (Frankle & Yang, 1992; Garrow, 1988; Olson, 1993; Stunkard & Wadden, 1992; & Wadden & VanItallie, 1992).

There should be criteria for selecting treatments to fit individuals based on classification of obesity (Bray, 1992) or percent of overweight (Brownell & Wadden, 1992). In Brownell and Wadden's system, individuals are categorized into levels, based on the percentage overweight:

- Level 1: 5% to 20% overweight
- Level 2: 20% to 40% overweight
- Level 3: 40% to 100% overweight
- Level 4: 100% overweight

For individuals in level 1 selection of the self-initiated and nonclinical programs would be appropriate. Level 2 individuals might benefit from the self-initiated, nonclinical, and some clinical programs with a behavioral management approach. Behavioral management programs to modify eating and exercise habits have been the most successful with moderately obese individuals (Brownell & Wadden, 1992) and the losses tend to be better maintained (Foreyt & Goodrick, 1993).

For level 3 individuals, clinical programs that are hospital based and those that manage very low-calorie diets may be the best to assist with their weight control attempts. Surgery may be the best approach for individuals in level 4. Private counseling and residential programs are also acceptable.

Several components are important regardless of type of program selected. The program needs to provide adequate nutritional/diet information. In addition, the individual needs to be introduced to a daily diet based on desired weight goals and exercise. Many dietary aids and books exist in the public domain. In addition to program support women should be encouraged to obtain additional information that is relevant and appropriate and will help them to self-monitor their dietary intake, body weight, and exercise regimen.

Assisting individuals to maintain weight loss is also important. The Federal Trade Commission defines long-term weight loss as a period of 2 years (Perri et al., 1992). Exercise is the single most important predictor in maintenance of weight loss (Blair, 1993). Blair et al. (1989) in a follow-up of a healthy cohort of men and women found that age-adjusted all-cause mortality was higher in less fit individuals. Perri et al. (1992) developed a problem-solving model for obesity treatment that includes a phase for initial weight loss and a phase for weight maintenance. Within this model they propose strategies that address the interaction of psychological, social, and physical factors that affect successful weight loss treatment.

Finally, feminist researchers suggest that health care professionals provide services that allow women the opportunity reevaluate information about appropriate body size and weight loss regimens. This evaluation is designed to assist them to reject all forms of treatment as ineffective (Berg, 1993). The focus of feminist therapy is on assisting women to develop positive self-esteem and an enhanced body image regardless of size. Feminist researchers and therapists suggest emphasizing the positive effects of weight. For instance, results of a study of 2285 of postmenopausal women revealed that women with higher BMIs had lower rates of hip fractures (Berg, 1993). However, encouraging women to accept a larger body size may have negative consequences. It may influence women who have the ability to lose weight to abort efforts designed to achieve small weight losses. These small weight losses may have a positive effect on the reduction of health risks. Future research studies should explore factors that determine successful medical outcomes for overweight women who elect to remain at a body size that may be associated with health risks.

Implications

The high prevalence of obesity in the United States and the associated chronic diseases contribute to a high portion of the health care dollar. Estimates are that the health care costs associated with obesity are over $70 billion a year (Thomas, 1995). An increase in the prevalence of obesity will influence future health care costs. Major implications for public health include the need to assist individuals to control their weight. Weight control includes prevention of weight gain as well as treatments for weight loss.

The major implication of the above research is for health professionals to comprehend the extent of the increase in the rates of obesity and the long-term impact of the obesity on the health of women specifically and the public in general. Health professionals must be aware of the long-term implications of obesity treatment. Recognition that obesity treatment warrants ongoing attention will enable the practitioner to develop the necessary skills to assist women to control their weight. Successful management will require a multifactorial approach to problem solving. Long-term success includes helping women to develop a lifestyle that sustains a balance between energy intake and energy expenditure.

In the area of education, health professionals need to be trained in the use of methods to collect accurate and reliable body composition data and techniques to assist women in monitoring dietary intake and planning an appropriate exercise regimen. Assessment of overweight individuals requires sensitivity and knowledge of the etiology of obesity. Assessments should include collection of cultural data and other factors that influence a woman's ability and motivation to engage in obesity risk reduction behavior.

Although genetics has a role in the development of obesity, environmental factors are major contributory factors. Data from cross-sectional and prospective studies on health risks associated with obesity in women demonstrate the importance of developing gender-specific weight loss interventions. Recognition that body size and values vary among ethnic racial groups will assist nurses and other health professionals to develop and implement culturally relevant weight control programs for women.

Prevention and treatment are equally important. Researchers concerned about the increase in obesity have suggested targeting children and adolescents as a strategic prevention measure (Melnyk & Weinstein, 1994; Young, 1993). Education programs should be developed to assist with the development of skills, health promotion behavior, and emotional management (Wilmore, 1993). Intervention efforts with children and adolescents may include counseling on the importance of adopting the recommended diet and exercise behavior. Self-monitoring techniques should be incorporated into counseling sessions with women in their early twenties to assist them to recognize the need to monitor their weight during the early years of their marriage and periods of gestation. These strategies may decrease rates of obesity during gestation and prevent obesity in their children. Nurses and other health professionals can assist individuals to find an acceptable and appropriate program in which they are willing to participate.

Future research studies should include efforts to obtain accurate data on ethnic minority groups including appropriate measures to obtain body composition and factors that influence the development and maintenance of obesity.

Research studies can be guided by questions that are designed to identify appropriate weight loss and maintenance strategies for all groups, especially those at high risk. Health professionals should conduct longitudinal studies to determine whether weight loss strategies in the obese can reduce the risk of obesity-related chronic disease and all-cause mortality.

References

Allan, J. D., Mayo, K., & Michel, Y. (1993). Body size values of white and black women. *Research in Nursing & Health, 16,* 323-333.

American Cancer Society. (1995). *Cancer facts and figures—1995.* Atlanta, GA: Author.

American Diabetes Association. (1993). *Diabetes 1993: Vital statistics.* Alexandria, VA: Author.

Anderson, J. J., & Felson, D. T. (1988). Factors associated with osteoarthritis of the knee in the first national Health and Nutrition Examination Survey (HANES I): Evidence for an association with overweight, race, and physical demands of work. *American Journal of Epidemiology, 128*(1), 179-189.

Berg, F. (1993). *Special report: Health risks of obesity.* Hettinger, ND: Obesity & Health, Healthy Living Institute.

Berg, F. (1994). America gains weight. *Healthy Weight Journal, 8*(6), 107-109.

Bernal, H., & Perez-Stable, E. J. (1994). Diabetes mellitus. In C. W. Molina & M. Aguirre-Molina (Eds.), *Latino health in the US: A growing challenge* (pp. 279-311). Washington, DC: American Public Health Association.

Bjorntorp, P. (1986). Fat cells and obesity. In K. D. Brownell & J. P. Foreyt (Eds.), *Handbook of eating disorders: Physiology, and treatment of obesity, anorexia, and bulimia* (pp. 88-98). New York: Basic Books.

Bjorntorp, P. (1993). Visceral obesity: A "civilization syndrome." *Obesity Research, 1,* 206-222.

Blair, S. N. (1993). Evidence for success of exercise in weight loss and control. *Annals of Internal Medicine, 119* (7, Pt. 2), 702-706.

Blair, S. N., Kohl, H. W., & Paffenbarger, R. S. (1989). Physical fitness and all-cause mortality: A prospective study of healthy men and women. *Journal of the American Medical Association, 262,* 2395-2401.

Bouchard, C. (1991). Current understanding of the etiology of obesity: Genetic and non-genetic factors. *American Journal of Clinical Nutrition, 53,* 1561s-1565s.

Bouchard, C. (1994). The genetic link: Are we born to be overweight? *Weight Control Digest, 4* (2), 329, 332-334, 338.

Bray, G. (1984). The role of weight control in health promotion and disease prevention. In J. D. Matarazzzo, S. M. Weiss, J. A. Herd, N. E. Miller, & S. M. Weiss (Eds.), *Behavioral health: A handbook of health enhancement and disease prevention.* Philadelphia: Wiley.

Bray, G. (1985). Complications of obesity. *Annals of Internal Medicine, 103,* 1052-1062.

Bray, G. A. (1989). Classification and evaluation of the obesities. *Medical Clinics of North America, 73,* 161-184.

Bray, G. A. (1992). Pathophysiology of obesity. *American Journal of Clinical Nutrition, 55,* 488S-492S.

Brolin, R. E. (1992). Critical analysis of results: Weight loss and quality data. *American Journal of Clinical Nutrition, 55,* 577S-581S.

Brown, P. J. (1992). Cultural perspectives on the etiology and treatment of obesity. In A. J. Stunkard & T. A. Wadden (Eds.) *Obesity: Theory and therapy* (2nd ed, pp. 179-193). New York: Raven Press.

Brownell, K. D., & Wadden, T. A. (1992). Etiology and treatment of obesity: Understanding a serious prevalent and refractory disorder. *Journal of Consulting and Clinical Psychology, 60* (4), 505-517.

Burke, G., Savage, P., Manolio, T., Sprafka, J., Wagenkneecht, L., Sidney, S., et al. (1992). Correlates of obesity in young black women: The CARDIA study. *American Journal of Public Health, 82*(12), 1621-1625.

Castiglia, P. (1989). Obesity in adolescence. *Journal of Pediatric Health Care, 3,* 221-223.

Croft J. B., Strogatz D. S., James S. A., Keenan N. L., Ammerman A. S., Malarcher, A. M., & Haines, P. S. (1992). Socioeconomic and behavioral correlates of body mass index in black adults: The Pitt County study. *American Journal of Public Health, 82,* 821-826.

Curb, J. D., Aluli, N. E., Kautz, J. A., et al. (1991). Cardiovascular risk factor levels in ethnic Hawaiians. *American Journal of Public Health, 81,* 164-167.

Dawson, D. A. (1988). Ethnic differences in female overweight data from the 1985 National Health Interview Survey. *American Journal of Public Health, 78,* 1326-1329.

DiPietro, L., Anda, R. F., Williamson, D. F., & Stunkard, A. J. (1992). Descriptive symptoms and weight change in a national cohort of adults. *International Journal of Obesity, 16,* 745-753.

Douglas, J. O., & Milligan, S. E. (1994). Race, ethnicity, and health: Diabetes and hypertension. *Ethnicity and Disease, 2,* 152-153.

Dowling, H. J., & Pi-Sunyer, X. (1993). Race-dependent health risks of upper body obesity. *Diabetes, 42,* 537-543.

Flatt, J. P. (1993). Alcohol promotes fat storage. *Obesity and Health, 7* (6), 107-108.

Folsom, A. R., Cook, T. C., Sprafka, J. M., Burke, G. L., Norsted, S. W., & Jacobs, D. R. (1991). Differences in leisure-time physical activity levels between blacks and whites in population-based samples: The Minnesota Heart Survey. *Journal of Behavioral Medicine, 14,* 1-9.

Folsom, A. R., Kaye, S. A., Sellers, T. A., Hong, C., Cerhan, J. R., Potter, J. D., et al. (1993). Body fat distribution and 5-year risk of death in older women. *Journal of the American Medical Association, 269* (4), 483-487.

Foreyt, J. P., & Goodrick, G. K. (1993). Factors common to successful therapy for the obese patient. *Medicine and Science in Sports and Exercise, 23,* 292-297.

Foreyt, J. P., Brunner, R. L., Goodrick, K. G., Cuter, G., Brownell, K. D. & St. Joer, S. T. (1995). Weight fluctuation links to stress. *International Journal of Eating Disorders.*

Frankle, R. V. & Yang, M. (Eds). (1992). *Obesity and weight control: The health professional's guide to understanding and treatment.* Gaithersburg, MD: Aspen.

Ganley, R. M. (1989). Emotion and eating in obesity: A review of the literature. *International Journal of Eating Disorders, 8* (3), 343-361.

Garfinkel, L. (1985). Overweight and cancer. *Annals of Internal Medicine, 103,* 1034-1036.

Garrow, J. S. (1988). *Obesity and related diseases.* New York: Churchill Livingstone.

Goldstein, D. J. (1992). Beneficial health effects of modest weight loss. *International Journal of Obesity, 16,* 397-415.

Greenberg, E., Vessey, M., & McPherson, K. (1985). Body size and survival in premenopausal breast cancer. *British Journal of Cancer, 51,* 691-697.

Haffner, S. M., Stern, M. P., Hazuda, H. P., Pugh, J., & Patterson, J. K. (1986). Upper body and centralized adiposity in Mexican Americans and non-Hispanic whites. Relationship to body mass index and other behavioral and demographic variables. *International Journal of Obesity, 10,* 493-502.

Hall, S. K., Cousins, J. H., & Power, T. G. (1990). Self-concept and perceptions of attractiveness and body size among Mexican-American mothers and daughters. *International Journal of Obesity, 15,* 567-575.

Harris, M. I. (1990). Noninsulin-dependent diabetes mellitus in black and white Americans. *Diabetes/Metabolism Reviews, 6* (2), 71-90.

Harrison, G. G. (1985). Height-weight tables. *Annals of Internal Medicine, 103,* 989-994.

Heckler, M. (1985). *Report of the Secretary's task force on black and minority health.* U.S. Department of Health and Human Services. Washington, DC: U.S. Government Printing Office.

Henderson, K. A. (1990). The meaning of leisure for women: An integrative review of the litera-ture. *Journal of Leisure Research, 22* (3), 228-243.

Higgens, M., Kannel, W., Garrison, R., Pinsky, J., & Stokes, J., 3d. (1988). Hazards of obesity: The Framingham experience. *Acta Medica Scandinavica Supplement, 723,* 23-36.

Horm, J., & Anderson, K. (1993). Who in American is trying to lose weight. *Annals of Internal Medicine, 119* (7, Pt. 2), 672-676.

Hubert, H. B., Feinleib, M., McNamara, P. M., & Castelli, W. P. (1983). Obesity as an independent risk factor for cardiovascular disease: A 26-year follow-up of participants in the Framingham heart study. *Circulation, 67,* 968-977.

Hyman, F. N., Sempos, E., Saltsman, J., & Glinsmann, W. H. (1993). Evidence for success of caloric restriction weight loss and control: Summary of data from industry. *Annals of Internal Medicine, 119* (7, Pt. 2), 681-687.

Istvan, J., Zavela, K., & Weidner, P. (1992). Body weight and psychological distress in NHANES I. *International Journal of Obesity, 16,* 999-1003.

Kahn, H. S., & Williamson, D. F. (1991). Is race associated with weight change in US adults after adjustment for income, education, and marital factors. *American Journal of Clinical Nutrition, 53,* 1566S-1570S.

Kales, A., Vela-Bueno, A., & Kales, J. D. (1987). Sleep disorders: Sleep apnea and narcolepsy. *Annals of Internal Medicine, 106,* 434-443.

Keenan, N. L., Strogatz, D. S., James, S. A., Ammerman, A. S., & Rice, B. L. (1992). Distribution and correlates of waist-to-hip ratio in black adults: The Pitt County study. *American Journal of Epidemiology, 135,* 678-684.

Keesey, R. E. (1989). Physiological regulation of body weight and issue of obesity. *Medical Clinics of North America, 73,* 15–28.

King, A. C., Blair, S. N., Bild, D. E., Dishman, R. K., Dubbert, P. M., Marcus, B. H., et al. (1993). Determinants of physical activity and interventions in adults. *Medicine and Science in Sports and Exercise, 24,* S221-S236.

Kral, J. G. (1985). Morbid obesity and related health risks. *Annals of Internal Medicine, 103*(6, Pt. 2), 1043-1047.

Kuczmarski, R. S. (1992). Prevalence of overweight and weight gain in the U.S. *American Journal of Clinical Nutrition, 55,* 495S-502S.

Kuczmarski, R. S., Flegal, K. M., Campbell, S. M., & Johnson, C. L. (1994). Increasing prevalence of overweight among U. S. adults: The National Health and Nutrition Examination surveys, 1960 to 1991. *Journal of the American Medical Association, 272,* 205-211.

Kumanyika, S. (1987). Obesity in black women. *Epidemiologic Reviews, 9,* 31-50.

Kumanyika, S. (1989). Association between obesity and hypertension in blacks. *Clinical Cardiology, 12,* 72-77.

Kumanyika, S. (1993). Special issues regarding obesity in minority populations. *Annals Internal Medicine, 119*(7, Pt. 2), 650-654.

Kumanyika, S. (1994a). Obesity in minority populations: An epidemiologic assessment. *Obesity Research, 2,* 166-182.

Kumanyika, S. (1994b). Racial and ethnic issues in diet and cancer epidemiology. In M. M. Jacobs (Ed.), *Diet and cancer: Markers, prevention, and treatment* (pp. 59-70). New York: Plenum Press.

Kumanyika, S., & Adams-Campbell, L. (1991). Obesity, diet, and psychosocial factors contributing to cardiovascular disease in blacks. In E. Saunders & A. Brest (Eds.), *Cardiovascular disease in blacks: Cardiovascular clinics* (pp. 47-73). Philadelphia: Davis.

Kumanyika, S., Morssink M., & Agurs T. (1992). Models for dietary and weight change in African-American women: Identifying cultural components. *Ethnicity and Disease, 2,* 166-175.

Kumanyika, S., Obarzanek, E., Stevens, V. J., Hebert, P. R., & Whelton, P. K. (1991). Weight loss experience of black and white participants in NHLBI sponsored clinical trials. *American Journal of Clinical Nutrition, 53,* 1631S-1638S.

Kumanyika, S., Wilson, J. F., & Guilford-Davenport, M. (1993). Weight-related attitudes and be-haviors of black women. *Journal of the American Dietetic Association, 93,* 416-422.

Kushner, R. F., Kunigk, A., Alspaugh, M., Andronis, P. T., Leitch, C. A., & Schoeller, D. A. (1990). Validation of bioelectrical-impedance analysis as a measurement of change in body composition in obesity. *American Journal of Clinical Nutrition, 52,* 219-223.

Lapidus, L., & Bengtsson, C. (1988). Regional adiposity as a health hazard in women: A prospective study. *Acta Medica Scandinavica Supplement, 723,* 53.

Levy, A. S., & Heaton, A. W. (1993). Weight control practices of U.S. adults trying to lose weight. *Annals of Internal Medicine, 119* (7, Pt. 2), 661-666.

Liebel, R. L., Rosenbaum, M., & Hirsch, J. (1995). Changes in energy expenditure resulting from altered body weight. *New England Journal of Medicine, 332* (10), 621-622.

Lukaski, H. C., & Bolonchuk, W. W. (1988). Estimation of body fluid volumes using tetrapolar bioelectrical impedance measurements. *Aviation, Space, and Environmental Medicine, 59,* 1163-1169.

Manson, J. E., Colditz, G. A., Stampfer, M. J., Willett, W. C., Rosner, B., Monson, R. R., et al. (1990). A prospective study of obesity and risk of coronary heart disease in women. *New England Journal of Medicine, 322,* 882-889.

Markham, B. S. (1987). Anatomic and metabolic aspects of adipose tissue. *Perspectives in Plastic Surgery, 1*(2), 158-172.

Marx, J. (1994). Obesity gene discovery may help solve weighty problem. *Science, 266* (2), 1477-1478.

Massara, E. B. (1980). Obesity and cultural weight valuations. *Appetite, 1,* 291-298.

Massara, E. B. (1980). *Que Gordita!: A study of weight among women in a Puerto Rican community.* New York: Ames Press.

Melnyk, M. G., & Weinstein, E. (1994). Preventing obesity in black women by targeting adolescents: A literature review. *Journal of American Dietetic Association, 94* (5), 536-540.

Meyer, J. M., & Stunkard, A. J. (1992). Genetics and human obesity. In A. J. Stunkard & T. A. Wadden (Eds.). *Obesity: Theory and therapy* (2nd ed, pp. 137-149). New York: Raven Press.

Miller, A. B. (1988). Cancer and obesity. In R. T. Frankle & M. Yang (Eds.), *Obesity and weight control: The health professional's guide to understanding and treatment* (pp. 445-446). Gaithersburg, MD: Aspen.

National Center for Health Statistics. (1988). Schoenborn: Health promotion and disease prevention: United States, 1985. *Vital and Health Statistics* (Series 10, No. 163, DHHS Publication No. PHS 88-1591). Washington, DC: U.S. Government Printing Office.

National Heart, Lung and Blood Institute. (1993). *Obesity and cardiovascular disease. Data fact sheet.* Bethseda, MD: NHLBI Education Programs, Information Center.

National Institutes of Health. (1992). *Opportunities for research on women's health* (DHHS Publication No. 92-3457). Washington, DC: Office of Research on Women's Health.

National Institutes of Health. (1995). Consensus development conference statement. Health implications of obesity. *Annals of Internal Medicine, 103,* 1073-1077.

Nickens, H. W. (1991). The health status of minority populations in the United States. *Western Journal of Medicine, 155,* 27-32.

Olson S. (1993). Obesity. In B. J. McElmurry & R. S. Parker (Eds.), *Annual review of women's health* (pp. 199-242). New York: National League for Nursing Press.

Perri, M. G., Nezu, A. M., & Viegener, B. J. (1992). *Improving the long-term management of obesity: Theory, research and clinical guidelines.* New York: Wiley.

Pi-Sunyer, F. (1990). Obesity and diabetes in blacks. *Diabetes Care, 13* (Suppl.), 1144-1149.

Pi-Sunyer, F. (1993). Medical hazards of obesity. *Annals of Internal Medicine, 119* (7, Pt. 2), 655-660.

Rand, S. W., & Kuldau, J. M. (1990). The epidemiology of obesity and self-defined weight problem in the general population: Gender, race, age, and social class. *International Journal of Eating Disorders, 9,* 329-343.

Ravussin, E., & Swinburn, B. A. (1992). Energy metabolism. In A. J. Stunkard & T. A. Wadden (Eds.), *Obesity: Theory and therapy* (2nd ed., pp. 97-123). New York: Raven Press.

Saunders, E. (1991). *Cardiovascular disease in blacks.* Philadelphia: Davis.

Schapira, D. V., Kumar, N. B, Lyman, G. H., & Cox, C. E. (1990). Abdominal obesity and breast cancer risk. *Annals of Internal Medicine, 112,* 182-186.

Schatzkin, A., Palmer, J. R., Rosenberg, L., Helmrich, S. P., Miller, D. R., Kaufman, D. W., et al. (1987). Risk factors for breast cancer in black women. *Journal of the National Cancer Institute, 78* (2), 213-217.

Schotte, D. E., & Stunkard, A. J. (1990). The effects of weight reduction on blood pressure in 301 obese patients. *Archives of Internal Medicine, 150,* 1701- 1704.

SeChrist, K. R., Walker, S. N., & Pender, N. J. (1987). Development and psychometric evaluation of the exercise benefits/barriers scale. *Research in Nursing and Health, 10,* 357-365.

Sichieri, R., Everhart, J. E., Roth, H. P. (1990). Low incidence of hospitalization with gallbladder disease among blacks in the United States. *American Journal of Epidemiology, 131*(5), 826-835.

Sjostrom, L. (1992). Impacts of body weight, body composition, and adipose tissue distribution on morbidity & mortality. In A. J. Stunkard & T. A. Wadden (Eds.), *Obesity: Theory and therapy* (2nd ed., pp. 13-41). New York: Raven Press.

Sobol, J., & Stunkard, A. (1989). Socioeconomic status and obesity: A review of the literature. *Psychological Bulletin, 105* (2), 260-275.

St. Jeor, S. T. (1993). The role of weight management in the health of women. *Journal of the American Dietetic Association, 93,* 1007-1012.

Stunkard, A. J. (1992). Talking with patients. In A. J. Stunkard & T. A. Wadden, (Eds.), (pp. 355-363). *Obesity: Theory and therapy* (2nd ed.). New York: Raven Press.

Stunkard, A. J. & Wadden, T. A. (Eds.). (1992). *Obesity: Theory and therapy,* 2nd ed. New York: Raven Press.

Summerson, J. H., Konen, J. C., & Dignan, M. B. (1989). Race-related differences in metabolic control among adults with diabetes. *Southern Medical Journal, 85* (10), 953-956.

Terry, R. D., & Bass, M. A. (1984). Obesity among Eastern Cherokee Indian women: Prevalence, self perceptions, and experience. *Ecology, Foods, & Nutrition, 14,* 117-127.

The Nation's Health. (1993, April). Survey finds Americans backsliding on many healthy habits. Washington, DC: American Public Health Association, 8, 12.

Thomas, P. R. (1995). (Ed.). *Weighing the options: Criteria for evaluating weight-management programs.* Washington, DC: National Academy Press.

Thomas, S., & Donnellan, M. (1991). Correlates of anger symptoms in women in middle adulthood. *American Journal of Health Promotion, 5* (4), 266-272.

Thomas, V. G., & James, M. D. (1988). Body image, dieting tendencies, and sex role traits in urban black women. *Sex Roles, 18* (9/10), 523-529.

Trials of Hypertension Prevention Collaboration Research Group. (1992). The effects of non-pharmacologic interventions on blood pressure of persons with high normal levels. *Journal of the American Medical Association, 267,* 1213-1220.

U.S. Department of Health and Human Services. (1991). *Healthy people 2000: National health promotion and disease prevention objectives* (DHHS Publication No. PHS 91-50213). Washington, DC: U.S. Government Printing Office.

U.S. Department of Health and Human Services. (1993). *Health United States 1992 and Healthy People 2000 review* (DHHS Publication No. PHS 93-1232). Hyattsville, MD. Author.

U.S. National Commission on Diabetes. (1975). Report of the National Commission on Diabetes to the Congress of the United States. (U.S. Department of Health, Education, and Welfare Publication No. 76-1021, 1). Bethesda, MD: Author.

U.S. Public Health Service. (1988). *The Surgeon General's report on nutrition and health* (DHHS Publication No. 88-50210). Washington, DC: Author.

VanItallie, T. B. (1985). Health implications of overweight and obesity in the United States. *Annals of Internal Medicine, 103,* 983-988.

VanItallie, T. B., & Lew, E. A. (1992). Assessment of morbidity and mortality risk in the overweight patient. In T. A. Wadden & T. B. VanItallie (Eds.), *Treatment of the seriously obese patient* (pp. 3-32). New York: Guilford Press.

Verreault, R., Brisson, J., Deschenes, L., & Naud, F. (1989). Body weight and prognostic indicators in breast cancer: Modifying effect of estrogen receptors. *American Journal of Epidemiology, 129,* 260-268.

Wadden, T. A. & Letizia, K. A. (1992). In T. A. Wadden & T. B. VanItallie (Eds.), Predictors of attrition and weight loss in patients treated by moderate and severe caloric restriction. *Treatment of the seriously obese patient* (pp. 383-410). New York: Guilford Press.

Wadden, T. A., & Stunkard, A. J. (1985). Social and psychological consequences of obesity. *Annals of Internal Medicine, 103,* 1062-1067.

Wadden, T. A., & Stunkard, A. J. (1992). Psychosocial consequences of obesity and dieting: Research and clinical findings. In A. J. Stunkard & T. A. Wadden (Eds.), (pp. 163-177). *Obesity: Theory and therapy* (2nd ed., pp. 13-41). New York: Raven Press.

Wadden, T. A., & VanItallie (Eds.). (1992). *Treatment of the seriously obese patient.* New York: Guilford Press.

Walcott-McQuigg, J. A. (1992). *Self-presentation and minority women: Exploring psychosocial factors that influence health practices of African-American women.* Unpublished dissertation. University of Illinois at Chicago.

Walcott-McQuigg, J. A. (1993). Exploring the relationship between stress and weight control behavior in African-American women. *Journal of the National Medical Association., 87*(6), 427–432.

Walcott-McQuigg, J. A. (1994). *Exploring weight management health practices of Hispanic women* (Research Report No. 2-5-38206). Washington, DC: American Nurses Foundation.

Walcott-McQuigg, J. A., Sullivan, J., Dan, A., & Logan, B. (1995). Exploring psychosocial factors influencing weight control behavior in African-American women. *Western Journal of Nursing Research., 17*(5), 502–520.

Westrate, J. A., Dekker, J. Stoel, M., Begheijn, L., Deurenberg, P., & Hautvast, J. G. A. J. (1990). Resting energy expenditure in women: Impact of obesity and body-fat distribution. *Metabolism, 39* (1), 11-17.

White, C. C., Powell, K. E., Hogelin, G. C., et al. (1987). The behavioral risk factor surveys: IV The descriptive epidemiology of exercise. *American Journal of Preventive Medicine, 3* (6), 304-309.

Williamson D. F. (1993). Descriptive epidemiology of body weight and weight change in U.S. adults. *Annals of Internal Medicine, 119* (Pt. 2), 646-649.

Williamson, D. F., Kahn, H. S., & Byers, T. (1991). The 10-y incidence of obesity and major weight gain in black and white US women aged 30-55 y. *American Journal of Clinical Nutrition, 53,* 1515S-1518S.

Williamson, D. F., Kahn, H. S., Remington, P. L., & Anda, R. F. (1990). The 10-year incidence of overweight and major weight gain in U.S. adults. *Archives of Internal Medicine, 150,* 665-672.

Williamson, D. F., Serdula, M. K., Anda, R. F, Levy, A., & Byers, T. (1992). Weight loss attempts in adults: Goals, duration, and rate of weight loss. *American Journal of Public Health, 82,* 1251-1257.

Wilmore, J. H. (1993). Determining an optimal body weight: Overweight versus obesity. *Weight Control Digest, 3* (6), 297, 300-303.

Wing, R. R. (1992). Obesity and weight gain during adulthood: A health problem for United States women. *Women's Health Issues, 2* (2), 114-122.

Wing, R. R. (1993). Obesity and related eating and exercise behaviors in women. *Annals of Behavioral Medicine, 15* (2/3), 124-134.

Winston, M. (1988). Heart disease: A review. In R. T. Frankle & M. Yang (Eds.), *Obesity and weight control: The health professional's guide to understanding and treatment* (pp. 393-411). Gaithersburg, MD: Aspen.

Wood, P. D., Stefanick, M. L., Williams, P. T., & Haskell, W. L. (1991). The effects on plasma lipoproteins of a prudent weight reducing diet with or without exercise. *New England Journal of Medicine, 325,* 461-466.

Young, E. (1992). Marked caloric restriction and organ response in normal-weight and obese experimental animals. In T. A. Wadden & T. B. VanItallie (Eds.), *Treatment of the seriously obese patient* (pp. 107-135). New York: Guilford Press.

Young, T. K. (1993). Diabetes mellitus among Native Americans in Canada and the United States: An epidemiological review. *American Journal of Biology, 5,* 399-413.

Bibliography

Allan, J. D. (1994). A biomedical and feminist perspective on women's experiences with weight management. *Western Journal of Nursing Research, 16* (5), 524-543.

Anda, R. F, Remington, P. L., Williamson, D. F., & Binkin, N. J. (1989). Dietary and weight control practices among persons with hypertension: Findings from the 1986 behavioral risk factor surveys. *Journal of American Dietary Association, 89,* 1265-1268.

Sobol, J. (1991). Obesity and socioeconomic status. *Medical Anthropology, 13,* 231-247.

CHAPTER 16

Mental Disorders

Deborah Antai-Otong

Issues Affecting Women's Mental Health

Historically, women's mental health care has focused on their responses to reproduction and hormonal changes. Additionally, their self-worth and identity have coincided with external factors, such as caregiving, rather than internal factors, such as intelligence and coping styles. The contemporary woman is more educated, sophisticated and familiar with her rights and needs as a consumer. More than ever, women have enormous responsibilities as mothers, wives, career women, single parents, and so forth. Women tie their ability to handle these demands to various factors, such as coping skills, self-esteem, health status, culture, socioeconomic and educational level, availability of relationships, and community resources. Increased responsibilities place tremendous physical and psychological demands on women, putting them at risk of developing an array of mental health problems.

There is a growing need to focus on women's internal resources and strengths for helping them cope with today's stressors and societal transitions. Additionally, there is a paradigm shift in women's mental health care that centers on helping women define themselves internally rather than depending solely on external influences. Women's mental needs can be met by health care providers who recognize their global concerns in various health care settings. Women are more likely than men to seek preventive health behaviors, including mental health care, suggesting that they recognize their problems and are more likely to collaborate with others for assistance.

Health care providers in the front line of health care are more likely to collaborate and form partnerships with women to develop positive gender-specific treatment outcomes. Addressing women's health concerns involves recognizing and responding to their mental and physical health needs. Understanding the profound psychological, sociologic, and biologic differences between men and women is critical to developing gender-based plans of care.

This chapter focuses on the complexity of women's mental health, the importance of women's mental health issues, causative factors, health-related concerns, societal and political responses, and major treatment strategies.

The Magnitude of Mental Health Issues

There has been a recent public outcry since the National Institutes of Health admitted that most of their studies had excluded women. Moreover, they applied their research findings to women, overlooking gender differences in health care needs. Since this revelation, advocacy for gender-specific holistic care of women has become a priority (Hamilton, 1993; Johnson, 1992; Morse, 1995).

Previous studies reported that women outlive men for various reasons. However, current studies show they are no longer immune from diseases associated with stressful lifestyles, such as heart disease and lung cancer. Gender-based research studies have contributed to identifying women at risk for physical and mental illnesses.

Several factors, including the health provider's definition and perception, influence the importance of women's mental health problems and delineation of normal physiologic functions as health rather than illness, society's acceptance of women's help-seeking behaviors, and the impact of various stressful roles on health (Johnson, 1992; Nathanson, 1975). Health is generally defined as a holistic state of physical, mental, and social well-being and more than a mere absence of disease. Mental health refers to an ability to cope with stress effectively. A woman's ability to manage stress usually depends on the intensity and appraisal of the stressor, self-esteem, coping skills, supportive relationships, and available resources. Inability to cope or manage stress typically threatens personal integrity and mental health.

Women's Developmental Milestones

Understanding the perplexity of helping women throughout their lives requires appreciation of stressors that emerge during developmental milestones. Although normal stress is often overwhelming, it provides opportunities for growth and increased self-esteem. Providing appropriate treatment outcomes for women starts with understanding gender-specific developmental responses.

Adolescence generates immense cognitive, personality, and physiologic development. Normally, this developmental stage confronts the youth with stressors arising from peer pressures, impulsivity, and parental and separation conflicts. Moral development, identity, cultural mores, sexuality, career choice, and independence from parents also challenge the female adolescent.

Adolescence also heralds a stage of tremendous neuroendocrine transition that contributes to secondary sexual development. *Menarche*, or beginning of menstruation, is a major pubertal change. Adolescence ends as the young woman moves into early adulthood with a sense of identity, an ability to form meaningful and intimate relationships, and some idea of career choice.

As a woman enters *early adulthood* she is assumed to enter a developmental stage of maturity with a sense of who she is, where she is going, and with whom. A woman's lifestyle often centers on career development, sexuality in marriage and other intimate relationships, childbearing, and increased sense of freedom and independence. Career choices and financial responsibilities present many stressors. Additionally, marital and relationship turmoil arises with time along with the stress of pregnancy, childbirth and parenting or nurturing young children, or the decision not to have children.

Stressors in *middle adulthood* depend on the stage of career development, age of children, states of marital or other intimate relationships, and financial stability. Other stressors include entry of mothers into the workplace, which requires balancing jobs, childrearing, homemaking, and marital partner. Continued disparity between division of household chores is a major source of distress for the working woman.

Our youth-oriented society also places tremendous pressure on women to attach their self-esteem to "staying young and thin." Physiologic changes caused by pregnancy and normal aging often threaten a woman's self-esteem and integrity. Healthy self-esteem and coping behaviors plus quality relationships enable women to manage these stressors effectively. Physiologic changes may add additional demands on middle-aged women who may also undergo diminished sexual performance. Change in body function and image is often distressful and decreases self-esteem. Menopause is an example of a major biologic transition during this period.

Many women describe *menopause* as an unpleasant stage of their lives, whereas others report that it did not affect their lives. Because of neuroendocrine changes, some women experience anxiety and depression during menopause.

Late adulthood is considered to begin at age 65. Mental health depends on successful resolution of previous developmental milestones. Retirement, healthy adult relationships, adult children and grandchildren, financial security, and health are major stressors (Antai-Otong, 1995).

Many factors determine women's mental health as including their "connection" or relationships with others. Women who "participate" or interact in mutually sensitive and supportive relationships experience a sense of power, self-value, and clarity of their emotions and thoughts.

Mental health problems usually appear when women are not involved in meaningful relationships, lack confidence and self-esteem, experience neuroendocrine changes, and, consequently, fail to manage stress effectively. Inability to mediate stress often leads to major mental disorders (Miller & Stiver, 1993). A paradigm shift in addressing women's problems from a relational perspective is critical to understanding their responses to stress and encouraging their participation in the treatment process. Managing stress requires a positive self-regard and confidence or high self-esteem, healthy coping skills, quality support systems, and ability to use relationships as a buffer in times of great stress.

Epidemiologic studies (Kessler, McGonagle, Zhao, et al., 1994) show that nearly one third of U.S. citizens have had or will have a mental disorder at some time in their lives. Women tend to suffer more from anxiety and depressive disorders than men, whereas men tend to suffer more from alcohol and other substance misuse than women. The most common mental disorders are anxiety disorders, followed by mood disorders, and alcohol and other substance misuse. Women may also experience schizophrenia and dissociative and substance use disorders (substance use disorders are discussed in Chapter 13). Depression, followed by anxiety, is a major reason that women seek mental health services (Kendler, Walters, Neale, et al., 1995).

Major Mood Disorders

Major mood disorders include major depressive episodes, bipolar disorders, hypomania, and dysthymic disorder.

Prevalence

Depression is a serious health problem for women. During her lifetime a woman will experience depression twice as often as a man. One in 10 women will suffer severe depression. Epidemiologic studies reveal that the prevalence of depression in women may be as high as 26% and only 12% in men (Kendler, Neale, Kessler, Heath, & Eaves, 1992; Regier et al., 1993; Weissman et al., 1993). The National Comorbidity Survey revealed that women often suffer from three or more mental disorders compared with two or three for men. Depression often accompanies other serious mental disorders, such as borderline personality, dissociative, eating, and substance use and anxiety disorders (Kessler et al., 1994).

Bipolar I and II disorders occur less frequently than major depressive episodes, affecting approximately 0.5% and 0.8% of adults, respectively. Few gender differences exist between men and women for bipolar I disorders, but bipolar II disorders are more common in women. Men are more likely to present with symptoms of mania during their first episode, whereas women are more likely to experience a depressive episode. Several depressive episodes often precede manic episodes (American Psychiatric Association [APA], 1994; Kaplan, Sadock, & Grebb, 1994; Weissman, Bruce, Leaf, Florio, & Holzer, 1991).

Causative Factors

Most mental disorders, including major mood disorders, are multifaceted and include biologic, psychosocial, and environmental factors. Depression is more than the normal passing "blues" or sad mood that most people experience throughout their lives. Sometimes it is difficult to distinguish normal sadness or "blues" from depression. Discerning symptoms of sadness and a major depressive episode is vital to achieving positive treatment outcomes.

Major depressive episodes in women arise from various biologic and cognitive factors and from alterations in complex neurobiologic processes including neurotransmitters, the neuroendocrine system, brain changes arising from separation and loss, and the circadian cycle. These alterations produce biologic or neurovegetative symptoms such as sleep, appetite, cognitive, and energy disturbances.

A major depressive episode with postpartum onset is a multifaceted disorder. It differs from postpartum "blues," which is a normal, mild, and time-limited mood state that emerges within the first few weeks postpartum in almost 80% of women (Stowe & Nemeroff, 1995).

The postpartum period is a particularly vulnerable time. Studies report increased incidences of mental disorders and acute psychiatric hospitalizations during this period. Postpartum depressive symptoms frequently emerge within 6 to 9 weeks postpartum. Approximately 8% to 12% of women experience this disorder.

The duration of symptoms depends on severity and ranges from 3 to 14 months. Manifestations of this disorder range from mild to some severe depressive symptoms or major depressive episode with psychotic features (O'Hara, Zekoski, Phillips, Wright, 1990; Stowe & Nemeroff, 1995).

As with other depressions, a major depressive episode with postpartum onset is often associated with alterations in complex biochemical and neuroendocrine processes (Owens & Nemeroff 1994), history of mood disorders, psychosocial stressors, and a lack of quality support systems (Stowe & Nemeroff, 1995).

Depression is also associated with other neuroendocrine changes including premenstrual syndrome and menopause.

Premenstrual syndrome (PMS) is an array of symptoms that parallels the luteal phase of the menstrual cycle. Approximately 4% of menstruating women experience this syndrome. Mood and anxiety disturbances are thought to arise from ovarian steroid hormones that affect the synthesis, release, and reuptake of neurotransmitters (eg, serotonin, norepinephrine) at both presynaptic and postsynaptic receptors and other neuroendocrine processes (Bancroft, Cook, Davidson, Bennie, & Goodwin, 1991; Yatham 1993). Depression, anxiety, labile mood, and irritability, for at least two menstrual cycles, are major symptoms occurring during the premenstrual phase. Medical and psychiatric conditions may exaggerate or trigger these symptoms (Fava et al., 1992; Kaspi, Otto, Pollack, Eppinger, & Rosenbaum, 1994; Pearlstein, 1995; Rivera-Tovar & Frank, 1990; Rubinow, 1992).

Menopause is a normal physiologic transition into the climacteric and refers to an absence of menses for a year and a follicle-stimulating hormone level of more than 25 IU/L (Andrews, 1994). A direct link between menopause and mood disturbances remains controversial. The role of estrogen in euthymic (a normal mood) women also remains unclear. Menopause alone does not account for depression during this stage of a woman's life. Often other developmental and social issues confront women during menopause and may cause depressive symptoms. Natural menopause usually does not produce adverse mental health problems (Matthews, Wing, Kuller, Costello, & Caggiula, 1990). Treatment of depression during menopause varies. Estrogen replacement that increases presynaptic serotonin reduces depressive symptoms and reduces the breakdown of norepinephrine and monoamine oxidase. Additionally, researchers surmise progesterone to increase monoamine levels and reduce brain stimulation by elevating gamma-aminobutyric acid levels by opening chloride channels at the receptor site (Pearlstein, 1995; Sherwin & Suranyi-Cadotte, 1990). Hormone replacement therapy (eg, estradiol) shows promise in treating women experiencing menopausal mood disturbances (Hay, Bancroft, & Johnstone, 1994; Sherwin, 1991; Wiklund, Karlberg, & Mattsson, 1993).

Cognitive Factors

Cognitive factors arise from the woman's perception of herself, others, and the world. Depression is often linked to negative cognitions of self, others, and the world and underscored by a sense of powerlessness and learned helplessness. Cultural and social influences contribute to formation of self-concept. Women are often revered for meeting the needs of others. Self-esteem and identity are based on meeting the needs of or pleasing others with disregard for personal needs. Despite technologic advances, women continue to be perceived as less than equal to men. They often base relationships on providing emotional support rather than receiving it. The basis of self-esteem and a woman's capacity to network enhance worth and maintain relationships. The need to "connect" and relate to others through relationships often limits a woman's capacity to express anger and aggression and avoid controversy. These efforts are used to maintain relationships, resulting in relinquishing control or power and internalizing anger. A sense of helplessness and powerlessness often follows, placing women at risk of developing depression. These influences produce distorted perceptions of situations, interactions with others, and self-concept.

Social or Environmental Factors

These factors include trauma or abuse, major losses, and social expectations. Prevalence studies relate increased depression in women to prior trauma and abuse. Trauma and abuse, including domestic violence, incest, date rape, and sexual assault, increase the risk of developing serious mental disorders including acute and chronic anxiety and depression, posttraumatic stress, and dissociative, substance use, personality, and eating disorders (Cole & Putnam, 1992; Kessler, Sonnega, Bromet, Hughes, & Nelson, 1995; von der Kolk, 1991).

Another environmental factor is a woman's social status. Society places tremendous demands on a woman to do well in multiple roles. Women's entry into the workplace reflects society's trend toward the need for two-income families to sustain a comfortable lifestyle. Additionally, the number of homes headed by single women continues to grow, further increasing the presence of women in the work force. Motherhood confronts women with major stressors that include balancing and coping with the demands of the job, significant other, and child care. Concerns about adequate day care, job constraints, children's illnesses, finances, and a healthy relationship with her partner continue to confront the woman who is often taking care of others at the risk of not taking care of herself.

Additional societal pressures arise from our male- and youth-oriented culture that further demeans women for aging. Social and cultural demands for a youthful appearance daunt a woman's self-esteem, suggesting that her worth diminishes with age (Johnson, 1991). A lack of validation through various social systems and a culture that expects submissive behavior and sustained youth contribute to frustration, devaluation, self-depreciation, anxiety, and depression.

Depression in women is a major health problem. Distinguishing major causative factors and symptoms is critical to identifying and treating women at risk of depression.

Specific Mood Disorders

In the *Diagnostic and Statistical Manual of Mental Disorders* (*DSM-IV*), the diagnosis of *mood disorders* refers to major depressive episodes, manic episode or bipolar and hypomanic episodes, or bipolar I and II disorders (APA, 1994). Mixed episode, dysthymic disorder, and depressive episode not otherwise specified are examples of other mood disorders. In this chapter, major mood disorders discussed include major depressive episode, bipolar disorders I and II, hypomanic episode, and dysthymic disorder.

A *major depressive episode* includes the presence of at least five of the following symptoms:

- depressed mood
- significant loss of interest in pleasure
- sleep disturbances
- significant weight loss (eg, 5% of body weight in a month)
- psychomotor retardation or agitation
- decreased energy
- feelings of worthlessness
- impaired concentration
- recurrent thoughts of dying or death

Symptoms persist for more than 2 weeks and reflect a change in a previous level of functioning with either a depressed mood or loss of interest in things previously perceived as pleasurable.

A *manic episode* or bipolar I disorder is described as a mental disorder manifested by an aberrant, elevated, expansive, or irritable mood enduring for at least a week. During this period three of the following symptoms also exist:

- exaggerated self-esteem or delusions of grandeur
- decreased need for sleep
- talkativeness
- "racing thoughts"
- distractibility
- increased goal-directed activity or psychomotor agitation
- increased engagement in pleasurable activities, such as shopping sprees and credit card abuse

Primary manifestations of *hypomanic episode* include an obvious period of a continual expanded, expansive, and irritable mood for at least 4 days, strikingly different from nondepressed mood. The *DSM IV* delineates bipolar II disorders as recurrent major depressive episodes with hypomanic episodes (APA, 1994).

Dysthymic disorder is an episodic, milder, and chronic form of depression. Women under age 64 tend to have a higher rate of this disorder, which frequently begins in adolescence and persists for decades. It is manifested by chronic sleep and appetite disturbances, low energy, feeling "down or low," lack of interest in previously pleasurable activities, feelings of helplessness, a lack of motivation, and low self-esteem.

Mood disorders are diagnosed when presenting symptoms do not arise from physical properties of psychoactive substance(s) or underlying general medical conditions. In-depth physical and mental examinations are imperative to rule out medically and substance-induced conditions.

Treatment Strategies

Psychiatric disorders mimic many medical conditions. Having a complete physical examination, including current medical problems, is essential for women. A history of medications, menstrual cycle and sexual activity, and previous surgeries is necessary. Psychiatric and substance use histories are also critical along with a current mental status examination, past and present psychiatric history, and level of dangerousness, including history of self-destructive behaviors. Current support system, level of functioning, and available resources must also be identified during the early stage of treatment.

Treating mood disorders depends on the nature and severity of presenting symptoms, causative factors, health status, and previous responses to treatment. Treatment may range from psychotherapeutic interventions to a combination with various somatic interventions. Brief or short-term strategies that integrate principles of behavior and cognitive therapy may be used to help in challenging distorted cognitions and learned helplessness. Assertiveness and conflict resolution training can help build effective communication skills and self-esteem. Additionally, suicide is also a risk in clients experiencing depression. The client's level of dangerousness must be assessed continuously throughout treatment. Marital, family, and group therapies may be used to deal with depression and relationship problems. Somatic treatment is the most common treatment for major depressive episodes. Antidepressants, electroconvulsive therapy, and light therapy are examples of somatic interventions for major depressive episodes. Manic type bipolar disorder is often treated with antimanic agents, such as valproic acid, carbamazepine, lithium, and neuroleptics during acute phases.

Anxiety Disorders

Discerning normal anxiety from anxiety disorders is vital to defining appropriate interventions. *Normal anxiety* is an innate and protective emotion that is an integral part of daily living. It is a mental and physical condition whose major manifestations result from autonomic nervous system arousal. In contrast, anxiety disorders depict inappropriate responses by virtue of their severity or progression.

Prevalence

Anxiety disorders are the most common disorders, occurring in about 15% of all clients in medical or surgical settings. Anxiety is second to depression as the most frequent cause of women seeking mental health services. Women are two to three times more likely to suffer anxiety disorders than men, with most of them experiencing severe symptoms (Kessler et al., 1994; Kessler et al., 1995). Furthermore, anxiety disorders are more often comorbid in women than in men (eg, anxiety disorders and mood disorders).

Causative Factors

Low to moderate levels of anxiety are expected when a threat or potential threat occurs. Persistent anxiety is potentially debilitating and associated with a variety of anxiety and medical disorders. Major causative factors of anxiety disorders include alterations in complex biologic processes, trauma, stress, and other psychosocial influences.

Biologic factors include alterations in brain systems that regulate moods and emotions. Various neurotransmitter systems (eg, serotonergic and GABA) and neuroanatomic structures, such as the limbic system, the thalamus, locus coeruleus, and reticular-activating system, play a major role in anxiety and anxiety disorders.

Specific Anxiety Disorders

Major anxiety disorders delineated in *DSM IV* (APA, 1994) include panic disorders with and without agoraphobia, agoraphobia without history of panic disorder, specific phobia, social phobia, obsessive-compulsive disorder, posttraumatic stress disorder, acute stress disorder, generalized anxiety disorder, and anxiety disorder not otherwise specified. Anxiety disorder caused by a general medical condition and a substance-induced anxiety disorder are diagnosed when the history and physical findings link anxiety with these conditions. Major anxiety disorders experienced by women include panic disorders and posttraumatic stress disorders.

Panic Disorders

The lifetime prevalence of panic disorders is 1.5% to 3.0% and 3% to 4% for panic attacks. Women are usually two to three times more often affected than men. Research studies suggest that these figures are related to underdiagnosing in men (Katerndahl & Realini, 1993; Kendler et al., 1995).

Major symptoms of panic disorder are comparable to other major anxiety disorders delineated by *DSM IV* criteria. These include autonomic arousal states, such as palpitations, diaphoresis, shakiness, chest pain, dizziness, and paresthesia. Symptoms usually emerge abruptly during a panic attack. Thoughts or situations may trigger other anxiety disorders.

Posttraumatic Stress Disorder

Posttraumatic stress disorder, like other anxiety disorders, is a complex mental disorder. As its name infers, it arises from exposure to profound stress, such as war, sexual assault, and incest, which are outside the range of normal human experiences. Manifestations include intrusive memories, avoidant behaviors, panic attacks, and hypervigilence accompanied by intense autonomic nervous system arousal (APA, 1994).

A lifetime prevalence of this disorder in women ranges from 1.3% to 12.3%; it occurs in 17.9% to 30.7% of women exposed to trauma compared with 6% to 14% in men exposed to trauma (Breslau, Davis, Andreski, & Peterson, 1991; Kessler et al., 1995; Resnick, Kilpatrick, Dansky, Saunders, & Best, 1993).

Treatment Strategies

Major treatment for anxiety disorders includes a variety of somatic interventions, such as antidepressants, anxiolytic or antianxiety agents, and antiobsessional agents. Psychosocial interventions including cognitive-behavioral approaches and psychotherapies have also been effective in treating anxiety disorders.

Women are at greater risk of having more than one mental disorder at a time. Unfortunately, anxiety and mood disorders may also accompany other serious mental health problems including schizophrenia and dissociative and substance use disorders.

Schizophrenia

Schizophrenia is a serious and chronic psychotic mental disorder. Major psychotic symptoms include positive (type I) and negative (type II) symptoms. Hallucinations, loose associations, bizarre behavior, incoherence, and delusions are examples of positive symptoms. Negative symptoms include affective flattening, apathy, attention disturbances, impoverished speech, and impaired social interactions. Positive symptoms are more responsive to traditional neuroleptic or antipsychotic agents and positive treatment outcomes than negative symptoms.

Prevalence

The prevalence of schizophrenia between men and women is comparable. Major gender differences include the onset and progress of illness. Women usually experience a milder and less severe course (eg, positive symptoms) with fewer psychotic episodes than men. They also respond better to treatment and maintain better social functioning than men because they have fewer negative symptoms. This premise is also linked with more positive treatment outcomes in women than men (Angermeyer, Kuhn, & Goldstein, 1990; Goldstein & Tsuang, 1990; Perry, Moore, & Braff, 1995). Only one third of the women have their initial psychotic break and subsequent hospitalization before age 25. The peak age for onset of schizophrenia in women is 25 to 35 compared with 15 to 25 years for men (Pulver et al., 1992).

Causative Factors

Schizophrenia is one of the most researched and discussed mental disorders. Recent studies show that many biologic factors including alterations in neurotransmitters such as dopamine, neuroanatomic changes, and psychosocial stressors cause this complex disorder.

Treatment Strategies

Somatic treatment of schizophrenia includes use of neuroleptics or antipsychotic agents. Psychosocial interventions include supportive therapy, medication groups, and psychological education with the client and family. Because women are more likely to have higher functioning social skills, they are more responsive to a combination of medications and psychosocial interventions than some men.

Dissociative Disorders

Dissociative disorders are unconscious attempts to protect against conscious awareness of painful emotional experiences. Dissociation acts as a defense against traumatic experiences. It enables women to mentally remove themselves from a painful event as it occurs while delaying the "working through process." Delayed resolution of trauma frequently results in a lack of self-identity or distortion of identity. Major *DSM IV* dissociative disorders include dissociative amnesia, dissociative fugue, depersonalization, and dissociative identity disorder formerly called multiple personality disorder (APA, 1994). Because women suffer a significantly high incidence of trauma, dissociative identity disorder is the most common dissociative disorder among women. Therefore, the following section briefly discusses dissociative identity disorder.

Dissociative Identity Disorder

Dissociative identity disorder is commonly called multiple personality disorder. This multifaceted chronic and progressive mental disorder is associated with early childhood traumas, both physical abuse and sexual (frequently incestuous) abuse. It is commonly associated with borderline and other serious personality disorders. Dissociative identity disorder means a failure to merge thoughts, feelings, behaviors, and memories into a logical and full sense of consciousness. Amnesia or fugue states, depersonalization, and derealization are manifestations of dissociative identity disorder (APA, 1994; Kaplan et al., 1994; Putnam, 1991). Self-mutilation, intentional self-injury without the purpose of suicide, frequently accompanies dissociative disorders (Brodsky, Cloitre, & Dulit, 1995; Dulit, Fyer, Leon, Brodsky, & Frances, 1994; Shearer, 1994, von der Kolk et al. 1991).

Prevalence

Controlled studies show that 0.5% to 2% of clients entering psychiatric hospitals meet criteria for dissociative identity disorder. Women are more likely to be diagnosed with this disorder than men. This disorder is usually diagnosed during the late teens and young adulthood. The median age is 30 years although the clients report a 5- to 10-year history of symptoms (Putnam, 1991).

Treatment Strategies

Effective treatment of dissociative identity disorder encompasses several approaches, including psychotherapy. Psychotherapy can be used to identify various personalities or "alters"; it can engage each alter in a contract designed to reduce self-destructive behaviors. Major treatment issues also include establishing a trusting relationship, providing consistent and firm boundaries between the therapist and client, and enhancing self-esteem and coping skills. Ultimate treatment goals include reintegration and resolution of the personality and trauma.

The Future of Women's Mental Health

Political and Societal Impact on Women's Health Care

Women are the greatest users of health care. Historically, they have not been active participants in their treatment. Acceptance of this passive role reflected society's perception of women's health care needs. Women demand greater participation in their care and control over their physical and mental well-being. Appreciating issues unique to women's mental health provides many challenges and opportunities for health care providers. As we approach the next century, health care policies affecting women's health must reflect gender differences. Moreover, greater understanding of significant psychological and biologic differences between men and women will come only when policymakers integrate these differences into legislative agendas. Legislative agendas must identify women at risk, increase access for the uninsured, and provide gender-sensitive preventive services. Policymakers must also be willing to allocate research funds to support legislative concerns for women's health care.

Research

It is well known that researchers generalized most studies comprising male subjects to women. An outcry from the public sector and various health providers has pushed research using women to the forefront. Developing empirical studies that reflect gender-specific mental health issues continues to be a concern of researchers. Areas that show expansion include research that deals with addiction, the impacts of early childhood traumas, acute and chronic depression, and the role of female health care providers in developing effective gender-specific treatment strategies (Bolen, 1993; Cyr & Moulton, 1993; Derry & Gallant, 1993; Kendler et al., 1995; Pearlstein, 1995; Stowe & Nemeroff, 1995).

Health care providers need more research to identify preventive measures that promote mental health in women. Limited outcome studies examine specific interventions and the effects of cognitive therapy and psychopharmacology on acute and chronic forms of depression. Other areas of interest include exploring the role of gender-specific therapists on treatment outcomes. We also need more studies that compare traditional relapse prevention programs with those that address women's issues, such as shame, a need to care for others, and depression. The paucity of gender-specific assessments and interventions challenges health care providers to develop research that addresses women's health care.

Summary

As we move into the next century, women's health care concerns will continue be a priority for health care providers. Women's health care often involves a balance between physical and mental health. Appreciating gender differences helps in developing partnerships that address individual needs and facilitate positive treatment outcomes.

References

American Psychiatric Association. (1994). *The diagnostic and statistical manual of mental disorders* (4th ed.). Washington, DC: Author.

Andrews, M. C. (1994). Primary care for postreproductive women: Further thoughts concerning steroid replacement. *American Journal of Obstetrics and Gynecology, 170,* 963-996.

Angermeyer, M. C., Kuhn, L., & Goldstein, J. M. (1990). Gender and the course of schizophrenia: Differences in treatment outcomes. *Schizophrenia Bulletin, 16,* 293-307.

Antai-Otong, D. (1995). *Psychiatric nursing: Biological and behavioral concepts.* Philadelphia: Saunders.

Bancroft, J., Cook, A., Davidson, D., Bennie, J., & Goodwin, G. (1991). Blunting of neuroendocrine responses to infusion of L-tryptophan in women with premenstrual mood changes. *Psychological Medicine, 21,* 305-312.

Bolen, J. D. (1993). The impact of sexual abuse on women's health. *Psychiatry Annals, 23,* 446-453.

Breslau, N., Davis, G. C., Andreski, P., & Peterson, E. (1991). Traumatic events and posttraumatic stress disorder in urban population of young adults. *Archives of General Psychiatry, 48,* 216-222.

Brodsky, B. S., Cloitre, M., & Dulit, R. A. (1995). Relationship of dissociation to self-mutilation and childhood abuse in borderline personality disorder. *American Journal Psychiatry, 152,* 1788-1792.

Cole, P. M., & Putnam, F. W. (1992). Effect of incest on self and social functioning: A developmental psychopathology perspective. *Journal of Consulting and Clinical Psychology, 60,* 174-183.

Cyr, M. G., & Moulton, A. W. (1993). The physician's role in prevention, detection, and treatment of alcohol abuse in women. *Psychiatric Annals, 23,* 454-462.

Derry, P., & Gallant, S. (1993). Motherhood issues in the psychotherapy of employed mothers. *Psychiatric Annals, 23,* 432-437.

Dulit, R. A., Fryer, M. R., Leon, A. C., Brodsky, B. S., & Frances, A. J. (1994). Clinical correlates of self-mutilation in borderline personality disorder. *American Journal of Psychiatry, 151,* 1305-1311.

Fava, M., Pedrazzi, F., Guaraldi, G. P., Romano, G., Genazzani, A. R., & Facchinetti, F. (1992). Comorbid anxiety and depression among patients with late luteal phase dysphoric disorder. *Journal of Anxiety Disorders, 6,* 325-335.

Goldstein, J. M., & Tsuang, M. T. (1990). Gender and schizophrenia: An introduction to synthesis of findings. *Schizophrenia Bulletin, 16,* 179-183.

Hamilton, J. A. (1993). Feminist theory and health psychology: Tools for an egalitarian, woman-centered approach to womens' health. *J. Women Health, 2,* 49–54.

Hay, A. G., Bancroft, J., & Johnstone, E. C. (1994). Affective symptoms in women attending a menopausal clinic. *British Journal of Psychiatry, 164,* 513-516.

Johnson, K. (1991). *Trusting ourselves: The complete guide to emotional well-being for women.* New York: The Atlantic Monthly Press.

Johnson, K. (1992). Pro: Women's health: Developing a new interdisciplinary specialty. *Journal of Women's Health, 2,* 95-99.

Kaplan, H. I., Sadock, B. J., & Grebb, J. A. (1994). *Kaplan and Sadock's synopsis of psychiatry* (7th ed.). Baltimore: Williams & Wilkins.

Kaspi, S. P., Otto, M. W., Pollack, M. H., Eppinger, S., Rosenbaum, J. F. (1994). Premenstrual exacerbation of symptoms in women with panic disorder. *Journal of Anxiety Disorders, 8,* 131-138.

Katerndahl, D. A., & Realini, J. P. (1993). Lifetime prevalence of panic disorder. *American Journal of Psychiatry, 150,* 246-249.

Kendler, K. S., Neale, M. C., Kessler, R. C., Heath, A. C., & Eaves, L. J. (1992). A population-based twin study of major depression in women. *Archives of General Psychiatry, 49,* 257-266.

Kendler, K. S., Walters, E. E., Neale, M. C., Kessler, R. C., Heath, A. C., & Eaves, L. J. (1995). The structure of the genetic and environmental risk factors for six major psychiatric disorders in women. *Archives of General Psychiatry, 52,* 374-383.

Kessler, R. C., McGonagle, K. A., Zhao, S., Nelson, C. B., Hughes, M., Eshleman, S., Wittchen, H-U., & Kendler, K. S. (1994). Lifetime and 12-month prevalence of DSM-III-R psychiatric disorders in the United States: Results from the National Comorbidity Survey. *Archives of General Psychiatry, 51,* 8-19.

Kessler, R. C. Sonnega, A. Bromet, E., Hughes, M., Nolson., C. B. (1995). Posttraumatic stress disorder in the national comorbidity survey. *Archives of General Psychiatry, 52,* 1048–1060.

Matthews, K. A., Wing, R. R., Kuller, L. H., Costello, E. J., & Caggiula, A.W. (1990). Influences of natural menopause on psychological characteristics and symptoms of middle-aged healthy women. *Journal of Consulting and Clinical Psychology, 58,* 345-351.

Miller, J. B., & Stiver, I. P. (1993). A relational approach to understanding women's lives and problems. *Psychiatric Annals, 23,* 424-431.

Morse, G. G. (1995). Reframing women's health in nursing education: A feminist approach. *Nursing Outlook, 43,* 273-277.

Nathanson, C. A. (1975). Illness and the feminine role: A theoretical review. *Social Science and Medicine, 9,* 57-62.

O'Hara, M. W., Zekoski, E. M., Phillips, L. H., & Wright, E. J. (1990). Controlled prospective study of postpartum mood disorders: Comparison of childbearing and nonchildbearing women. *Journal of Abnormal Psychology, 99,* 3-15.

Owens, M. J., & Nemeroff, C. B. (1994). The role of serotonin in the pathophysiology of depression: Focus on the serotonin transported. *Clinical Chemistry, 40,* 288-295.

Pearlstein, T. B. (1995). Hormones and depression: What are the facts about premenstrual syndrome, menopause, and hormone replacement therapy. *American Journal of Obstetrics and Gynecology, 173,* 646-653.

Perry, W., Moore, D., & Braff, D. (1995). Gender differences on thought disturbance measures among schizophrenia patients. *American Journal of Psychiatry, 152,* 1298-1301.

Pulver, A. E., Liang, K-Y., Brown, C. H., Wolyniec, P., McGrath, J., Adler, L., Tam, D., Carpenter, D., & Childs, B. (1992). Risk factors in schizophrenias: Season of birth, gender, and familial risk. *British Journal of Psychiatry, 160,* 65-75.

Putnam, F. W. (1991). Recent research on multiple personality disorder. *Psychiatric Clinics of North America, 14,* 489-502.

Regier, D. A., Narrow, W. E., Rae, D. S., Manderscheid, R. W., Locke, B. Z., & Goodwin, F. K. (1993). The de facto US mental and addictive disorders service system: Epidemiologic catchment area prospective 1-year prevalence rates of disorders and services. *Archives of General Psychiatry, 50,* 85-94.

Resnick, H. S., Kilpatrick, D. G., Dansky, B. S., Saunders, B. E., Best, C. L., (1993). Prevalence of civilian trauma and posttraumatic stress disorder in a representative national sample of women. *J. Consulting Clinical Psychology, 61,* 984–991.

Rivera-Tovar, A. D., & Frank, E. (1990). Late luteal phase dysphoric disorder in young women. *American Journal Psychiatry, 147,* 1634-1636.

Rubinow, D. R. (1992). The premenstrual syndrome: New views, *JAMA, 268,* 1908–1912.

Shearer, S. L. (1994). Dissociative phenomena in women with borderline personality disorder. *American Journal of Psychiatry, 151,* 1324-1338.

Sherwin, B. B. (1991). The impact of different doses of estrogen and progestin on mood and sexual behavior in postmenopausal women. *Journal of Clinical Endocrinology Metabolism, 72,* 336-343.

Stowe, Z. N., & Nemeroff, C. B. (1995). Women at risk for postpartum-onset major depression. *American Journal of Obstetrics and Gynecology, 175,* 639-645.

von der Kolk, B. A., Perry, J. C., & Herman, J. L. (1991). Childhood origins of self-destructive behavior. *American Journal Psychiatry, 148,* 1665-1671.

Weissman, M. M., Bland, R., Joyce, P. R., Newman, S., Wells, J. E., & Wittchen, H-U. (1993). Sex differences in rates of depression: Cross-national perspectives. *Journal of Affective Disorders, 29,* 77-84.

Weissman, M. M., Bruce, M. L., Leaf, P. J., Florio, L. P., Holzen, C. III. (1991). Affective disorders. In: L. N. Robins, D. A. Reger (Eds.) *Psychiatric disorders in America: The epidemiologic catchment area study.* (pp. 53–80). New York: Free Press.

Wiklund, I., Karlberg, J., & Mattsson, L. A. (1993). Quality of life of postmenopausal women on a regimen of transdermal estradiol therapy: A double-blind placebo-controlled study. *American Journal of Obstetrics and Gynecology, 168,* 824-830.

Yatham, L. N. (1993). Is 5HT$_{1A}$ receptor subsensitivity a trait marker for late luteal pahase dysphoric disorder? A pilot study. *Canadian J. Psychiatry, 38,* 662–664.

Bibliography

Sandberg, D. A., & Lynn, S. J. (1992). Dissociative experience, psychopathology and adjustment, and child and adolescent maltreatment in female college students. *Journal of Abnormal Psychology, 101,* 717-723.

Simeon, D., & Hollander, E. (1993). Depersonalization disorder. *Psychiatric Annals, 23,* 382-388.

Cultural Diverseness and Women's Health

CHAPTER 17

African American and Caribbean Women

Marilyn H. Gaston
Kelly Garry

Overview

This chapter examines the health status of African American and Caribbean women. The analysis includes an historical perspective of the population; a look at socio-economic factors such as education, occupation, and income; a look at the role of cultural beliefs and practices; and finally, a review of specific mortality and morbidity data.

Caribbean women are included in this review because of their African heritage and migration patterns to the United States. Unfortunately, data limitations prevent an extensive review but what information is available can provide some perspective on their status. Caribbean categories included are primarily Haitians, Dominicans, and Jamaicans.

Historical Perspective of African American and Caribbean Women

African American women were brought to North America as slaves beginning in 1619. In 1790, when the first census was taken, African Americans numbered about 760,000. By 1860, at the start of the Civil War, the African American population had increased to 4.4 million, but their percentage, as compared to the total population, had dropped to 14% from 19%. Most were slaves, with only 488,000 counted as "freemen" (U.S. Department of Commerce, 1993).

By 1900, the African American population had doubled and reached 8.8 million. In 1950, it had reached 15 million and by 1990 it had doubled again to 30 million or 12% of the total population. Over one-half of the African American population was female, 16 million or 53%.

The African American population increased an average of 1.4% annually between 1980 and 1992 compared to 0.6% for the Caucasian population and 0.9% for the total population. Eighty-four percent of the growth was from natural increases, such as excess births over deaths. Immigration, which has increased substantially since 1980 for the African American population, has also been a factor (Bennett, 1993).

The 1965 Immigration Law changed the prevailing system that had favored Europeans and enabled large-scale immigration from the Caribbean region. As a result, Caribbean immigrants constituted almost one third of the foreign-born population in New York City in 1989. The 1980 census reported 517,000 Caribbean immigrants in New York City, which does not account for undocumented immigrants (Graham, 1989). The country sending the most immigrants to New York between 1975 and 1980 was the Dominican Republic with 35,860, followed by Jamaica with 23,600, Guyana with 15,720, Haiti with 13,840, and Trinidad and Tobago with 10,640 (Graham, 1989). Currently, approximately 3% of African Americans are foreign born, mainly comprised of non–Spanish-speaking Caribbean people and French/Creole-speaking Haitians (Graham, 1989).

The migration process tends to have a traumatic impact on Caribbean women because of the radical changes in their social milieu. Most migrate after they have begun to establish their families and to rear children, leaving spouse and children behind in their native country. The resulting separation requires major sacrifices and changes in families to facilitate the migration of these women. Once in the United States, the quest for family unification tends to be a major priority. This quest entails a high degree of anxiety, guilt, and stress, all of which may have serious health implications.

The number of minorities will continue to increase into the year 2000. In 1993, Caucasians made up 74% of the total population, African Americans 12%, Hispanic Americans 10%, Native Americans 1%, Asian and Pacific Islanders, 3%. By the year 2030, it is estimated that Caucasians will make up 60%, African Americans 13%, Hispanics 18%, Native Americans 1%, and Asian and Pacific Islanders 8% (U.S. Bureau of the Census, 1993).

Socioeconomic Status of African American and Caribbean Women

Many of the disparities in health outcomes between African Americans and other populations have resulted from the fact that although they are only 12% of the total population, they make up 35% of the unemployed and 40% of the poor. This supports the need to look at socioeconomic factors as they relate to health issues. These factors include but are not limited to education, occupation, and income. There is an association between poor health outcomes and socioeconomic data.

Education

The nature of one's schooling partly determines the types of occupational opportunities, the amount of money earned, and one's lifelong socioeconomic status. Poor young women of color have experienced serious inequities in schooling and educational opportunities. This has an impact on health through poor socioeconomic status but also through limited knowledge of sound health promotion and disease prevention practices.

Since 1940, progress has been made for African Americans in attaining a high school diploma. In 1940 only 7% of African Americans had completed high school. By 1992, the proportion had increased to 68% (Bennett, 1993). However, the high school drop-out rate is increasing, especially for African American girls. African American girls have a high school drop-out rate twice that of both Caucasian girls and African American boys. Many factors come into play, but the most profound is teenage pregnancy.

If a poor female student of color remains in school she is typically tracked in vocational, general, or special education programs. The communities in which poor female students of color reside often offer few or no programs of support or challenge. The link between schooling and job opportunity is crucial. Female students who manage to graduate from high school and to enroll in higher education programs are most frequently clustered in lower cost 2-year colleges (Gordon-Bradshaw, 1987).

High school completion rates and college attendance have improved; in 1992, 12% of African American women and 11% of African American men had at least a bachelor's degree (Bennett, 1993). Unfortunately, college completion rates have continued to decline since 1975 for both African American men and women.

In New York City, based on 1980 data, the regional average for Caribbean women's elementary educational attainment was 5.2%, for high school 32%, and for college 4.7%. Haiti and Trinidad and Tobago had the lowest level of elementary educational attainment at 3.0% (Graham, 1989).

Occupation

Women of every racial group increased their labor force participation rates between 1980 and 1990. In 1980 and 1990, African American women and Asian and Pacific Islander women had the highest labor force participation rates. For African American women it increased from 53% to 60% during 1980 and 1990 (Bennett, 1993).

In 1992, 13.9 million African Americans 16 years old and over were in the labor force. African Americans made up 11% of the total labor force. African American men had an annual average labor force participation rate of 70% compared to 58% for African American women in 1992 (Bennett, 1993).

Nearly 30% of African American women are employed in technical, sales, and administrative support jobs, such as cashiers, secretaries, and typists. Fifty percent of African American women are employed in service occupations such as nursing aides, orderlies and attendants, cooks, janitors, and cleaners. One-fourth of all African American professionals are teachers, mainly elementary school teachers (Bennett, 1993). African American women continue to hold jobs that as a whole do not command much earning power.

Caribbean women are more likely to have jobs in low-paying service occupations (eg, laborers and factory workers). These occupations often have hazards such as exposure to toxins, irradiation, anesthetic gases, and infectious agents. A significant number of Caribbean women, 30%, are employed in the allied health care field with the majority working as nurses aides (Graham, 1989).

Income

The income of African American women is affected by educational and occupational opportunities and also by family composition. In 1989, the median income for all African American families was $22,430. However, in that same year, the median income for African American female-headed households was only $12,520. In 1980, the median family income for Caribbean households was $15,645 compared to $17,361 for African American households. The households headed by women of Caribbean families had higher median income, $10,971, compared to African American families with $7625 (Graham, 1989).

The number of African American families maintained by women has increased steadily since 1970. The proportion is higher for African American women than any other group of women. Between 1970 and 1990, African Americans had the greatest increase in the proportion of families maintained by women, increasing from 27.4% in 1970 to 43.7% in 1990 (Bennett, 1993).

In 1990, 32% of all African Americans and 36% of all African American women were living in poverty. The percentage of African Americans living in poverty since 1973 has remained at 30% to 33%, three times that for Caucasians (Leigh, 1994). For Caucasians it has remained at 9% to 11%.

Single parent, female-headed households, 44% of all African American households in 1990, lived in poverty to a greater degree than the entire African American population. Forty-eight percent of all African American female-headed families had incomes below the poverty level in 1990. Seventy-eight percent of the 2 million African American families in poverty were maintained by single African American women (U.S. Department of Commerce, 1993).

Education, occupation, and income are all determinants of economic status and provide some indication as to who may be most at risk to live at or below the poverty level. Half the nation's poor in 1990 were either children under 18 years (40%) or elderly (10.9%). Children continue to be overrepresented among the poor. Unfortunately, African American children are disproportionately represented. For children younger than 18 years, the poverty rate in 1990 was 15.9% for Caucasian children, 38.4% for children of Hispanic origin, and 44.8% for African American children (U.S. Dept. of Commerce, 1993).

Despite willingness to work and strides in education, African American women remain the lowest paid and least rewarded for their contributions in the workplace. African American women most exemplify the feminization of poverty, with a rate of poverty three times that of her Caucasian counterparts. African American women are also most likely to be caretakers, nurturers, and heads of households for children and extended family. Unfortunately, it is not surprising that with these indicators the status of African American and Caribbean women's health is also compromised.

The poverty rates of African American women directly influence health outcomes. Inadequate diets, dangerous work environments, poor housing, lack of access to primary and preventive health care, inadequate health systems to handle stress, anger, and depression all result in many of the poor health outcomes observed across all life cycles.

Cultural Implications Affecting Health Care

In addition to socioeconomic factors, cultural beliefs and practices can affect the health status of women by influencing their use of health care services, confidence and acceptance of recommended prevention and treatment strategies, and global beliefs regarding their body, illness, religion, and so forth. For example, prayer, consultation with ministers, and reliance on home remedies can be common solutions used to treat illness. It may be difficult for some African American women to perform routine breast self-examination if they were taught "not to touch their private parts."

There can be cultural barriers to care are that lead to lack of respect shown by providers and mistrust, fear, and anger on the part of clients. In addition, there is a lack of culturally sensitive, culturally relevant health information of a kind that could promote behavioral change.

An analysis of the Caribbean community in New York found that although the various nationality groups have a diversity of cultures, the following similarities exist (Graham, 1989):

- Health beliefs and folk medical practices of the population are by-products and expressions of their cultural heritage that have an impact on their childbearing experience.
- An interplay exists between aspects of culture such as family roles and expectations and religious factors that influence the use of prenatal care services.
- Lack of access to medical care in the immigrants' country of origin forces a reliance on folk medical systems and these practices may be continued in the new country.

A study of the pattern of health service use by immigrant communities demonstrated an underutilization of services caused by the following (Graham, 1989):

- reliance on self-management and folk medicine
- lack of orientation to preventive health
- limited health education
- fear of deportation
- lack of culturally sensitive providers
- financial barriers
- language barriers
- lack of value by providers for folk health practices and home remedies
- weak linkages between health care systems and ethnic and immigrant organizations

However, emergency rooms were overutilized as their only source of care. Lack of coverage and the anonymity of emergency service promoted their use.

Inability to speak English is another obstacle in accessing health care services. The Caribbean population is multilingual; they are Spanish speaking, French/Creole speaking, and Dutch speaking. The language barrier is accentuated because these groups have English as a second language. Varying accents and dialects of the English language tend to also create communication barriers. For example, within the Haitian population of New York, 3.8% do not speak English and 16.1% do not speak it well (Graham, 1989).

Mortality and Morbidity of African American and Caribbean Women

Mortality

All people in the United States regardless of race or ethnic background are living longer and healthier lives. When the nation was founded, the life expectancy was 35 years and at the turn of the century it had risen to 45 years for Caucasian women. However, for African American women it was less than 40 years. This disparity in health outcomes was present then and has remained, even though the gap has narrowed from 15 years in 1900 to 5 years in 1990 (National Center for Health Statistics, 1992).

This gap can also be recognized through the identification of excess deaths. The term "excess deaths" expresses the difference between the number of deaths actually observed in a minority group and number of deaths that would have occurred in that group if it had experienced the same death rates as the Caucasian population.

The 1985 Report of the Secretary's Task Force on Black and Minority Health revealed that African Americans suffered a significant amount of excess mortality (U.S. Department of Health and Human Services [DHSS], 1985). Analysis of 1991 mortality data makes evident a continuing disparity in the burden of death and illness experienced by African American persons compared with Caucasian persons.

Overall, the number of deaths among African Americans has continued to be in excess of what would be expected if the death toll for African Americans and Caucasian persons were equal. The same causes identified in the 1985 report continued to contribute significantly to this excess mortality in heart disease, cancer, diabetes, homicide, cirrhosis, infant mortality, and now human immunodeficiency virus/acquired immunodeficiency syndrome (HIV/AIDS) (DHHS, 1994b). Cardiovascular disease is the number one killer if all age groups are aggregated. However, the number one cause of death varies widely by age group and also varies geographically. For example, for African American women aged 15 to 25, homicide is the number one cause of death, whereas in New York and New Jersey, AIDS is the number one cause of death for that age group (Villarosa, 1994).

Infant and Maternal Mortality

The disparity in health outcomes between African American women and Caucasian women is obvious at the beginning of the life cycle with differences in infant and maternal mortality rates. The gap between infant mortality rates for

Caucasian and African American babies has widened for each sex since 1980, even though the infant mortality rate per 1000 live births has decreased for each group.

In 1980, 5646 African American female infants died. Of these, 54.8% were considered excess deaths. In 1991, comparable calculations show that the excess mortality rate had risen to 59.5% for African American female infants. The Caucasian female mortality rate was 6.3/1000 live births versus 14.8/1000 for African American female infants (DHHS, 1994b).

In 1991, the African American maternal mortality rate was three times that of Caucasian women (14.2/100,000 live births to 5.1/100,000) Most of the deaths are preventable. The epidemic of teenage pregnancy contributes significantly to poor maternal and infant outcomes. The maternal death rate is 35% higher for mothers aged 15 to 19 years and 60% higher for mothers 14 years and under (U.S. Public Health Service, 1990).

Increasing poverty and growing barriers to utilization of prenatal services early and throughout pregnancy by poor African American women are evidenced by the increasing number of women seen with late or no prenatal care. These barriers extend beyond the inability to pay for prenatal services and include obstacles that the overall state of poverty imposes (ie, lack of resources for transportation and child care and inadequate information). Inadequate prenatal care is a reflection of these multiple barriers (Obey et al., 1991).

The decreasing infant mortality rate is a reflection of better tertiary care. However, increasing incidence of low-birth weight nationally, especially for African American babies, reflects decreasing access to quality primary health care and poor prenatal care. All the factors are not well delineated because middle-class African American women have higher rates of low-birth weight babies when compared to middle-class Caucasian women (Schoendorf et al., 1992).

Infant mortality in Caribbean countries remains high, especially in Haiti; however, some Caribbean countries, notably Trinidad and Tobago, have a lower rate than the African American rate in the United States (Buvinic & Leslie, 1981). In Caribbean neighborhoods in the United States, infant mortality rates are usually high. People from the Caribbean live in areas of the city that have a shortage of doctors, nurses, and other health care professionals (Pollnais, 1991). In addition, lack of U.S. citizenship is a barrier to the use of maternal child health services by pregnant Caribbean women, as well as an obstacle to entitlement benefits such as Aid for Families with Dependent Children and Medicaid.

A study on Reproductive Health Experience of Immigrant Caribbean women in New York City, 1980—1984, found that Caribbean women had a lower proportion of births among mothers 19 years of age and younger compared to African American women. In contrast, Caribbean women had a higher proportion of older mothers (over age 30) compared to African Americans (Graham, 1989).

Heart Disease

Heart disease is the number one killer for all Americans. The rate of death from heart disease has decreased for all Americans, including African American women. However, the gap remains and the rate of death for African American women in

1990 was the same as the rate for Caucasian women in 1970 (Figure 17-1) (National Center for Health Statistics, 1992). African American women were 25% more likely to die from heart disease than Caucasian women (National Center for Health Statistics, 1992).

Deaths from cardiovascular disease contributed more to the excess for African American women 45 to 69 years of age than under the age of 45. For the age group 45 to 69, cardiovascular disease accounted for 32% of the excess mortality for African American men compared to 54% for African American women (DHHS, 1994b).

African American women are more likely to die from heart disease than Caucasian women because they have more risk factors. Risk factors include hypertension, obesity, high cholesterol level, diabetes, smoking, and inadequate exercise. The more risk factors an individual has, the greater the risk of dying from cardiovascular disease. Having three risk factors—smoking, high blood pressure, and high blood cholesterol level—can boost the risk to eight times that of women who have no risk factors. Research shows that African American women are more likely to have hypertension, obesity, and diabetes and to consume high-fat and high-cholesterol diets (National Heart, Lung and Blood Institute, 1992).

Hypertension plays a major role in the continuing problem of cardiovascular disease. It is more common and more severe in African American women, who have a higher incidence of hypertension than Caucasian women, Hispanic women, Caucasian men, and African American men. The risk is also high during the reproductive years from ages 25 to 34. Forty-four percent African American women were found to be hypertensive, more than double the rates for Mexican American women (20%) and Puerto Rican women (19%) and more than triple the rate among Cuban American women (14%) (National Center for Health Statistics, 1992).

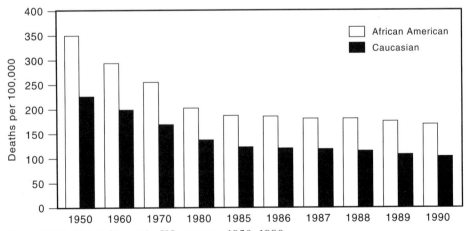

Figure 17-1. Heart disease in U.S. women, 1950-1990.

Studies are beginning to show that hypertension is being documented in African American teenage girls. With the increasing incidence of obesity at younger ages—10 and 11 years—the incidence of cardiovascular disease will be seen with greater frequency in teenage girls.

Cancer

Cancer is the number two cause of death overall for both African American and Caucasian women and the leading cause of death among women aged 35 to 50. Historically, most of the deaths were from breast cancer; however, with the dramatic increase in lung cancer this pattern has changed. Deaths from lung cancer have increased 600% over the past 30 to 40 years. In the past 10 years death from lung cancer has increased 36% for Caucasian women and 26% for African American women (National Center for Health Statistics, 1992) (Figure 17-2).

Breast cancer is also a major cause of death for African American women. African American women have lower incidence rates than Caucasian women but higher death rates at every stage of diagnosis (DHHS, 1994a). Poor women have the lowest survival rates for breast cancer (Ayanian, 1993). Recently released results from a National Cancer Institute study indicate that African American women are more than twice as likely as Caucasian women to die from breast cancer. The 5-year survival rate for African American women was only 62% compared with 79% for Caucasian women.

Much of this increase in mortality is attributed to the fact that breast cancer in African American women more often reaches an advanced stage before it is diagnosed. Some evidence that breast tumors may be more aggressive in African American women was provided, but the most important conclusion of the study is that early screening for breast cancer is essential (Eley et al., 1994).

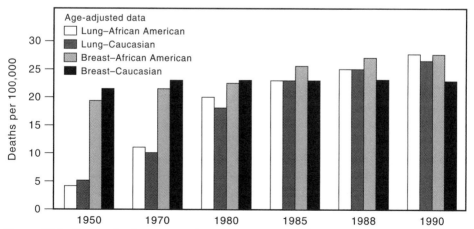

Figure 17-2. Cancer deaths among African American and Caucasian women in the United States, 1950-1990.

These results are important in light of the current controversy regarding routine mammograms in women under age 50. The guidelines should recommend mammograms earlier for African American women. In addition, these results are important because current data show that African American women have fewer mammograms and are being diagnosed later after metastases have occurred. Data from the National Breast and Cervical Cancer Early Detection Program indicate that the percentage of screening mammograms provided in 1993 was 48.4% for Caucasian women and 14.7% for African American women (Leigh, 1994). Poor women receive mammograms at half the rate as nonpoor women and 43% are diagnosed after metastasis.

The rate of cervical cancer is higher in African American women than in any other group. African American women continue to have cervical cancer at three times the rate of Caucasian women and a mortality rate that is twice the rate of Caucasian women. These mortality outcomes clearly reflect the difference in access to preventive and primary health care and the difference in use of Papanicolaou (Pap) smears.

Rates for carcinoma in situ reach a peak for both African American and Caucasian women between 20 and 30 years of age. After the age of 25, the incidence of invasive cancer in African American women increases dramatically with age, whereas in Caucasian women the incidence rises more slowly (DHHS, 1994a). The incidence of cervical cancer has been estimated to have been decreased 70% by screening. However, a large proportion of women, particularly elderly African American women and middle-aged poor women, have not had regular Pap tests. If women appropriately had Pap tests, death from cervical cancer could almost entirely be prevented (Runowicz, 1994).

Cerebrovascular Disease (Stroke)

Cerebrovascular disease or stroke in U.S. women is decreasing for both groups, but it continues to be the third leading cause of death for both groups. Strokes occur in African American women at almost twice the rate as they do in Caucasian women. African American women are 86% more likely to die from stroke than Caucasian women. Hypertension greatly increases the risk of stroke (National Institute of Neurologic Disorders & Stroke, 1994).

Diabetes

Diabetes is a major health problem in the African American community. It was uncommon among African Americans at the turn of the century, but now is the fourth leading cause of death for African American women and sixth for African American men. Diabetes is more common in women in general and African American women in particular. It is double that of the nonminority population. African American women have 50% more diabetes than Caucasian women, with a greater frequency of complications such as cardiovascular disease, stroke, kidney failure, and blindness and a higher death rate (National Center for Health Statistics, 1992).

A report issued by the National Center for Health Statistics in 1987 noted that the prevalence of diagnosed diabetes in African Americans increased fourfold in two decades, double the rate of increase among Caucasian Americans. The prevalence of non–insulin-dependent diabetes mellitus is 60% higher than in Caucasians. African Americans have higher rates of diabetes at all adult age levels, and among those 65 to 74 years of age, one in four has diabetes. Among African American women, diabetes is epidemic: one in four African American women older than 55 has diabetes, double the rate in Caucasian women. African American women are three times more likely to be blind as a result of diabetes and have twice as many amputations. Eighty-three percent are obese compared to 62% of Caucasian women and 45% of African American men (National Institute of Diabetes and Digestive and Kidney Diseases, 1992).

Homicide

Homicide is a major cause of death among African American women under the age of 44. In 1991, homicide rates were nearly five times as high for African American females (13.9) as for Caucasian females (3.0), (deaths per 100,000 resident population). Homicide is the number one cause of death in female African Americans aged 15 to 24 years except in those cities where AIDS is the number one cause of death (National Center for Health Statistics, 1992).

African American and other minority women have consistently experienced higher death rates than Caucasian women and for homicide by a family member or friend, even higher rates than Caucasian men. Among African American women, 47% are murdered by acquaintances and 43% by "family members" (Stark, 1990).

Homicide is a major cause of death in African American infants 6 to 12 months of age and in elderly African American women over the age of 85.

Most homicides are preceded by a history of assault and are embedded in a larger pattern of economic, social, and sexual control by men and poor self-esteem by women.

In 1990, the rate of domestic homicides among African Americans was eight times greater than that of Caucasians.

HIV/AIDS

Currently, AIDS has replaced homicide as the leading killer of African Americans aged 25 to 44. Women account for approximately 11% of AIDS cases in the United States. Fifty-three percent of women with AIDS are African American, and most live in urban areas (Centers for Disease Control and Prevention, 1992). HIV/AIDS accounted for 12.8% of the total excess deaths for African American women under 45 years of age compared with 7.6% for African American women aged 45 to 69 (DHHS, 1994b). African American children account for more than 50% of all children with AIDS (U.S. Public Health Service, 1990). The rate of death for African American women with AIDS in 1991 was more than nine times that for Caucasian women. African American women are among the fastest growing groups of HIV-infected individuals. Between 1987 and 1991, the rate increased annually by 26% for African American women and 19% to 21% for Caucasian men, African American men, and Caucasian women. Intravenous drug use and unprotected heterosexual intercourse account for much of this growth. Important contributing factors such as the inequity of power within heterosexual relationships, sexual behaviors, and awareness of risks make these women particularly prone to HIV infection. In addition, pregnancy and child care issues may make their problems even more complicated (Bing & Soto, 1991).

Morbidity

Depression

Depression is the leading diagnosis of mental disorder in women. Risk factors for depression include unhappy marriages, poverty, maternal stress, reproductive events, personality, family roles and intimate relationships, work roles or lack of work, spouse absence, social isolation, victimization, and health problems (U.S. Public Health Service, 1992).

Minority women are affected to a great degree by depression, and it is aggravated by such factors as racial prejudice, lower educational and income levels, low-status/high-stress employment, immigration and acculturation, larger family sizes, marital dissolution, single parenthood, and poor health (Commonwealth Fund Women's Health Survey, 1993). In particular, African American women face a number of mental health-related issues based on their position in life in this society (ie, their historical, cultural, and structural position; their experience with racial and sexual discrimination; and their socioeconomic status). Many of these mental health issues are reflected in increased risk for stress, alcoholism, drug abuse, and suicide. However, depression is the most common, being twice as common in African American women as in Caucasian women (McGrath, Kieta, Strickland, & Riesso, 1990).

The family patterns that influenced Africans were significantly changed by slavery, and new patterns developed that emphasized blood ties and the extended family. African American women have been viewed as the backbone of the family and not always economically dependent on the man. The structure of this relationship has contributed to the higher rate of divorce among African Americans (Bennett, 1993).

High levels of depressive symptoms are reported in women with insufficient personal support, lack of childrearing assistance, and those experiencing chronic stress, particularly stress caused by inadequate financial resources (Belle, 1990).

An analysis of social class and racial differences in depressive symptomatology in a random sample of 1645 adults showed that African American women, the aged, the poor, and those with the least formal education had the highest rates of depressive symptomatology. The highest depression scores were found in women (24%) in contrast to men (13%). African American women had significantly higher scores (34%) compared to Caucasian women (21%). When socioeconomic status was controlled, no significant racial difference was noted in these depression scores. The most significant indicators of depression were gender and socioeconomic status (Warhert, Holzer, & Schwab, 1983).

Data show that major depression morbidity is beginning earlier in African American girls. An analysis of 677 junior high students' responses to the Center for Epidemiologic Studies Depression Scales showed that 4.4% had major depressive disorders with the prevalence being highest among African American girls (11%)

and lowest among African American boys (1.67%) and Caucasian girls (4.4%) (Garrison et al., 1989). Of significance is that adolescent depression also extends into the adult years (Kandel & Davies, 1986).

Lupus Erythematosus

Lupus erythematosus is an immune disease that can affect many parts of the body such as the joints, skin, kidneys, lungs, heart, or brain. Lupus is a serious health problem that mainly affects young women. However, lupus is three times more common in African American women than in Caucasian women (Graham, 1994).

Signs of lupus include the following (National Institutes of Health, 1991):

- red rash or color change on face, often in the shape of a butterfly across the bridge of the nose
- painful or swollen joints
- unexplained fever
- chest pain upon breathing
- unusual loss of hair
- pale or purple fingers or toes from cold or stress
- sensitivity to the sun
- low blood count

A study done by Siegel and Lee, which covered a 10-year period from 1956 to 1965, showed that the higher frequency in new cases of lupus among African American women was attributed to low socioeconomic status, adverse environmental conditions, and poor access to clinics for treatment (Graham, 1994). A more recent study by Dr. Matthew Liang defines four determinate factors of health status in minorities: socioeconomic status, nutritional status and dietary practices, environmental and occupational exposures, and stress and coping patterns. He also states that influence factors can be associated with low income, education, access to health care, understanding of what symptoms mean and when medical attention is needed, social supports, nutrition, housing conditions, and employment opportunities (Graham, 1994).

Obesity

Obesity is a major health problem for African American women in the United States. Among adults the prevalence of obesity in African American women is greater than among Caucasian women or among men of either race. African American women suffer more from overweight-associated conditions resulting in significantly higher rates of morbidity and mortality compared with Caucasian women. Mortality rates from coronary heart disease, stroke, hypertensive disease, and diabetes are substantially higher among African American women than among Caucasian women (National Center for Health Statistics, 1992).

Obesity is inversely related to low family income and low educational attainment in African American and Caucasian women with the relationship to education in African American women having the strongest correlation. African American women in rural areas are more overweight than those in urban areas and African American women living in the southern region are more overweight than those living in other regions (Gillum, 1987).

Data from the National Health Interview Survey indicate that fewer African American women perceived themselves to be overweight compared with Caucasian women (46% versus 51%) despite the excess prevalence of obesity in African American women. Of those who perceived themselves overweight, 75% of African American women and 67% of Caucasian women said they were trying to lose weight. This indicates that cultural norms for desirable weight may vary by race (National Center for Health Statistics, 1978).

Obesity is also associated with diets of poverty, which are high in fat and cholesterol and low in fruits and vegetables. Studies have also shown that African American girls are more likely than Caucasian girls to be overweight during infancy and childhood (Gartsidy, Khonry, & Glueck, 1984).

Summary and Recommendations

The gaps in health status between African American and Caucasian women continue to widen with ongoing and significant disparities in mortality and morbidity and poor health outcomes across all life cycles. This is related to many factors:

- increasing poverty
- lack of access to primary and preventive health care
- inadequate health care systems to handle stress, anger, and depression
- racial and sexual discrimination
- inadequate education
- inadequate modification of risky behavior
- increasing epidemic of teenage pregnancy
- violence
- HIV/AIDS

Poverty is the most powerful single determinant of negative outcomes, one that must be examined more completely. The outcomes of racial and ethnic differences within the context of the socioeconomic impact are also important to understand so that more effective interventions and outcomes can be realized. The disparities in health outcomes are complex and multifactorial. These factors require further definition and investigation of the degree of impact in combination or alone. It is critical that more complete demographic data be obtained so that all women are not aggregated but are analyzed based on their specific ethnic, economic, and age categories. Gender identification must stand out so that African American women do not fall under the rubric of "Black" and be included with African American men. Data on African American women are frequently combined with all the data on "women" or all the data on "Black." Once these major descriptions are delineated, then the impact of health status will be seen more clearly. Without the delineation, it is impossible to develop effective policies, conduct competent research, and deliver effectual interventions to deal with the health status issues of African American women.

Health care services must become more accessible for African American women. A concerted effort must be made to improve the primary care infrastructure so that poor and vulnerable women have access to health education, preventive services, and services providing early diagnosis and early intervention.

The need for continuing health education cannot be overlooked. This is essential for health promotion and disease prevention. This will empower women to take care of their own health. Every opportunity to educate must be used.

It is also important to extend beyond the patient and mobilize women in the community (churches, jobs, neighbors) to provide support to educate on health care issues and increase compliance. We use support groups after a woman has breast cancer diagnosed. We should do the same to put prevention and early diagnosis into practice. There are model programs that use support groups to help women receive preventive care services such as mammograms, blood pressure screens, and cholesterol screens. There are also model programs on preventing teenage pregnancy that encourage young women to sign pacts with each other and commit to themselves and their group members. Whatever the particular issue, the goals are to allow group members to assist each other in making health a priority and to provide continuous support so that it becomes a habit.

Lastly, but most importantly, young African American girls must be taught how to develop a lifelong habit of health. This education should begin early, in kindergarten, if possible. Programs that begin early, provide education and support, and enhance self-esteem will succeed in addressing the continuing disparities in health outcomes that can be prevented.

References

Ayanian J. Z., Kobler, B. A., et al. (1993). The relation between health insurance coverage and clinical outcomes among women with breast cancer. *New England Journal of Medicine, 329,* 326-331.

Belle, D. (1990). Poverty and women's mental health. *American Psychologist, 45,* 385-389.

Bennett, C. E. (1993). *The black population of the United States.* March 1992, U.S. Bureau of the Census, Current Population Reports, P20-471. Washington, DC: U.S. Government Printing Office.

Bing, E. G., & Soto, T. (1991). Treatment issues for African-Americans and Hispanics with AIDS. *Psychiatric Medicine, 9* (3), 455.

Buvinic, M., & Leslie, J. (1981). Health care for women in Latin America and the Caribbean. *Studies in Family Planning, 12* (3), 112-115.

Centers for Disease Control and Prevention. (1992). *HIV/AIDS Surveillance.* Atlanta, GA: Author.

Commonwealth Fund Women's Health Survey. (1993). New York: Louis Harris and Associates.

Eley, J. W., Hill, H. A., Chen, V. W., et al. (1994). Racial differences in survival from breast cancer: Results of the National Cancer Institute Black/White Cancer Survival Study. *Journal of the American Medical Association, 272,* 947-954.

Garrison, C. Z., Schluchter, M. D., Schoenbach, J. S., & Kaplan, B. K. (1989). Epidemiology of depressive symptoms in young adolescents. *Journal of the American Academy of Child and Adolescent Psychology, 28,* 343-351.

Gartsidy, P. S., Khonry, D., & Glueck, C. (1984). Determinants of high-density lipoprotein cholesterol in blacks and whites. *American Heart Journal, 108,* 641-53.

Gillum, R. (1987). Overweight and obesity in black women: A review of published data from the National Center for Health Statistics. *Journal of the National Medical Association, 79,* 865-871.

Gordon-Bradshaw, R. H. A social essay on special issues facing poor women of color. *Women and Health, 12,* 3–4, Fall—Winter, 243–259.

Graham, R. (1994, July-September). Lupus...knowing the facts: African American women and lupus. *Vital Signs, X,* 62.

Graham, Y. (1989). Maternal and child health profile of the Caribbean population in New York City, establishing new lives. *Selected reading on Caribbean immigrants in New York City.* New York: Caribbean Research Center, Medgar Evers College, City University of New York.

Kandel, D., & Davies, M. (1986). Adult sequelae of adolescent depressive symptoms. *Archives of General Psychiatry, 43,* 255-262.

Leigh, W. (1994). *The health status of women of color.* Washington, DC: Joint Center for Political and Economic Studies.

McGrath, Kieta, Strickland, & Riesso (Eds.). (1990). *Women and depression. Risk factors and treatment issues.* American Psychological Association.

National Center for Health Statistics. (1978). *Characteristics of persons with hypertension, United States.* Vital and Health Statistics Series (DHEW Publication No. 79-1549). Washington, DC: U.S. Government Printing Office.

National Center for Health Statistics. (1992). *Health, United States, 1991.* Hyattsville, MD: U.S. Department of Health and Human Services.

National Heart, Lung and Blood Institute. (1992). *The healthy heart handbook for women* (NIH Publication No. 92-2720). Washington, DC: National Institutes of Health.

National Institute of Diabetes and Digestive and Kidney Diseases. (1992). *Diabetes in black Americans.* (NIH Publication No. 93-3266). Washington, DC: Author.

National Institute of Neurologic Disorders and Stroke. (1994). *Stroke Research Highlights.* Washington, DC: Author.

National Institutes of Health. (1991). *What black women should know about lupus.* (NIH Publication No. 91-3219). Washington, DC: NIAMS Task Force on Lupus in High Risk Populations.

Obey, C. Tia-Hoagbey, B., Skovhold, C., et al. (1991). Prenatal care use and health insurance status. *Journal of Health Care for the Poor and Underserved, 2,* 270-293.

Pollnais, E. (1991). A case for prenatal care in Brooklyn's Caribbean immigrant communities. *Caribbean Sun, 1,* 7-8.

Runowicz, C. (1994, July-September). Women's health care: Prevention is the key. National Black Women's Health Project. *Vital Signs, X,* 52.

Schoendorf, K. C., Card, J. R., Hogue, Kleinman, J., & Cowley, D. (1992). Mortality among infants of black as compared with white college-educated parents. *New England Journal of Medicine, 326,* 1522-1526.

Stark, E. (1990). Rethinking homicide: Violence, race, and the politics of gender. *International Journal of Health Services, Section on Health and Social Policy, 20,* 3-26.

U.S. Bureau of the Census. (1993). *Social and economic characteristics, 1990* (CP-2-1). Washington, DC: U.S. Government Printing Office.

U.S. Department of Commerce, Economics and Statistics Administration. (1993). *We the American blacks.* Washington, DC: Author.

U.S. Department of Health and Human Services. (1985). *Report of the Secretary's task force on black and minority health.* Washington, DC: Author.

U.S. Department of Health and Human Services. (1994a). *Clinician's handbook of preventive services.* Washington, DC: U.S. Government Printing Office.

U.S. Department of Health and Human Services. (1994b). *Excess deaths and other mortality measures for the black population.* Washington, DC: Author.

U.S. Public Health Service. (1990). *Healthy people 2000: National health promotion and disease prevention objectives.* Washington, DC: Author.

U.S. Public Health Service, Region VIII, Office on Women's Health. (1992). *Minority women dimensions in health.* Final Report, June 18-20, 1992, p. 12. Washington, DC: PHS Coordinating Committee on Women's Health Issues.

Villarosa, L. (1994). *Body and soul: The black women's guide to physical health and emotional well-being.* New York: Harper Collins.

Warhert, G., Holzer, C., & Schwab, J. (1983). An analysis of social class and racial differences in depressive symptomatology: A community study. *Journal of Health and Social Behavior,* 291-297.

CHAPTER 18

Asian and Pacific Island Women

Vivian T. Chen

Introduction

As the fastest growing ethnic minority group (U.S. Bureau of the Census, 1992a; 1993b; 1993c), the Asian and Pacific Islander (API) population remains the most misunderstood, underrepresented, underreported, and understudied ethnic population when it comes to health status (Chen, 1993; Kroll & Bradigan, 1993). The absence of national longitudinal incidence and prevalence rates on API women is alarming when reviewing the body of health research publications. For the most part, when research data are found on APIs and women it has been limited. The lack of health-related data bases creates barriers to establishing an accurate assessment of the health care needs of APIs. This lack of population-based health data perpetuates a cycle of ignorance, including the denial of access to culturally appropriate health care and lack of health objectives. Unfortunately, national policy is driven by these national data bases.

Historically, when minorities are classified and included in public health research, minority samples are typically of African Americans. When other ethnic or racial populations are included in studies, they are generally lumped into the "other" category. Over the last 10 years, efforts to learn more about minority populations have resulted in the expansion of the minority classification to include Hispanics/Latinas and sometimes other ethnic populations. Limited as it is, a growing body of literature on various API subgroups provides some preliminary insights on their health status. The trends found ties close to racial, sexual, and cultural experiences in the United States. The APIs are bimodally distributed socioeconomically and quite heterogenous as a group.

This chapter pieces together the scanty health status data on API women in historical, economic, and cultural perspectives. Finally, areas where public policy can be enhanced are proposed.

Background

The lack of information on the history of APIs drives the general absence of health data. To discuss the overall health status of API women requires the presence of data to portray each life cycle adequately. The inability to perform a rigorous examination of research findings is perhaps the most troubling aspect of this review. This is attributed to the absence of national data and methodologic flaws found in the studies. Many studies reported were limited in sample size, did not represent subgroup differences, were gender specific (mostly male), or were geographically restricted. Given the dearth of available data on APIs, it is disconcerting that, nevertheless, generalizations and policy decisions are being made. Without sufficient API data, a clear understanding or meaningful conclusion about the health status and needs of the over 60 subethnic groups with over 500 dialects/languages cannot be drawn. An historical perspective on the immigration of Asians and Pacific Islanders may provide insight to the current perceptions and limited practices.

For so long the stereotypical portrayal of the API population has been that of the "model minority." It has been suggested that this myth emerged after the 1965 Watts riots as a means to pit minority groups against each other (Hu-DeHart, 1992), providing a rationale for policymakers not to be concerned about the welfare of the API population. After all, APIs are a small number and considered healthy, successful, and wise. This enviable stereotype also assumes that their health status is as good, especially when looking at aggregate data for the entire API population. This is a logical assumption given that health status has been shown to be strongly associated with socioeconomic status. Perhaps a positive stereotype should not be of concern. However, benign neglect is another form of discrimination. It also implies that people of color should be as "successful" as the "model minority." It is thought that APIs have reached ultimate success.

API women have faced additional stereotypes that influence mental and physical well-being. Positive and negative stereotypes such as being docile, accommodating, passive/demure, "neuter gender," submissive, exotic/erotic, and terms such as "dragon lady," " Suzy Wong," "China Doll," "Hula Miss," and so forth have contributed to a myriad of images. Most of these stereotypes leave the API women feeling less than empowered. Models of docility and subservience coupled with stereotypes of being sexless and exotic are difficult roles for API women to assume.

By not knowing or recognizing the impact of these stereotypes and data inconsistencies that limit health policy, programs, and research, the health status of API subgroup populations will continue to be compromised. Fortunately, through the efforts of API community leaders and researchers, dispelling the "model minority" has raised national consciousness among many policymakers. The current discussions on the reclassification of racial and ethnic categories are an example of an effort to understand the importance of race and ethnicity on health status.

Demographics: Immigration Patterns

Since 1980, the API population has more than doubled from 3,726,440 (1.6%) of the United States population to 8,451,000 (3.3%) (Lin-Fu, 1993), representing an increase of over 108%, with women comprising 51%. Among the 3.7 million API women reported, 1,979,000 (53%) are between the ages of 15 and 44 years. This represents 45.6% of the total API population. But the journey of the APIs to this country is filled with human sacrifice.

Early immigration patterns over 140 years ago (eg, Chinese sojourner in the mid-19th century) tended to favor men for the labor markets. As many as eight generations of API families have lived in the United States. As history has shown, however, anti-Asian laws (eg, antimiscegenation laws such as the Cable Act of 1922, anti-Asian exclusion acts that prohibited citizenship and established immigration quotas and sterilization laws in the South to prohibit Asian women from having children) inhibited APIs from flourishing.

Immigration of Asian (particularly Chinese) women into this country was prohibited by law until after 1943, despite marital status to a spouse already in the United States. The laws were designed to prevent the establishment of families and a second generation of United States citizens with Asian parentage. When Chinese men first arrived in this country in the mid-1800s, they were "recruited" as laborers during the gold rush and in effect replaced the declining African American slavery market. As cheap labor, they immigrated to the West Coast to work in the mines and on the railroads. They served as the "new Negro" class and were called "nagurs" by the Caucasian majority (Hu-DeHart, 1993). After this period of history, the notion of a "Yellow Peril" stigmatized the Chinese as less than acceptable, diseased, and heathens. Immigration of the Chinese was forbidden until 1942 and citizenship not granted until 1952.

Japanese women from 1900 to 1919 entered this country as "picture brides" as arranged by families and strictly monitored by their government (Ichioka, 1979). Korean women entered similarly as a means to prevent Asian men from marrying Americans. Early immigration patterns of API immigrants began from China, followed by Japan, Korea, the Philippines, and the remaining Pacific Rim countries. When the immigration laws changed in 1965, the National Origins Act that established immigration quotas for each country was also changed. This law enabled the reunification of families and allowed those with selected skilled occupations to immigrate. Ten years later the immigration of Southeast Asians began. The *Civil Rights Issues Facing Asian Americans in the 1990s* provides accounts of the bigotry, hatred, and violence that have been and still are experienced by APIs (U.S. Commission on Civil Rights, 1992).

Over 200 years of Native Hawaiian history exists, but it is not well known. Pacific Islanders have immigrated from over 22 territories and nations with up to 1000 languages (Ponce, 1990). The poor health status of Native Hawaiians and Pacific Islanders is largely associated with their socioeconomic status. Native Hawaiians have experienced traumatic social changes that have threatened their traditions and survival as a distinct group. Statehood has resulted in loss of land and political power, causing the population to be disproportionately represented in the lower income brackets. Nearly 20% of the Native Hawaiian and Pacific Islander families, compared to the national average of 12.5%, earn less than $15,000 per year.

The current demographic data reflect much of the diversity found within and across API subgroups in health care issues and needs, cultural response to illness, and treatment and patterns of disease. Clearly, much of the subethnic variation found among APIs is tied to the length of time in this country and educational attainment. As noted in the *Healthy People 2000 Cross-cutting Progress Review* for *Asians and Pacific Islanders* (U.S. Public Health Service, 1994), 7.5% of the API women have less than 5 years of elementary school education compared to 2.5% of Caucasian women. The educational attainment level of API women receiving college degrees differed widely among subethnic groups. Subgroup variations ranged from less than 3% of Cambodian women to 48% for Japanese American women ever receiving a college degree (U.S. Bureau of the Census, 1990).

Although aggregate findings on API women's educational attainment are above the national average in receiving a 4-year college degree, the higher educational attainment does not reflect proportionately better income for APIs as noted in the United States Bureau of Census 1990 figures. APIs earn 71 cents for every dollar a Caucasian American earns despite parity in levels of educational attainment (Hubler, 1992). In fact, APIs have raised serious concern for the glass ceiling of APIs (Ohata, 1993; Wong & Nagasawa, 1991). An alarming 6.2% of API women, or three times that of the general population (2.1%), have 0 to 4 years of elementary education. About 15.6% of APIs work in service occupations that include poor pay and limited or no health insurance coverage.

Only 6.5% of the trained API physicians are primary care providers and only 15% reside geographically on the West Coast where the majority of the API populations reside. This geographic mismatch in the supply of potentially culturally competent providers heightens the problems of access to health care services for APIs. If subgroup representation is to be accomplished, then programs that recruit additional API health professionals and providers who are linguistically and culturally capable must be trained to meet the needs of the newer API populations such as the various Southeast Asian subgroups and Hawaiian, Samoan, Thai, and Tongan populations.

Despite the reported higher number of family members found in the API family (5.7% of the API families have six or more persons compared to the national average of 1.9%), the figures represent multiple family members or extended family members residing under one roof who contribute to the family earnings (U.S. Bureau of the Census, 1990). This cultural lifestyle presents a distorted image of the API family by which the term family is culturally defined by the API as extended. Erroneous assumptions are made regarding the "high economic success" or higher wage earnings of the API family when traditional families in the United States are typically deemed as the immediate family.

In fact, 12% of the API families and 9% of married couple families compared to the national average of 10% and close to 6%, respectively, were reported below the poverty threshold in 1990. However, significant subpopulation disparity exists where seven subethnic groups exceed the national average of 13% below poverty. The seven subgroups reported as below the poverty rate represent Laotian (66%), Hmong (63.6%), Cambodian (42.6%), Vietnamese (25.7%), Chinese (14.0%), and Korean (13.7%). Close to one-fourth (21%) of the API population have no health insurance and do not know how to obtain other financial assistance (Lin, 1990).

The data also strongly suggest a relationship between recent immigration (within the last 15 years) and lower socioeconomic status (educationally and financially). The increases found in the API figures also indicate that 74% of the APIs in this country are foreign born. The increase in population is attributed to the adoption of the

Immigration Act of 1965, Indochina Migration and Refugee Assistance Act of 1975, and changes in the census race definitions in the 1970s, by which enumeration of APIs has become better defined in the census process. Fifty-six percent of the APIs do not speak English "very well," with 36% linguistically isolated. Language proficiency coupled with negotiating a fragmented health care delivery system creates further alienation or lack of access to health care. Bilingual access and culturally competent health care are cited by the Asian American Health Policy Forum (AAHPF) (formerly Asian American Health Forum [AAHF]), the National Asian Pacific Families Against Substance Abuse, and the Association of Asian and the Pacific Islander Community Health Organization (AAPCHO) as major obstacles to the API community.

The API population increases are found in California, Hawaii, New York, Illinois, and Texas. Fifty-four percent of the API population resides on the West Coast. Yet, only 10 federally funded community health centers are funded nationally by the Public Health Service to provide comprehensive multilingual and cultural primary health care services to predominantly API populations. Only three are funded in California, three in Hawaii, one in New York, and none in Texas or Illinois. When 66% of the API population resides in these five states, it is not surprising that this has raised concern about the lack of bilingual and culturally appropriate access to health care from the API community organizations and Asian Caucus. The absence of these funded delivery sites is documented by the AAPCHO (1993) and the portions of the Minority Health Care Improvement Act report (Fuentes, 1991).

The incorporation of traditional cultural beliefs, values, and practices will vary depending on the individual's geographic, spiritual, socioeconomic, and subethnic background. Clearly, more research and data must be generated to determine the various risk factors associated with API subethnic populations.

Overall Health Status

According to the U.S. Public Health Service (1990), only 8 of the 336 established objectives are targeted for APIs. The intent of the objectives is to establish some baseline markers for meeting the national goal to improve the health status of all Americans. The sparse number of objectives is a direct result of unavailable or insufficient data from which an objective with a baseline figure can be established. Of the 13 objectives targeted for women in *Healthy People 2000 Objectives*, specific reference to API women is not found. Furthermore, the use of aggregate data perpetuates the myth that APIs are healthier because it masks the small numbers within smaller subethnic API populations. The Office of Research on Women's Health (ORWH) published *Opportunities for Research on Women's Health*, which presents a comprehensive review of leading health concerns faced by women and recommendations for research based on available data (ORWH, 1992). Again, because of the lack of available data, API women are mentioned infrequently despite having their top three mortality rates from heart disease, malignant neoplasms (cancer), and cerebrovascular disease. Given the importance of these objectives in funding decisions at the state and national levels, a number of leading health concerns faced by API women are discussed next.

Cancer

Health, United States 1992 (U.S. Public Health Service, 1993) reported malignant neoplasms death rates for API women aged 45 years and over (age-adjusted) to be 216/100,000 compared to 382/100,000 for all races. The aggregation of figures prevent a close review. Much attention is being paid to breast cancer and other cancers that affect women. Breast cancer is by far the most common cancer among API women. Caucasian and Native Hawaiian women are at highest risk for developing breast cancer (Leigh, 1994). The highest breast cancer mortality rates are for Hawaiian women (115/100,000) compared to all populations, including African Americans (ORWH, 1992). Breast cancer rates for other API women are: Chinese (58/100,000), Japanese (57/100,000), and Filipino (45/100,000). Unfortunately, a number of Public Health Regional Office sanctioned reports (Region X Women's Health Conference background papers) and health objectives view API women to be at "low risk" based on the limited data. Hawaiian women along with African Americans, Native Americans, and Mexican American women are considered to have high incidence rates requiring increased prevention strategies and efforts (ORWH, 1992). Higuchi et al. (1993) report race as a predictor for Japanese women in terms of cancer death among women with localized disease. In a case-controlled study on migration patterns and breast cancer among API women, it is noted that API women born in the West have a sixfold gradient in breast cancer risk (60%) (Ziegler et al., 1993).

California data reveal the second and third leading cancers among APIs are lung and cervical, respectively (California Department of Health Services, 1990). Risk factors contributing to the high rates are diet, smoking, and health education. Nonsmoking is as important a predictor for developing lung cancer in Asian women (second-hand smoke). A population-based cancer study examined the colorectal cancer incidence rates in Chinese Americans and Chinese in the People's Republic of China. The study indicates that older Chinese American women have colon cancer rates three to four times the rates of their counterparts in China and male/female ratio differences (Whittemore, 1989).

Underutilization of cancer screening is cited; only one-third of the Asian female immigrants ever had a Pap smear and only 30% had a mammogram. Among API women aged 45 years and older, only 47% reported ever having a mammogram. Late diagnosis and high recurrence rates explain some problems in diagnosis (Centers for Disease Control and Prevention [CDC], 1990b). A California cancer screening study conducted in 1990 on Vietnamese women reported that 50% had never had a breast examination or mammogram, close to 60% had not had a Pap smear, and 70% had never had a rectal examination. There are reports of late diagnosis and high recurrence rates for breast cancer in API women (Pham & McPhee, 1992).

Cervical cancer comprises about 3% of all cancers in American women, with an estimated 6000 deaths a year. Among API women, cervical cancer rates are highest for Hawaiian women at 14/100,000, followed by Chinese (11/100,000) and Filipino (8.8/100,000) compared with Caucasian women at 8.8/100,000 (CDC, 1988). Additionally, the esophageal cancer rate among Chinese women is 1.6 times higher than that for Caucasian women. The incidence of pancreatic cancer among Chinese women is 20% higher than the general population (Koo & Ho, 1990). Higher rates of lung cancer may be attributed to higher rates of smoking among certain API subgroups. Thirty-four percent of the Hawaiian women surveyed in the Moloka'i Heart Study, a population-based study conducted in Hawaii, were smokers, compared with the National Household Interview Survey figure of 31% of the U.S. women (CDC, 1990b). Smoking among API women appears to be increasing (Hu et al., 1991).

Most studies conducted by the National Cancer Institute have excluded subethnic sampling to determine differences. A number of population-based studies are underway in Hawaii and China but are limited in gender, foreign population, or sample size. The Secretary for Health and Human Services' National Breast Cancer Strategy (National Institutes of Health, 1993) identifies a blueprint to reduce the high rates. Unfortunately, these plans are general and do not adequately address the subethnic differences within cultures to appropriately ensure culturally competent programming for non-Caucasian populations. National strategies must provide a baseline or outline to ensure minimum efforts are made across ethnic and cultural populations.

Hepatitis B

The chronicity of APIs infected with hepatitis B virus (HBV) is well documented. API populations from China, Korea, Philippines, Southeast Asia, and the Pacific have a prevalence rate of 8% to 22% compared to that of less than 2% in North American populations. The most common mode of HBV transmission is perinatal (13% of all births); with 48% of all hepatitis B surface antigen (HBsAg)-positive women of API descent; about 8% result in hepatitis B-carrier babies. Over 11% of Southeast Asians in the United States are known to have a positive HBsAg. The transfer of the HBV from an HBsAg-positive carrier to the infant occurs. Carriers become infected during early childhood or during their teenage years. When this occurs, chronic hepatitis B, cirrhosis, and primary liver cancer can develop later in life. The prevention of perinatal transmission has been an important public health effort as evidenced by the CDC guidelines regarding early screening and testing of pregnant women, particularly those of Asian descent (CDC, 1988). Appropriate administration of the immunoprophylaxis should be provided the HBsAg-positive mother and infant.

Figures are limited on the vaccination coverage of infants born to HBsAg-positive API women. The use of multilingual and culturally appropriate materials to educate and train women and prevent this disease has been slow and efforts are regionalized. Vaccines are limited to pregnant women and outreach is hampered by insufficient state and county funds. Funding for vaccinations of older API children have not been available but are proposed in the Comprehensive Children's Immunization Initiative. Public health policy to provide alternative vaccine schedules for API infants in the Pacific is also needed. Given that the API female population is young and at greater risk, public health efforts to reduce the higher incidence rates in this population must be made.

Maternal and Child Health

Based on limited data, infant mortality rates for API women tend to be at or lower than rates of Caucasian women. It is believed that early prenatal care (in the first trimester of pregnancy) increases the chances of optimal outcomes. The prevention of problem pregnancies (such as complications with diabetes, fetal abnormalities) can be averted through early intervention. The current health care delivery system tends to overlook the need for culturally appropriate care and understanding. The API infant mortality rate in 1984 was 8.8/1000 live births compared to 8.6 for Caucasians.

Pregnancy outcomes are hampered when birth and death records are misclassified, particularly among API populations (Hahn et al, 1992; Lin-Fu, 1987). Hahn et al. noted the highest percentage of misclassified API infants were for Filipinos (79%), followed by Japanese (49%) and Chinese (33%). Misclassification for APIs occurred 43% of the time compared to African Americans at 4% and Caucasians at 1%. It is not surprising to find that the general data being reported reflects API infants not to be at risk.

Low birth weight is considered to account for two-thirds of infant deaths. Although this may be a result of lack of prenatal care, substance abuse, smoking, low socioeconomic status, or little education, it does not always consider cultural factors as well. Low birth weights reported in 1988 by the National Center for Health Statistics indicate subgroup differences compared to Caucasian births at 5.7% (Table 18-1). The fact that certain subethnic API populations, particularly Cambodian women, have "lighter" babies (Gann, Nghiem, & Warner, 1989) complicates the "average or appropriate" weight scales when defined by mainstream populations. Despite the reporting limitations, it is clear that infant mortality rates are highest among Native Hawaiians at 11.4/1000 live births compared to Caucasians at 8.4/1000 live births. Preterm birth was one-third greater for native born Filipinos (11.5%), Hawaiians (10.8%), and other Asians (9.8%) than Caucasians (8.0%). Similar rates were found among foreign born populations from the Philippines (10.8%), Hawaiians (11.8%), and other Asians (10.9%) (Singh & Yu, 1993). Singh and Yu's (1993) review of pregnancy outcomes among API women confirm that variation within API subgroups exist and that the API population as a whole reflects substantial heterogeneity. The higher maternal risk profile of the "other Asian" women indicate higher rates of perinatal, infant, neonatal, and postneonatal mortality rates.

The AAPCHO (1993) cited from a California study that late or no prenatal care ranged from 25% to 59% among new immigrant groups, whereas older immigrant groups tended to range from 3% to 5%. Table 18-2 includes specific figures by ethnic group for reported late or no prenatal care in the first trimester of mothers with live births.

Table 18-1. Group Differences in Rates of Low Birth Weight Infants

Subethnic Group	Percent
Filipinos	7.2
Hawaiian	7.0
Other API	6.4
Japanese	6.2
Chinese	4.6

Adapted from NCHS 1988

Table 18-2. Percentage of API Women Who Received Late or No Prenatal Care in the First Trimester

Subethnic Group	Percent
Chinese	3.6
Japanese	2.7
Filipino	4.7

adapted from NCHS 1992a

In another similar study of Southeast Asian women living in California (AAP-CHO, 1990), the following subgroups reported late or no prenatal care—Samoan (59%), Laotians (48%), Cambodian (47%), and Vietnamese (32%).

The obstetric utilization practices of the API women vary among cultures. For many Southeast Asian women, cultural practices of inhibition require the API woman not to expose her genitals because it is humiliating. Because of these types of cultural beliefs, some Southeast Asian women do not seek or underutilize prenatal care. Fullerton, Palinkas, and Cavero (1991) examined maternal risk factors among low-income Mexican American, Caucasian, and Southeast Asian women in an urban and rural community with nurse midwifery services. Southeast Asian women were older and had more children but had fewer prenatal visits and used less analgesia/anesthesia during delivery (Fullerton et al., 1991). A comparative study examining Asian and non-Asian women's reproductive health practices and their hospital case notes revealed underutilization of cervical smears, later prenatal care, lack of health care knowledge about procedures such as amniocentesis, breast self-examination, and poor communication skills as factors for poor pregnancy outcomes (Firdous & Bhopal, 1989). During menopause, it is noted that small-boned Asian women and heredity pose greater risk factors for developing osteoporosis (Papazian, 1991). However, only one study was found and data remain limited.

Thalassemia

Thalassemia (α, β, and hemoglobin E) affects primarily persons of Mediterranean, Asian, and African decent. Classified in the group of genetic blood disorders, thalassemia affects the production of a major globin chain of normal hemoglobin. Carriers can manifest symptoms ranging from nonsymptomatic to severe anemia. In the United States, little has been known about the prevalence of this disorder in APIs. It is because of this lack of available data that needed genetic screening of API women is not being conducted routinely. Prevalence rates in Asian countries range from 3% to 7% in China to as high as 44% among individuals from Thailand. In the United States, local or regional studies have indicated prevalence rates of α-thalassemia-1 to be 9% (South Cove Community Health Center, 1989) and 8% to 27% (AAPCHO, 1990) among Southeast Asian refugees. β-Thalassemia prevalence rates ranged similarly with 8% found among Vietnamese. Hemoglobin E studies in the United States are on Southeast Asians in California. Reported prevalence rates were 1% among Vietnamese, 28% among Laotians, and 36% among Cambodians (South Cove Community Health Center, 1989).

Asian women are affected by this disorder as carriers during pregnancy and subsequently if a negative pregnancy outcome occurs. Screening for thalassemia is an invasive process, and new immigrants and refugees culturally do not permit venipuncture for blood drawing. Screening should be incorporated into medical protocol when other medical testing and screens are being conducted and health education provided to API women. The national prevalence rates for thalassemia are higher than those for sickle cell disease. Given the high prevalence rates among APIs, a national program should be designed to address this genetic disorder, similar to the National Sickle Cell program. Although figures are nonexistent, some Asian subgroups are also at risk for lupus erythematosus.

Mental Health

Leading mental health disorders cited by community health centers and researchers (Chung & Kagawa-Singer, 1993; Luu, 1989; Mollica & Jalbert, 1989; Mollica & Lavelle, 1988) include high prevalence of anxiety, depression, posttraumatic stress, low self-esteem, hopelessness, and despair, particularly among Southeast Asian refugee women. Much of the published research reported the psychosocial and psychophysiologic adjustment of Southeast Asian women given the premigration violence experienced through torture, multiple rape, witnessing executions or deaths of family members, war, and active genocide. The rapes, as reported, were so brutal that it often led to deformation or mutilation of the genitals (Mollica & Jalberta, 1989).

Other medical disorders associated with sexual abuse included infertility, miscarriage, venereal disease, pregnancy, menstruation disorders, and persistence of severe chronic abdominal and pelvic pain. Many were kidnapped and sold into prostitution (Burton, 1983). The cultural mores of these women required them to remain silent because they believed they were to blame for "creating or causing" the trauma. Victims of rape for this API subgroup remained silent because virginity is a prized cultural value for single Asian women and fidelity for married Asian women. The inability to express their experience to overcome the shame, stigma, and feeling of isolation has led a number of Southeast Asian women to commit suicide. The abuse of Asian women in part was perpetuated by racial stereotypes of Asian women. Adjustments for many recent immigrant and refugee families in male-female or superordinate-subordinate roles have created family conflict. The extent of premigration trauma and camp experience is a strong predictor of psychological distress among Southeast Asian refugees (Bernier, 1992; Chung & Kagawa-Singer, 1993; Matsuoka, 1990).

Suicide rates among the Chinese American women over 45 years of age and for Japanese women aged 75 and over are higher than for Caucasian women of the same age groups. The etiology for these rates are unknown. *Health United States* (U.S. Public Health Service, 1993) reported API women 65 years and over having a suicide rate of 9.8% compared to 6.3% for all races during the 1988 to 1990 period. Use of mental health services is foreign to the API immigrant or refugee and generally deemed a matter to be handled by the family. Kitano & Chi (1985) attribute strong community norms and family support as a means to confine episodes of mental illness until conditions become intolerable. Low utilization rates by APIs of alcohol, drug, and mental health services may be a result of culturally inappropriate care (Hatanaka, Watanabe, & Ono, 1975; Hu et al., 1991; True, 1975). Subethnic differences in use are noted between Japanese Americans, Southeast Asians, and Filipinos. Studies are limited and require methodologic rigor and representative sampling.

National efforts to train API mental health providers must be increased as well as programs designed to address the linguistic and cultural needs of the API women. Assessment tools must consider the varying cultural norms, values, and beliefs. Because many APIs are willing to seek health care, the integration of mental health services in the health care delivery system is needed.

Tuberculosis

Until the 1980s, tuberculosis (TB) rates were on a steady decline. TB is a pulmonary and systemic disease that primarily enters through the lung. The TB bacillus is spread by airborne transmission. The higher rates of TB in this country have been of such concern that the disease is one of the objectives identified in the *Healthy People 2000 Objectives* for Asian and Pacific Islanders (U.S. Public Health Service, 1990). The baseline incidence rate among APIs in 1989 was 17.6% or five times that of the overall United States population. This represents a 10.2% increase since 1985 (CDC, 1989). The large influx of Southeast Asian refugees to the United States during the 1980s contributed to the increased prevalence rate of TB; over 11% of the new cases reported or 22,201 new cases in 1985 were among APIs. The difference in age groups affected is notable in that API victims tend to be 25 to 44 years of age and the Caucasian population with TB tends to be the elderly.

In 1989, 9.3% of the CDC reported cases were in children under 15 years of age. The current epidemic of acquired immunodeficiency syndrome (AIDS) has contributed to a more recent increase in TB cases, including drug-resistant TB (isoniazid resistant). The Southeast Asian refugees have a rate of 250/100,000 as compared to the 9/100,000 found in the total United States population. An estimated 25% of Southeast Asian immigrants are isoniazid resistant. The CDC estimates that 39% of API cases were preventable for those under 35 years of age. Of all reported cases in 1989, 96% are foreign born. Specific figures by gender are not provided (CDC, 1990a).

Substance Abuse

Limited incidence and prevalence rates on the alcohol and drug behavior of APIs are available. The nonexistence of national probability samples, culturally competent treatment services, and cultural attitudes hamper the understanding of the APIs' alcohol and other drug behavior. In a review of national data bases none provide API-specific treatment data or incidence and prevalence rates. Sue (1987) reviewed the etiology of alcohol use and abuse for APIs and found the data to be limited in scope, nonrepresentative, and contradictory. On of the few studies that report alcohol use and abuse among Asian Americans notes the high abstinence rates for some subgroups geographically (National Institute on Alcohol Abuse and

Alcoholism, 1991). Studies by other researchers have reported findings that are limited to specific geographic areas, age, drug or alcohol behavior, or subethnic samples among API populations (Zane & Kim, 1994). Few reported studies have distinguished specific gender differences. Studies have been designed to examine the hypothesis that low consumption rates are based on genetics and physiology (also known as "Oriental flushing") or cultural values. Unfortunately, the studies reflect the behavior of small numbers, specific subethnic groups (Chinese, Japanese, or Korean), or foreign Asian populations (Taiwan). Although the physiologic reaction to alcohol may account for low use rates, cultural values may play a more significant role in the underreporting of alcohol use. Cultural norms to protect the family result in the lower treatment rates. Admissions to treatment facilities are generally in the late stage of alcoholism and to private facilities (Kitano & Chi, 1985). In terms of drug use, specific data on API women are limited to youth or geographic samples. More use of Valium, codeine, and Quaalude was found in a study conducted by Wong (1985) on Asian youth in San Francisco.

Cultural norms and values also encourage moderate drinking and discourage assertive, independent drunken behavior. The Western value structure encourages individualism, whereas the Eastern culture emphasizes consideration for others, contribution to society, and less emphasis on self. Alcohol use is known to manifest aggressive behavior. As for drug prevalence rates, the data are as limited. The emergence of API treatment programs over the last 10 years is reflected by the growth in the membership of the National Asian Pacific American Families Against Substance Abuse.

The newer immigrant and refugee populations are just beginning to be examined. Anecdotal information reported by the health care providers in API health centers indicate increased amounts of alcohol being consumed by male API refugees. After the political unrest in many of the API countries, API men have come to this country believing in the American dream for unlimited opportunities and find themselves either unemployed or in low-paying service jobs. Once again, because the API family is patriarchal, dependence on the man to provide for the family poses increased pressure. Depression, adjustment problems, and poor socioeconomic status increase the pressure to self-medicate the pain. Alcohol abuse has contributed to the increased domestic violence against API women. The acceptance of the Southeast Asian women for being beaten by a husband is culturally tied.

For APIs, the increase in substance use can be related to a variety of factors including self-identity, acculturation, employment stresses, or difficulties in the home environment. Increased use by Pacific Islanders can be tied to the rapid social change and resultant effects of family disintegration and chaos. Anecdotal and clinical evidence suggests that Pacific Islanders are at greater risk of alcohol-related safety and health problems (eg, violence, injury from drunk driving, fetal alcohol syndrome) and hidden use among women, middle-aged, and elderly groups. Women are able to hide their alcohol and other drug problems if they work exclusively at home or if no one expects them to have a problem. API researchers such as Kitano and Chi (1985), Sue (1987), and Akutsu, Sue, Zane and Nakamura (1989) point out the absence of reliable and culturally appropriate research on APIs and encourage the development of large-scale probability samples, particularly with subethnic distinctions.

Cardiovascular Disease

The reduction of heart disease deaths to no more than 100/100,000 is among the health objectives established in *Healthy People 2000* (U.S. Public Health Service, 1990). From 1985 to 1990, heart disease, malignant neoplasms, and cerebrovasular diseases continued to be among the top three ranked causes of death for API women. The reported age-adjusted death rate for API women 45 years and over between 1988 and 1990 was 209/100,000 (U.S. Public Health Service, 1993). For all age categories, API women have lower death rates when compared to women of all races. The heart disease mortality rate among Native Hawaiian women is 244/100,000 (Mokuau et al., 1992). It is reported that hypertension is a major risk factor for stroke, coronary heart disease, and cerebrovasular disease, yet health education and targeted API programming are limited. Hypertension is defined as an average systolic blood pressure greater than 140 mm Hg or an average diastolic blood pressure greater than 90 mm Hg. For a number of subethnic API populations, hypertension incidence rates are high. For instance, Filipino women over 50 years of age who live in California have a higher incidence rate (65%) than African Americans (63%) (CDC, 1991). In a population-based study conducted on Native Hawaiians, 24% of the Native Hawaiian female population had hypertension. Native Hawaiians (pure blood) and Japanese Americans have the highest incidence rates of heart disease (Papa Ola Lokahi, 1992). Filipino, Pacific Islanders, Japanese, and Chinese have higher death rates from cerebrovascular disease than other API groups (Curb et al., 1991). Age-adjusted death rates for API women aged 45 years and over that were attributed to cerebrovascular diseases were 81/100,000 compared to 94/100,000 for all races from 1988 to 1990 (U.S. Public Health Service, 1993).

Diabetes

Diabetes mellitus is caused by chronic abnormal glucose metabolism that affects the circulatory system, heart, and kidney. In 1989, SEER (Surveillance, Epidemiology, and End Results) incidence rates for diabetes were two to three times higher for Filipinos, Japanese, Koreans, and Chinese living in Hawaii than for Caucasian non-minorities. American-born Japanese, Chinese, and Filipinos have higher death rates from diabetes than their counterparts. Diabetes among elderly Native Hawaiians, Filipinos, Chinese, and Koreans is sometimes double and triple the rate for Caucasians. Japanese Americans have more than twice the incidence of diabetes than those living in Japan. Subethnic variation within the API population is noted by King and Rewers (1993) in findings from a project that was to assemble standardized estimates of abnormal glucose tolerance in adults in diverse communities. The diabetes mortality rate for Native Hawaiian women is close to 30/100,000, well over the rate of 9.6/100,000 for all women.

Obesity

Pacific Island women (Native Hawaiian and Samoan) are reported to be the most obese in the world and second to Pima Indians in terms of low longevity. High-fat diets and sedentary lifestyles are contributors to the high rates. Obesity is generally associated with hypertension, cardiovascular disease, diabetes, and potentially cancer. Traditional diets of high fiber, complex carbohydrates, and ratio of polysaturated/saturated fatty acids are prevalent in API populations. However, the abundance of fast foods and high-fat meals in the United States has carried over into the API lifestyle. Eating disorder studies are limited and contradictory (Lucero et al., 1992).

HIV/AIDS

For individuals reported with human immunodeficiency virus (HIV) and AIDS from the API community, 2273 adult and pediatric cases were reported to CDC in September 1993. API women had the highest percentage (14.5%) of increase in newly diagnosed AIDS cases compared to African Americans (10.7%), as reported during this period by CDC and noted in the first National Congress on the State of HIV/AIDS in Racial and Ethnic Communities held in September 1994. The average rate of increase among women of color was 10.7% compared to 10.1% for Caucasian women. In 1990, the AAHPF noted that the primary routes of transmission within the API female population were heterosexual (35%), blood transfusion (31%), intravenous (16%), and other (17%). Of the 0.5% reported API female cases, 2.6% were in women aged 15 to 44 (CDC, 1990a). Among the API pediatric cases, 47% involved prenatal transmission from an HIV-infected mother. The largest Asian population affected by AIDS is Filipinos, followed by Japanese, Chinese, and Vietnamese.

Fear, denial, and lack of education are considered the primary reasons for the increase. API women believe that HIV/AIDS is contracted by Caucasians, men, or homosexuals or that it can be contracted by casual contact (eg, toilet seats). Recommendations from the National Congress on the State of HIV/AIDS in Racial and Ethnic Communities (1994) provided a forum for minority populations to share cultural beliefs and values as well as to identify the leading health policy recommendations to prevent HIV/AIDS in the API community. More funding for multilingual prevention and health education materials was identified as a top priority. Additionally, the members of the Asian Pacific Institute of the Congress identified the lack of trained API professionals to provide care to the API women and lack of data as major obstacles to preventing the deadly disease.

Health Beliefs, Values, and Practices

A number of cultural strengths have been cited for various subgroups of API women throughout this chapter. The inner strength of API women, especially the immigrants and refugees (Japanese Americans and Indochinese women) who experienced adverse treatment or left their native homes for political reasons, are embodied with mixed cultural values and beliefs and challenged by Western practices. Although each subethnic population has its own cultural norms, values, and beliefs, many APIs still follow the philosophy of yin–yang that prescribes the individual's lifestyle practices to achieve balance and harmony. The importance of food in the Asian culture is often closely linked to Asian cultural values and beliefs. If one experiences an illness, it is often thought to be a result of imbalance in "hot" and "cold" and that the body must restore balance through consumption of appropriate foods, alternative medicine, and medicines.

In addition to the maintenance of balance and harmony, one believes in the predestined events as well as in spiritual occurrences. Among some API cultural groups, a negative health outcome (eg, birth defect) is considered retribution for having sinned themselves or for the sins of a parent or relative of another generation. A fatalistic approach to disease is not uncommon to API women. For some API populations, "illness" is not a part of the vocabulary. In fact, formal health care for the elderly is unfamiliar and self-treatment or family treatment is preferred. The religious beliefs of the API women embody generations of Buddist, Hindu, Christian, and East Asian philosophies. Placing a higher value on helping others, including contribution to society, is a common belief.

Most API women follow a traditional hierarchy of gender (patriarchal) and age. Men are considered the dominant figures in terms of discipline and earnings within the API family. The API women are traditionally responsible for the welfare of the children and home. This superordinate-subordinate role prescribes the specific role of family members. Family needs and contribution to society above one's self-promotion are cultural values. For APIs who have resided in this country for many generations, the women have faced conflict between the Eastern and Western concepts (eg, feminist) that tend to equalize roles and encourage more assertive behavior for women and children.

Having respect for the hierarchy is an important element of the API culture. Respect for authority, elders, teachers, and leaders is often practiced. Respect for authority transcends into the health care arena where the health care provider is viewed as an authority figure. Questioning the word of this authority figure would be deemed disrespectful. For traditional non–English-speaking or limited English-speaking API women, receipt of health care is through an interpreter, typically by a family member. For more recent immigrant and refugee families, the complex interpreting of medical terminology may rely on a youngster. Cultural beliefs not to expose portions of the body between the waist and knees, especially the genital area, create conflicts for the API women and the interpreter. Discussion on positive outcomes and matters that can be controlled is translated to the API women. Unfavorable news (eg, breast cancer) is not always relayed to the patient especially when remedies to the problem may not be available.

Implications for Practice, Research, and Policy

The previous sections attempted to provide an overview on the health status of API women. The limitations of this review only heighten the importance for more research to be conducted on APIs and increased access to care for this population. Although a number of these articles provide insight to the health status of API women, the body of work does not provide a comprehensive picture. Most studies were methodologically flawed and limited to a specific disease or a specific API subgroup. Comparison groups tended to be limited and nonexistent; study samples were small (eg, the Health and Nutrition Examination Survey contains only 250 APIs out of 4000 participants) and lacked gender breakdown. Articles were based on case studies or personal perceptions and accounts of their experiences. No study was national in scope or representative. Data concerns were identified in the *Healthy People 2000 Cross-cutting Progress Review on Asian and Pacific Islander Work Group Report* (USPHS, 1994).

The paucity of reliable national data on the subethnic differences within the API populations is of serious concern and requires immediate attention. Concern has been raised by the three national API public health advocacy organizations since 1990. When national data samples are used and serve as the basis for determining and establishing national funding policies, the collapsing or aggregation of API data results in the masking of high need, including the urgent health education, prevention, and service needs of subethnic API groups. Serious implications arise given that a number of diseases can be controlled and prevented (eg, TB, hepatitis B, thalassemia, breast cancer, AIDS) when data are available to demonstrate need. Through appropriate data, the health status of the API population can be improved and economic cost to society reduced.

Programming that considers the socioeconomic, linguistic, and cultural values, beliefs, and practices of the API women would enhance the well-being of the API woman and overall health care delivery system. Five primary barriers preventing APIs easy access to health care delivery systems are: perceptive, cultural, linguistic, structural, and financial. The "model minority" stereotype portrays APIs as healthy. There is a bimodal distribution between those that fit this stereotype and those APIs suffering from poverty, unemployment or underemployment, substandard or inadequate housing, inadequate health services, and insufficient social services. The current emphasis on delivery of health care via Western medicine ignores the recent influx of APIs and their reliance on traditional Oriental health practices. APIs tend to view health as a whole body, spiritual, and mind relationship with consequences occurring when these are out of balance. Their health problems are influenced by dietary habits, unhealthy risk behaviors, and psychological trauma from their immigration experience. Language is also a major barrier. Development of culturally appropriate research, services, education, and prevention programs are warranted as is an increase of API health providers for each subethnic population.

References

Akutsu, P., Sue, S., Zane, N., & Nakamura, C. (1989). Ethnic differences in alcohol consumption among Asians and Caucasians in the United States: An investigation of cultural and physiological factors. *Journal of Studies on Alcohol, 50* (3), 261-267.

Asian/Pacific AIDS Coalition. (1994). *U.S. national Asian and Pacific Islander HIV/AIDS agenda.* (Conference Paper from National Congress on the State of HIV/AIDS in Racial and Ethnic Communitees. September 15–18, Washington, DC.)

Association of Asian Pacific Community Health Organizations. (1993). *Health problems of Asians and Pacific Islanders, fact sheets* [Unpublished data]. Oakland, CA: Author.

Bernier, D. (1992). The Indochinese refugee: A perspective from various stress theories. *Journal of Multicultural Social Work, 2* (1), 15-30.

Burton, E. (1983). Surviving the flight of horror: The story of refugee women. *Indochinese Issues, 34,* 1-7.

Centers for Disease Control. (1988). Recommendations of the Immunization Practice Advisory Committee. Prevention of perinatal transmission of hepatitis B virus: Prenatal screening of all pregnant women for hepatitis B surface antigen. *Morbidity and Mortality Weekly Report, 37,* 341–346.

Centers for Disease Control. (1990a). *HIV/AIDS Surveillance Report.* Atlanta, GA: Author.

Centers for Disease Control. (1990b). *National health interview survey, 1990.* Hyattsville, MD: National Center for Health Statistics.

Chen, M. (1993). Status report on the health status of Asian Americans and Pacific Islanders: Comparison with *Healthy People 2000* objectives. *Asian American and Pacific Islander Journal of Health, 1*(1), 37-55.

Chi, I., Lubben, J., & Kitano, H. (1989). Differences in drinking behavior among three Asian American groups. *Journal of Studies on Alcohol, 50* (1), 15-23.

Chung, R. C., & Kagawa-Singer, M. (1993). Predictors of psychological distress among Southeast Asian refugees. *Social Science and Medicine, 36* (5), 631-639.

Curb, J. D., Aluli, N. E., et al. (1991). Cardiovascular risk factor levels in ethnic Hawaiians. *American Journal of Public Health, 81*(2), 164-167.

Firdous, R., & Bhopal, R. (1989). Reproductive health of Asian women: A comparative study with hospital and community perspectives. *Public Health, 103* (4), 307-315.

Fuentes, J. (1991). *Region IX draft response to request.*

Fullerton, J. T., Palinkas, L., & Cavero, C. (1991). Nurse-midwifery services in one multiethnic, underserved community. *Journal of Health Care for Poor and Underserved, 2* (2), 293-306.

Gann, P., Nghiem, L., & Warner, S. (1989). Pregnancy characteristics and outcomes of Cambodian refugees. *American Journal of Public Health, 79* (9), 1251-1257.

Hahn, R. A., Mulinare, J., & Teutsch, S. M. (1992). Inconsistencies in coding on racial and ethnic groups. *Journal of the American Medical Association, 267,* 259-263.

Hatanaka, H., Watanabe, B., & Ono, S. (1975). The utilization of mental health services in the LA area. In W. Ishikawa & N. Archer (Eds.), *Service delivery in Pan Asian communities* (pp. 33-39). San Diego: Pan Asian Coalition.

Higuchi, C. M., Serxner, S. A., et al. (1993). Histopathological predictors of breast cancer death among Japanese in Hawaii. *Cancer Epidemiological Biomarkers, 2* (3), 201-205.

Hu, T. W., Snowden, L., et al. (1991). Ethnic populations in public mental health: Services choice and level of use. *American Journal of Public Health, 81*(11), 1429-1434.

Hubler, S. (1992, August 17). '80s failed to end economic disparity, census shows. *Los Angeles Times,* Part A, p.1.

Hu-DeHart, E. (1993). From yellow peril to model minority: The Columbus legacy and Asians in America. In *The New World.* Washington, DC: Smithsonian.

Ichioka, Y. (1979). Amerika Nadeshiko: Japanese immigrant women in the United States, 1900–1924. *Pacific Historical Review, 48,* 339-357.

King, H., & Rewers, M. (1993, January). Global estimates for prevalence of diabetes mellitus and impaired glucose tolerance in adults. In WHO Ad Hoc Diabetes Reporting Group, *Diabetes Care,* 157-177.

Kitano, H., & Chi, I. (1985). Asian Americans and alcohol: The Chinese, Japanese, Koreans and Filipinos in Los Angeles. In *Alcohol use among U.S. ethnic minorities* (NIAAA Research Monograph 18, DHHS Publication No. ADM 89-1435, pp. 373-382). Washington, DC: U.S. Department of Health and Human Services.

Koo, L. C., & Ho, J. E. (1990). Worldwide epidemiological patterns of lung cancer in nonsmokers. *International Journal of Epidemiology, 19* (Suppl. 1), S14-23.

Kroll, S., & Bradigan, T. (1993). Medline search strategies for literature on Asian Americans/Pacific Islanders. *Asian American and Pacific Islander Journal of Health, 1*(1), 56-62.

Leigh, W. (1994). *The health status of women of color.* Washington DC: Women's Research and Education Institute.

Lin, S. (1990). Health status of the Asian and Pacific Islander Americans. Presented Asian American Health Policy Forum Conference, San Francisco.

Lin-Fu, J. (1987, March). Meeting the needs of Southeast Asian refugees in maternal and child health and primary care programs. *MCH Technical Information Series,* 2-7.

Lin-Fu, J. (1993). Asian and Pacific Islander Americans: An overview of demographic characteristics and health care issues. *Asian American and Pacific Islander Journal of Health, 1*(1), 20-36.

Lucero, K., Kicks, R. A., et al. (1992). Frequency of eating problems among Asian and Caucasian women. *Psychology Reports, 71*(1), 255-258.

Luu, V. (1989). The hardships of escape for Vietnamese women. In Asian Women United California (Eds.), *Making waves: An anthology of writing by and about Asian American women* (pp. 60-72). Boston: Beacon Press.

Matsuoka, J. (1990). Differential acculturation among Vietnamese refugees. *Social Work, 35* (4), 341-345.

Mokuau, N., et al. (1992, May). Heart disease among native Hawaiian women: Impact of risk factors and recommendations for change. Presented at the 4th National Forum on Cardiovascular Health, Pulmonary Disorders and Blood Resources, National Heart Lung and Blood Institute. Bethesda, MD: Author.

Mollica, R. F., & Jalbert, R. R. (1989). *Community of confinement: The mental health crisis on site two: Displaced persons' camps on the Thai-Kampuchean border.* Boston Committee on World Federation for Mental Health.

Mollica, R. F., & Lavelle, J. (1988). Southeast Asian refugees. In Comas-Diaz & Griffith (Eds.), *Clinical guidelines in cross-cultural mental health* (pp. 262-303). New York: Wiley.

National Center for Health Statistics. (1989). *SEER (Surveillance, Epidemiology, and End Results) Data.* Hyattsville, MD: Author.

National Institute on Alcohol Abuse and Alcoholism and National Institute on Alcoholism in Japan. (1991). *Alcoholism consumption patterns and related problems in the United States and Japan: Summary report of a joint United States-Japan alcohol epidemiologic project.* Washington, D.C: U.S. Government Printing Office.

National Institutes of Health, Office of the Secretary. (1993). *Secretary's conference to establish a national action plan on breast cancer.* Proceedings, December 14-15, 1993. Bethesda: MD: Author.

Office of Research on Women's Health. (1992). *Report on the National Institutes of Health: Opportunities for research on women's health.* (NIH Publication No. 92-3457). Bethesda, MD: Author.

Ohata, C., & API American Advisory Committee. (1993). Employment of Asians and Pacific Islanders in the National Institutes of Health. Division of Equal Opportunity Office of the Director. Unpublished data.

Papazian, R. (1991). Osteoporosis treatment advances. *Current issues in women's health*, Food and Drug Administration Consumer Special Report. Washington, DC: Food and Drug Administration.

Papa Ola Lokahi. (1992). *Native Hawaiian health data book 1992.* Honolulu:.

Pham, C., & McPhee, S. (1992). Knowledge, attitudes, and practices of breast and cervical cancer screening among Vietnamese women, *Journal of Cancer Education*, 7(4):305.

Ponce, N. (1990). Asian and Pacific Islander health data: Quality issues and policy recommendations. Unpublished material in AAHF *Policy Papers.* San Francisco: AAHF.

Singh, G., & Yu, S. (1993). Pregnancy outcomes among Asian Americans. *Asian American and Pacific Islander Journal of Health, 1*(1), 63-79.

South Cove Community Health Center (1989). Unpublished figures.

Sue, D. (1987). Use and abuse of alcohol by Asian Americans. *Journal of Psychoactive Drugs, 19* (1), 57-66.

True, R. (1975). Mental health services and a Chinese American community. In W. Ishikawa & N. Archer (Eds.), *Service delivery in Pan Asian communities* (pp. 15-22). San Diego, CA: Pan Asian Coalition.

U.S. Commission on Civil Rights. (1992). *Civil rights issues facing Asian Americans in the 1990s* (pp. 332-279). Washington DC: U.S. Government Printing Office.

U.S. Bureau of the Census. (1990). *1990 Census Profile* (No. 7). Washington, DC: U.S. Government Printing Office.

U.S. Bureau of the Census. (1992). The Asian and Pacific Islander Population in the United States. *Current population reports, population characteristics.* Washington, DC: U.S. Government Printing Office.

U.S. Bureau of the Census. (1993a). *We the American...Asians*. Washington DC: U.S. Government Printing Office.

U.S. Bureau of the Census. (1993b). *We the American...Pacific Islanders*. Washington DC: U.S. Government Printing Office.

U.S. Bureau of the Census. (1993c). *We the Asian and Pacific Islander Americans*. Washington DC: US Government Printing Office.

U.S. General Accounting Office. (1990). *Asian Americans, a status report*. Washington, DC: Author.

U.S. Public Health Service. (1990). *Healthy people 2000: National health promotion and disease prevention objectives*. Washington, DC: U.S. Government Printing Office.

U.S. Public Health Service. (1993). *Health United States 1992 and Healthy People 2000 review*. (DHHS Publication No. 93-1232). Hyattsville, MD: Author.

U.S. Public Health Service. (1994). *Progress Report for Asian and Pacific Islander Americans*. Published internally.

Whittemore, A. S. (1989). Colorectal cancer incidence among the Chinese in North America and the People's Republic of China: Variation with sex, age and anatomical site. *International Journal of Epidemiology, 18* (3), 563-568.

Wong, H. Z. (1985). Substance use and Chinese American youths: Preliminary findings on an interview survey of 123 youths and implications for services and programs. Unpublished manuscript. San Francisco, CA: The Richmond Area Multi-Services, Inc..

Wong, P., & Nagasawa, R. (1991). Asian American scientists and engineers: Is there a glass ceiling for career advancement? *Chinese American Forum, 6* (3), 3-6.

Zane, M., & Kim, J. (1994). Substance use and abuse among Asian Americans. In N. Zane, D. Takeuchi, & K. Young (Eds.), *Confronting critical health issues of Asian and Pacific Islander Americans* (pp. 316-343). Thousand Oaks, CA: Sage.

Ziegler, R. G., Hoover, R. N., et al. (1993). Migration patterns and breast cancer risk in Asian-American women. *Journal of National Cancer Institute, 85* (22), 1819-1827.

Bibliography

Butynski, W., & Canova, D. M. (1988). Alcohol problem resources and services in state supported programs, FY87. *Public Health Reports, 103*(6), 611-620.

Hsu, F. L. K. (1970). *Americans and Chinese*. New York: Doubleday.

National Cancer Institute. (1992). *Interim Report: Research focusing on women* (p. 74). Bethesda, MD: Division of Cancer Prevention and Control.

CHAPTER 19

Latino/Hispanic Women

Aida L. Giachello

Introduction

The terms "Latino" and "Hispanic" refer to persons who consider themselves Mexicans, Mexican Americans, Puerto Ricans, and Cubans, or those who are born or descended from those born in Central or South America, Spain, or selected locations in the Caribbean. The terms "Latino" and "Hispanic" encompass people who come from more than 20 countries (Figure 19-1). There is tremendous heterogeneity among Latinos despite the fact that they share a common language and selected aspects of the Spanish culture. For example, some Latinos are U.S. citizens, others are not; some are newly arrived, yet others have been in the United States for many years or are native to the Southwest. Some speak only Spanish, some are bilingual in English and Spanish, and others speak only English. Diversity is evident in levels of acculturation and assimilation, socioeconomic status, living conditions, and migration status. This diversity among different subgroups of Latinos is also reflected in health beliefs, attitudes and knowledge, health status, and patterns of health services utilization. The terms Latino and Hispanic are used in this chapter interchangeably, referring to the same group.

Latinos are one of the fastest growing population groups in the United States. In March 1993, there were 22.8 million Latinos in the United States, representing 8.9% of the total U.S. population (U.S. Bureau of the Census, 1994). This does not include the 3.5 million persons in Puerto Rico or the number of undocumented workers (estimated at 3–6 million). The largest groups in the U.S. are listed in Table 19-1.

In 1990, Latino women comprised 49.2% of the total Latino population in the United States (National Council of La Raza [NCLR], 1993). Mexican American women are the largest subgroup, representing 61% of the Latino female population, followed far behind by women of Central or South American origin (14%), Puerto Ricans (12%), women of other Hispanic nationalities (8%), and Cubans (5%).

Despite the rapid population growth, little is known about the health needs, health status, and health services use of Latino women. The limited information available reveals a large disparity in their socioeconomic and health characteristics compared to Latino men or to non-Latino women in the United States. Giachello (1995b) and others (Bracho de Carpio, Carpio-Cedraro, & Anderson, 1993) have argued that urban poverty and the limited culturally appropriate health services available to Latino women are the strongest factors associated with Latino

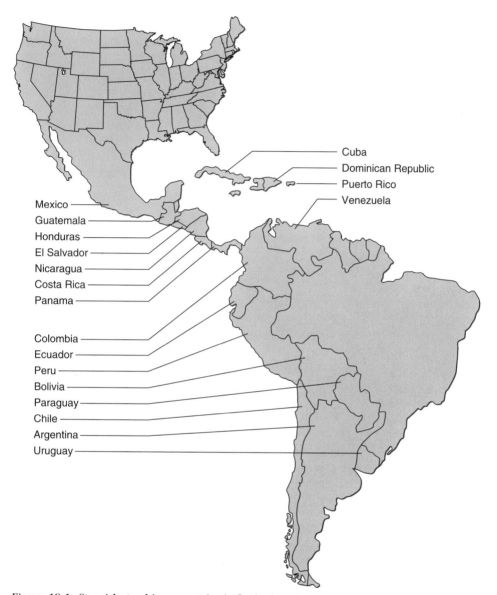

Figure 19-1. Spanish-speaking countries in Latin America.

women's poor health status. Latino women experience a series of racial and social inequalities. Many poor Latino women are undereducated, experience employment and housing discrimination, and are geographically concentrated in
inner city areas.

Latino women experience a series of financial, cultural, and institutional barriers to obtaining health services and unequal treatment once they enter the medical
care system (Giachello, 1994a). Giachello (1985, 1994a, 1995b) has argued that so-

Table 19-1. Percentage of Latinos in the United States by Country of Origin

Nationality	Percent
Mexican/Mexican American	64.3
Puerto Rican	10.6
Cubans	4.7
Central and South American origin	13.4
Other Hispanic/Latino nationalities	7.0

Source: U.S. Bureau of the Census. (1994). The Hispanic population in the United States, March 1993. *Current population report* series (P20–475). Washington, DC: U.S. Government Printing Office.

cioeconomic factors (eg, health insurance) appear to be the strongest determinants of gaining entry into the formal medical care system. Once Latino women enter the medical care system, they find that health services are often middle-class oriented and may be designed around policies and practices that reflect underlying biases and attitudes toward women in general and women of color in particular. The health care system in the United States has limited flexibility to meet the needs of populations who may have different illnesses, cultural practices, or languages. Even though acculturation among Latino women does occur, in the form of adopting the predominant behavior patterns and language, structural assimilation (gaining access to American institutions, including the medical care system for prevention, screening, and treatment) continues to be difficult (Giachello 1988, 1994a, 1995a). These circumstances lead to differential health and medical treatment for Latino women, who therefore do not benefit to the greatest possible extent from state-of-the art preventive and treatment services.

This chapter first provides an overview of the sociodemographic and economic characteristics of Latino women. It then discusses Latino women's health within the context of women's general health and social needs. Furthermore, the chapter summarizes selected data on morbidity, mortality, and issues of access to health care as they affect Latino women, as well as issues of acculturation and health. The chapter concludes with findings and recommendations for programs, policy, and future research. Because of the great diversity of Latino women, caution is needed because most of the limited research data available refer to Mexican or Mexican American women. Limited information is available on Latino women of different national origins.

Changing Demographics and Economic Conditions of Latino Women

The Latino female population as a whole is expected to increase by one fourth, from 8.6% of the total female population in the United States in 1990 to 10.7% in 2010 (NCLR, 1993). Hispanics are one of the youngest population groups in the

United States with a median age of 26.7 in 1993 compared to 34.4 for non-Latinos (U.S. Bureau of the Census, 1994, p. 2). The median age among the Hispanic subgroups, regardless of gender, varies substantially. In 1993, the Cuban population had the highest median age (43.6 years), followed far behind by those from Central and South America (28.6 years). Mexican Americans and Puerto Ricans had the lowest median ages (24.6 and 26.9 years, respectively) (U.S. Bureau of the Census, 1994).

In 1993, 38% of the Latino female population was under the age of 20. Age structure is an important factor in the study of Latino women's health because it determines the medical services most in need and in demand (ie, family planning, prenatal care, and pediatric services.)

Although Latinos are usually classified as a young population, since 1970 the Latino elderly population (aged 65 and older) has grown 61%, a rate well above the rate of the total elderly population growth in the United States. According to projections by the Bureau of the Census, the increase in the total number of Latino elderly will account for 25% of the total Latino population growth over the next 20 years (U.S. Bureau of the Census, 1994).

Latino women suffer from a series of social and economic disadvantages reflected in low education levels, low income, high unemployment, and a high level of poverty. Latinos have the lowest level of education of any racial or ethnic group. Close to half the Latino population 25 years and older (53%) had 4 years or more of education in 1993. This percentage is even lower for the Mexican population (46%) (U.S. Bureau of the Census, 1994). A recent report on Latino women prepared by the National Council of La Raza (NCLR) indicates that only 7 in 10 Hispanic women aged 16 to 19 were in school compared with 8 in 10 Caucasians and 3 in 4 African Americans (NCLR, 1994, p. 1). Hispanic women continue to be less likely to have a high school diploma than Caucasian women and are least likely to complete college. Only 1 in 12 Hispanic women in 1990 completed college compared to one-fifth of Caucasian and one-eighth of African American women. This is critical because education not only enables Latino women to better meet their socioeconomic needs and the needs of those who depend on them, but also better educated women are more likely to have better health status, more control of their reproductive health, and better living conditions and life opportunities (NCLR, 1994, p. 2).

In part because of their low levels of education Hispanic women have a lower average income than either Caucasian or African American women (NCLR, 1994, p. 6). Giachello (1995b, pp. 125-127) argues that high poverty rates for Latino women are linked to several factors (Display 19-1). These factors lead them to seek public assistance from the government. Those who are recipients of Aid to Families with Dependent Children find it difficult to become financially independent because they confront a series of barriers to self-sufficiency. Some of these barriers according to NCLR (1993) are:

- family responsibilities
- lack of basic skills and relevant job training
- cost and logistics of transportation
- housing costs
- lack of child care and health insurance

DISPLAY 19-1
Factors Affecting Poverty Rates Among Latino Women

- Latino women low median earnings. Latino women's earnings were much lower ($10,813) than those of Latino men ($14,706) and non-Latino women ($14,046) in 1992. This may be related to their disproportionate representation in low-paying occupations (U.S. Bureau of the Census, 1994; Giachello, 1995a, p. 124). A shift in job creation from manufacturing to the service sector has resulted in a decrease in jobs with higher pay for Latino women (NCLR, 1994).

- High poverty rate among Latino married-couple families (26% versus 11.7% for total U.S. population). Among Latino two-parent families the incidence of poverty in 1993 was 26.4% for those of Mexican origin, 32.5% for Puerto Ricans, 15.4% for Cubans, and 27.0% for those of Central and South American origin (NCLR, 1994).

- Latino women low participation in the labor force. In 1993, the labor force participation of Latino women was lower overall compared to non-Latino women (51.9% as opposed to 57.6%). The percentage of Latino women in the labor force varies by national origin, the highest being for women of Central or South American origin, and the lowest prevailing among Puerto Rican women (57.2% and 46.2%, respectively) (U.S. Bureau of the Census, 1994).

- High prevalence of families headed by a woman. These families are at greater risk of poverty. The proportion of Latino families maintained by a woman with no husband present has increased from 15% in 1970 to 22% in 1990 (NCLR, 1993). In 1992, the percentage of Latino families below the poverty level headed by a woman was 48.8%. This percentage is nearly twice as high as for all Latino families below the poverty level (26.2%) and non-Latino families headed by a woman (33.3%). The percentage of families living below the poverty line with female-headed households in 1992 varies from 46% for Mexican families to 60.3% for Puerto Ricans. The percentage of poverty among this type of family for persons of Central and South American origin was 51.3%. The NCLR report (1994) states that a major reason for the poverty of female-headed families is the failure of noncustodial fathers to fulfill their economic responsibilities. In 1989, only about one-half of all single mothers obtained child support. Latino women were much less likely to receive child support, possibly because of the lower income of Latino fathers (NCLR, 1993, 1994).

- High unemployment. In 1993, the unemployment rate for Latino women was 11%. This was twice as high as for non-Latino women (5.4%). The female rate of unemployment varies by national origin, with women of Central or South American origin experiencing the highest levels of unemployment (14.4%) and Cuban women the lowest (7.3%) (NCLR, 1993, 1994).

- Increases in adolescent pregnancy and parenthood. In 1993, 17.4% of all live births to Latino women were to adolescents (under 20 years of age), compared to 9.5% for Caucasian women and 22.9% for African Americans (Ventura, 1995). Among all Latino women giving birth in 1993, Puerto Rican women had the highest percentage of births to adolescents (22.3%). The percentages for other Latino teen women were: 18.2% for Mexican Americans, 6.8% for Cubans, and 9.9% for mothers of Central or South American origins (Ventura, 1995, p. 45). Increasingly, teenage mothers do not marry the father, choosing instead to raise their children on their own, sometimes with the assistance of parents, and often with some financial support from the government. Therefore, single teenage parents and their children are most likely to live in poverty (Giachello, 1994b).

In summary, low earnings, low education, high unemployment, low participation in the labor force, family composition, and single parenting are associated with poverty among Latino women. Poor Latino women experience inadequate housing, poor nutrition, poor sanitation, and high rates of physical, emotional, and sexual abuse (Giachello, 1995b). They tend to live in ghetto areas where there is a sense of despair and a lack of hope, and where they are engaged in daily survival with limited knowledge about opportunities available to them. Poor Latino women also experience the worst health status, reflected in a higher incidence of chronic diseases, higher mortality rates for certain health conditions such as breast and cervical cancer and acquired immunodeficiency syndrome (AIDS), and poorer survival rates for these and other conditions (Cooper, Steinhauer, Miller, David, & Schatzkin, 1981; Haan, Kaplan, & Camacho, 1987; Miller, 1987; U.S. Department of Health and Human Services, 1986, 1990; Woolhandler et al., 1985). Latino women with the worst health status and poorest access to health care live in poor communities, where living conditions are not only unhealthy, but where health problems such as communicable diseases (ie, tuberculosis, sexually transmitted diseases [STDs]), the use of alcohol and other drugs, and violence are much more prevalent. Poor women experience a disproportionate share of these problems, suggesting a strong association between poverty and poor health.

Several policies of the U.S. government have had negative and long-lasting effects on the well-being of a number of population groups, particularly women of color. According to McKenzie et al. (1992), and summarized by Bracho-De Carpio and Carpio-Cedraro (1993), between 1980 and 1990 severe cuts were made in federal programs in the areas of maternal and child health, community clinics, employment and housing assistance, and Title X funds (that provide contraceptive services for poor women). In an effort to reform health care and balance the budget, several federal and state initiatives are under consideration (eg, welfare reform, Contract with America, Personal Responsibility Act, Medicaid block grant, Medicaid and Medicare managed care, and California's proposition 187). Some people may feel that these proposals jeopardize the well-being of vulnerable populations such as racial and ethnic minorities and poor women. However, others may see these proposals as necessary economic measures with positive consequences over the long term. Regardless of the motives for such policies, the social, economic, and physical well-being of disadvantaged groups is presently and will continue to be at risk well into the future.

Research on Latino Women's Health: Understanding the Problem

Despite the fact that the U.S. Latino population continues to increase at a faster rate than that of any other population, little effort has been made by the government, academic institutions, and the private sector to provide empirical health data on the population of Hispanics as a whole. Even less information is available on issues relevant to Hispanic women. Until recently, the prevailing norm in research has emphasized research on men, with insufficient focus on the illnesses and diseases that affect women in general and women of color in particular (Office of Research on Women's Health [ORWH], 1992). Latino women tend to be excluded as subjects and topics in major studies; their relatively low numbers in the population have been used as an excuse to exclude them from surveys and data collection systems.

Epidemiologic data are lacking on such significant factors as mortality, morbidity, and survival rates for certain illnesses (eg, cancer). In public health, we lack data bases (or registries) in key areas related to chronic disease and mental health, making the task of data collection and analysis more difficult. Therefore, we depend on utilization and mortality data, when available. In addition, hospital utilization data lack Hispanic identifiers in all states (Arrom, 1993). An added difficulty is the small number of studies conducted among the Latino female population as a whole and the even smaller number that address Latino women by national origin. When available, the data seldom provide information on cultural, national, and lifestyle differences that may affect the health of Latino women. Nor do the data allow for differences in levels of education and literacy, levels of acculturation and assimilation, immigration history, or socioeconomic status, all of which have been shown to affect the rates and types of certain diseases and ease of access to the health care system.

Furthermore, social and biomedical research is conducted within a social and cultural context. Thus, it can be argued that the limited research on women of color reflects the values and attitudes of mainstream society toward women in general and women of color in particular, which may reinforce the social, economic, and political disadvantages of this group in our society. This argument is based on facts and deficiencies found in conducting research on Latino women and other women of color (Display 19-2).

Data on Latino women's health and social needs are extremely limited. Research on this population has sometimes included methods of observation and criteria for validating facts and theories that intentionally or unintentionally justify preconceived ideas and stereotypes of Latino women and other women of color, and reflect traditional sociocultural patterns of power, status, and privilege (Hixson, 1993).

Because of the severe limitation of data on Latino women's health, assumptions have to be made at times based on observations and anecdotal stories, which may lead to poor formulation of hypotheses, poor program planning and implementation, and poor formulation of public policies. In reference to this issue, Antonia C. Novello, MD, former U.S. Surgeon General stated:

> When we talk about improving data collection strategies, it means responsiveness to all ethnic groups and subgroups and accountability to the truth. It means that our population of 22 million people needs to be accounted for and counted in. It means getting comprehensive data, identifying what is and is not appropriate, and making accurate assessments and reasonable predictions about the real status of Hispanic/Latino health. Developing a comprehensive research agenda goes hand in hand with collecting better data. We cannot expect to understand where we are headed and where we ought to be in terms of health until we understand first, where we are today. It means finding a way by which we benefit from what science has to offer by tailoring its benefits to our needs. It means focusing on the diseases that kill us and putting priorities on research aimed at Hispanics/Latinos and other minorities... (U.S. Office of the Surgeon General, 1993, p. 11).

DISPLAY 19-2

Facts and Deficiencies in Research on Latino Women and Other Women of Color

- Most research has been done on men. There is failure to mention that studies are single sex or have highly unbalanced sex ratios, or that women of color have been excluded.

- The research activity on people of color and on women of color have not involved a careful and diligent search of available facts (Hixson, 1993).

- The research on minority women's health traditionally has had limited or no utility in understanding or solving important health and social issues for women. Topics of significance for women of color are ignored.

- A research problem is formulated for men or women (in general) only, but this limitation is not explicitly noted.

- The limited research on Latino women has been done by non-Latinos who belong to either the middle class or have a middle-class orientation in conducting research.

- Most research studies on Latino women have not included a representative of this population as part of the research team and when they do seldom are they included in a leadership role (Principal Investigators, Co-Investigators, Project Directors).

- Most research on Latino women has not had culture- or gender-specific relevance. Gender variables are not explored or incorporated into the theory being studied or in the interpretation or analysis of the data.

- Situations in which women of color act outside of prescribed sex roles are defined for the purpose of the study as deviant behavior or problems (eg, female-headed households). Situations in which they conform to prescribed roles are assumed to be nonproblematic (ASA, 1990) (eg, unpaid household and childrearing).

- On highly sensitive gender-related questions, efforts are not made to ensure that interviewers are of the sex and cultural background that will yield the least bias in eliciting responses (ASA, 1990).

- Latino women and other women of color are arbitrarily excluded from studies because of financial constraints, convenience, language barriers, lack of familiarity, or personal preference of the investigator; or the topic is presumed not to be relevant to women of color.

- In behavioral research, the research hypotheses and overall research design tend to stress a cultural deficit model.

- Research on minority health tends to emphasize genetic and cultural factors as solely responsible for minority poor health and ignores socioeconomic, political, and environmental influences.

- Little intervention research has been conducted on Latino women, and even fewer clinical trials have included or focused on Latino women, hampering effective intervention in the lives of Latino women (Giachello, 1993). The overall lack of data available to measure the health status of the variety of Latino female populations may lead to hypotheses and conclusions that are wholly inadequate in addressing each Latino female population's specific health needs (Ramirez, Valdez, & Carter-Pokras, 1994).

Issues of Social Inequalities and Women's Health

Latino women's health needs to be viewed within the culture of the American society and within the context of women's general health, well-being, and social status. It is important to keep in mind that the culture of a society socializes the individual on how to think, act, and feel toward illness. It determines our health attitudes and behaviors and defines the roles of the participants. The doctor, the patient, and medicine are all part of the culture, which consists of a vast system of knowledge beliefs, techniques, roles, values, ideologies, attitudes, customs, and rituals that interlock to form a mutually reinforcing and supporting system. In addressing Latino women's health, factors related to religion, social norms, environment, physical and mental health, and spiritual and social well-being must be integrated and equally considered.

Barriers to Health Care

In addition to problems arising from discrimination, urban poverty, and the lack of cultural competency among health care practitioners, Latino women confront a series of problems in gaining access to the medical care system in the United States (Giachello, 1994a, 1995a). Access refers to the entry into the system for either preventive and maintenance health care or for the treatment of illness. Lack of access to health care results from financial, cultural, and institutional barriers. In a recent review of the literature, Giachello (1994a) summarized the barriers to health care that Latinos overall confront based on a number of indicators, which are discussed briefly in the sections that follow:

1. Whether or not a person has a regular source of care
2. Lack of health insurance coverage and other financial barriers
3. Cultural and institutional inconveniences in obtaining care

Regular Source of Care

Studies consistently document that Latinos are less likely than any other racial or ethnic group to be linked to a regular source of care such as a family doctor or a public or private clinic (Anderson, Giachello, & Aday, 1986; Giachello, 1994a; Robert Wood Johnson Foundation [RWJF], 1983, 1987; U.S. General Accounting Office [GAO], 1992; Valdez, Giachello, Rodriquez-Tias, Gomez, & La Rocha, 1993). In 1989, approximately 35% of all Latinos did not have a regular source of medical care. This percentage was even higher among those with low family income (Aday, Anderson, & Fleming, 1980) and among Latino children and adolescents (Garcia, Salcedo, & Giachello, 1985). The 1982–1984 Hispanic Health and Nutritional Examination Survey (HHANES) data indicate that within Latino subgroups the proportion of those having a regular source of care varies by gender and age group. For instance, only 56% of Mexican American men aged 20 to 30 years reported a regular source of care compared to 69% for those aged 31 to 45 and 78% for those aged 46 to 74. Mexican American women consistently reported higher linkages with a regular source of care (78% for those aged 20–30) (Estrada, Trevino, & Ray, 1990).

When a regular source of care is reported, poor and uninsured Latinos tend to use public health care facilities or hospital outpatient clinics. They are also most likely to be disproportionately linked to facilities with limited medical services outside regular office hours or that provide emergency treatment (Anderson et al., 1986; Garcia et al., 1985; Giachello & Arrom, 1989). As a result, Latinos tend to use the hospital emergency room disproportionately.

Lack of Health Insurance

The high cost of care and the lack of health insurance make it difficult for Latino women to have access to a broad array of health services, especially for primary care (Estrada et al., 1990). In 1990, 35% of all Latinos did not have health insurance (NCLR, 1992; U.S. GAO, 1992; Giachello, 1994b; Valdez et al., 1991). Recent analyses of the problem have indicated that lack of health insurance among Latinos is related to employment status, type of industry, and income. A U.S. GAO (1992, p. 12) report indicates that 78% of Latino family members under the age of 65 who were uninsured lived in families with an adult worker. It also found that uninsured Latinos were more likely than Caucasians and African Americans to work in industries that are less likely to provide health insurance coverage, such as construction and agriculture (U.S. GAO, 1992; Valdez et al., 1991).

Lack of health insurance coverage varies by gender, by type of occupation, and by income. In 1990, 52% of working Latino women below the poverty level did not have health insurance coverage (NCLR, 1993). Those Latino working women below the poverty level were least likely to report employment-based health insurance coverage, even if they work full-time year round.

Research on uninsured Latinos by gender summarized by Giachello (1995a, p. 151) also indicates differences in coverage among subpopulations. The 1982–1984 HHANES found that 34% of Mexican American men in the study reported no health insurance compared to 28% for Cuban American men and 30% for Puerto Rican men. The percentages for Latino women were 34% for Mexican American, 25% for Cuban American, and 17% for Puerto Ricans (Solis et al., 1990). The problem of lack of insurance coverage is even more severe among Latino children and adolescents (Bloom, 1990; Giachello & Aponte, 1989; Rodriguez-Trias & Ramirez de Arellano, 1994).

Type of health insurance coverage varies among racial and ethnic groups and among Latinos of various national origins. Using data from the 1989 Current Population Survey, Treviño, Moyer, Burciaga Valdez, and Stroup-Benham (1991) found that Mexican Americans (43.7%) and Puerto Ricans (43.6%), followed closely by African Americans (45.4%), were least likely to have private health insurance. Furthermore, Puerto Ricans were most likely of all racial and ethnic groups to report Medicaid coverage (32.5%), followed by African Americans (23.3%), Mexican Americans (13.7%), and Cuban Americans (11.9%), compared with the total U.S. population (8.3%) (Treviño et al., 1991).

The high percentage of Puerto Ricans on Medicaid programs was explained by the high prevalence of Puerto Rican poor families that are female-headed households and are thus more likely to be eligible for Medicaid coverage. The low prevalence of Medicaid coverage among Mexican Americans was explained by the difference in Medicaid eligibility criteria across states (National Coalition of Hispanic Health and Human Services Organization [COSSMHO], 1990; U.S. GAO, 1992; Treviño et al., 1991) and by the fact that many states exclude families with two parents from the Medicaid program, regardless of whether they meet the income requirements.

Having insurance coverage, however, does not guarantee Latino women equal access to the health care system because of inequities in benefits packages, providers' discretion in deciding which health insurance company to accept, increased search costs from private cost-containment efforts (eg, deductibles and copayments), and poor quality of care. Even the presence of insurance (public or private) may not provide adequate coverage for the needs of Latino women. More than half of private health insurance plans do not cover pre- or postnatal care, both critical time periods for insuring a child's future health. Of employment-based insurance plans, only 9% cover preventive care, 15% cover eyeglasses, and 32% cover dental care (COSSMHO, 1992; Valdez et al., 1991). Similar inadequacies are also found in public programs (COSSMHO, 1990). Valdez et al. found that Latinos appear particularly vulnerable to these weaknesses in the current system of financing medical care (Valdez et al., 1991, p. 4).

The current trend toward managed care is an area of great concern. Managed care plans offer incentives to physicians and other health care providers to encourage them to provide minimum care by restricting referrals to more expensive specialty medical care and limiting hospitalization (Giachello, 1995b). This type of health care financing will limit medical services to routine care and will restrict access to state-of-the-art services, diagnostic screening, and more specialized care.

In summary, Latino women are least likely to be able to afford medical care and most likely to have no health insurance. The situation has become more acute in the last decade and appears to be more severe among certain subgroups, such as children and adolescents, and those with lower income. Among Latino ethnic groups, Mexicans and Mexican Americans are most likely to be uninsured. When health insurance is reported, Puerto Ricans are most likely to be covered by government-sponsored programs such as Medicaid. Furthermore, recent data indicate that Latinos are not obtaining the full benefit from their health insurance plans and that those under managed care plans may be denied needed specialized services and hospitalization.

Cultural and Institutional Barriers to Health Care

Latino women confront a host of other inconveniences in obtaining care. The lack of linkage with a regular source of health care and the high cost of services force many Latino women turn to public facilities for routine care. There they confront inadequate bilingual or bicultural services, long waiting times between calling for an appointment and the actual visit, and long waits once they get to the facility (Giachello, 1994b). Other barriers are related to the fact that these services are too bureaucratic and fragmented, have complicated forms to be filled out, and are organized around the convenience of the health care providers rather than the consumers. Furthermore, few providers locate their practices in Latino communities, leading to shortages of health care professionals.

Additional barriers that Latino women confront are related to cultural and gender differences. Providers may lack knowledge and sensitivity about Latino culture and women's health, particularly the health of women of color. Most services available are aimed at reproductive health, following a middle-class orientation and a maternal and infant model.

The lack of knowledge about Latino culture and women's health may result in stereotypes that have a negative impact on the provider–consumer relationship and the quality of care. Some stereotypes that prevail among non-Latino providers view Latino women as superstitious, present oriented, uninterested in preventive examinations, and noncompliant (Gregory, 1978). A 1988 mail survey done in Chicago documented providers' knowledge, attitudes, and practices toward Latino patients/clients (Aponte & Giachello, 1989). The study found that more than half the health care providers who responded to the questionnaire reported not knowing about Latino health status and about the heterogeneity of the Latino population.

The language barrier is another factor that influences the provider–consumer relationship, and communication may be further complicated by the use of technical medical jargon that confuses the Latino woman. Usually the responsibility for interpretation in a health or mental health facility falls to anyone who is bilingual, such as an employee, family member (eg, child), or friend; usually this person has no formal interpretation training (Putsch 1985). This may lead to inaccuracies, failure to disclose information, violation of confidentiality, and failure of the provider to develop rapport with the patient.

Prejudice against Latinos arising from this communication gap may also maintain and reinforce the social distance between provider and consumer (Aponte & Giachello, 1989; Giachello, 1995a; Quesada & Heller, 1977). The 1988 Chicago survey found that 50% of health care providers stated that Latinos should learn English instead of expecting bilingual services to be provided.

Most recently, it has been argued that communication barriers can be reduced or eliminated with the use of interpreters (Giachello 1994b, 1995b). Unfortunately, this may not be the case because interpreters require a great deal of skill to describe and explain terms, ideas, and processes regarding patient care (Putsch, 1985).

In summary, Latino women experience a number of barriers that are related to cultural and gender differences and the way in which the medical care system is organized. These barriers lead women to noncompliance and poor adherence to treatment. Latinos as a whole underutilize medical services (Giachello, 1994a). For example, they are less likely to see a physician or to be hospitalized within a year or to use preventive health services. Utilization studies show differences among Latinos of different national origins and by gender with Puerto Ricans and Cubans reporting the highest use of formal medical care and Mexican Americans the least use (Giachello, 1994a). Latino women reported higher use than Latino men, particularly for general preventive services, but lower use for mental health services (Giachello, 1994a).

The Health Status of Latino Women

The barriers that Hispanic women confront in gaining access to the medical care system occurs at a time in which their health and medical needs are the strongest.

Despite the fact that Latino women live longer than Latino and non-Latino men, they experience chronic conditions and disabilities, and their health status is negatively associated with their length of time in this country.

Life Expectancy

In 1991, life expectancy for Latino women was higher compared to Latino men (77.1 versus 69.6 years) but lower compared to Caucasian non-Latino women (79.2 years) (ORWH, 1992) (Table 19-2). These statistics seem positive, but according to the National Institutes of Health (ORWH, 1992), we need to interpret them with caution considering the increase of certain diseases that women in general are experiencing as they get older. For example, osteoporosis and Alzheimer's disease are increasing among women in general. Women and women of color in particular also experience more acute symptoms of illnesses, chronic conditions, and short- and long-term disabilities arising from health problems (ORWH, 1992). The higher life expectancy rate should not be used as an excuse for not focusing on women's health and on the health of women of color (Giachello, 1995a; ORWH, 1992).

Leading Causes of Death

In 1992, the leading cause of death among Latino women was heart disease, which claimed 19,829 lives (Table 19-3) (National Center for Health Statistics [NCHS], 1995). Malignant neoplasm (cancer) was the second major cause of death for Latinas, with 7235 deaths for that year. In 1992, these two leading causes of death accounted for 49% of all deaths to Latino women. The third and fourth leading causes of death among Latinas in 1992 were cerebrovascular disease and diabetes mellitus, respectively. The remaining leading causes of deaths for Latino women were as follows (NCHS, 1995):

- accidents and adverse effects
- pneumonia and influenza
- conditions originating in the perinatal period
- chronic obstructive pulmonary diseases, including asthma
- congenital anomalies
- human immunodeficiency virus (HIV) and acquired immunodeficiency syndrome (AIDS)

Table 19-2. Life Expectancy by Gender and by Racial/Ethnic Groups, 1989

	Men (years)	Women (years)
Total population	71.8	78.6
Caucasians	72.7	79.2
African Americans	64.8	73.5
Hispanics/Latinos	69.6	77.1

Source: Office of Research on Women's Health. (1992). *Summary report*. Hunt Valley, MD: Author.

Table 19-3. Leading Causes of Death of the Hispanic Population by Gender and for All Ages

Causes of Death	Percent of Total Death	
	Female	Male
Diseases of heart	27.4	21.8
Malignant neoplasms	22.0	16.1
Cerebrovascular diseases	6.6	3.9
Diabetes mellitus	5.1	2.7
Accidents and adverse effects	4.7	10.9
Pneumonia and influenza	3.2	2.7
Conditions originating in the perinatal period	2.6	—
Chronic obstructive pulmonary disease	2.3	—
Congenital anomalies	2.1	—
Human immunodeficiency virus	2.0	7.7

Source: *Advance report of final mortality statistics,* National Center for Health Statistics, 1995.

Although cerebrovascular disease ranked as the third leading cause of death among Latino women, it represented the seventh leading cause of death for Latino men. Diabetes mellitus was the fourth leading cause of death for Latino women in 1992, but it ranked tenth among the leading cause of deaths for Latino men (NCHS, 1995).

Heart Disease

We know little about heart disease among women and about its effects and symptom manifestation, because most studies have been done on men. Health care providers are more likely to recognize symptoms of heart disease in men than in women and to be more knowledgeable about the effectiveness of various medical treatments or interventions on men than on women. Because of this discrepancy, health care providers tend to assume that these complaints by women are imaginary or stress related. Therefore, anecdotal evidence and direct observation seem to indicate that health care providers are more apt to refer women complaining of certain symptoms to a mental health worker rather than to screening, diagnosis, or treatment for heart-related conditions.

Heart disease usually develops over a long period of time. Studies indicate that high blood pressure and a high serum (blood) cholesterol concentration combined with obesity and smoking are major factors. These factors have serious implications for Latino women because they are most likely to be obese and to suffer from diabetes mellitus (NCLR, 1993).

Cardiovascular Conditions

Two main risk factors associated with cardiovascular conditions are cholesterol level and hypertension. A diet high in unsaturated fats and low in fiber is one of the causes of elevated cholesterol levels. Latino women appear less likely to have high serum cholesterol levels than non-Latino African American or non-Latino Caucasian women (Giachello, 1995b). The 1982–1984 HHANES indicated that cholesterol levels were higher for non-Latino Caucasian women (28.3%) than for non-Latino African American women (25.0%) or for the three Latino subgroups surveyed (Estrada et al., 1990). The HHANES data indicated that Cuban women (16.9%) were less likely than Mexican American (29%) or Puerto Rican women (22.7%) to have high cholesterol (Estrada et al., 1990). Overall, Latino data are unavailable because HHANES data cover only the major Latino subgroups in certain geographical areas.

Hypertension is also a risk factor for cardiovascular and cerebrovascular disease. Available data suggest that Latino women are less likely than non-Latino women to suffer from hypertension. According to HHANES, 43.8% of African Americans and 25.1% of non-Latino Caucasians between the ages of 20 and 74 were hypertensive. Among the three Latino subgroups studied, the prevalence was lowest for Cuban women (14.4%), followed by Puerto Rican women (19.2%) and Mexican American women (20.3%) (National Heart, Lung and Blood Institute [NHLBI], 1992). Yet these numbers may be deceptive because hypertension increases with age and the relative youth of the Latino population may lead to an underestimation of the extent of the problem.

Cancer

The leading external factor contributing to the rise in the number of preventable cancer cases among women is cigarette smoking. The American Cancer Society (1991) reports that smoking is responsible for approximately 76% of lung cancer deaths among women and is a major cause of heart disease and other pulmonary conditions such as colds, chronic bronchitis, and emphysema. Although Hispanic women are less likely to smoke than Caucasian and African American women, there have been dramatic increases as a result of heavy marketing by the tobacco industries in Latino communities, targeting Latino youth and women (Maxwell & Jacobson, 1989). A Denver study covering 1970 and 1980 documents a doubling of lung cancer rates among Latino women and men. During this period, lung cancer among Latino women grew by 109% compared to 95% for Caucasian women (Maxwell & Jacobson, 1989).

The other three most frequently reported types of cancer among women are cervical, colorectal, and breast (Giachello, in press). The incidence of breast cancer among Latino women is lower compared to Caucasian non-Latinos but they are more likely than Caucasian women to die of breast cancer. The differences in survival rates reflect the stage at which breast cancer is diagnosed and treated; early diagnosis and treatment are considered critical for survival (Giachello, in press). Latino women, particularly Mexican Americans, are more likely to develop cervical cancer than uterine cancer (Giachello, in press). However, uterine cancer survival rates are slightly better for Mexican American women than cervical cancer survival rates.

Finally, the relatively high prevalence of cancer among Latino women is related to the fact that Latino women are less likely than Caucasian women to have received common types of cancer screening. Financial, cultural, and other barriers to access and system problems related to the delivery of health services have been major obstacles to prevention, screening, and treatment.

Diabetes Mellitus

An estimated 1.3 million Latinos (11.8% of an estimated total 11 million Americans) over the age of 21 are afflicted with diabetes mellitus (American Diabetes Association, 1992; U.S. House of Representatives Select Committee on Aging, 1992). Diabetes mellitus is a chronic condition characterized by abnormal metabolism. Diabetes affects the circulatory system and is frequently associated with conditions such as arteriosclerosis (hardening of the arteries), kidney failure, vision loss, and amputations. Diabetes mellitus was the fourth leading cause of death among Latino women in 1992. The diabetes mortality rate for Latinos is twice the rate for non-Latino Caucasians (American Diabetes Association, 1992; U.S. House of Representatives Select Committee on Aging, 1992).

In a recent summary of the research literature, Giachello (1994b, 1995b) documented that Mexican Americans and Puerto Ricans experience 110% to 120% higher diabetes rates compared to Caucasians. The rate for Cuban Americans ranges from 50% to 60%. Mexican Americans and Puerto Ricans also have two to three times greater risk of non–insulin-dependent diabetes (NIDDM) than non-Latinos (American Diabetes Association, 1992; U.S. House of Representatives Select Committee on Aging, 1992). Data from the NCHS Health and Nutrition Examination Survey (HANES II) and 1982–1984 HHANES show that 42% of Mexican Americans, 40% of Puerto Ricans, and 58% of Cubans who had diabetes did not know they had the disease. The prevalence of undiagnosed diabetes was higher among Puerto Ricans and Mexican Americans than among Caucasians. The prevalence of diabetes is related to low socioeconomic status, which in turn correlates with lack of insurance and hesitation to visit a physician (U.S. GAO, 1992).

One study found that 10% of Mexican American women over the age of 45 were diabetic compared to the national rate of 3.7% (Manley, Lin-Fu, Miranda, Noonan, & Parker, 1984). Mexican American and Puerto Rican women are more than twice as likely as non-Hispanic Caucasian women to have diabetes. About 15% of Mexican American and 16.2% of Puerto Rican women 45 to 74 years of age have diabetes compared to 5.8% of non-Hispanic Caucasian and 11.4% of non-Hispanic African American women (Flegal et al., 1991). Latino women have three times the risk of developing diabetes and greater metabolic severity than non-Latino Caucasians. Gestational diabetes, which occurs only during pregnancy, is another risk factor for NIDDM. Women who have had gestational diabetes have a 30% to 40% chance of developing NIDDM. Latinos' increased risk may be due to genetic predisposition, age, diet, obesity, family history of diabetes, and sedentary lifestyle.

Because adherence to a diabetes treatment regimen requires monitoring by health care providers and family support, treatment poses particular challenges for Hispanics. In addition to the cultural barriers discussed earlier in the chapter, a clinical approach that focuses on the individual rather than the family may also make adherence to treatment for Latino women more difficult. Recent pilot studies indicate that to improve the health status of diabetic Latinos, it is not enough merely to increase the client's self-care skills and knowledge about the illness. It is also necessary to increase the health care provider's knowledge and the standard of diabetes treatment by reinforcing clinical guidelines for control and good management of diabetes (Lipton, Losey, Giachello, & Mendez, in press).

HIV/AIDS

Women show the fastest growing AIDS incidence rate. AIDS has become a leading cause of death among all women of childbearing age and the leading cause of death for women aged 25 to 44 (Centers for Disease Control and Prevention [CDC], 1995a; Kochanek & Hudson, 1994). In 1985, women accounted for 7% of all cases; in 1994, the number jumped to 18% (CDC, 1995a).

By 1994, Latino women represented 20% of all accumulated AIDS cases among women in the United States. Equally alarming are indications that Latino women are eight times more likely to acquire AIDS than non-Latino Caucasian women (Holmes, Karon, & Kreiss, 1990; Selick, Castro, & Pappaioanou, 1988). The majority of female Latino AIDS exposures were through intravenous drug use (46%) or through heterosexual contact with intravenous drug users (43%) (CDC, 1995a). Latino women are also at risk for HIV transmission from bisexual men, given the higher level of bisexuality found among Latino men (CDC, 1993a). Furthermore, high levels of seropositive status have been found among various subpopulations of Latino women, including intravenous drug users, women of childbearing age, those applying for military service, and others. This has given rise to expectations of dramatic increases in female Latino AIDS cases (CDC, 1990b; Smith et al., 1991; Stricof, Kennedy, Nuttell, Weisfuse, & Novick 1991; Novick et al., 1991).

Giachello (1991) argues that Latino women are often diagnosed only in later stages of HIV infection, This is a result, in part, of a lack of access to medical care and health education. Women who are diagnosed with HIV or AIDS are then excluded from most clinical trials (Giachello, 1991). Women present a different symptomatology for AIDS from men, and so face a higher risk of misdiagnosis and exclusion from health insurance benefits for AIDS. Women with AIDS have therefore been found to have a much lower life expectancy than men. Whereas men with AIDS may survive from 24 to 36 months, the average life expectancy of women, from the time of diagnosis, is only 3.5 to 6 months.

Bracho de Carpio, Carpio-Cedraro, and Anderson (1993) further argue that urban poverty increases the vulnerability for HIV infection and decreases the capability of prevention among individuals, particularly among Latino women. When analyzing the prevalence of HIV/AIDS in certain geographical areas, such as New York City (Bronx), Chicago (Logan Square, Humboldt Park, and West Town), Texas (Houston, Dallas, and San Antonio, border counties Cameron, Hidalgo, Webb, and the City of El Paso, which is the fourth poorest city in the United States), these researchers found that HIV/AIDS was most prevalent among Latino women living in areas of extreme poverty. They recommend that the primary strategy needed to combat AIDS is confronting "poverty itself."

Sexually Transmitted Diseases

The STDs remain a serious health issue for the Latino population in the United States. Although significant reductions have occurred in the number of cases of primary and secondary syphilis and gonorrhea in the past 8 years, the rates of these health problems continue to be substantially higher for Hispanics than Caucasian non-Hispanics (NCLR, 1995). A recent report by NCLR (1995) found that in 1993 Latinos were five times as likely to contract primary and secondary syphilis as Caucasian non-Latinos (6.0 and 1.2/100,000 population, respectively) (NCLR, 1995, p. 5). In 1993, Latinos were three times as likely to contract gonorrhea as were non-Latino Caucasians (90.4 and 28.6/100,000 population, respectively). Latino women are most likely to be less aware of symptoms and are less likely to seek medical treatment because of financial and system barriers, until symptoms are either visible or produce pain.

In 1991, the highest male/female primary and secondary syphilis ratio per 100,000 was among Hispanics (1.7), compared to Caucasians (1.5), and African Americans (1.3) (CDC, 1993b). Despite a decline between the years 1985 and 1986, syphilis infection rates have since steadily increased among Latino and African American women, while decreasing numbers of syphilis cases are reported in Caucasians (CDC, 1990a). Latino and African American adolescents aged 15 to 19 years also recorded high increases of syphilis infection. Latino teenaged girls, for example, recorded increases in primary and secondary syphilis infection from 17 cases per 100,000 population in 1986 to 22 cases per 100,000 in 1987, with only slight decreases in infection rates in the years thereafter (Hispanic Health Council [HHC], 1989).

Chlamydia and *Trichomonas* infections are most elevated among adolescent Latinos as compared with other populations (Eager, 1985). In one study, for example, the highest rate of *Chlamydia* infection was found among Latino teenagers aged 15 to 17 (Smith, 1988). Among Latino women of all ages, a South Texas study recorded that approximately 10% of its female Latino participants were infected with *Chlamydia* (Gleeney, Glassman, Cox, & Brown, 1988).

The health consequences related to STDs, including pelvic inflammatory disease, infertility, ectopic pregnancy, stillbirth, spontaneous abortion, as well as congenital problems and blindness in infants born to STD-infected mothers, are well known. An additional source of concern is the recent connection made between STD infection and infection with HIV (Moran, Aral, Jenkins, Peterman, & Alexander, 1989; Turner, 1989).

Mental Health Issues

The ORWH indicates that mental disorders are among the health problems that are more prevalent in women than in men. For example, the rate of affective disorders is almost twice as high for women, about 7%, compared to 3% in men. In elderly women, the prevalence of depression is 3.64% as opposed to 1% in men (ORWH 1992, p. 9).

Latino women are at higher risk of developing depression, psychoses, and other serious mental illnesses. In a national women's health survey conducted by Louis Harris and Associates, 53% of Hispanic women reported severe depression compared to 37% of non-Hispanic Caucasian and 47% of non-Hispanic African American women (COSSMHO, 1994, p. 2; Commonwealth Fund Women's Health Survey, 1993). This same study indicates that Mexican American women are more than twice as likely as men to exhibit high levels of depressive symptoms. For example, 18.7% of Mexican American women aged 20 to 74 exhibit high levels of depressive symptomatology compared to 8.0% of Mexican American men (COOSMHO, 1994; Commonwealth Fund Women's Health Survey, 1993).

According to several researchers (Amaro, 1987; Leon, Mazur, Montalvo, & Rodriguez, 1984; Treviño & Rendón, 1994), the prevalence of mental illnesses among Latino women may be the result of a number of factors:

- low socioeconomic status
- high incidence of poverty
- stress associated with single parenting
- gender roles
- low educational achievement
- migration and the process associated with acculturation
- language and other cultural differences
- domestic violence
- discrimination caused by racism, sexism, and classism

Despite their high risk for mental illness, studies indicate that Latinos in general use mental health services less frequently than other groups. Among the explanations provided by the mental health literature and summarized by Treviño and Rendón (1994) are:

- lack of recognition of mental illnesses
- lower frequency and severity of mental illnesses
- use of alternative or traditional treatment for mental illnesses (eg, use of curanderos)

However, lack of access to mental health services, particularly financial and cultural barriers, may be the strongest explanation for Latino women's lower use of mental health services. Furthermore, therapeutic interventions are most likely to focus on psychological dynamics within a middle-class framework, rather than by addressing social and environmental conditions that predispose women to stress and mental illness.

Violence

Violence has emerged as a major public health issue in the 1990s. It is a serious problem in our streets and in our homes, and manifests itself in different ways.

Gang-Related Violence

One type of violence is that associated with gang-related activities. Homicide, for example, is one of the leading causes of death among Hispanic children and youth between the ages of 1 and 14. It is also the second leading cause of death among adolescents and young adults aged 14 to 24 (NCHS, 1995).

Traditionally, we have associated gang-related activities and violence as a problem affecting young men. Unfortunately, regardless of ethnicity, this behavior has increased among young women, including Latino women. It is not clear what are the strongest determinants of gang membership for women. Some of the psychosocial factors for both young men and women may be related to:

- low self-esteem
- inadequate recreational activities
- poor academic performance
- lack of or limited parental supervision
- peer pressure
- need for acceptance among the peer group

It has been argued that increased participation in gang-related activities is associated with a high degree of acculturation of minority youth into the mainstream society, producing conflict between the youth value system and those of the parent place of birth or origin.

Workplace Violence

A second type of violence and abuse experienced by women is that associated with the workplace. Violence is a major contributor to fatal injuries occurring in the workplace (Illinois Department of Public Health [IDPH], 1995, p. 1). With the increased participation of women in the work force, this type of violence is on the rise. Those most affected work in offices and in social services agencies. They are usually victimized during the daytime and assaulted in public buildings (IDPH, 1995).

Incidences of homicide in the workplace often occur during a robbery, because the woman is a witness to a crime, or because it is a crime of passion. Another kind of violence that affects women in the workplace is related to sexual harassment, where issues of power and abuse of power come into play, and emotional abuse as well, where women may be mistreated verbally and otherwise (IDPH, 1995).

Domestic Violence

One of the most serious problems women experienc is domestic abuse. Women may be battered by their spouse, children, or other relatives (as in the case of elder abuse). Often, the public perception of the woman in such cases is that she is masochistic (she has a psychological need to be beaten and, therefore, provokes the husband or sexual partner) or that she is deserving of the abuse. Furthermore, women may experience pressure to conform from members of the extended family or may find no way out because of limited financial resources, low self-esteem, or depression.

Domestic violence may occur as a result of the family experiencing social stressors, including financial difficulties. Alcohol and other drugs are usually involved. This may also be related to issues of power and control, especially in the case men who think they have the right to abuse women and children.

Issues of Acculturation and Latino Women's Health

As Latinos immigrate into the United States, they gradually begin to adopt the values and behaviors of the mainstream culture. Some Latinos may engage in a conscious effort to acculturate (eg, learning the English Language). This may be a result of their strong need to adjust to the new environment, to be socially accepted, or to be able to take advantage of the social and economic opportunities available to them. Even when acculturation does occur, structural assimilation (gaining access to the American institutions, including the health care system) is still difficult.

The process of acculturation has influenced the way in which Latino women deal with health and illness behaviors. It has increased women's level of awareness about health (eg, breast and cervical cancer screenings). However, recent research is beginning to document some of the negative consequences of acculturation to immigrant health. This has been particularly true in the area of pregnancy outcomes (see Display 19-3 later in this chapter). As Latino women adopt the mainstream health behaviors, patterns, and expectations, they lose or decrease some of their traditional self-care practices and support systems, which in fact maintain or improve their health status.

There is limited empirical work regarding acculturation, behavioral risk factors, and health outcomes among Latino women. The knowledge and dominance of the English language and place of birth are usually used as the principal markers of acculturation. Although acculturation and its measurement are poorly understood (Zambrana & Ellis, 1995), the findings on the negative effects of acculturation are interesting and important.

Briefly, this section summarizes some selected health behaviors for which the research literature documents differences in health status and health behaviors of Latino women according to levels of acculturation and assimilation.

Smoking

Tobacco consumption among Latino women is generally found at lower rates than among non-Latino women (Carrillo & Torres, 1988). Smokers comprise only 13% of Latino women, whereas 23% of all women in the United States are current smokers (NHLBI, 1992). Latino women giving birth in 1993 smoked less (5%) compared to Caucasian women (18.6%) and African American women (12.7%) (NCHS, 1995). Within Latino subgroups, Puerto Rican mothers smoke more (11.2%) than Mexicans (13.7%), South and Central Americans (2.3%), and Cubans (5%) (NCHS, 1995). Furthermore, Ventura (1993) found that U.S.-born Latino mothers smoke more than foreign-born Latino mothers.

An increase in cigarette smoking among young U.S. Latino women is primarily a result of heavy marketing by the tobacco industry in Latino neighborhoods. For example, many companies sponsor most of the neighborhood cultural festivities, such as the Mexican's Cinco de Mayo event, Mexican Independence Day, the Puerto Rican Parade, and so forth.

The rise of cigarette consumption from foreign- to U.S.-born Latinos has a serious impact on the health status of Latino women. This population is now at a greater risk for heart and lung disease, hypertension, cancer, and undesirable outcomes of pregnancy.

Alcohol Consumption

The available literature on levels of alcohol use and abuse among Latinos indicates great variance across gender, levels of acculturation, and national origin. However, Latinos in general have been found to drink less than non-Latinos. Within the Latino population, women tend to drink much less than men (Arredondo, Weddige, Justice, & Fitz, 1987; Christian, Zobeck, & Martin, 1985; Holck, Warren, Smith, & Rochat, 1984). Among women giving birth in the United States, U.S.-born Latino women were twice as likely to drink than foreign-born Latino women (Ventura, 1993).

One factor that may have an important impact on levels of alcohol consumption is acculturation. Holck et al. (1984) found, for example, that although non-Latino women were three times more likely to drink than Latino women, the rate of drinking increased with increasing levels of education (an indicator of acculturation level). When controlling for education, no significant ethnic variations in alcohol consumption were revealed. As more Latino women find employment, particularly in traditionally male-dominated, high-stress occupations, the pattern of alcohol consumption may be expected to change. In addition, the number of alcoholic women may increase, given the longer life expectancy of women (Giachello, 1991).

A study comparing drinking levels between female-headed and two parent families found that women in female-headed households record higher rates and quantities of alcohol consumption. Female-headed or single parent status was a more significant factor than age, education, income, or acculturation (Stroup, Trevino, & Trevino, 1988). As more Latino women are unable to depend on their immediate or extended families, the stress of being a single parent is further compounded by the lost value of family. Unfortunately, the risk for alcohol use among these women seems ever more present.

Illicit Substance Abuse

Studies on Latino women and substance abuse are extremely limited. Available studies that were summarized by Giachello (1991, 1994a, 1995a) indicate that illicit drug use is limited among Latinos and Latino subpopulations. Further data suggest that Latino women in general are less likely to use illicit drugs than Latino men and African American or Caucasian women. For example, 37.8% of Latino men and 26.9% of Latino women reported ever using illicit drugs; percentages for Caucasian and African American women were 34.8% and 29.6%, respectively.

The literature suggests that Caucasians may be more likely to use illicit drugs on an experimental basis, whereas African Americans and Latinos are more likely to use them regularly (NCLR, 1995). This pattern of use is more likely attributed to socioeconomic factors rather than cultural factors. Latinos were also more likely to report current use of psychotherapeutic drugs such as sedatives, tranquilizers, stimulants, or analgesics than Caucasians or African Americans (NCLR, 1995). Some new evidence shows that, for certain types of drugs (eg, crack), the proportion of Latino users is increasing relative to Caucasian and African American users. Data by Latinos of national origin indicate that Puerto Ricans and Mexicans are equally likely to use cocaine. Recent studies from New York City and data from CDC HIV/AIDS testing and counseling centers document high numbers of Latino women who are intravenous drug users.

According to HHANES, some of the demographic characteristics of Latino drug users were that they spoke English, had higher levels of income and education, and were most likely born in the United States (NIDA, 1987).

Pregnancy and Birth

In 1993, the estimated birth rate (number of live births per 1000 population) for the Latino population was 26 compared to 14.2 for the non-Latino population (NCHS, 1995). The birth rates among Latino women by national origin were as follows: 27.4 for Mexican Americans, 21.9 for Puerto Ricans, 10.5 for Cubans Americans, and 26.9 for Central and South America women (NCHS, 1995). Birth rates clearly indicate that Latino women, particularly the Mexican cohort, are the most prolific ethnic group in the United States. They begin having children at a younger age and continue until their older years, with variations by national origin (NCHS, 1995). Selected characteristics of Latino women who gave birth in 1995 indicate that over 50% of Latino mothers are foreign born. The fertility rate in 1993 for Hispanic women was 106.9 births per 1000 women aged 15 to 44. The rates for Hispanic subgroups ranged from 114.8 for Mexican women to 55.5 for Cuban women.

These high birth and fertility statistics indicate that it is especially important to study the effects of acculturation on pregnancy outcomes. The incidence of births to unmarried Latino women is increasing, particularly among adolescent Latinos. Also, Latino adolescents born in the United States have a considerably higher percentage of teen pregnancy (see Giachello, 1994a for a comprehensive review of the research literature in the area of perinatal health). One of the biggest drawbacks of acculturation is that these women are removed from the social support systems so largely depended on by Latino women in their country of origin. These networks encourage pregnant women to conform to family practices. Lamberty (1994) summarized some of these traditional behaviors that benefited the pregnancy outcomes of foreign-born Latino women (Display 19-3). Although Latino women born outside the United States are more likely to receive prenatal care late in pregnancy, interestingly, they are less likely to have babies of low birth weight. These data suggest that the many aspects of Latin culture, including those discussed above, may largely contribute to healthier pregnancy outcomes. Further research would certainly be worthwhile.

In summary, data on acculturation into the mainstream society, measured by English language dominance and place of birth, indicate that the health status of Latinos declines as they adopt new behaviors that may be detrimental to their health. However, the measures of acculturation are not refined enough to allow research a better understanding of the dynamics involved. Zambrana & Ellis (1995) argue that the assumption of linear acculturation does not examine the multidimensionality of the process of cultural adaptation and how this process may nega-

DISPLAY 19-3
Cultural Explanations for Benefits to Health

- Persons with low levels of acculturation maintain their indigenous culture's dietary practices, which leads to better nutrition (less sodium, less fat, more fruits and vegetables, etc).

- Value systems of the indigenous culture promote healthy lifestyles (no/little smoking or alcohol consumption).

- Migrants bring with them or join extended family support networks that buffer the stress generated by the host culture. Apparently, the longer the individual lives in the United States, the more their family and social supports appear to weaken.

- Selective migrant processes. Those that immigrate are healthier.

tively affect an individual health. More research is needed to develop a clear understanding of the impact of acculturation (including many ways to measure it) and to document whether the adoption of high-risk behaviors is more related to the poverty and low socioeconomic status of minority groups.

Summary

Latino women are experiencing serious health problems, and access to health care continues to be difficult for them. Furthermore, the process of adaptation and acculturation of immigrants to the American society may worsen their health.

Latinos with the worst health status and with the poorest access to medical services live in extreme poverty. The proposed welfare reform in Congress may further eliminate health and social programs for poor women and children. All of these suggest a strong association between poor health and poverty.

In examining Latino women's health we need to acknowledge that traditionally women's emotional, social, legal, and medical needs have been neglected in our society. Women as a group must continue their efforts to obtain social justice and equality, particularly in health care.

Recommendations

Health care providers and policymakers must give the proper attention to the special needs of Latino women in all aspects, particularly in the area of health. They must consider the tremendous diversity of this population, in terms of national origin, age, socioeconomic status, level of education, assimilation and acculturation into the mainstream society, and geographic distribution.

Long-term institutional and structural changes are needed to deal effectively with the health problems of Latino women. Social changes must occur in our society to minimize poverty and to improve levels of education and income among Latinos. We cannot properly address the health needs of Latino women unless we address the social and economic inequalities that women confront in this society.

More research and data are needed on Latino women's health. Despite a gradual increase of data on Latino women, tremendous gaps exist. We do not have sufficient epidemiologic data on their health status and on their health service use patterns. Likewise, there is little information on the health status of women from Central or South American origins. Research needs to be conducted with the active participation of Latino women in the planning and implementation process, ideally with a Latino woman as Principal Investigator or Project Director.

There is a need to study health care finances and issues of managed care as they relate to health outcomes and access to health care services for Latino women, particularly specialized services and hospitalization, for those enrolled in managed care plans. Part of this process should include analyses of the marketing strategies being used by representatives of managed care organizations in recruiting Latino women.

Efforts should be made to reduce sociocultural barriers to health care for Latino women. Some of the aspects to be examined are:

- financial barriers (eg, cost of services, health insurance coverage—private as opposed to government sponsored)
- characteristics of the regular source of health care (eg, private as opposed to public)
- inconveniences of health care (eg, clinic hours, appointment system, staff composition)

Because Latino teens are increasingly becoming sexually active, more programs are needed to educate Latino adolescents of both sexes about issues of sexuality, family planning methods including abstinence, and the social and medical implications of teen pregnancy. More importantly, Latino youths, particularly females, need assistance to increase their communication, decision-making, and negotiation skills regarding when, how, and under what circumstances they will become sexually active.

More programs are needed at the community level that could provide the necessary support (eg, mental health programs, training programs, day-care services) and financial assistance to Latino women who are female heads of households. Help is needed to break the cycle of poverty for women and their children, and to reduce the level of stress that results from these and other factors.

Policies, programs, and funding for HIV/AIDS must be responsive to the needs of Latino women. Funds for prevention and education should be directed to the Latino communities. Despite the fact that we are now in the second decade of the HIV/AIDS epidemic, Latino communities are just beginning to be exposed to HIV/AIDS education and prevention activities. Many Latino women, particularly the poor or migrants, or those living in small communities in the Midwest, have not been reached at all. For these populations already lacking access to medical care in general, HIV and AIDS is not a "chronic manageable disease" but a fatal condition.

Prevention and education remain the only effective tools in the fight against AIDS; they are inexpensive and cost-effective ways to fight the epidemic. In addition to prevention and early detection of HIV, we need a continuum of care policy that in a holistic way will combine treatment and rehabilitation.

More alcohol and drug treatment programs are needed for Latino women addicted to drugs. There are practically no culturally appropriate, gender-specific, and affordable programs for female adolescents and adult women who are dependent on alcohol and other drugs. There is a need to strongly advocate for more treatment slots for pregnant women with alcohol and drug addiction. These women tend to be excluded from drug treatment programs.

Public health and social policies that promote the prosecution of women who use alcohol and drugs during the pregnancy should be reexamined. A series of legal and ethical controversies have emerged regarding alcohol and drug use during pregnancy. There has been an increasing debate on whether women who use drugs during their pregnancy should be criminally prosecuted for their conduct. Criminalization of drug use during pregnancy may lead pregnant Latino women who are drug users to either delay their entry into the medical care system or not to use the system at all for prenatal care because of fears of prosecution or of removal of the child after birth. These actions would neither serve the baby nor the mother's health.

Finally, Giachello (1995a) provides a series of specific policy recommendations aimed at changing the culture that prevails in the health care delivery system so health services will be more relevant and culturally sensitive to women of color.

References

Aday, L. A., Anderson, R. M., & Fleming, G. V. (1980). *Health care in the US: Equitable for whom?* Beverly Hills, CA: Sage.

Amaro, H. (1987). Hispanic women and mental health. *Psychology of Women Quarterly, 11,* 93-40.

American Cancer Society. (1991). *Cancer facts and figures for minority Americans.* Washington, DC: Author.

American Diabetes Association. (1992). *Diabetes 1991 vital statistics.* Washington, DC: Author.

American Sociological Association (ASA; 1990). Sex biases in sociological research. *Journal of the American Sociological Association.*

Anderson, R. M., Giachello, A. L., & Aday, L. A. (1986). Access of Hispanics to health care and cuts in services: A state-of-the-art overview. *Public Health Reports, 101,* 238-252.

Aponte, R., & Giachello, A. L. (1989). *Health care provider's knowledge, attitudes, and practices about Hispanics in Chicago: Analyses of a 1988 citywide survey.* Chicago: Hispanic Health Alliance.

Arredondo, R., Weddige R. L., Justice, C. L., & Fitz, J. (1987). Alcoholism in Mexican-Americans: Intervention and treatment. *Hospital and Community Psychiatry, 138,* 180-183.

Arrom, J. O. (1993, March 13). *Issues of research and data regarding Hispanics/Latinos in the Midwest.* Paper presented at the Surgeon General's Regional Meeting on Hispanic/Latino Health. Chicago: Midwest Hispanic AIDS Coalition.

Bloom, B. (1990). Health insurance and medical care: Health of our nation's children, United States. 1988. *Advance data from vital and health statistics* (p. 188). Hyattsville, MD: National Center for Health Statistics.

Bracho de Carpio, A., Carpio-Cedraro, F., & Anderson, L. (1993, September 27). *Latino female poverty and HIV prevention: An overspoken and undeveloped link.* Presented at the UCLA Latino Health Services Research Conference.

Carrillo, E., & Torres, M. I. (1988). *Risk factor prevalence among Hispanics; A literature review.* Presented at the COSSMHO Conference, New York, NY.

Centers for Disease Control and Prevention (1990a). *Sexually transmitted disease report.* Atlanta, GA: National Center for Infectious Diseases.

Centers for Disease Control and Prevention. (1990b). *HIV/AIDS surveillance report: U.S. AIDS cases reported through June 1990.* Atlanta, GA: Center for Infections Diseases, Division of HIV/AIDS.

Centers for Disease Control and Prevention. (1993a). *HIV/AIDS surveillance report: U.S. AIDS cases reported through September 1993*. Atlanta, GA: Center for Infectious Diseases, Division of HIV/AIDS.

Centers for Disease Control and Prevention (1995a). *HIV/AIDS surveillance report: U.S. AIDS cases reported through December 1994*. Atlanta, GA: Center for Infectious Diseases, Division of HIV/AIDS.

Christian, C. M., Zobeck, T. S., & Martin, H. J. (1985). Self-reported drinking behavior among Mexican-Americans: Some preliminary findings. *U.S. Public Health Conference on Records and Statistics*. Washington, DC: U.S. Public Health Service.

Cooper, R., Steinhauer, M., Miller, W., David, R., & Schatzkin, A. (1981). Racism society and disease: An exploration of the social and biological mechanisms of differential mortality. *International Journal of Health Services, 11* (3).

Eager, R. (1985). Epidemiology and clinical factors of *Chlamydia trachomatis* in black, Hispanic and white adolescents. *Western Journal of Medicine, 143,* 457-462.

Estrada, A. L., Trevino, F. M., & Ray, L. A. (1990). Health care utilization barriers among Mexican-Americans: Evidence from HHANES 1982–84. *American Journal of Public Health, 80* (12 Suppl.), 27-31.

Flegal, K. M., Ezzati, T. M., Harris, M. I., et al. (1991). Prevalence of diabetes in Mexican Americans, Cubans, and Puerto Ricans from the Hispanic Health and Nutrition Examination Survey, 1982–1984. *Diabetes Care, 14* (Suppl. 3), 628-638.

Garcia, R., Salcedo-Gonzalez, I., & Giachello, A. L. (1985). *Access to health care and other social indicators among Hispanics in Chicago*. Chicago: Latino Institute.

Giachello, A. L. (1985). Hispanics and health care. In P. Cafferty & W. McCready (Eds.), *Hispanics in the U.S.: The new social agenda*. Brunswick, NJ: Transaction Books.

Giachello, A. L. (1988). *Self-care behavior among Hispanics, blacks and whites in the United States: Analysis of national data*. Doctoral dissertation, University of Chicago, Chicago, IL.

Giachello, A. L. (1991, Summer). Women and substance abuse and HIV/AIDS. *Common ground*. Chicago: Illinois Prevention Resource Center.

Giachello, A. L. (1993). *Issues of recruitment and retention of Hispanic/Latino women in clinical studies*. Testimony presented at public hearings, Office of Research on Women's Health, March 29-30.

Giachello, A. L. (1994a). Maternal/perinatal health issues. In C. W. Molina & M. Aguirre-Molina (Eds.), *Latino health in the U.S.: A growing challenge*. Washington, DC: American Public Health Association.

Giachello, A. L. (1994b). Issues of access and use. In C. W. Molina & M. Aguirre-Molina (Eds.), *Latino health in the U.S.: A growing challenge*. Washington, DC: American Public Health Association.

Giachello, A. L. (1995a). Cultural diversity and institutional inequality. In D. L. Adams (Ed.), *Health issues for women of color: A cultural diversity perspective*. Thousand Oaks, CA: Sage.

Giachello, A. L. (1995b). Latino women. In M. Bayne-Smith (Ed.), *Race, gender, and health*. Thousand Oaks, CA: Sage.

Giachello, A. L. (in press). Cancer among women of Central and South American origins. In *Cancer and women of color*. Special Publication of the National Cancer Institute. Washington, DC: U.S. Department of Health and Human Services.

Giachello, A. L., & Aponte, R. (1989). *Health status and access issues of Hispanic children and adolescents in Chicago: Analyses of a 1984 citywide survey*. Chicago: Hispanic Health Alliance.

Giachello, A. L., & Arrom, J. O. (1989). *Access to health care among Hispanics, blacks and whites in the Northwest Side of Chicago*. Chicago: Hispanic Health Alliance.

Gleeney, K., Glassman, S., Cox, S., & Brown, H. (1988). The prevalence of positive test results for *Chlamydia trachomatis* by direct smear from fluorescent antibodies in a South Texas family planning population. *Journal of Reproductive Medicine, 33* (6), 457-462.

Gregory, K. (1978). Transcultural medicine: Treating Hispanic patients. *Behavioral Medicine, 5,* 22-29.

Haan, M., Kaplan, G., & Camacho, T. (1987). Poverty and health: Prospective evidence from the Alameda County study. *American Journal of Epidemiology, 125* (6).

Hispanic Health Council. (1989). *Puertorriquenas: Sociodemographics, health and reproductive issues among Puerto Rican women in the United States. A fact handbook*. Hartford, CT: Author.

Hixson, J. (1993). *Racism in research*. Paper presented at the annual meeting of the National Association of Perinatal Addiction Research and Education, Chicago.

Holck, S. E., Warren, C. W., Smith, J. C., & Rochat, R. W. (1984). Alcohol consumption among Mexican-Americans and Anglo women: Results of survey along the US-Mexican border. *Journal of Studies in Alcohol, 45,* 49-154.

Holmes, K. K., Karon, J. N., & Kreiss, J. (1990). The increasing frequency of heterosexuality acquired AIDS in the Unites States. *American Journal of Public Health, 80* (7), 858-863.

Illinois Department of Public Health, & Howe, H. L. (1995). *Gender differences in assaults and violent acts in the workplace United States, 1993* (Series 95, p. 3). Springfield, IL: Illinois Department of Public Health, Division of Epidemiologic Studies.

Kochanek, K. D., & Hudson, B. L. (1994). Advance report of final mortality statistics. *Monthly Vital Statistics Report, 43* (6 Suppl.). Hyattsville, MD: National Center for Health Statistics.

Lamberty, G. (1994). *Infant mortality experience of Hispanics.* Paper presented to the National Advisory Committee on Infant Mortality.

Leon, A., Mazur, R., Montalvo, E., & Rodriguez, M. (1984). Self-help support groups for Hispanic mothers. *Child Welfare, 63,* 261-268.

Lipton, R., Losey, L., Giachello, A. L., & Mendez, J. (in press). Factors affecting diabetes treatment and patient education among Latinos: Results of a preliminary study in Chicago. *Journal of Medical Systems.*

Manley, A., Lin-Fu, J., Miranda, M., Noonan, A., & Parker, T. (1984). *Special health concerns of ethnic minority women.* Commissioned paper. Rockville, MD: Health Resources and Services Administration.

Maxwell, B., & Jacobson, M. (1989). *Marketing disease to Hispanics: The selling of alcohol, tobacco, and junk foods.* Washington DC: Center for Science in the Public Interest.

McKenzie, N., Bilofsky, E., & Sharon, L. (1992, Summer). Women and the health care system. *Health/PAC Bulletin.*

Miller, S. (1987). Race in the health of America. *The Milbank Quarterly, 65* (Suppl. 2).

Moran, J. S., Aral S. O., Jenkins W. C., Peterman, T. A., & Alexander, E. R. (1989). The impact of sexually transmitted diseases on minority populations. *Public Health Reports, 104* (6), 560-565.

National Center for Health Statistics. (1995). Advance report of final mortality statistics, 1992. *Monthly Vital Statistics Report, 43* (6), Suppl., March 22. Hyattsville, MD: Author.

National Coalition of Hispanic Health and Human Services Organizations. (COSSMHO; 1990). *And access for all Medicaid and Hispanics.* Washington, DC: Author.

National Coalition of Hispanic Health and Human Services Organizations. (COSSMHO; 1992). *The state of Hispanic health.* Washington, DC: Author.

National Council of La Raza. (1992). *Health promotion fact sheet: Hispanic women's health status.* Washington, DC: Author.

National Council of La Raza. (1993). *State of Hispanic America 1993: Toward a Latino anti-poverty agenda.* Policy Analysis Center, Office of Research, Advocacy, and Legislation. Washington, DC: Author.

National Council of La Raza. (1994). *What the 1990 census tells us about women: A state factbook.* Washington, DC: Author.

National Council of La Raza. (1995). Injecting drug use and HIV/AIDS in the Hispanic community. Fact sheet. Washington, DC: Author.

National Heart, Lung and Blood Institute. (1992). *Fact sheet on cardiovascular conditions on minority population.* Bethesda, MD: Author.

National Institute on Drug Abuse (NIDA; 1987). *Use of selected drugs among Hispanics: Mexican Americans, Puerto Ricans, and Cuban Americans. Findings from the Hispanic health and nutrition examination.* Washington, DC: Author.

Novick, L., Glebatis, D., Stricof, R., et al. (1991). Newborn seroprevalence study: Methods and results. *American Journal of Public Health, 81* (Suppl.), 15-21.

Office of Research on Women's Health. (1992). *Summary report.* Hunt Valley, MD: Author.

Putsch, R. W., III. (1985). Cross-cultural communication: The special case of interpreters in health care. *Journal of the American Medical Association, 254,* 3344-3348.

Quesada, G., & Heller, P. (1977). Sociocultural barriers to medical care among Mexican-Americans in Texas: A summary report by the Southwest Medical Sociology Ad Hoc Committee. *Medical Care, 15,* 93-101.

Ramirez, A. G., Valdez, R. B., Carter-Pokras, O. (1994). Cancer. In C. W. Molina & M. Aguirre-Molina (Eds.), *Latino health in the US: A growing challenge.* Washington DC: American Public Health Association.

Robert Wood Johnson Foundation. (1983). *Update report on access to health care for the American people. Special Report, 1.* Princeton, NJ: Author.

Robert Wood Johnson Foundation. (1987). *Access to health care in the United States: Results of a 1986 survey. Special Report, 2.* Princeton, NJ: Author.

Rodriguez-Trias H., & Ramirez de Arellano, A. B. (1994). The health of children and youth. In C. W. Molina & M. Aguirre-Molina (Eds.), *Latino health in the U.S.: A growing challenge*. Washington, DC: American Public Health Association.

Selick, R. M., Castro, K. G., & Pappaioanou, M. (1988). Racial/ethnic differences in the risk of AIDS in the United States. *American Journal of Public Health, 78,* 1539-1544.

Smith, P., Mild, J., Truman, B., et al. (1991). HIV infection among women entering the New York State correctional system. *American Journal of Public Health, 81,* 35-39.

Smith, P. B., Phillips, L. E., Faro, S., McGill, L., & Wait, R. B. (1988). Predominant sexually transmitted diseases among different ages and ethnic groups of indigent sexually active adolescents attending a family planning clinic. *Journal of Adolescent Health Care, 9,* 291-295.

Solis, J. L., et al. (1990). Acculturation, access to care, and use of preventive services by Hispanics: Findings from HHANES 1982–1984. *American Journal of Public Health, 80* (12 Suppl.), 27-31.

Stricof, R. L., Kennedy, J. T., Nuttell, T. M., Weisfuse, I. V., & Novick, L. F. (1991). HIV seroprevalence in a facility for runaway and homeless adolescents. *American Journal of Public Health, 81,* 50-53.

Stroup, M., Trevino, F. M., & Trevino, D. (1988). Alcohol consumption patterns among Mexican-American mothers and children from single and dual-headed households. *American Journal of Public Health, 80* (Suppl.), 36-41.

Treviño, F. M., Moyer, M. E., Burciaga Valdez, R., & Stroup-Benham, C. A. (1991). Health insurance coverage and utilization of health services by Mexican Americans, mainland Puerto Ricans, and Cuban Americans. *Journal of the American Medical Association, 265* (2), 233-237.

Treviño, F. M., & Rendón, M. I. (1994). Mental illness/mental health issues. In C. W. Molina & M. Aguirre-Molina (Eds.), *Latino health in the U.S.: A growing challenge*. Washington, DC: American Public Health Association.

Turner, C. F. (1989). Research on sexual behaviors that transmit HIV: Progress and problems. *AIDS, 3* (Suppl. 1), 563-569.

U.S. Bureau of the Census. (1986). Projections of the Hispanic population: 1983 to 2080 (series P-25, No. 995). Washington, DC: Author.

U.S. Bureau of the Census (1994). The Hispanic population in the United States, March 1993. *Current population reports* (series P-20, No. 475). Washington, DC: U.S. Government Printing Office..

U.S. Department of Health and Human Services. (1986). Reports of the Secretary' Task Force on Black and Minority Health (Vols. 1-8). Washington, DC: U.S. Government Printing Office.

U.S. Department of Health and Human Services. (1990). *Health status of the disadvantaged chartbook 1990* (Publication No. HRSA-HRS-P-DV 90-1). Washington, DC: U.S. Government Printing Office.

U.S. General Accounting Office. (1992). *Hispanic access to health care: Significant gaps exist* (GAO/PEMD 92-6). Washington, DC: U.S. Government Printing Office.

U.S. Office of the Surgeon General. (1993). *One voice, one vision–Recommendations to the Surgeon General to improve Hispanic/Latino health*. Surgeon General's National Hispanic/Latino Health Initiative. Washington, DC: U.S. Government Printing Office.

U.S. House of Representatives Select Committee on Aging. (1992). Diabetes: Threat to the health of Hispanics. A Congressional report based on public hearings. Washington, DC.

Valdez, R. B., Morganstern, H., Brown, E. R., Wyn, R., Wang, C., & Cumberland, W. (1991). Insuring Latinos against cost of illness. *Journal of the American Medical Association, 269* (7), 889-894.

Valdez, R. B., Giachello, A. L., Rodriguez-Trias, H., Gomez, P., & de La Rocha, C. (1993). Improving access to health care in Latino communities. *Public Health Reports, 103* (5), 534-538.

Ventura, S. J. (1993). Maternal and infant health characteristics of births to US and foreign-born Hispanic mothers. Presented at the 121st Annual Meeting of the American Public Health Association. October 24-28, 1993, San Francisco.

Ventura, S. J., Martin, J. A., Taffel, S. M., Mathews, T. J., Clarke, S. (1995). Advance report of final natality statistics, 1993. *Monthly Vital Statistical Report, 44*(3 Suppl.). Hyattsville, MD: National Center for Health Statistics.

Woolhandler, S., Himmelstein, D., Silber, R., Bader, M., Harnly, M., & Jones, A. (1985). Medical care and mortality: Racial differences in preventable deaths. *International Journal of Health Services, 15* (1).

Zambrana, R. E., & Ellis, B. K. (1995). Contemporary research issues in Hispanic/Latino women's health. In D. Adams (Ed.), *Health issues for women of color: A cultural diversity perspective*. Thousand Oaks, CA: Sage.

CHAPTER 20

American Indian Women

Linda Burhansstipanov
Martha Tenney
Connie Dresser

Many positive, culturally relevant, constructive efforts are occurring throughout Indian Country that are likely to increase the number of well women and well communities. Increasingly, native peoples are finding ways to celebrate and enhance wellness. This chapter addresses the demographic "reality" of Native American women's health and identifies selected cultural strengths and ways that people have incorporated these strengths into current successful interventions that affect Indian women's health and wellness. It is our intent to identify the positive strengths and celebrate what is right as Indian women are reclaiming their wellness.

Overall Health Status of American Indian Women

Before describing American Indian women's health, the following is a brief summary of selected Indian demographics. Approximately 1.9 million people (0.8% of the U.S. population) were self-identified as American Indians and Alaska Natives on the 1990 U.S. Census (U.S. Bureau of the Census, 1992a) In 1988, the Bureau of Indian Affairs *Federal Register* listed and recognized approximately 500 tribes of Native People in the United States. There are 314 federal reservations and trust lands, 217 Alaska Native village statistical areas, 12 Alaska Native regional corporations, and 17 tribal jurisdiction statistical areas (previously referred to as the "historic areas of Oklahoma, excluding urbanized areas") (U.S. Bureau of the Census, 1992b). The 1990 Census indicates that only 19.8% of all American Indians live on federal reservations and approximately two-thirds of the population reside in urban areas. The median age of the American Indian population is 26 years (U.S. median age is 33 years) (U.S. Bureau of the Census, 1993). From 1986 to 1988, the life expectancy at birth for nine of the Indian Health Service (IHS) areas (including Alaska) was 70.1 years, which is 4.9 years less than the 1987 estimate of 75.0 for "U.S. All Races" population (U.S. Department of Health and Human Services [DHHS], 1992b).

Although many Native Peoples continue to acknowledge the traditional perspective of respect for Indian women, the well-being of Indian women dropped significantly during this century. The leading causes of death for 1987 to 1989 (DHHS,

1993) for American Indian women follow (the numbers in parentheses represent the mortality rate per 100,000 women):

- diseases of the heart (97.8)
- malignant neoplasms (73.1)
- accidents (43.9)
- diabetes mellitus (26.7)
- cerebrovascular diseases (24.0)
- chronic liver disease and cirrhosis (21.1)
- pneumonia and influenza (17.9)
- certain conditions originating in the perinatal period (8.4)
- chronic obstructive pulmonary diseases and allied conditions (8.4)
- nephritis, nephrotic syndrome, and nephrosis (8.3)

According to the IHS Indian Women's Health Care Consensus Statement, Indian women suffered disproportionately from diseases related to lifestyle and premature deaths, and the significant Indian women health issues were cancer, diabetes, obstetric/gynecologic issues, alcoholism and substance abuse, family violence, elderly care issues, and access to care.

Cancer

American Indians and Alaska Natives continue to experience low cancer incidence rates in comparison with other racial groups such as Caucasian Americans, African Americans, and Asians. However, within the last few generations, cancer has become the leading cause of death for Alaska Native women and is the second leading cause of death among American Indian women (DHHS, 1992a; Valway, Kileen, Paisano, & Oritz, 1992).

According to the New Mexico Surveillance, Epidemiology, and End Results (SEER) Registry (1977–1983), American Indian women *living in New Mexico and Arizona* have incidence rates for stomach, cervix uteri, primary liver, and gallbladder cancers that are higher than for the U.S. female population. American Indian women experience excessive mortality rates from cervical and gallbladder cancers when compared with SEER Caucasian American female rates (DHHS, 1992c).

Although cancer incidence and mortality rates appear to be lower among American Indian women than most other racial groups, the survival from all cancer sites combined among American Indian women is the *poorest* of any other racial or ethnic group, for example, African Americans, Caucasian Americans, and Hispanics (Horner, 1990). Compared with non-Indian peoples in the Southwest, even when cancer is diagnosed in early stages (ie, stage II), when stage at diagnosis and treatment are considered, survival from cancer for American Indians is poor (Samet, Key, Hunt, & Goodwin, 1987). Such assessments are made in light of statistical limitations in cancer data for Native Americans, which could result in significant underreporting of both incidence and mortality rates and survival percentages.

There is great variation in cancer sites depending on the tribe and geographic regions. In general, the most common cancer mortality sites (1977–1983) among

American Indian women are: lung (18.1), colon and rectum (9), breast (9), stomach (5.8), cervix (5.5), pancreas (4.6), kidney and renal pelvis (2.7), liver (2.0), and oral cavity/pharynx (1.8) (Burhansstipanov & Dresser, 1993). Despite the data limitations, when the data are broken down by Native American subgroup, a dramatically different picture emerges. For example, Alaska Native women had the highest age-adjusted (1970 standard) mortality rates (ie, number of cases per 100,000) of any racial or ethnic group (eg, Caucasian Americans, African Americans) for cancers of the colon and rectum (27.2), cervix uteri (12.5), pancreas (10.3), oral cavity/pharynx (6.3), gallbladder (6.3), and kidney and renal pelvis (4.4) (Burhansstipanov & Dresser, 1993).

In general, Native Americans in the southwestern part of the country have lower cancer mortality rates than do Indians living in the northern part of the country (Valway et al., 1992). However, there are significant variations in the cancer rates for different tribes and IHS areas. For example, the age-adjusted cervical cancer mortality rate for Indian women in the Phoenix IHS area was 12.8 and for Indian women in Billings IHS area 10.7. In comparison, the "U.S. All Races" (1988) rate was 2.7 (DHHS, 1994). Another example of regional variability is illustrated in Figure 20-1.

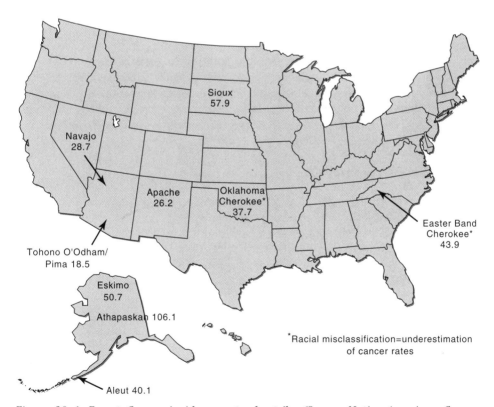

Figure 20-1. Breast Cancer incidence rates by tribe. (Source: Native American Cancer Research Program, AMC Cancer Research Center, Denver, Colorado)

Diabetes

Diabetes is the eighth leading cause of mortality among American Indians, both sexes. However, it is the fifth leading cause of death among American Indian women and is the third most frequent reason for medical visits to IHS outpatient clinics nationally (DHHS, 1991). Diabetes among some tribes is five times the rate of Caucasian Americans. The Pima Indians of Arizona have the highest incidence of non–insulin-dependent diabetes mellitus (NIDDM or type II) in the world (Chamberlain, 1990). By age 35, over 50% of the adult Pima population have NIDDM. Of the Indian people who were diagnosed with diabetes in 1987 in Oklahoma IHS facilities, 63.1% were women (Clark, 1988). Complications from diabetes are also present among the tribes. In a 1987 study of Navajo pregnancies, 6.1% were identified as having gestational diabetes as compared with 1% to 3% for Caucasian Americans and African Americans. Among the mothers who developed gestational diabetes, approximately 60% will develop overt diabetes within 16 years after delivery (Massion et al., 1987; DHHS, 1991). According to the 1987 study, approximately half (51.3%) of the diabetes-related amputations performed in Oklahoma were to Indian women and there was a 70% probability that after a leg amputation, a diabetic will have the second leg amputated within 5 years (Dye, Henderson, & Jones, 1990). The incidence of end-stage renal disease (ESRD) in Native Americans attributable to diabetes rose 16.8% per year from one 3-year period (1984–1986) to the next 3-year period (1987–1989) and the age-adjusted incidence of ESRD for Native Americans was 2.8-fold that for Caucasian Americans (Lee et al., 1994).

The IHS Indian Women's Round Table Steering Committee identified model programs, such as "Three Sisters" at Winnebago and the Dialysis Unit at Turtle Mountain, which had effectively educated Native communities about the complications of diabetes. To effectively prevent diabetes, they suggest that community-based programs need to teach about commodity foods, poverty diets, exercise, and conscientious foot care.

Obstetric/Gynecologic Issues

The American Indian and Alaska Native birth rate for 1987 through 1989 was 28.8 births per 1000 women, which was 81% higher than the "U.S. All Races" birth rate for 1988 of 15.9, and nearly double the rate for the U.S. Caucasian population (14.7) (DHHS, 1993). Forty-five percent of Indian mothers were under age 20 when they had their first child compared with 24% of "U.S. All Races" mothers who were under age 20 (DHHS, 1993; IWRT Final Report, 1991). The infant mortality rate for American Indians and Alaska Natives was 11.0 in 1987 to 1989 (the Caucasian American rate was 8.5) (DHHS, 1993). The leading cause of infant death (birth to under 1 year of age) for American Indians and Alaska Natives (1987–1989) was sudden infant death syndrome with a rate of 2.8 deaths per 1000 live births, as compared with U.S. Caucasian rate of 1.2 (DHHS, 1993). However, the leading reason for female outpatient visits to IHS facilities and tribal and contracted health services was prenatal care (DHHS, 1993).

American Indian women are reported to have more sexually transmitted diseases (STDs) than the general population (DHHS, 1991). STD rates are an indicator for "unsafe sex" and transmission of human immunodeficiency virus (HIV). The numbers of American Indians and Alaska Natives who are infected with HIV are growing every day. Of the over 360,000 U.S. cases of acquired immunodeficiency syndrome (AIDS) (December 1993), 818 are American Indian and Alaska Natives. It is not known how many additional Native people are infected with HIV (National Native American AIDS Prevention Center, 1994). Native women are contracting AIDS at a higher rate than Caucasian women. Although women represent 6% of the AIDS cases among Caucasian Americans, American Indian women represent 14% of AIDS cases among Native Americans (Centers for Disease Control and Prevention, 1993).

Alcoholism

Today's Native woman, aged 15 to 24 experiences an age-specific alcoholism death rate that exceeds the Indian male rate by 40% (Indian Women's Health Care Round Table [IWHCRT], 1991). It has been estimated that 95% of American families are affected either directly or indirectly by a family member's alcohol abuse (Rhoades, Hammond, Welty, Handler, & Amler, 1987). Approximately 75% of all unintentional injuries and accidents are alcohol related, and 54% of those injuries and accidents involve motor vehicle crashes (DHHS, 1993). Table 20-1 lists alcoholism mortality rates.

Fleming, Manson, and Engs (1990) identified the following reasons to explain why Indian women become alcohol and drug abusers:

- cultural disruption
- loss of social controls
- prejudice
- poverty
- role reversals
- peer group dynamics
- familiar socialization
- decreased self-worth and alienation

Another frequently cited reason for alcohol and drug abuse is having been a victim of sexual abuse.

Table 20-1. Alcoholism Mortality Rates Among Native Women

Age Group	American Indian ♀	U.S. Caucasian ♀
15–24	3.1	0.1
25–34	21.2	1.1
35–44	39.7	3.3
45–54	68.0	6.8
55–64	71.7	10.0
65–74	38.8	7.9
75–84	14.4	4.2
85+	19.4	1.1

Family Violence

Family violence is not a Native American tradition. Violence has probably evolved from a combination of the following:

- cultural role changes
- values related to Christian influence
- off-reservation boarding school policies that contribute to deterioration of the family structure
- introduction of alcohol
- history of oppression

These factors influence appropriate behavior choices (IWHCRT, 1991). According to the Indian Adolescent Health Survey, approximately 9% of the Indian young women had been sexually abused and 8% had been physically abused (Office of Technology Assessment, 1990). According to the IHS Indian Women's Health Care Round Table Consensus Statement, family violence, substance abuse, and child neglect increase dramatically during the beginning of each month when the welfare or land lease checks are received (IWHCRT, 1991). The majority of family violence (eg, spousal abuse, child abuse, incest) is alcohol related. Since fiscal year 1987, injury prevention services have increased by 162% and in fiscal year 1991, nearly 50,000 services were provided (DHHS, 1993). Although many of those services involve motor vehicle accidents and a variety of other accidents, the numbers of family abuse victims were also included within those data.

Elder Issues

According to almost every tribes' traditional social structures, elders are cherished as resources of vast knowledge and experience. It is expected that they will help educate the young about tribal practices, histories, and ceremonies, information that is verbally passed from one generation to another (Burhansstipanov & Dresser, 1993). Elders are the greatest wealth and natural resource among Indian peoples. Unfortunately, some contemporary Indian communities have adapted the popular American culture's negative attitudes toward the old...to be disrespectful, pushed aside for younger, more aggressive individuals, and therefore, "neglect" people who by their wisdom and experience are great treasures to the cultures. This contemporary attitude is unacceptable within traditional Indian cultures and is currently being challenged within many tribal communities.

Perhaps the most impressive example of "remembering" the respect that is due to elders has been exemplified by the development of a national center. Early in 1994, the Administration on Aging funded the Native Elder Health Care Resource Center (NEHCRC) to be a national resource center for older American Indians, Alaska Natives, and Native Hawaiians, with special emphasis on culturally competent health care. Its mission is to promote the health and well-being of older American Indians, Alaska Natives, and Native Hawaiians by increasing cultural competence among health care professionals and paraprofessionals who plan, administer, and provide relevant services to these populations. The NEHCRC is located at the National Center for American Indian and Alaska Native Mental Health Research in Denver, Colorado. Telecommunications and print media are used to increase awareness of and access to program activities, information resources, faculty, and fellow participants. The NEHCRC's work focuses on four themes:

- ascertaining health status and conditions
- improving practice standards
- increasing access to care
- mobilizing community resources

To obtain information or become involved within the NEHCRC computer network, the information specialist of NEHCRC can be contacted at the Department of Psychiatry, Campus Box A011-13, 4455 East Twelfth Avenue, Denver, Colorado 80220, (303) 372-3250 and fax (303) 372-3579.

Access to Care

The IHS was established under the Transfer Act of 1954 (Public Law 83-568). This act mandated that "all functions, responsibilities, authorities, and duties relating to the maintenance and operation of hospital and health facilities for Indians be administered by the Surgeon General of the U.S. Public Health Service." The IHS is responsible for providing medical services to American Indians and Alaska Natives living in the 33 reservation states.

Although American Indians and Alaska Natives are eligible to receive comprehensive health services free of charge from the IHS, over half of Native Peoples do not use IHS services. For those who do not take advantage of IHS facilities, the more common reasons are that they have medical insurance or that no IHS facility is accessible. For example, American Indians or Alaska Natives living in California (which is a reservation state and the state with the second largest number of Native Peoples) cannot use IHS facilities because there is no IHS hospital or clinic within the state. Individual Indian clinics receive small amounts of funding to provide services to Indians. Another example is in Colorado. Although 43% of the American Indian and Alaska Native population of Colorado lives in Denver, these Native Peoples are unlikely to use IHS facilities because the closest services are located on the Ute Reservation, 390 miles from Denver.

Although the IHS has the primary role of providing services, the IHS lacks sufficient budget, personnel, facilities, and resources to provide quality, comprehensive health care services *without collaboration* from other agencies and states. For example, breast cancer screening was assessed via the Survey of American Indians and Alaska Natives (SAIAN), as a subset of the National Medical Expenditure Survey by the Agency for Health Care Policy and Research. The SAIAN found that only 23% of the subjects reported ever having had a mammogram (Agency for Health Care Policy and Research, 1991). As of May 10, 1993, *nationwide* the IHS had a total of 14 dedicated mammography machines and only two IHS areas had contracts for mobile mammography services (Gwilt, 1993). Obviously, access to screening is an issue.

Budgetary and resource constraints within IHS result in additional problems related to access to state-of-the-art care. Many follow-up tests and services are not available from local IHS service units. The official federal policy is to place Indian patients on a "priority list" to transport them for follow-up services ("contract health services") as monies are available *as determined by Congress*. However, IHS policies are restricted by budgetary constraints that create frustrating situations for both providers and patients. For example, during January 1994 a Cheyenne woman (a 6-year breast cancer survivor) was diagnosed with what appeared to be tumorous growths on her knees. She needed to be referred to diagnostic services to another IHS facility. Compliant with IHS policy, she was placed on a priority list for contracted health services and was told that transportation monies would probably be available in about 9 months for her to receive those follow-up services. It is widely known that early treatment is essential for effective cancer treatment (Burhansstipanov & Tenney, 1995).

Economics, Culture, Health Beliefs, Values, and Practices

The 1990 Census indicates that 31% or 603,000 American Indians are living below the poverty level (national poverty rate is 13%). In 1989, 51% of the 437,431 American Indians residing on reservations and trust lands were living below the poverty level (U.S. Bureau of the Census, 1993) More than 20% of American Indian housing units on reservations and trust lands lacked complete plumbing facilities (eg, an indoor toilet).

World View

For Native American women, pride and strong cultural identity are the roots of health beliefs, values, and practices. Perhaps the easiest way to exemplify the world view is to paraphrase Cecelia Fire Thunder (Oglala Sioux Tribe) when she describes the way Native People pray. According to Fire Thunder, "First you pray for our brothers and sisters of all colors and from all four directions, from all continents. Second you pray for Native People, the people of your nation, your tribe, your clan, your band. Then you pray for your family and loved ones. Lastly you pray for yourself." All people are part of the balance and the relationships with Earth, Moon, Sky, and Spirits. Also apparent within this prayer is that women are the caretakers of others within the family and community. They frequently need to be reminded of how important it is for them to take care of themselves so that they may continue in this role of caretaker.

Wellness Beliefs

Native Americans do what they wish to do. "It is Indian people who are ultimately responsible for their own communities, and it is Indian people who will determine what level of health Indian people will achieve and maintain" (Stanford Center for

Research in Disease Prevention, 1992). Since 1985, Locust has prepared and disseminated summaries of tribal-specific health beliefs. Tribes have unique belief systems from one another. However, according to Locust (1985) *most* tribes have
common beliefs that influence health promotion programs (Display 20-1).

Indian culture must also be somewhat understood before the Indian woman can
be fully appreciated. According to Bennett (1992), "being Indian is more than checking the box for ethnic origin. It is a way of life, a way of being. The love for family, respect for your elders, spirituality, self-determination, integrity, pride,
understanding, protecting the environment, humor, and socializing are all the
essence of being Indian."

Traditional Lifestyles That Promote Health

During "wellness" discussions among Native Peoples, a common theme or concept
is "becoming healthy again." This concept refers to the many healthy lifestyles that
were practiced by different tribes, which helped prevent disease and promote health.
American Indians and Alaska Natives have traditionally cherished good health and
longevity. Health and the well-being of each tribal member was believed to determine the community's productivity (Reichard, 1963). A person in good health and
well-being was *in a state of beauty or harmony*. In this state, all parts of the body
functioned perfectly and exalted feelings of well-being were felt. A person not in a
"state of harmony" was considered either *sick or ill*. *Sickness* could be physical,
mental, social, spiritual, or environmental in nature. Physical sickness included

DISPLAY 20-1
Common Health Beliefs Among Native American Tribes

- Native Americans believe in a supreme creator.
- A person is a threefold being made up of the body, mind, and spirit.
- The spirit existed before it came into a physical body and will exist after the body dies.
- Plants and animals, like human beings, are part of the spirit world. The spirit world exists side by side and intermingles with the physical world.
- Wellness is harmony in body, mind, and spirit.
- Unwellness is caused by disharmony among the body, mind, and spirit.
- Natural unwellness is caused by the violation of a sacred or tribal taboo.
- Unnatural unwellness is caused by witchcraft (or "one who is on the bad side").
- Each of us is responsible for our own wellness.

colds, burns, skin rashes, conditions associated with the menstrual cycle and pregnancy, broken bones, and other similar occurrences. *Illness*, considered more serious than sickness, was disharmony caused by domestic strife, mental anguish, bad dreams, or misfortune (Levy, 1963). Illness came about slowly, lingered for a long time, and had no discernible cause or meaning (Clements, 1932).

Numerous tribes integrated health and sickness concepts with their basic religious precepts. These concepts defined their social origins, relationships with the Creator and the nature of the cosmos. Tribes believed that the Creator and the Spirits made the worlds and aided them in overcoming numerous environmental and social hardships. In addition, each act was related to a spiritual event that occurred in the past and therefore deserved its proper respect in the present. *Performing prescribed behaviors guaranteed them spiritual, social, and physical well-being* and trouble, of any kind, was a direct consequence of a breach of the "prescribed order" (Levy, 1963). Native Americans believed that either transgressions of prescribed behavior or evil spirits caused a person's disharmony, and that disharmony of any kind affected the entire community by removing the person from his or her functioning role (Reichard, 1963).

Theories of illness led to logical methods of curing. Some tribes believed that illness came from the meat of animals that had not been treated with proper respect (Swanton, 1931). Other tribes believed illness was the consequence of mistreating animals and that certain plants would counteract the conditions (Swanton, 1928). A person who could heal the body and spirit of others was revered. Native People believed that the healer was given power from the spirits and herbal medicines (Keely et al., 1982) because he or she had learned to control or counteract the negative powers from the human or spiritual world that caused illness. The healer often used song or chant to conquer negative spirits; thus, the healer's spoken words had incredible power at a time when Indian tribes had no written language (Reichard, 1963).

Most Native American tribes have communicated their attitudes about health and illness to younger generations through ceremonial participation and storytelling. As a result, the old attitudes about health, illness, and healing are held by most Native People today. However, some non-Native health care providers who treat the illnesses of these tribal communities do not know about or understand these attitudes. Many non-Native health care providers do not understand that the actions and reactions of their Native American patients are influenced by their cultural and religious beliefs (Levy, 1963).

Social Structure

Native cultures have strong social structures. The family is the focal point of most activities and practices. Within the family unit, the historical as well as contemporary perspective views a woman as highly esteemed because she gives the gift of life. The woman is typically the caretaker of the family who places the needs of family members before her own. Likewise, the man is traditionally viewed as the protector of the home and the local tribal community. Children are viewed as blessings from the Creator and are included in almost every tribal activity rather than being kept at home to be watched by nonfamily persons. Elders are respected for their wisdom and leadership. Each of these family member roles can be constructively integrated within a health program or project (Burhansstipanov & Dresser, 1993).

Cultural Strengths in Action: Defining What Works in Indian Country

Throughout Indian Country, the growing wellness and empowerment movement is based on the many cultural strengths of Native women. This section looks at the way that Native American people—especially women—have used these cultural strengths to enhance the promotion of well-being to others, thus defining "what works."

Cultural Strengths as Resources for Appropriate Interventions

The Traditional Perspective

Traditional perspectives of Native women have included many roles and responsibilities, such as peacekeeper, educator, healer, comforter, nurturer, gatherer, mother, elder, leader, and homemaker. A growing number of health programs are specifically focused on Indian women. The emphasis of these programs is that the woman be the *model* for her daughters, sisters, and other members of the community and that she practice good health behaviors so that she will be around to influence her family and community. In general, Indian women tend to be less responsive to health or wellness messages that are geared to the individual woman's well-being. For example, a health message such as, "You need to have an annual Pap smear," tends to have little impact on health behavior. Within the cultural context described earlier, this message can be interpreted to be somewhat "selfish" for the woman to think only of herself rather than what her children, family, and community need. An example of a cultural message is one delivered by a grandchild, "Grandmother, please take care of yourself and have your health tests so that I can continue to learn from you."

In general, there is a tremendous amount of variability among the 500+ federally recognized tribes in the U.S. and, as a result, women's *roles within each tribe differ*. Naturally, even within the same tribe, women will have their own personalities and characteristics. Even so, it has been demonstrated that when the women accept and promote a concept, their influence is reflected within the home and community.

Intergenerational Education

The wisdom of the elders in Native American communities is highly regarded. Intergenerational education typically works well within Indian community, such as Indian teens teaching about HIV and AIDS to elders, or elders teaching younger women about tobacco cessation. Likewise, Natives teaching Natives is more easily accepted than are non-Natives who wish to implement health programs within the community. Non-Natives can be well accepted within Indian community, but the non-Natives need to establish trust between themselves and the community, usually requiring an investment of time and patience.

Talking Circles

Talking Circles are traditional cultural practices to provide a forum that is designed to heal, resolve, and support participants. Only honesty and truth are allowed within the Circle and individuals are able to express their thoughts and feelings about an issue without fear of interruption or aggression. Talking Circles may be limited to people who share the same experience, such as victims of abuse or assault. Other Talking Circles may be with students sharing their challenges (ie, dealing with the challenges of being the only Indian in a college program). Many Talking Circles help heal the spirit and the heart so that the individual can let go of former grievances and move on to a more positive place in life. Other Talking Circles are being used as support groups, for example, for cervical cancer survivors (Center for American Indian Research and Education; see list of additional resources).

Traditional Healing

Traditional healing is still practiced and respected by most Native cultures. Traditional healing involves treating the body, mind, and spirit of the individual in addition to the symptoms and physical manifestations. Diseases that are regarded to be "white man's diseases" (eg, diabetes or cancer) usually do not have traditional treatments because the diseases did not exist in sufficient numbers or were not recognized to warrant a treatment until recent years. Traditional healers and medical doctors occasionally work cooperatively with one another and are greeted with great welcome and relief by Native patients (Burhansstipanov & Dresser, 1993).

Storytelling

Storytelling is the traditional manner of recording Indian heritage (Caduto & Bruchac, 1991). Storytelling can also be used as a manner of support. It has been used to help others who experience a particular problem. For example, the Native American Cancer Research Consortium of California and Colorado has been working with Native American cancer survivors to share their stories of living through a cancer diagnosis and continuing to have a productive life. Another contemporary use of stories has been to compare the HIV/AIDS virus with traditional monsters and then to stress positive and disease-preventing behaviors.

Song

Song is one of many ways to communicate and pray with the Creator. A "sing" is also used for prevention when it is known that an individual will come into contact with objects or malignant forces (Burhansstipanov & Dresser, 1993). Music has a powerful healing role among most Native cultures. The drum is more than a symbol among Native People and likewise, drum groups are highly regarded for their ability to communicate with the Creator.

Diet and Food Selection

Before European influence, the traditional diet of most Northern American Indian tribes included a variety of foods that they gathered, hunted, or caught during each season of the year. At that time, there were several distinct methods of attaining foods, such as the woodsmen of the eastern forests, the hunters of the plains, the Navajo sheep herders, the Pueblo farmers, the desert dwellers, the northern fishermen, and the seed gatherers (Bosley, 1959).

When food was abundant, Native people ate large quantities for satiety, the excess of which was stored as body fat; however, the active lifestyle (hunting, fishing, food gathering, festive and ceremonial activities) kept their bodies lean. The traditional consumption pattern consisted of one meal eaten in late morning. The food was cooked and eaten out of a single pot, most often with their fingers or bread. During the remainder of the day, stews were kept simmering over a fire, and dried foods were eaten as snacks (Burhansstipanov & Dresser, 1993).

Traditional American Indian diet did not include "fry bread" or any other contemporary foods that are made with lard or cow products, such as beef, milk, or butter. The types of foods consumed in the past (ie, before contact with Europeans) were based on availability and included foods that were primarily low in fat, such as fish and game (eg, deer, antelope, buffalo), corn, squash, beans, rice, and roots. High-fat foods included seeds, nuts, and occasionally high-fat protein foods like bear or whale (for Alaska Natives) (Burhansstipanov & Dresser, 1993).

Over the last 30 years, the traditional foods consumed by the ancestors of American Indians and Alaska Natives have been replaced by processed and commercially prepared foods, the variety and quality of which have been limited. Foods traditionally prepared over slow fires have been replaced with pan or deep-fat frying cooking methods. Although today's Native American populations are encouraged to incorporate more of their traditional foods in their diet (Burhansstipanov & Dresser, 1993; DHHS, 1993), these cultures have been slow to adopt the healthier habits. This may be due in part to the availability of traditional foods or the time it takes to prepare them (Burhansstipanov & Dresser, 1993).

As of 1990, 19.8% of all Native Americans lived on one of 215 Federal reservations (Gwilt, 1993). In a 1990 report evaluating the Department of Agriculture's Food Distribution Program, it stated that approximately 65% to 70% of Native Americans living on reservation received either food commodities or food stamps. A typical Food Distribution Program on Indian Reservations (FDPIR) household included an average of 3.2 persons; 40% of the families were one or two person households, and 8.5% were single parent homes. The households generally included children and adults aged 60 and over. The average level of education attained was the 10th grade. Over 50% of the adults in FDPIR households worked, were looking for work, or were laid off and were looking for work. Most of the households were poor by conventional standards and experienced transportation difficulties (Burhansstipanov & Tenney, 1995).

Most FDPIR participants had to rely on food purchases, home food production, and other USDA programs, in addition to the program commodities to meet their dietary needs. When asked about the amounts of food provided by the program, seven of eight households said they had enough; others did not have enough to eat 1 day out of every 5 or 6 days. Although most households (except for some of those who live in the North and Southwest) had adequate food preparation and storage facilities (eg, running water, electricity, and refrigeration), more than half of all households had one adult with one or more nutrition-related health problems; and more than one of four households had at least one member on a special diet (Burhansstipanov & Tenney, 1995).

Because this is a supplemental food source, participation in the FDPIR program does not guarantee Native Americans nutrient-dense foods, proper nourishment, or compliance with the 1990 dietary guidelines. It was not intended to provide a 30-day supply of food. Rather, recipients are expected to purchase a portion of their monthly food supply. For Native Americans participating in the Food Stamp program, the purchasing power of the stamps depends on reasonable food prices on and off the reservations, accessibility to grocery stores with an ample nutrient-dense food supply, and the appropriate use of the stamps by participants. These situations pose problems for Native People who are dependent on commodities or live in remote areas of the country. Too often Native Americans supplement food commodities items with foods from the local grocery store, convenience store, or vending machines that increase their intake of refined sugar and fats (sodas, sweets and desserts, fatty hamburgers, and processed white bread products) rather than fiber, vitamins, and minerals (Burhansstipanov & Tenney, 1995). This may occur because healthier foods are not available or are available in limited quantities (Burhansstipanov & Dresser, 1993), or people make poor food choices.

Physical Fitness and Exercise

In the past, survival required gathering and hunting sufficient amounts of food to feed people and animals on a daily basis and to store sufficient amounts to last through the winter. Most tribes, such as Plains Indians migrated to different geographic regions during the seasons of the year. For example, there would be a summer gathering place to interact, trade, and visit with other tribes. A winter location would be selected to provide access to water, firewood, and protection from the winds and winter storms. While migrating, people walked and after attaining horses, rode and hunted and gathered food while in transit. All of this resulted in regular daily physical activity. In addition, traditionally, American Indian tribes participated in competitive sports that required excellent cardiovascular fitness. Common Native sports included walking, dancing, lacrosse, and foot races. These running events were of varying lengths, but many exceeded contemporary marathons (26 miles). Today most cultures, including Native Americans, are less physically active because of modern conveniences. An example of a proactive fitness model is the *100-mile clubs* that are comprised of Native people of all ages, including elderly women, who document the number of miles walked.

Cultural Strength in Numbers—Organized Efforts

Indian Health Service Prevention Efforts

Since the early 1990s, the IHS has supported and implemented workshops with traditional healers and spiritual leaders regarding the prevention of HIV/AIDS transmission during ceremonies, such as the Sun Dance. The goals of these workshops were to increase the collaboration and respect among traditional healers and Western doctors as well as offer an opportunity for healers and providers to learn new information. For example, during ceremonies, skin is pierced and there is the possibility of contact with contaminated blood among Sun Dance participants and the spiritual leader. During the workshop, sterilization and other disease prevention techniques are reviewed and practiced by the healers.

Condom use is being promoted by more Indian communities, primarily by HIV educators, health educators, community health representatives, and nurses. Condom use reduces the risks of unplanned pregnancy, STDs, and HIV exposure. In the past, condoms were not greeted with much acceptance and although many Native communities continue to be resistant, an increased number of people self-report using condoms.

Four Worlds Institute

The Four Worlds Development Project in Alberta, Canada has the goal to implement a full and complete spiritual offensive to eliminate forever, by the year 2000, alcohol and drug abuse, child sexual abuse, incest, family violence, and abuse of women. Phil Lane Jr., the coordinator of the project, has emphasized that the abuse of women must "stop on this planet before any of the other issues can be addressed . . . . It is said the eagle of humanity flies with two wings towards its goal of love, honor and equality. One wing is man and the other is woman. Until those two wings are entirely equal the eagle will not fly to its promised destiny" (Allison, 1993). The Four Worlds Development Project has many unique features. For example, it is rooted in Native cultural perspectives and reliant on continued advice of Native elders. It balances cultural and scientific knowledge with a holistic and interdisciplinary approach—searching out and using innovations in education and development from around the world to assist Native communities. Four Worlds works with associated programs in many Native communities or organizations across Canada to develop models of holistic development from which others can learn. It also provides valuable networking, linking ideas and human and financial resources for those who need them. Four Worlds Development is a powerful working model of how university-based knowledge can be combined with American Indian perspectives, with implications for assisting developing communities anywhere in the world.

HIV Minority Congress

During August 1994, more than 100 American Indians and Alaska Natives participated in the National Congress on the State of HIV/AIDS in Racial and Ethnic Communities and prioritized issues relevant to Native American people and specifically to Native women. Among the recommendations were to provide unique and culturally acceptable services specific to the needs of women, for example, support for elders so that they can continue to support their family members during the course of the HIV-related illness and beyond. This Congress plans to meet annually.

Diabetes Camps

Both youth health camps and adult diabetes camps teach self-care skills (healthy eating, exercise, and family education) to control diabetes. Participants are encouraged to help prevent diabetes in their own families by teaching their children and grandchildren to stay active (Keely, Martinsen, Hunn, & Norton, 1992). The IHS has initiated a series of diabetes-related workshops and conferences that focus on improved eating habits, exercise, appropriate foot care, and so on. Culturally relevant diabetes education materials have also been developed with IHS support.

Network for Cancer Control Research Among American Indian and Alaska Native Populations

The Network for Cancer Control Research (NCCR) was originally organized in April 1990 and is comprised of approximately 22 steering committee members, of whom at least two-thirds are Native American. The network meets regularly to address the issue of Native Americans and cancer. The mission of the NCCR is to improve the health of American Indian and Alaska Native peoples by reducing cancer morbidity and mortality to the lowest possible levels and to improve cancer survival through cancer control research. The NCCR is primarily supported by the Special Populations Studies Branch of the National Cancer Institute.

Cultural Strength in Numbers—Native Women's Voices

Women in Politically Powerful Roles

As a result of the magnitude of Indian health and economic problems, Indian women have begun to reassert themselves within Indian communities. The most obvious illustration of this is the number of Indian women who now hold positions on tribal councils. In the early 1980s, only a handful of women were in such a strong political position. However, according to the Bureau of Indian Affairs in 1994, about 25% of the tribal councils include at least one woman.

Indian Health Service Women's Round Table

In 1991, the IHS gathered an Indian Women's Health Care Round Table meeting to discuss the above list of Native women-oriented health outcomes and develop a consensus statement for Indian women's health care. The result was the publication "Indian Women's Health Care Consensus Statement." Significant health issues identified in this report were described earlier. At least two additional conferences have been convened since that time to continue the discussion regarding how to address the identified issues.

Indian Women's Wellness Conferences

Concern over the demise of contemporary Indian women's health resulted in the University of Oklahoma organizing the first national gathering designed for Indian women to discuss the health and well-being of indigenous women. This gathering has grown from 300 participants in 1990 to over 2000 Indian women in 1995. Approximately 60% of the conference participants are lay members of the communities and Indian outreach workers (eg, community health representatives). About 35% are Native professional and paraprofessionals (eg, MD, DrPH, PhD, MPH, MSW, RN, NP, and health educators). The remaining 5% are men and non-Native people who work with or are interested in working with Indian communities on wellness programs. Examples of topics suggested by participants to be included in the 1995 workshops include but are not limited to the following: motivation, domestic violence, traditional healers, relationships, boarding school survivors, grief, parenting, parenting teens, two-spirited (lesbian) peoples, communication, youth life path, rituals/ceremonies, rites of passages, mother-daughter workshops.

Among the highlights of the annual gathering is a culturally relevant health fair. Each year, more than 550 women participate in screening during the health fair. These screenings include but are not limited to mammography, diabetes, obesity, dietary analysis, behavioral health risk assessments, and high blood pressure screening. These health fairs provide the opportunity to determine the impact of access to screening and cultural relevance of screening messages. For example, many of the mammogram users have never been screened before this gathering. When asked about this phenomenon, respondents typically make one of two statements: 1) there are no mammography services available in their local area; or 2) they did not realize that Indian women developed breast cancer (eg, the need for culturally relevant breast cancer informational materials). The need for elders to participate in cancer screening is emphasized in both workshops and general sessions of the conference to promote access and cultural relevance of the need for such screening.

Regional wellness conferences have emerged from these national meetings. Since the introduction of the "Wellness and Women" national gathering, tribal communities have organized 60 to 70 local and regional conferences throughout the United States and Canada.

Implications for Practice, Research, and Policy

The first sections of this chapter looked at the "reality" of Native American woman's history and her path to current health outcomes. The 1990 Census data have been helpful to document this "reality" so that important culturally appropriate interventions can be developed. It should be noted, however, that significant statistical and data limitation issues should be considered that are also a "reality" for the present.

Statistical and Data Limitation Issues

Public health practitioners are accustomed to examining national databases to determine significant health problems. However, national databases have limitations that affect *most* underserved populations (eg, Native Hawaiians, Vietnamese, Hispanic) and include one or more of the following: racial misclassification, undercounting, coding errors (universal to people of all races), inclusion of insufficient numbers of the racial group to formulate conclusions, and data collection in selected geographic regions that cannot be generalized to Native Peoples in other areas (Burhansstipanov & Dresser, 1993).

As of September 1994, there was discussion in process regarding how to use racial and ethnic identifiers. The original Office of Management and Budget Directive 15, developed in 1977–1978 is being revisited for more appropriate identifiers. A description of this discussion can be found in the *Federal Register* Notice, June 9, 1994, entitled, "Standards for the Classification of Federal Data on Race and Ethnicity." The appendix of that issue of the *Federal Register* has the 1978 version of the current standards.

Researchers need to be careful about generalizing data collected from one region of the country to Native people in another section of the country. For example, the SEER national database, which is recognized as being representative of the U.S. population, identifies an age-adjusted lung cancer incidence rate of 7.3 for American Indians (both sexes) (Burhansstipanov & Dresser, 1993). However, those data are primarily collected from American Indians living in Arizona and New Mexico and cannot be generalized to other areas. These two states include tribes such as the Navajo, Apache, and 19 Pueblo tribes—tribes that have significantly lower numbers of self-reported cigarette smokers as compared with tribes in other areas. Obviously, tribes that have a higher number of habitual cigarette smokers are more at risk for tobacco-related maladies than are southwestern tribes and those tribes are not represented in the Arizona and New Mexico databases. Table 20-2 compares the age-adjusted lung cancer incidence rates for women from selected from different geographic tribes.

The shift from denying to acknowledging one's heritage and ancestry creates data problems for the researcher or program planner. For example, an individual may have self-identified himself as "Caucasian" on the 1980 U.S. Census, but as "American Indian" on the 1990 U.S. Census. The researcher or program planner who is attempting to use Census data has no way to determine if the individual is of high blood quantum, which may be of interest if genetic cancers are the focus of one's research project. Likewise, the researcher, provider, or program planner does not know whether the individual practices Native American cultural behaviors or Caucasian cultural practices—both of which influence health outcomes.

Some of these issues are being aggressively examined by organized groups such as the NCCR among American Indians and Alaska Native populations (described earlier).

Recommendations for Practice: In Search of the "Perfect" Model for Native Women Wellness

The rich history, diversity, and cultural strengths of Native American communities defined in this chapter ensure that a variety of models or intervention strategies for Native American women may be effective. However, research models that work in

Table 20-2. Comparison of Age-Adjusted Lung Cancer Incidence Rates Among Native American Tribes

Tribe	Incidence Rate
Southwestern	
Apache	8.3
Navajo	4.6
Tohono O'Odham	17.0
Pima	17.0
Non-Southwestern	
Eastern Band Cherokee	35.2
Oklahoma Cherokee	16.4
Sioux	34.1
Alaska Native	
Aleut	101.7
Athapaskan	111.3
Eskimo	53.2

From Nutting, P. A., et al. (1993). Cancer incidence among American Indians and Alaska Natives, 1980 through 1987. *American Journal of Public Health, 83*(11), 1589.

other communities may not be successful with Native American peoples. For example, the Health Belief Model has successfully been used in diverse communities (Hochbaum, 1959; Rosenstock 1966). However, acceptance in one community or with one population does not mean the model will be accepted in another. The Health Belief Model includes "perceived susceptibility" that may be reflected in a needs assessment survey with an item such as, "I believe that I can develop breast cancer." However, during a survey being implemented at a large Indian women's gathering, as soon as the interviewer verbalized this statement, the Indian participant exclaimed alarm and immediately exited the facility. The interview obviously was terminated on her departure. Among several tribes, to make such a statement is to invite the cancer spirit into one's body. This woman who rushed from the interviewer's area had immediately contacted her traditional healer to begin a cleansing ceremony because the interviewer had exposed her to the cancer spirit. It is clear that a cultural understanding is the best beginning for culturally appropriate enhancement of wellness for women. There is no "perfect model," but recommendations on where to begin are suggested.

Display 20-2 is a summary of recommendations for working with American Indian men and women. It includes suggestions that relate to the entire community, rather than focusing on Indian women alone. The most important suggestion is to work in a collaborative relationship with members of the local community in leadership roles and initially develop a relationship based on mutual respect rather than mutual assumptions. This type of a relationship takes time to develop. Many researchers and policymakers attempt to initiate such a relationship after reviewing a request for application, which has a grant submission date within 60 days.

DISPLAY 20-2

Summary List of Recommendations for Public Health Practitioners, Health Educators and Researchers Working with Native Communities

- Allow "up-front" time to develop collaborative relationship(s) among Native Peoples and technical professionals.
- Hire and include American Indians in all phases of the research or service program.
- Allow sufficient time (approximately 3–6 mo) to obtain a Tribal Council Resolution that supports your project.
- Consider the Native organization as the primary recipient of the grant and the academic/research organization(s) as the subcontractor(s).
- Work with Native Americans to adapt materials and procedures for cultural appropriateness.
- Work with Native Americans to develop procedures and protocols that are culturally acceptable.
- Share project/research information via publications and media which are used by Native community members (eg., *Indian Times Newspaper,* Indian radio stations).
- Involve gatekeepers who have access to the "*moccasin telegraph*" (word-of-mouth communication).
- Include members of the target community in developing publications and determining dissemination plans.
- Develop dissemination plans which include apprising Native community of preliminary as well as final results, findings, and conclusions.
- Allow time for Native community members to review findings and conclusions before publication. This will prevent misinterpretation.
- Be respectful of cultural norms (eg, modesty).
- Use community development and community-driven models
- Provide mechanism for "empowerment" or continuation of the project after funding ceases.
- Emphasize benefits (health and other) to the family rather than one's own health.
- Involve elders in leadership roles.
- Involve "gatekeepers" and community health representative (CHRs). They are helpful in providing credibility to the project and ensuring that messages get to the community.
- Include members of local tribal community as coauthors on publications. Sign an agreement with local Native people that findings from your research will be given to the local tribal community as soon as feasible and before publication.
- Keep demographic and other types of information in mind while preparing strategies.
- Always keep the community in mind—interventions should empower the community, enhance capacity building, and provide services or something perceived as a benefit to the community. This approach is much more dynamic and rewarding to all rather than simply surveying the community.
- Be conscious of issues of confidentiality.
- Be aware and respectful of tribal council protocol and their agenda versus the researchers' agenda.
- Become aware of unpublished but notable ongoing community-driven activities.

Optimal rapport and trust typically take longer and need to be based on something of greater importance than a request for application alone.

Among the challenges facing the health educator or researcher who approaches an American Indian or Alaska Native community with hopes of initiating a health promotion or wellness project is community distrust and suspicion. Unfortunately, the health educator, program planner, or researcher must "pay for the sins of previous researchers" and many well-intentioned professionals are immediately confronted with accusations. Researchers have typically invaded Native American communities, studied the people and their behaviors "like we were guinea pigs," failed to share results or findings of the study with the community, and published a paper in a professional journal that included inaccurate interpretations of the communities' cultures, practices, and beliefs. From the Native perspective, these are examples of "using" Indian people in the name of research. Unfortunately, often the community does not see the benefits of or their contributions to the research. This pattern, which has occurred repeatedly throughout Indian Country, is the primary basis for the recommendations included within Display 20-2 (Burhansstipanov & Tenney, 1995).

Another pattern has been to publish specific information about tribal participants without having reviewed the description with tribal leaders or verifying that confidentiality of participants has been protected. Researchers have on occasion become excited about their research findings and delved into explanations for a particular finding (eg, HIV diagnoses) and begun to analyze the data for related behaviors. When discussing the specific behavior or health outcome, the paper may include statements such as, "Of the HIV-positive Bonsai Tribal members, almost all of the infected individuals had traveled to urban areas within the previous 2 years." Unbeknownst to the researcher, the tribal community is so small, that community members know who has and who has not traveled to the city within the last 2 years, and the identity of the HIV-positive individuals is no longer confidential information. Obviously this was not the intent of the researchers, but had selected members of the community been given the opportunity to participate in writing or reviewing the article, ideally, such a violation of confidentiality would not occur (by the way, the Bonsai Tribe is simply a fictitious name used in this example).

For protection of confidentiality, the IHS produces publication "guidelines" specifying that tribes should not be specifically identified in papers, but rather the general region where the tribe is located, such as "a southwestern tribe" or "a northwestern tribe."

When researchers and health care workers begin to work with tribes, most erroneously assume that the tribes will welcome them with open arms and immediately recognize the importance of the professional. Although this occasionally happens, it frequently does not. Researchers and providers sometimes call the tribal office and request to be placed on the agenda of the next tribal council meeting. This is a good plan, but it should be recognized that there are many priorities within each tribal community and, on average, it takes about 3 months to get on the tribal council agenda. In some councils, once the item is included, it may require that a member of the tribe present the issue rather than the professional. Some council meetings are open for people to observe. However, for others, people are *invited* to observe tribal council meetings and the researcher may or may not be allowed to be present for that discussion.

Professionals need to realize that community-driven and community-based efforts are currently going on within the Native American communities. However, most of these efforts are not described in juried publications. It is imperative that the provider first determine what the local community is doing well rather than assuming the community is doing nothing for the health and wellness of its peoples. An embarrassing situation emerges when the professional who is unaware of ongoing health promotion efforts assumes that such activities do not exist.

Health practitioners, researchers, and program planners need to be respectful of the resolution and policy developmental processes that are used throughout Indian Country. Approval of a resolution ensures that the tribal council or board of directors are informed and supportive of an issue/program/project and is a necessary step in community ownership and support of the issue. The resolution process also provides commitment from the Native organization that is unrelated to current political leadership within the tribal government. If there is no resolution, there is no formal commitment from the tribe to continue to support the issue/program/project once a new chairperson is elected.

Respect for the timing necessary for policy development is equally important. Resolutions are formally introduced and discussed during tribal council meetings or during board of director meetings (which are typically scheduled monthly). Some Indian communities require that a resolution be discussed at a minimum of two council meetings before being placed for a vote. Other communities allow resolutions to be introduced and voted on during the same meeting. Many communities require that resolutions be introduced by tribal members and nontribal members may or may not be allowed to be present while the resolution is being discussed. Although there is great variability among tribal governments, in general, a resolution must be in place before a new policy is adopted.

Conclusion

There is a strong wellness movement being initiated by women throughout Indian country, which is being supported by tribal leaders, urban Indian organizations, the IHS, and many other organizations and agencies. Although Indian Country continues to experience poverty and other psychosocial factors in disproportionate levels in comparison with other racial populations, more and more positive, constructive efforts are occurring throughout Indian Country that are likely to increase the number of well women and well communities.

References

Agency for Health Care Policy and Research. (1991, July). *National Medical Expenditure Survey, access to health care: Findings from the survey of American Indians and Alaska Natives* (DHHS Publication No. 91-0028). Washington, DC: U.S. Government Printing Office.

Allison, F. (1993, July 24). Four Worlds delegates commit to a complete spiritual offensive. *Herald Newspaper*.

Bennett, S. K. (1992). The American Indian: A psychological overview. In *Psychology of culture* (pp. 35-39). Needham Heights, MA: Allyn & Bacon.

Bosley, B. (1959). Nutrition in the Indian Health Program. *Journal of the American Dietetic Association*, 9, 905-909.

Burhansstipanov, L., & Dresser, C. M. (1993). *Native American monograph no. 1: Documentation of the cancer research needs of American Indians and Alaska Natives* (NIH Publication No. 93-3603). Bethesda, MD: National Cancer Institute.

Burhansstipanov, L., & Tenney, M. (1995). Native American health issues. *Current Issues in Public Health*, 1, 35-41.

Caduto, M. J., & Bruchac, J. (1991). *Native American stories*. Golden, CO: Fulcrum Publishing.

Centers for Disease Control and Prevention (1993). *HIV/AIDS surveillance report*. Atlanta, GA: Author.

Chamberlain, J. (1990). NIDDK researchers probe causes of diabetes, obesity. *The NIH Record*, XLII(24), 9.

Clark, B. (1988). *Diabetes mellitus among Oklahoma Indians in 1987*. Unpublished paper, Albuquerque, NM.

Clements, F. E. (1932). Primitive concepts of disease. In: *American archaeology and ethnology*, XXXII, 186-190, University of California Publications.

Dye, S. K., Henderson, Z., & Jones, D. (1990). *Standards of diabetic foot care*. Oklahoma City: Indian Health Service.

Fleming, C. M., Manson, S., & Engs, R. C. (1990). Indian women and alcohol. In R. C. Engs (Ed.), *Women, alcohol, and other drugs*. Iowa: Kendal/Hunt Publishing.

Gwilt, R. C. (1993, May 10). Letter in response to NCI queries regarding availability of breast cancer screening services.

Hochbaum, G. M. (1959). *Public participation in medical screening programs: A sociological study* (PHS Publication No. 572). Washington, DC: U.S. Public Health Service.

Horner, R. D. (1990). Cancer mortality in Native Americans in North Carolina. *American Journal of Public Health*, 80, 940-944.

Indian Women's Health Care Round Table Final Report. (1991). *Indian women's health care consensus statement*. Rockville, MD: Author.

Keely, P. B., Martinsen, C. S., Hunn, E. S., & Norton, H. H. (1982). Composition of Native American fruits in the Pacific Northwest. *Journal of the American Dietetic Association*, 81, 568-572.

Lee, E. T., Lee, V. S., Lu, M., Lee, J. S., Russell, D., & Yeh, J. (1994). The incidence of renal failure in NIDDM. *Diabetes*, 43, 572.

Levy, J. E. (1963). *Navajo health concepts and behavior: The role of the Anglo medical man in the Navajo healing process*. Window Rock, AZ: Navajo Area Indian Health Service.

Locust, C. S. (1985). *American Indian beliefs concerning health and unwellness* (Monograph Series). Tucson, AZ: University of Arizona, Native American Research and Training Center.

Massion, C., O'Connor, P., Gorab, R., Crabtree, B., Nakamura, R., & Coulehan, J. (1987). Screening for gestational diabetes in a high-risk population. *Journal of Family Practice*, 25(6), 569-576.

National Native American AIDS Prevention Center. (1994, September). *HIV policy guidelines*. Oakland, CA: Author.

Nutting, P. A., Freeman, W. L., Risser, D. R., Helgerson, S. D., Paisano, R., Hisnanick, J., Beaver, S. K., Peters, I., Carney, J.P., & Speers, M. A. (1993). Cancer incidence among American Indians and Alaska Natives, 1980 through 1987. *American Journal of Public Health*, 83(11), 1589.

Office of Technology Assessment. (1990). *Indian adolescent mental health* (Publication No. OTA-H-446). Washington, DC: U.S. Government Printing Office.

Reichard, G. A. (1963). *Navaho religion: A study of symbolism*. Princeton, NJ: Princeton University Press.

Rhoades, E. R., Hammond, J., Welty, T. K., Handler, A. O., & Amler, R. W. (1987). The Indian burden of illness and future health interventions. *Public Health Reports*, 102 (4), 361-368.

Rosenstock, I. M. (1966, July). Why people use health services. *Milbank Memorial Fund Quarterly*, 44, 94-127.

Samet, J. M., Key, C. R., Hunt, W. C., & Goodwin, J. S. (1987). Survival of American Indian and Hispanic cancer patients in New Mexico and Arizona, 1969–82. *Journal of the National Cancer Institute*, 79 (3), 457-563.

Stanford Center for Research in Disease Prevention. (1992). *Restoring balance: Community-directed health promotion for American Indians and Alaska Natives*. (Library of Congress Catalog Card Number 92-93511, p. xiii.) Stanford, CA: Author.

Swanton, J. R. (1928). *Religious beliefs and medical practices of the Creek Indians. Forty-Second Annual Report of the Bureau of American Ethnology*, 1924–25 (pp. 637—639). Washington, DC: U.S. Government Printing Office.

Swanton, J. (1931). *Source material for the social and ceremonial life of the Choctaw Indians.* (Bureau of American Ethnology Bulletin No. 103). Washington, DC: U.S. Government Printing Office.

U.S. Bureau of the Census. (1992a). *General population characteristics, from the Census Bureau tape, 1990 census.* Washington, DC: U.S. Government Printing Office.

U.S. Bureau of the Census. (1992b). *Total and American Indian, Eskimo, or Aleut populations for selected reservations and trust lands, by rank: 1990* (CPH-L-73). Washington, DC: U.S. Government Printing Office.

U.S. Bureau of the Census. (1993). *We the first Americans* (Publication No. 350-631, p. 3). Washington, DC: U.S. Government Printing Office.

U.S. Department of Health and Human Services, Indian Health Service. (1991). *Indian Women's Health Care Consensus Statement.* IHS Office of Planning, Evaluation, and Legislation, Tucson, AZ, p. 7.

U.S. Department of Health and Human Services. (1992a). *IHS trends* (p. 34). Washington, DC: U.S. Government Printing Office.

U.S. Department of Health and Human Services. (1992b). *Regional differences in Indian health* (DHHS Publication No. 0-324-746, p. 43). Washington, DC: U.S. Government Printing Office.

U.S. Department of Health and Human Services (1992c). *Report of the Special Action Committee, 1992: Program initiatives related to minorities, the underserved and persons aged 65 and over* (Appendix A). Washington, DC: U.S. Government Printing Office.

U.S. Department of Health and Human Services. (1993). *Indian Health Service: Trends in Indian Health—1993* (pp. 31, 37, 41, 50, 87, 99). Rockville, MD: Author.

U.S. Department of Health and Human Services. (1994). *Indian health service: Regional differences in Indian health—1993* (pp. 60, 63). Rockville, MD: Indian Health Service.

Valway, S., Kileen, M., Paisano, R., Ortiz, E. (1992). *Cancer mortality among Native Americans in the United States: Regional differences in Indian health, 1984–88 and trends over time, 1968–1987.* Rockville, MD: Indian Health Service.

Bibliography

Black, W. C., & Key, C. R. (1980). Epidemiologic pathology of cancer in New Mexico's tri-ethnic population. *Pathology Annual, 15,* 181-194.

Creagan, E. T., & Fraumeni, J. F. (1972). Cancer mortality among American Indians, 1950–67. *Journal of the National Cancer Institute, 49,* 956-967.

HIV and Minorities Congress. (1994, September 17). Summary paper *American Indian/Alaska Native recommendations for the breaking barriers.* Washington, DC: Building Bridges Conference.

Lanier, A. P., Bulkow, L. R., & Ireland, B. (1989). Cancer in Alaskan Indians, Eskimos, and Aleuts, 1969–83: Implications for etiology and control. *Public Health Reports, 104,* 658-664.

Mahoney, M. C., Michalek, A. M., Cummings, K. M., Nasca, P. C., & Emrich, L. J. (1989). Cancer surveillance in a Northeastern Native American population. *Cancer, 64,* 191-195.

Mao, Y., Morrison, H., Semenciw, R.. et al. (1986). Mortality on Canadian Indian reserves 1977—1982. *Canadian Journal of Public Health, 77,* 263-268.

Miller, B. A., Ries, L. A. G., Hankey, B. F., Kosary, C. L., & Edwards, B. K. (Eds.). *Cancer statistics review: 1973–1989* (National Cancer Institute Publication No. NIH 92-2789). Bethesda, MD: National Cancer Institute.

Native American Cancer Research Consortium (1994) is with the American Indian Clinic of Bellflower, CA and the AMC Cancer Research Center's Native American Cancer Research Program in Denver, CO.

Sorem, K. A. (1985). Cancer incidence in the Zuni Indians of New Mexico. *Yale Journal of Biology and Medicine, 58,* 489-496.

U.S. Department of Health and Human Services. (1991). *Healthy people 2000: National health promotion and disease prevention objectives—Full report, with commentary* (DHHS Publication No. PHS 91-50212, p. 39). Washington, DC: U.S. Government Printing Office.

Young, T. K., & Frank, J. W. (1983). Cancer surveillance in a remote Indian population in Northwestern Ontario. *American Journal of Public Health, 73,* 515-520.

Additional Resources

Adult Diabetes Camp: Acton K. PHS Indian Health Center. P.O. Box 280, St. Ignatius, MT 59865. (406) 745-1205 and Town W. Blackfeet Diabetes Program. P.O. Box 760, Browning, MT 59417. (406) 338-6307.

Center for American Indian Research and Education, 1918 University Avenue, Suite #2A, Berkeley, CA 94704, 510/843-8661.

Four Worlds Development Project, University of Lethbridge, Alberta, Canada, (403) 329-2065 or fax (403) 329-3081.

Keeley, Cherokee Nation Health Department, P.O. Box 948, Tahlequah, OK 74465. (918) 465-0671.

UNIT 5

Issues Affecting Women's Health

CHAPTER 21

Violence

Nancy E. Isaac
Deborah Prothrow-Stith

Introduction

Violence against women encompasses a variety of events, including physical assault, sexual assault, and homicide. Perpetrators of these acts may be strangers, acquaintances, intimate partners, and family members.

This chapter focuses predominantly on sexual assault and domestic violence. Although the term violence usually brings to mind physical acts of aggression, it is important to recognize from the outset that violence against women occurs along a continuum, from verbal aggression and sexual harassment all the way to homicide.

Nonphysical forms of violence can affect both the physical and mental health of women, and we must therefore be careful not to limit our attention to those acts resulting in observable injury. For example, a gun held to a woman's head may be used to intimidate and control her in ways that few people would not define as abusive. If the trigger is not pulled, or if the gun's chamber is empty, she will have no observable physical trauma and yet may suffer both psychological and physical sequelae (eg, depression, ulcer, migraines) resulting from this abuse.

Data Collection: Methodology and Issues

The collection of data on violence against women is complicated by the "hidden" nature of many of these crimes—victims may be reluctant to report them to authorities or may not think of them as criminal, in part because of self-blame. An understanding of the methodology behind current incidence and prevalence figures used in the literature and common discourse on violence against women is important. Therefore, we begin this section with a brief review of how violence against women is measured in official statistics.

Unfortunately, the United States still lacks a valid and reliable set of methods for the collection of national population-based incidence data on violence against women. In particular, the currently available data sources tend to undercount instances involving intimate partners (defined here as spouses, ex-spouses, boyfriends, and ex-boyfriends, although violence does also occur in lesbian relationships).

The two major sources of routinely collected information on violence against women are the National Crime Victimization Survey (NCVS) and the Uniform Crime Reports (UCR).

The NCVS is an ongoing survey of U.S. households regarding their experiences with crime victimization conducted by the Department of Justice. A given household is enrolled in the study for 3 years, during which time the experiences of all household members ages 12 and older are assessed every 6 months, usually in a structured telephone interview. The survey has several weaknesses with respect to its ability to count accurately women's experiences with violence.

First, the focus of the survey is on "crime." Yet many women who have been or are being victimized by people known to them may not understand that these events constitute crimes. Recent revisions in the NCVS (instituted in 1993) attempt to address this problem by including an extra question prompting for events perpetrated by someone at work or school, a neighbor or friend, a relative or family member, or by other people known to the respondent. Whether this adequately addresses the problem may become clearer in future reports on data collected using this revised strategy.

Also, until the 1993 revisions, the NCVS did not ask directly about "rape." Women were left to volunteer descriptions of events constituting rape under general questions about assaults or attacks. Therefore, it is widely recognized that the figures for rape incidence provided by the NCVS up through the early 1990s are underestimates.

Figures from interviews using a revised methodology are not yet available. However, even these updated methods may fail to capture many cases. To obtain accurate counts it is necessary to be explicit when inquiring about acts that constitute rape. Many women will not classify what has occurred to them as rape because of the still prevalent notion that "real" rapes involve attacks by strangers (Koss, 1985). The revised NCVS does not specifically define "sexual intercourse" for a respondent as including vaginal, anal, or oral penetration unless the woman first responds positively to a broader question about unwanted sexual acts and is subsequently uncertain whether the events constituted "sexual intercourse." This design may continue to create a bias toward underestimation in the NCVS data.

Another methodologic issue in counting violence against women involves the sensitivity of the method to women's privacy and safety needs. If an interview is conducted in the presence of others, whether in person or over the phone, a woman's ability to respond candidly (or even to participate in the study) may be severely compromised. If, for instance, her abusive partner is within listening distance, she may also be placed in danger by responding to questions about experiences with violence. Some preliminary analyses from the NCVS have illustrated this potential problem, finding that rates of reported spouse abuse and rape are both significantly lower when a woman's spouse is present during the interview (Coker, 1994).

Despite their tendency to undercount violence against women perpetrated by intimates, the NCVSs still find that women are more frequently victimized by nonstrangers than by strangers. Of the 2.5 million women who experience violence annually, as estimated by the NCVS, two of three were related to or knew their attacker (Bachman, 1994). According to the Bureau of Justice Statistics (1994), for the period from 1987 to 1991, the average annual rates of single-offender violent victimizations per 1000 population for women were (by offender status):

- intimates, 5.0
- other relatives, 1.0
- acquaintances, 8.0
- strangers, 5.0

Of the violence reported in the NCVS as occurring between intimates, women were the victim in over 90% of instances (Bureau of Justice Statistics, 1994).

The UCR are another source of official information on violence against women, but these data are even more limited for generalization than the NCVS. The UCR are police report data that most police departments in the country voluntarily submit to the Federal Bureau of Investigation for aggregation into a national data set. These data can tell us how many incidents of violence against women were *reported to the police*—a figure that is obviously biased by factors that inhibit women's willingness to report. These factors may be numerous and varied, including shame, stigma, previous bad experiences with the criminal justice sector, fear of reprisal from perpetrators, and language and cultural barriers.

Despite their limitations, the NCVS and the UCR are important because they are routinely collected data sets. They have some potential, therefore, to address trends over time. But they also highlight the relative state of ignorance from which we must form policy on this important topic.

Other individual studies that have contributed to our understanding of the incidence of violence against women are described under the following subsections on sexual assault and domestic violence.

Sexual Assault

The NCVS reports roughly 133,000 rape victimizations among women age 12 or older in the United States each year (Bachman, 1994). In these data, 55% of the perpetrators were known to the victim, and about half of all incidents were reported to the police.

Kilpatrick, Edmunds, and Seymour (1992) studied forcible rape as part of the National Women's Study, a national probability sample of 4008 adult women in the United States interviewed by telephone in 1990, 1991, and 1992 (three waves). The definition of forcible rape used in the study was consistent with most legal definitions: "an event that occurred without the woman's consent, involved the use of force or threat of force, and involved sexual penetration of the victim's vagina, mouth or rectum." The questions used explicit, anatomically correct language to describe these events. According to this study, an estimated 683,000 *adult* women are raped each year. It is important to note, however, that this study also found that 60% of the rapes reported to have occurred in women's lifetimes occurred at ages *younger* than 18. An estimated 12.1 million American women were reported to have experienced forcible rape at some point in their lives. Only 22% of victims reported that the perpetrator was a stranger, and only 16% of all rapes were reported to the police.

Domestic Violence

Only two large population-based studies have been designed to measure the extent of domestic violence in the United States. (Straus & Gelles, 1990; Straus, Gelles, &

Steinmetz, 1980). The 1985 National Family Violence Survey found that 3.4% of adult women had been *severely* abused by an intimate male partner in the past year (Straus & Gelles, 1990). This leads to an estimate of about 2 million severely abused women. According to the American Medical Association (1992a), experts agree that an estimate of 3 to 4 million is probably closer to reality, given the underestimation inherent in survey techniques on stigmatized topics. If more "minor" acts such as pushing and slapping are included, 11.6% of women report some form of physical violence in their relationship in the past year.

The Conflict Tactics Scales (CTS), which was developed by Straus for the national family violence surveys, has become the most widely used measurement tool in research on domestic violence (Straus, 1979). Although it does measure a range of "tactics" for resolving "conflict," including calm discussion, leaving, yelling, and various levels of physical violence, the CTS provides little in the way of contextual depth. In particular, it does not clarify either the triggers or the motivations for the violence.

Both the name and the phrasing of the questions in the CTS imply that all domestic violence occurs in the context of an active "conflict." Yet many battered women and batterers themselves have described instances where violence occurred outside of an actual conflict situation. For example, a man who is extremely jealous may imagine that his wife is off having an affair while she is actually out grocery shopping. When she returns, he may assault her the moment she opens the front door, even with her hands full of groceries. Framing such an incident as arising from a "conflict" may distort both our understanding of the causes of domestic violence and our ability to design appropriate intervention and prevention strategies.

Dating Violence

If our understanding of violence in relationships between adult intimates is limited, it is disconcerting to think that our knowledge about dating violence is far less.

Most studies of dating violence have been performed with relatively small samples, often in only one or a few schools in a limited geographic region, which limits the ability to generalize the findings. Sometimes these populations offer little or no variability on important characteristics of interest; a large portion of the research on dating violence describes Caucasian, middle-class, Midwestern populations only. The selection criteria for participants, and response rates, are not provided in many papers, making it difficult to assess potential sources of bias in the sampling.

Makepeace (1981) undertook the first study on dating violence, using a college population, and found that 21% of students admitted involvement in violent relationships and 62% personally knew of someone affected by such a relationship (Makepeace, 1981). Since that time, a variety of studies have been conducted in both college and high school populations. Findings for these two age groups have tended to be more similar than divergent.

Studies have estimated the prevalence of involvement in dating violence among high school students (as victim, perpetrator, or both) at anywhere between 12% and 39% (Bergman, 1992; Henton, Cate, Koval, Lloyd, & Christopher, 1983; O'Keefe, Brockopp, & Chew, 1986; Reuterman & Burcky, 1989; Roscoe & Callahan, 1985; Roscoe & Kelsey, 1986). Most of these studies have used definitions of violence based on the CTS (Straus, 1979), and have included the use of threats or verbal assault as "violence," but have excluded sexual violence. Bergman (1992), in one of the few studies that included sexual violence, found that 15.5% of female students had experienced sexual violence, the same proportion had experienced physical violence, and 24.6% had experienced either or both. The corresponding prevalences for male students were 4.4%, 7.8%, and 9.9%, respectively.

Most studies find that women are more likely than men to be victims of dating violence, and the few studies that have included a measure of injury found that women are more likely to suffer injuries as a result of such violence (Henton et al., 1983; Makepeace, 1986).

Homicide

According to the Department of Justice, approximately 1500 women are known to have been killed each year by male intimates (spouses, ex-spouses, or boyfriends), or about one-third of all women over age 14 who were killed (Bureau of Justice Statistics, 1994). Women comprise 70% of all intimate murder victims. However, for all homicide data, the victim–offender relationship is unknown in nearly 40% of cases. In addition, official statistics fail to address the extent to which others are sometimes killed in the context of domestic homicides—children, friends, new intimate partners, and even bystanders.

Contributing Factors

Much of the early research on both sexual assault and domestic violence sought to determine the traits of victims that put them at risk for attack. However, most reviews and larger studies have found few factors that discriminate victims from non-victims (Hotaling & Sugarman, 1986; Koss & Dinero, 1989).

The trait of women that has the most significant effect on their risk for violence is one that is entirely beyond their control, namely age. Younger women are at much greater risk for both sexual assault and domestic violence.

Kilpatrick et al. (1992) found that only 6% of lifetime rapes occurred when the victim was older than age 29, whereas 29% occurred to women younger than age 11 years, 32% among women aged 11 to 17, and 22% in the age category 18 to 24. The 1985 National Family Violence Survey found that women aged 18 to 24 were at three times the risk of severe husband-to-wife violence as were older women (Straus, 1990).

The previous focus on women's appearance, behavior, and attitudes, much of which smacked of victim blaming, has shifted largely to an approach that emphasizes predisposing traits in perpetrators and the socioenvironmental context of events. In one of the largest studies of nonincarcerated, undetected perpetrators of sexual assault, Koss & Dinero (1988) reported on a sample of approximately 3000 male college students from a nationwide survey of 32 institutions of higher learning. Traits they found to be associated with sexual aggression included childhood sexual experiences (both forced and unforced), greater hostility toward women, and acceptance of the use of force in intimate relationships. They also report that "the more serious the self-reported sexual aggression, the more likely that current behavior was characterized by frequent use of alcohol, violent and degrading pornography, and involvement in peer groups that reinforce highly sexualized views of women" (Koss & Dinero, 1989, p. 144). These findings have some interesting implications for preventive approaches that address social norms that objectify and denigrate women.

Hotaling and Sugarman (1986) performed what is the largest summary analysis of risk markers for domestic violence. Consistent risk markers among men included witnessing violence as a child or adolescent, alcohol abuse, lower educational level, and lower income.

Violence in the family of origin, usually measured as violence between the spouses or violent forms of child discipline, is a consistent correlate of both adult domestic violence and dating violence (Henton et al., 1983; Hotaling & Sugarman, 1986; O'Keefe et al., 1986; Reuterman & Burcky, 1989; Roscoe & Callahan, 1985). This finding is consistent with several theories of the causation of violence against women, particularly a social learning model, which holds that individuals learn what is acceptable and normative behavior from the environment around them—from family, peers, media, and broad social norms. Observing violence in the home of origin appears to increase the risk for men to become perpetrators and for women to become victims.

A factor that appears to be present in many instances of violence against women is substance use—most commonly, alcohol abuse. The National Family Violence Survey of 1985 found a clear trend of increasing prevalence of husband-to-wife violence as the level of drinking in the male partner increased (Kaufman Kantor & Straus, 1987). The highest prevalence of violence (19%) was among binge drinkers, a pattern found in other studies as well. It is important to note, however, that the prevalence among abstainers was not zero (it was 6%) and that the majority of binge drinking men did *not* commit violence. In other words, there is no one-to-one correlation of violence with drinking. The study found that drinking immediately preceded violence in only about one-fourth of cases overall, but in half of cases where the male partner was a high- or binge-level drinker.

Debate continues as to whether or not alcohol use "causes" violence against women or is largely an exacerbating factor (see, for instance, Flanzer, 1993 and Gelles, 1993). Men who are violent toward women frequently use intoxication as an excuse for their behavior, recognizing (consciously or not) that in American culture we tend to hold individuals less responsible for violence that occurs while under the influence of alcohol.

Health Consequences of Violence Against Women

Numerous studies have examined the short- and long-term health consequences of violence against women.

Physical Effects

Immediate physical trauma resulting from both domestic abuse and sexual assault most often affects the head, face, neck, and torso, primarily in the form of contusions, abrasions, and lacerations (Koss & Heslet, 1992; Stark et al., 1981). More severe episodes may result in fractures, brain injury, damage to internal organs, or even death. Sexual assault may lead to trauma to the vagina or rectum (Geist, 1988), and health risks associated with sexually transmitted diseases (including human immunodeficiency virus [HIV]) (Lacey, 1990; Murphy, 1990) and pregnancy. Both physical and sexual assault may have serious traumatic consequences for pregnant women and their fetuses (Bullock & McFarlane, 1989; McFarlane, Parker, Soeken, & Bullock, 1992; Satin, Hemsell, Stone, Theriot, & Wendel, 1991).

According to the 1985 National Family Violence Survey, 3% of battered women received medical attention for abuse-related injuries in the past year (Stets & Straus, 1990). Among women who experienced severe abuse, this figure was 7.3%. These figures may undercount the number of women with injuries serious enough to "require" medical attention because batterers may prevent women from seeking help. The National Women's Study reported that 24% of rape victims sustained minor injury and 4% sustained serious injury (Kilpatrick et al., 1992). However, a full 49% of victims reported that they feared serious injury or death during the rape, and 40% of women raped within the past 5 years were fearful of contracting HIV or acquired immunodeficiency syndrome (AIDS).

Longer-term somatic consequences of both domestic and sexual abuse that have been cited include chronic pelvic pain, gastrointestinal syndromes, back pain, and headache (Koss & Heslet, 1992). The incidence of such outcomes, and their relationship to violent victimization, is more difficult to assess than immediate effects. Temporal associations may become cloudy over time and lack of information in medical records may lead to a dependence on (potentially biased) subjective recall of violence and subsequent symptomatology.

Acute trauma such as rape and assault may also confer an elevated risk for disease, mediated by stress-induced changes in immune functioning (Cohen & Williamson, 1991; Cohen, Tyrell, & Smith, 1991). Investigation with respect to such long-term outcomes specifically following violence has been limited, however.

Psychological Effects

Psychological or behavioral sequelae of violent victimization that have been described in the research literature include posttraumatic stress disorder (PTSD), major depression, anxiety disorders, substance abuse, and eating disorders (Kilpatrick et al., 1989; Resnick, Kilpatrick, Dansky, Saunders, & Best, 1993; Siegel, Golding, Stein, Burnam, & Sorenson, 1990; Stark et al., 1981; Steiger & Zanko, 1990; Winfield, George, Swartz, & Blazer, 1990).

In a national sample of 4008 women, those who had experienced criminal victimization (physical or sexual assault) were much more likely to receive a lifetime (25.8%) or current (9.7%) diagnosis of PTSD than were noncrime victims (9.4% and 3.4%, respectively) (Resnick et al., 1993). The same study estimated that approximately 1.3 million women currently suffer from rape-related PTSD (Kilpatrick et al., 1992). A high prevalence of prior violent victimization (50–80%) has also been found among psychiatric patients with a range of presenting complaints (Carmen, Rieker, & Mills, 1984; Jacobson & Richardson, 1987).

Major depression is another common sequelae of violent victimization. Stets and Straus (1990) reported that 58% of severely abused women had high depression scores, compared to 21% of women not abused. In the National Women's

Study, 21% of all rape victims were experiencing a major depressive episode at the time they were interviewed compared to 6% of women who were not victims of crime (Kilpatrick et al., 1992). This study also found that 13% of rape victims had attempted suicide compared to 1% of other women.

Several studies have found high rates of prior or ongoing violence among alcoholic women (Miller, Downs, & Gondoli, 1989; Swett et al., 1991). For instance, in a study that compared alcoholic women with a random household sample of women, both moderate and severe husband-to-wife violence were more common in the alcoholic sample (Miller et al., 1989). One-fourth of alcoholic women had been kicked, hit, or hit with a fist, compared to only 5% of the household women. Spousal violence remained a strong predictor of group type even after control for alcohol problems in the spouse, income, parental violence, and parental alcohol problems.

Kilpatrick et al. (1992) found that among rape victims who developed PTSD, 20% had two or more major alcohol-related problems compared to 1.5% of women who had never been crime victims.

Social Effects

Violence also has the potential to affect women's social health. Sequelae described in the literature include difficulty functioning at work and reduced ability to enjoy sexual relations (Feldman-Summer, Gordon, & Meagher, 1979; Resick et al., 1981). Even more seriously, some studies indicate that violence may be a risk factor for homelessness (Bassuk & Rosenberg, 1988; Wood, Valdez, Hayashi, & Shen, 1990).

The health care costs associated with violent victimization have been estimated in several studies. Koss, Koss, and Woodruff (1991) found that women crime victims, as compared to non-victims, made twice as many physician visits in the past year (6.9 versus 3.5). Severity of victimization was the best predictor of yearly physician visits and total outpatient costs in an analysis that controlled for age, income, ethnicity, education, health status, and other life stressors. Most recently, Miller, Cohen and Rossman (1993) estimated the total costs (monetary, mental health, and quality of life) associated with rape, robbery, assault, and arson. Total victim costs per crime were $47,424 for rape and $14,738 for assault. Among survivors with physical injury, total costs were $60,376 for rape and $49,603 for assault. For both rape and assault, mental health costs were substantially larger than medical costs and accounted for a major portion of total costs.

Response of Health Care Practitioners and the Health Care System

Although response to rape in most medical settings has been formalized for some time through protocols and wide use of forensic rape kits, evidence suggests that women often do not seek medical attention and proper procedures are not always followed. Kilpatrick et al. (1992) found that only 17% of women had a medical examination after their attack. Among those women who had received rape examinations within the past 5 years, 55% of victims were not counseled about pregnancy testing or pregnancy prevention; 50% were not given information about testing for HIV; and 33% were not provided with information about testing for exposure to sexually transmitted diseases.

Structured response in health care settings to forms of violence against women other than rape, particularly domestic violence, is more recent. The notion that health professionals should be trained to identify and refer patients affected by domestic abuse began to gain real momentum in 1991 when the American Medical Association established its National Coalition of Physicians Against Family Violence. Since then, training programs and treatment protocols have proliferated.

Violence against women has begun to obtain a small foothold in formal health policy statements. For instance, the Joint Commission on the Accreditation of Healthcare Organizations (JCAHCO) passed regulations effective in January 1992 calling for all hospital emergency departments and hospital-affiliated outpatient care facilities to have protocols and training plans for response to all forms of family violence (JCAHCO, 1991). Similarly, the Council on Ethical and Judicial Affairs of the American Medical Association has outlined the ethical duty of physicians to diagnose and treat family violence (American Medical Association, 1992b).

Unfortunately, significant barriers exist in accomplishing change among health practitioners with regard to addressing violence against women. Violence has received scant attention in the training of most clinicians (Tilden et al., 1994). Lack of knowledge not only of physical sequelae but of the interpersonal dynamics and sociology of violence hinders the ability to motivate health professionals to improve standards of practice. So long as physicians view topics such as domestic violence as a "Pandora's box" (Sugg & Inui, 1992), attempts at policy revision may be thwarted by resistance among the rank and file.

Prevention and Intervention

Primary Prevention

Within the discipline of public health, prevention is viewed as consisting of three separate forms or stages: primary prevention, which is intended to prevent an adverse outcome ever from happening; secondary prevention, which focuses on reducing the occurrence of future adverse events in at-risk populations; and tertiary prevention, which aims to reduce the consequences of adverse events that have already occurred. Secondary and tertiary prevention are usually accomplished through a variety of intervention strategies.

Prevention of lung cancer provides a useful and easily understood model of these forms of prevention. Primary prevention of lung cancer can be largely accomplished by reducing the number of individuals who ever take up smoking, which is by far the leading cause of this cancer. In this way, the cancer is prevented from ever occurring. Secondary prevention targets current smokers to reduce or give up smoking, which is putting them at increased risk for lung cancer even if the cancer has yet to develop. Tertiary prevention involves improved medical treatments for cancers that have already emerged, such as early diagnosis and more successful chemotherapies.

The hallmark of a public health approach to violence is a focus on primary prevention. Because we take a predominantly feminist view of the causes of violence against women, believing that the control and subjugation of women is a root motivating factor in many cases, we believe that primary prevention of this violence lies in improving the status of women in society. A thorough discussion of the many strategies needed to accomplish such a social transformation is beyond the scope of this chapter. Sparks and Bar On (1985) discuss the primary prevention of sexual assault through community programs that might increase women's equality, and Swift (1985) provides a description of educational and media-based strategies that address sex-role socialization.

Items that need to be on the agenda include addressing gender stereotypes embedded in our social norms, providing job opportunities for women at compensation equal to that of men, and increasing the number of women in legislative office.

One means of teaching young women and men about harmful gender stereotypes is through media literacy. Both entertainment and advertising media often portray women as fitting one of two general stereotypes: the self-sacrificing helpmate or the seductive temptress. Men are often pictured as being valued for virility, power, and financial success. Media literacy can help young people to decipher and question these stereotypes for themselves. Adolescents may benefit from thinking critically about how media messages may play a role in supporting the notion that men are entitled to expect subservience from women or are entitled to objectify them. These messages do a disservice to both men and women.

Violence of many sorts is also commonly glamorized in advertising, television, films, and even games (particularly video arcade games). Most depictions of violence fail to show the pain, suffering, sorrow, and loss that are the consequences of violent acts. Because it is unlikely that our media will become a great deal less violent in the near future, helping young people to examine these messages critically is one way to counteract negative media influences.

Secondary and Tertiary Prevention

Family Violence

The most important source of both secondary and tertiary prevention of family violence is the shelter system. Shelters and safe houses provide women with the most crucial need of women and children in crisis—safety. In addition, shelters usually provide group counseling for women and referrals for legal, job training, and housing assistance. They may also provide specialized programs for children of abused women, and they often do educational outreach in the local community.

Shelters cannot take on the entire burden of keeping women safe from their abusers, however. A variety of legal remedies are available to women although the specifics of these interventions tend to vary from state to state.

The police are frequently the first professionals to respond to domestic violence; however, the 1985 National Family Violence Survey found that only 7% of all incidents and 14% of serious incidents are reported to police (Kaufman Kantor & Straus, 1990). In many states, the police are now mandated to arrest the primary aggressor if they have reason to believe that abuse has occurred. The research on mandatory arrest provides a complex picture of this strategy's effects (Schmidt & Sherman, 1993). It appears that arrest may have a beneficial effect where the perpetrator is employed and otherwise has a "stake" in society. For perpetrators who are unemployed, it appears that arrest may have the ability to exacerbate the violence.

One of the most frequently used legal remedies for domestic violence is the civil restraining or protective order. These orders are available in all states although their coverage and provisions may vary. Generally speaking, restraining orders include provisions that require the defendant to stop the abuse, vacate the home (if there is a common domicile), stay a certain distance from the plaintiff, and have no contact whatsoever with the plaintiff except as specified (eg, for child visitation). Restraining orders can also include orders to surrender custody of minor children, provide child and other financial support, and surrender weapons (particularly guns). Although a restraining order is clearly no guarantee of physical safety, it can provide women with breathing space to assess their situation and plan future actions. Seeking a restraining order may also empower a woman, particularly in the context of a judge who sends a clear message that the defendant's behavior is illegal and inappropriate, and not deserved by the plaintiff.

Many women who have been abused are entitled to file criminal charges, which could include assault, aggravated assault, kidnapping, property damage, or stalking, depending on the specifics of the case. Unfortunately, it is still relatively rare for men to receive jail sentences in the context of criminal convictions related to non-fatal domestic violence, so women must weigh carefully the pros and cons of this strategy.

One other intervention that can be applied in cases of domestic violence is batterer treatment. Most often, men enter batterer treatment as a requirement under probation.

Sexual Assault

Rape crisis centers operate on the front lines of response to women who are sexually assaulted, dealing not only with the immediate physical and psychological trauma, but also assisting women with long-term recovery. According to Kilpatrick et al. (1992), over 2000 organizations assist rape victims. Given what is known about the potential for physical and mental health sequelae following assault, these centers and their adjunct services have a crucial role in reducing the toll of future morbidity among victimized women.

Although rape continues to be the most underreported violent crime, and arrest rates are extremely low (McCall, 1993), the criminal justice sector has attempted to address these cases more sensitively. Sex crime units and victim–witness programs may at least reduce the extent to which victims are revictimized by the legal process. Rape shield laws and other legislative reforms may also prove of some benefit to victims, but the evidence that legislative initiatives have accomplished any general deterrent effect is lacking (Marsh, Geist, & Caplan, 1982).

Some "personal safety" and resistance strategies may also have some utility in preventing sexual assault (Furby & Fischhoff, 1986). Because women of college age have been found to be at high risk for sexual assault, many institutions of higher learning have started prevention programs. Orientation seminars may suggest to women (in a manner that is not victim blaming) that drinking excessively in the presence of male acquaintances or strangers who are also drinking may place women in a situation where they are more vulnerable to assault. Using escort services across campus late at night is another example of personal safety strategies that may be recommended.

However, there are those who criticize these forms of prevention as "victim control," unduly constraining the freedoms of women in society (Sparks & Bar On, 1985). These strategies do not address primary prevention and may only displace an instance of sexual assault from a less vulnerable target to a more vulnerable one.

Political and Societal Response

The most important new legislative response to the problem of violence against women was the passage of the Violence Against Women Act (VAWA) in 1994. Among the initiatives included in the VAWA are increased funding for shelters, training of law enforcement officials and judges, education and rape prevention programs, piloting and assessment of youth education on domestic violence, and a national domestic violence hotline.

Most legislation related to violence against women continues to be enacted at the state level, where topics of recent interest have included antistalking measures, restriction of gun access and licenses for individuals convicted of domestic violence crimes, and reclassification of certain crimes involving violence against women as federal offenses. Careful evaluations are required to determine the effectiveness of these formal social controls. Unfortunately, the continued deficit of thorough and accurate information on this problem described at the opening of this chapter tends to hinder attempts to evaluate programs or policies.

It also remains to be seen what effect such legislative changes and other prevention and intervention strategies (ie, increasing shelter spaces, disseminating media awareness campaigns) will have on social norms or informal social control, which may well remain the key to long-term reductions in the level of violence against women.

References

American Medical Association. (1992a). Council on Scientific Affairs. Violence against women. Relevance for medical practitioners. *Journal of the American Medical Association, 267,* 3184-3189.

American Medical Association. (1992b). Council on Ethical and Judicial Affairs. Physicians and domestic violence: Ethical considerations. *Journal of the American Medical Association, 267,* 3190-3193.

Bachman, R. (1994). *Violence against women. A national crime victimization survey report* (NCJ-145325). Washington, DC: U.S. Department of Justice.

Bassuk, E. L., & Rosenberg, L. (1988). Why does family homelessness occur? A case-control study. *American Journal of Public Health, 78,* 783-788.

Bergman, L. (1992). Dating violence among high school students. *Social Work, 37,* 21-27.

Bullock, L., & McFarlane, J. (1989). The birth-weight/battering connection. *American Journal of Nursing, 89,* 1153-1155.

Bureau of Justice Statistics. (1994). *Violence between intimates* (NCJ-149259). Washington, DC: Office of Justice Programs, U.S. Department of Justice.

Carmen, E., Rieker, P. P., & Mills, T. (1984). Victims of violence and psychiatric illness. *American Journal of Psychiatry, 141,* 378-383.

Cohen, S., & Williamson, G. M. (1991). Stress and infectious disease in humans. *Psychological Bulletin, 109,* 5-24.

Cohen, S., Tyrell, D. A., & Smith, A. P. (1991). Psychological stress and susceptibility to the common cold. *New England Journal of Medicine, 325,* 606-612.

Coker, A. (1994). *Adjusting NCVS estimates of rape and domestic violence* [Project abstract]. National Institute of Justice Family Violence Research Program. Washington, DC: Office of Justice Programs, U.S. Department of Justice.

Feldman-Summer, S., Gordon, P. E., & Meagher J. R. (1979). The impact of rape on sexual satisfaction. *Journal of Abnormal Psychology, 88,* 101-105.

Flanzer, J. P. (1993). Alcohol and other drugs are key causal agents of violence. In R. J. Gelles & D. R. Loseke (Eds.), *Current controversies on family violence.* Newbury Park, CA: Sage.

Furby, L., & Fischhoff, B. (1986). *Rape self-defense strategies: A review of their effectiveness.* Eugene, OR: Eugene Research Institute.

Geist, R. F. (1988). Sexually related trauma. *Emergency Medicine Clinics of North America, 6,* 439-466.

Gelles, R. J. (1993). Alcohol and other drugs are associated with violence—they are not its cause. In R. J. Gelles & D. R. Loseke (Eds.), *Current controversies on family violence.* Newbury Park, CA: Sage.

Henton, J., Cate, R., Koval, J., Lloyd, S., & Christopher, S. (1983). Romance and violence in dating relationships. *Journal of Family Issues, 4,* 467-482.

Hotaling, G. T., & Sugarman, D. B. (1986). An analysis of risk markers in husband to wife violence: The current state of knowledge. *Violence and Victims, 1,* 101-124.

Jacobson, A., & Richardson, B. (1987). Assault experiences of 100 psychiatric inpatients: Evidence of the need for routine inquiry. *American Journal of Psychiatry, 144,* 908-913.

Joint Commission on the Accreditation of Healthcare Organizations. (1991). Revised standards address possible victims of abuse. *Joint Commission Perspectives,* March/April, 10.

Kaufman Kantor, G., & Straus, M. A. (1987). The "drunken bum" theory of wife beating. *Social Problems, 34,* 213-230.

Kaufman Kantor, G., & Straus, M. A. (1990). Response of victims and the police to assaults on wives. In M. A. Straus & R. J. Gelles (Eds.), *Physical violence in American families: Risk factors and adaptations to violence in 8,145 families.* New Brunswick, NJ: Transaction.

Kilpatrick, D. G., Saunders, B. E., Amick-McMullan, A., Best, C. L., Veronen, L. J., & Resnick, H. S. (1989). Victim and crime factors associated with the development of crime-related post-traumatic stress disorder. *Behavior Therapy, 20,* 199-214.

Kilpatrick, D. G., Edmunds, C. N., & Seymour, A. K. (1992). *Rape in America: A report to the nation.* Arlington, VA: National Victim Center.

Koss, M. P. (1985). The hidden rape victim: Personality, attitudinal and situational characteristics. *Psychology of Women Quarterly, 9,* 193-212.

Koss, M. P., & Dinero, T. E. (1988). Predictors of sexual aggression among a national sample of male college students. *Annals of the New York Academy of Sciences, 528,* 133-147.

Koss, M. P., & Dinero, T. E. (1989). Discriminant analysis of risk factors for sexual victimization among a national sample of college women. *Journal of Consulting and Clinical Psychology, 57,* 242-250.

Koss, M. P., & Heslet, L. (1992). Somatic consequences of violence against women. *Archives of Family Medicine, 1,* 53-59.

Koss, M. P., Koss, P. G., & Woodruff, W. J. (1991). Deleterious effects of criminal victimization on women's health and medical utilization. *Archives of Internal Medicine, 151,* 342-347.

Lacey, H. B. (1990). Sexually transmitted diseases and rape: The experience of a sexual assault centre. *International Journal of Sexually Transmitted Diseases and AIDS, 1,* 405-409.

Makepeace, J. M. (1981). Courtship violence among college students. *Family Relations, 30,* 97-102.

Makepeace, J. M. (1986). Gender differences in courtship violence victimization. *Family Patterns, 35,* 382-388.

Marsh, J. C., Geist, A., & Caplan, N. (1982). *Rape and the limits of law reform.* Boston: Auburn House.

McCall, G. J. (1993). Risk factors and sexual assault prevention. *Journal of Interpersonal Violence, 8,* 277-295.

McFarlane, J., Parker, B., Soeken, K., & Bullock, L. (1992). Assessing for abuse during pregnancy: Severity and frequency of injuries and associated entry into prenatal care. *Journal of the American Medical Association, 267,* 3176-3178.

Miller T. R., Cohen M. A., & Rossman, S. B. (1993). Victim costs of violent crime and resulting injuries. *Health Affairs, 12,* 186-197.

Miller, B. A., Downs, W. R., & Gondoli, D. M. (1989). Spousal violence among alcoholic women as compared to a random household sample of women. *Journal of Studies on Alcohol, 50,* 533-540.

Murphy, S. M. (1990). Rape, sexually transmitted diseases and human immunodeficiency virus infection. *International Journal of Sexually Transmitted Diseases and AIDS, 1,* 79-82.

O'Keefe, N. K., Brockopp K., & Chew, E. (1986, November/December). Teen dating violence. *Social Work,* pp. 465-468.

Resick, P. A., Calhoun, K. S., Atkeson, B. M., & Ellis, E. M. (1981). Social adjustment in victims of sexual assault. *Journal of Consulting and Clinical Psychology, 49,* 705-712.

Resnick, H. S., Kilpatrick, D. G., Dansky, B. S., Saunders, B. E., & Best, C. L. (1993). Prevalence of civilian trauma and posttraumatic stress disorder in a representative national sample of women. *Journal of Consulting and Clinical Psychology, 61,* 984-991.

Reuterman, N. A., & Burcky, W. D. (1989). Dating violence in high school: A profile of the victims. *Psychology, A Journal of Human Behavior, 26,* 1-9.

Roscoe, B., & Callahan, J. E. (1985). Adolescents' self-report of violence in families and dating relations. *Adolescence, 20,* 545-553.

Roscoe B., & Kelsey, T. (1986). Dating violence among high school students. *Psychology, A Quarterly Journal of Human Behavior, 23,* 53-59.

Satin, A. J., Hemsell, D. L., Stone, I. C., Theriot, S., & Wendel, G. D. (1991). Sexual assault in pregnancy. *Obstetrics and Gynecology, 77,* 710-714.

Schmidt, J. D., & Sherman, L. W. (1993). Does arrest deter domestic violence? *American Behavioral Scientist, 36,* 601-609.

Siegel, J. M., Golding, J. M., Stein, J. A., Burnam, M. A., & Sorenson, S. B. (1990). Reactions to sexual assault: A community study. *Journal of Interpersonal Violence, 5,* 229-246.

Sparks, C. H., & Bar On, B. A. (1985). *A social change approach to the prevention of sexual violence against women.* Stone Center for Developmental Services and Studies, Work in Progress (Series No. 83-08). Wellesley, MA: Wellesley College, Stone Center for Developmental Services and Studies.

Stark, E., Flitcraft, A., Zuckerman, D., et al. (1981). *Wife abuse in the medical setting: An introduction for health personnel* (Monograph Series, No. 7). Rockville, MD: National Clearinghouse on Domestic Violence.

Steiger, H., & Zanko, M. (1990). Sexual traumata among eating-disordered, psychiatric, and normal female groups. *Journal of Interpersonal Violence, 5,* 74-86.

Stets, J. E., & Straus, M. A. (1990). Gender differences in reporting marital violence and its medical and psychological consequences. In M. A. Straus & R. J. Gelles (Eds.), *Physical violence in American families: Risk factors and adaptations to violence in 8,145 families.* New Brunswick, NJ: Transaction.

Straus, M. (1979). Measuring intrafamiliy conflict and violence: The Conflict Tactics Scales. *Journal of Marriage and the Family, 41,* 75-88.

Straus, M. A. (1990). New scoring methods for violence and new norms for the Conflict Tactics Scales. Appendix B. In M. A. Straus & R. J. Gelles (Eds.), *Physical violence in American families: Risk factors and adaptations to violence in 8,145 families.* New Brunswick, NJ: Transaction.

Straus, M. A., & Gelles. R. J. (1990). How violent are American families? Estimates from the National Family Violence Resurvey and other studies. In M. A. Straus & R. J. Gelles (Eds.), *Physical violence in American families: Risk factors and adaptations to violence in 8,145 families*. New Brunswick, NJ: Transaction.

Straus, M. A., Gelles, R. J., & Steinmetz, S. K. (1980). *Behind closed doors: Violence in the American family*. New York: Anchor/Doubleday.

Sugg, N. K., & Inui, T. (1992). Primary care physicians' response to domestic violence: Opening Pandora's box. *Journal of the American Medical Association, 267,* 3157-3160.

Swett, C., Cohen, C., Surrey, J., et al. (1991). High rates of alcohol use and history of physical and sexual abuse among women outpatients. *American Journal of Drug and Alcohol Abuse, 17,* 49-60.

Swift, C. F. (1985). The prevention of rape. In A. W. Burgess (Ed.), *Rape and sexual assault: A research handbook*. New York: Garland.

Tilden, V. P., Schmidt, T. A., Limandri, B. J., et al. (1994). Factors that influence clinicians' assessment and management of family violence. *American Journal of Public Health, 84,* 628-633.

Winfield, I., George L. K., Swartz, M., & Blazer, D. G. (1990). Sexual assault and psychiatric disorders among a community sample of women. *American Journal of Psychiatry, 147,* 335-341.

Wood, D., Valdez, R. B., Hayashi, T., & Shen, A. (1990). Homeless and housed families in Los Angeles: A study comparing demographic, economic, and family function characteristics. *American Journal of Public Health, 80,* 1049-1052.

CHAPTER 22

Homelessness

Carol Fennelly
Bernardine Lacey

The Magnitude of the Problem

Homelessness in America is one of the great tragedies of our land. Exactly how many Americans are homeless is not clear. Figures range from 250,000 to 3 million (Hibbs et al., 1994). A 1994 study from Columbia University gives the most comprehensive look to date at the problem. The study found that 13.5 million (7.4%) Americans have experienced literal homelessness (ie, sleeping in shelters, abandoned buildings, bus and train stations, etc.) in their lifetime, with 5.7 million (3.1%) people being homeless between 1985 and 1990. When the definition was expanded to include people who had been homeless and slept at a friend or relative's house, the numbers jumped to an astonishing 26 million (14%) people who had experienced homelessness in their lifetime, with 8.5 million (4.6%) people between 1985 and 1990 falling into the enlarged category (Link et al., 1994).

The study was based on a telephone survey of 1507 households, so, consequently, could not reach those already homeless or households too poor to have a telephone, the groups most prone to homelessness. Therefore, the study's authors considered the figures to be conservative.

That the estimates of homeless people vary so wildly speaks to the politically volatile nature and the lack of understanding of the problem. Advocates first came up with an estimate of 2 million in 1982 (Hombs & Snyder, 1982). By 1984 the Reagan Administration had released a study that estimated the number at 250,000 and, thus, began the debate.

For many years the battle over the numbers raged with advocates on one side and government officials on the other. Each side had its own obvious vested interest in raising or lowering the numbers. In recent years, most have agreed to disagree and have focused on solving the problem rather than quantifying it (Interagency Council on the Homeless, 1994).

The fact is that homeless people are virtually impossible to count. It is in their interest to remain hidden. If a homeless person can be found, he or she can be harassed, assaulted, or in the case of women, raped. So, they remain hidden in alleys, abandoned buildings, cars, countrysides, parks, or anywhere that will provide them privacy and safety (Hombs & Snyder, 1982; Link et al., 1994).

Demographic Factors

Homeless families make up about 40% of the homeless population. Most of those families are headed by single women. About 25% are children. Families with children have been reported as the fastest growing group of homeless people for a number of years (Ugarriza & Fallon, 1994; Wright & Weber, 1987).

It has been widely believed that single homeless men outnumber single homeless women by as much as 10 to 1. However, some have long suspected that in reality the ratio is about equal. The misconception grew because single women came to shelters and were seen on the streets in far fewer numbers than men.

In reality, when a women becomes homeless she is perceived as more vulnerable, less threatening, and more in need of protection. Family members and friends are more willing to make room for a women than a man. In addition, women down on their luck are often exploited by men who may offer housing in exchange for other favors. As a result, the extent of homelessness among women (single or otherwise) has been a problem largely hidden from public view.

The Columbia study is especially interesting because it refutes a number of previously held ideas. In addition to finding much higher numbers generally, it found the number of homeless women to be nearly as high as men. It says that 15.5% of men and 12.8% of women in the United States have experienced one or more types of homelessness during their lifetime (Link et al., 1994).

The study also challenges the notion that homeless people are mostly young, single, male, urban, and African American. Instead, it found homelessness to be equally distributed racially and geographically, and between men and women. It is not, however, equal in its economic distribution. Not surprisingly, the study found that homelessness disproportionately affects low-income and poorly educated people.

Single Homeless Women

In many cases, to speak of single homeless women as "single" is inaccurate. Many homeless women have children from whom they have been separated (Brickner, Scharer, Conanan, Savarese, & Scanlan, 1994). Many women have lost their children as a result of their homelessness. In some cases, social service workers convinced the woman that the child should be placed in foster care until more stable housing could be secured. At that point, the check from Aid to Families with Dependent Children (AFDC) was stopped and, along with it, the eligibility for assisted housing. In other cases, the child was given up voluntarily or taken from the mother as a result of her mental illness or substance abuse problems. Whether the separation is by choice or otherwise, the effect on the woman can be tragic and devastating.

Single women who end up in shelters and on the streets are among the most broken members of our communities. They are more alienated and disenfranchised, and there is a higher incidence of mental illness (Brickner et al., 1994; Wright, 1990). In short, friends, family, and society have turned them out and they are most alone. Whether their various pathologies have created their alienation or the alienation has caused their pathologies is not clear. What is clear is that this is the most difficult and hard to reach group among the homeless population (Slagg, Lyons, Cook, Wasmer, & Ruth, 1994).

In his 1988 landmark book, *Rachel and Her Children*, about homeless women in New York's welfare hotels, Jonathan Kozol wrote,

> Few of the people in the Martinique were inmates of those institutions that were emptied prior to the 1980s; but all are inmates of an institution now. And it is this institution, one of our own invention, which will mass-produce pathologies, addictions, violence, dependencies, perhaps even a longing for retaliation, for self-vindication, on a scale that will transcend, by far, whatever deviant behaviors we may try to write into their pasts. It is the present we must deal with, and the future we must fear (p. 21).

DELORES

A homeless woman, Delores, came to a shelter. At the time, not too much was known about traditional bag ladies because they were a fairly new phenomenon. Delores refused all assistance except a bed at night. Shortly after her arrival she began to develop a strong odor. She did not respond to repeated pleas to take a shower. The odor was so powerful that she could be smelled from outside the building. The other women in the shelter were ready to harm her. The shelter staff finally laid down an ultimatum—shower or leave. She left.

For the next several weeks she took up residence in an abandoned car outside the building. Men could be seen entering and leaving the vehicle. Although the shelter staff repeatedly offered to intervene, she refused. Finally one day she said she had had enough. By then the odor was nauseating. She was taken into the house and a tub of water was drawn. She asked for help undressing. While assisting Delores, the staff found that her socks were stuck to her feet. They put her in the tub with her socks on, thinking they could soak them off. What came off were two of her toes that had become gangrenous from frostbite.

She was rushed to the hospital, and waited 10 hours in the emergency room for treatment, while her feet oozed and dripped. Finally, after a screaming tirade from the shelter staff, she was seen. Then the hospital tried to discharge her. At the shelter's insistence, she was admitted. They further insisted on a mental health examination. After a week, she was finally involuntarily committed to a mental hospital.

Homeless Women With Children

Homeless women with children present different problems from those seen with single women. Likewise, the causes of their homelessness are different. A Ford Foundation study found that 50% of homeless women with children have left abusive situations (Homelessness Information Exchange, 1994a). Whereas most men say their homelessness is caused by unemployment, drug or alcohol dependency, or imprisonment, women report leading causes to be domestic violence and eviction (Homelessness Information Exchange, 1993a).

Women with children are routinely discriminated against in housing. Keeping housing when resources are limited can be difficult; finding it in the first place can be impossible. Public housing lists in most cities have at least a 10-year waiting list. Last year the Department of Housing and Urban Development reported a shortfall of 5.1 million units of affordable housing nationwide. It is this housing shortage that most acutely affects homeless women with children (Community for Creative Non-Violence, 1993).

In 75% of the cities surveyed by the U.S. Conference of Mayors in 1992, families with children were identified as the group of homeless people for whom shelters and other services are particularly lacking. In that same year, Washington State reported turning away 47,728 women with children (Homelessness Information Exchange, 1993b). Services for single homeless women are even scarcer (Brickner et al., 1994).

Many homeless women, single or with children, have been abused at some point in their history, either physically or sexually. Often their mental and physical health needs go unmet (Brickner et al., 1994). A medical system created to treat housed people offers no understanding of the unique problems of homeless people in general, and homeless women in particular, and is often insensitive and alienating (Ugarriza & Fallon, 1994).

MARY

Mary sought shelter for herself and her three children, ages 8, 5, and 3. The father of the children had been incarcerated for 6 months. Mary had supplemented her aid check with babysitting but was barely able to meet expenses.

Her youngest child was hit by a car and was hospitalized. To be with her son she had to give up babysitting, and eventually fell behind in the rent and was evicted.

Mary was obese and had a multitude of health problems that were exacerbated by the stress of eviction, her son's illness, and her husband's incarceration. Her blood pressure rose to dangerous levels and she was hospitalized.

Because she had no family in the area, and her husband's family was inappropriate, her children were placed in foster care. Because she was a Medicaid patient she was released from the hospital prematurely and her healing time took longer than it should have.

Without her children living with her, she stopped receiving her AFDC check and could not get back into housing. A year later, and 6 months after her husband was released from prison, the family was finally able to reunite.

Health-Related Concerns

Homeless people in general are sicker and suffer from more chronic diseases than housed people. Poor diet, poor hygiene, lack of access to adequate health care, and constant exposure to the elements exacerbate even the simplest injury or illness. What is a simple cut on a housed person can become a major infection on someone who is homeless. A cold can easily become pneumonia (Wright, 1990).

Health problems are often sighted as a factor contributing to homelessness. A national study stated that 13% of those surveyed said it was a factor in their becoming homeless (Homelessness Information Exchange, 1994b).

Chronic Health Problems

Homeless people suffer from at least one chronic health problem almost twice as often as housed people (Wright, 1990; Wright & Weber, 1987). On average, homeless people die 20 years earlier than housed people, and the death rate among homeless people is at least 3.1 times higher than the standard mortality rate (Hibbs et al., 1994; Williams, 1991).

With the exception of obesity, stroke, and cancer, homeless people are far more likely to suffer from every category of chronic health problem. For example:

- Homeless people suffer from hypertension two to four times more often than the general population.
- Gastrointestinal disorders (including hernias, colitis, ulcers, diarrhea, gastritis) are found in homeless people two to three times more often than in housed people.
- Peripheral vascular disease including gout, varicosities, chronic edema, gangrene, ulcerations, phlebitis, thrombosis, chronic edema, and cellulitis of the extremities, are found 10 to 15 times more often in homeless people.
- Neurologic disorders from migraine headaches and neuritis to Parkinson's disease, peripheral neuropathy, multiple sclerosis, and quadriplegia are present in homeless people at a rate fives time higher than the general population. This figure does not include seizure disorders, which appear in nondrinking homeless people 22 to 25 times more frequently than among housed people.
- Anemia, ear disorders, liver disease, and genitourinary problems also appear at a more frequent rate among homeless people (Wright, 1994; Wright & Weber, 1987).
- Human immunodeficiency virus (HIV) and acquired immunodeficiency syndrome (AIDS) have risen among homeless people in some areas to as high as 20% (Williams, 1991). Nationally the rate of AIDS among the homeless population appears to be more than 10 times that in the general population (Wright, 1994).

Like the homeless population in general, homeless women suffer from illnesses at a higher rate and, in some cases, a significantly higher rate than housed women.

Among the general population, women tend to have higher rates of less serious illnesses, and men have higher rates of more serious diseases, and, thus, a shorter life expectancy. However, in the homeless population these figures shift in a startling way. Homeless women tend to have the same rate of serious disease and illness as homeless men, with these exceptions:

- Women do not exhibit as high a rate of hypertension, tuberculosis, or trauma as men.
- Women show higher rates of eating disorders.
- Women show higher rates of endocrinologic disorders and diabetes.
- Women are more likely to have genitourinary disorders.
- There is a higher rate of mental illness among women.
- There is a lower rate of alcoholism, but an equal rate of drug abuse among homeless women (Ugarriza & Fallon, 1994; Wright, 1994; Wright & Weber, 1987).

Pregnancy and Sexually Transmitted Diseases

The rate of pregnancy among homeless women is about the same as or a little higher than that of the general public. Should a homeless women become pregnant, she faces a host of problems. These are high-risk pregnancies because of a lack of prenatal care, poor nutrition, the tendency of homeless women to be substance addicted, and the uncertain life of homelessness. There is a higher rate of low birth weight infants and infant mortality among babies born to homeless mothers (Brickner et al., 1994; Wright, 1994).

Although most shelters are single-gender facilities, homeless women find ways to remain sexually active. Homeless women are frequently diagnosed with sexually transmitted diseases and, in fact, it is one of the most common diagnoses of many health clinics for homeless people (Brickner et al., 1994; Wright & Weber, 1987).

Both HIV and AIDS are growing concerns among homeless women. High-risk behavior makes them more prone to contact. Most homeless women have contracted the virus through intravenous drug use (Brickner et al., 1994; Wright, 1994).

Mental Illness

No discussion of health and homeless women would be complete without an examination of the high rate of mental illness in this population. Most studies reveal that mental illness is a factor for many homeless women (Ugarriza & Fallon, 1994). As a result, outreach becomes even more difficult. There is a high rate of undiagnosed physical illness among this group, which has led to an unexpectedly high rate of mortality from infectious causes and suicide (Brickner et al., 1994).

The process of deinstitutionalization began in the 1960s. Although it was a well intentioned move to provide more humane mental health care to patients, it went wildly off track. By the early 1980s, the actual deinstitutionalization process had ended. After that time, mentally ill people usually did not even make it to the door of the institution and, so, remain lost in America (Lamb, Bachrach, & Kass, 1992; Torrey, 1988).

In 1988, Dr. E. Fuller Torrey (1988, p. 50), one of the nation's leading experts on homeless mentally ill people, wrote this in his book *Nowhere to Go*:

1. There are at least twice as many seriously mentally ill individuals living on streets and in shelters as there are in public mental hospitals.
2. There are increasing numbers of seriously mentally ill individuals in the nation's jails and prisons.
3. Seriously mentally ill individuals are regularly released from hospitals with little or no provision for aftercare or follow-up treatment.
4. Violent acts perpetrated by untreated mentally ill individuals are increasing in number.
5. Housing and living conditions for mentally ill individuals in the community are grossly inadequate.
6. Community mental health centers, originally funded to provide community care for the mentally ill so these individuals would no longer have to go to state mental hospitals, are almost complete failures.
7. Laws designed to protect the rights of the seriously mentally ill primarily protect their right to remain mentally ill.

8. The majority of mentally ill individuals discharged from hospitals have been officially lost. Nobody knows where they are (Torrey, 1988, p. 5).

Trauma and Violence

The leading cause of death and disability among homeless people is trauma and violence (Hibbs et al., 1994; Wright & Weber, 1987). Because of the vulnerability of homeless women, they are at greater risk of facing violence through robbery, assault, and rape. The heightened rates of mental illness and substance abuse among this population increase their chances of falling victim to random abuse and violence (Brickner et al., 1994).

JOAN

Joan, a homeless severely mentally ill women went to a clinic for health care. She was tested for the HIV virus and results were positive.

The staff of the clinic wrestled with how to deal with the situation. Joan obviously needed to be informed of her condition, but her ability to absorb and process the information properly and appropriately were in question.

After she was told and informed of the risks and dangers of her disease, she went back to the streets and spread the word. Two weeks later she was found in an alley. She had been beaten to death.

Societal and Political Responses

Most homeless people lack health insurance and receive their primary health care in emergency rooms of hospitals when they have reached a health crisis (Hibbs et al., 1994; Ugarriza & Fallon, 1994). Staff in clinics and infirmaries frequently see patients who come from emergency rooms with prescriptions they have no way of filling and inappropriate instructions such as "get plenty of bed rest," or "keep feet elevated."

Often a medical crisis provides an opportunity to reach out to a homeless woman and turn her life around. A crack-addicted homeless woman came to a shelter with a broken leg. The staff had a chance to intervene in her life and she received not only treatment for her physical trauma, but for her addiction as well. She has been drug free for 3 years, is gainfully employed, and living on her own.

A health crisis can also provide an opportunity to educate and screen. Unfortunately because most medical care is received at impersonal public health facilities or emergency rooms, a lack of continuity of care means the opportunity is missed (Brickner et al., 1994; Hibbs et al., 1994).

In an ideal situation, health clinics attuned to the needs of homeless women will provide birth control education, substance abuse counseling, mental health evaluations, physical examinations and routine tests, education and screening for sexually transmitted diseases, hygiene counseling, and general relationship building. However, most health care for homeless women is crisis oriented, so again, these opportunities are missed (Brickner et al., 1994; Ugarriza & Fallon, 1994).

Two short case histories illustrate both the inadequacy of the health care system, its insensitivity to issues relative to homeless people, and the low priority given to this population.

GWEN

A homeless woman, Gwen, who stayed in a shelter, had grown increasingly weak and emaciated. She finally agreed to go to the clinic. She looked pale and her blood pressure was barely detectable.

The clinic staff called an ambulance because they believed she was too sick and fragile to be transported by car to the hospital. At the hospital Gwen was given an IV and released in the middle of the night with a note that said, "Eat more bran flakes for your constipation."

Miraculously, she managed to walk the 3 miles back to the shelter, where she awaited the clinic staff in the morning.

The staff found a bed in a small private facility that provided medical care to homeless people and was run by a religious group. A work-up at the facility showed cancer of the esophagus. Gwen died 6 weeks later.

SANDRA

Sandra was a resident of a women's shelter. One day she requested medical care. A doctor from the clinic was summoned and reported finding Sandra in bed with a bowl beside her.

She demonstrated for the doctor what happened when she tried to eat or drink. Whatever she consumed immediately came back up through her nose. On examination, she was found to have a large cancer of the oral cavity. She reported that when she had gone to the emergency room the previous day she had been given an antibiotic and sent back to the shelter.

These stories are not merely anecdotal. In fact, such tales can be heard in every city in the nation, and far too often. It was these too frequent experiences that inspired a joint effort between Howard University School of Nursing and the large shelter operated by the Community for Creative Non-Violence in Washington, D.C. It was felt that if students in medical training were sensitized to the nuances of homeless medicine, constituents would receive better care in the long run. The project was enormously successful.

Strategies for Intervening

Although life is made more comfortable by providing health care, good health cannot be sustained absent from adequate housing, nutrition, and peace of mind. Ending homelessness is the only solution to securing good health for homeless women.

Having said that, there is little disagreement about several issues. Even though the estimates of the numbers of homeless and substance addicted may vary, the numbers clearly are too high and increased substance abuse treatment is needed.

The shortfall of affordable housing nationwide clearly affects women in the most profound way, particularly women with children. The downsizing of Housing and Urban Development and the decimation of that agency's budget has ensured that this problem will grow in the future. However, even if the agency's budget and mission were to remain the same, a look at public housing would be in order. It is important that whatever replaces existing programs include service-enhanced housing.

Homeless women, particularly those who are single, have for many years posed a problem for providers because of their high rate of mental illness. The process of deinstitutionalization began in earnest during the 1960s with the Supreme Court ruling that declared that unless one is a danger to oneself or others, one cannot be held involuntarily in a mental institution. Although this was good human rights law, it has been transformed into nothing more than fiscal policy (Lamb et al., 1992; Torrey, 1988). The result has been disastrous. We need to rethink these policies, and revisit the commitment laws they generated.

Job training is critical to ending homelessness among women. Many have no job skills and have never been directed to that possibility. Existing training programs have been unsuccessful because there are no jobs at the end of the training. Further, it is necessary that these jobs provide a living wage to foster independence. A look at day care options must go hand in hand with any discussion about job training and placement for homeless women. It is obvious one cannot exist without the other.

In the current political climate, with a bloated deficit and reduced revenues, most advocates agree these solutions are only distant dreams. Increasingly, trends in both federal and state governments are toward cost-cutting measures that are likely to reduce existing social programs. This may leave many unable to keep up, fit in, and manage, leading to growing numbers of homeless people in the future.

Current anti-homeless sentiment in communities across the nation is manifesting itself in a variety of ways and is making the search for solutions even more difficult. For example, local governments are passing increasingly restrictive forms of legislation and neighborhoods are organizing to keep homeless people and programs from moving in.

Many advocates are quietly wondering if homelessness is a solvable problem. They believe that too many people have been outside for too long to ever bring them inside again. This is a frightening thought. For homeless women, the prospect is even more grim. They are a population traditionally underserved, misunderstood, and alienated. The future promises more of the same.

In the early 1980s, Bob Hayes, founder of the National Coalition for the Homeless, said the answer to homelessness was, "Housing, housing, housing." At the time, he was correct, but not now. The problem is far more complex and will require a major investment of money, energy, and political will to solve.

References

Brickner, P., Scharer, L., Conanan, B., Savarese, M., & Scanlan, B. (1994). *Under the safety net*. New York: Norton.

Community for Creative Non-Violence. (1993). *Housing fact sheet*. Washington, DC: Author.

Hibbs, J., Benner, L., Klugman, L., Spencer, R., Macchia, I., Melllinger, A., & Fife, D. (1994). Mortality in a cohort of homeless adults in Philadelphia. *New England Journal of Medicine, 332*(5),304–309.

Hombs, E., & Snyder, M. (1982). *Homelessness in America: A forced march to nowhere*. Washington, DC: Community for Creative Non-Violence.

Homelessness Information Exchange. (1993a). *Women and homelessness. Fact sheet*. Washington, DC: Author.

Homelessness Information Exchange. (1993b). *Homeless families with children. Fact sheet*. Washington, DC: Author.

Homelessness Information Exchange. (1994a). *Domestic violence—A leading cause of homelessness. Fact sheet*. Washington, DC: Author.

Homelessness Information Exchange. (1994b). *Health and homeless families. Fact sheet*. Washington, DC: Author.

Interagency Council on the Homeless. (1994). *Priority: Home! The federal plan to break the cycle of homelessness*. Washington, DC: Author.

Kozol, J. (1988). *Rachel and her children*. New York: Crown.

Lamb, R., Bachrach, L., & Kass, F. (1992). *Treating the homeless mentally ill: A report of the Task Force on the Homeless Mentally Ill*. Washington, DC: American Psychiatric Association.

Link B., Susser, E., Stueve, A., Phelan, J., Moore, R., & Struening, E. (1994). *Life-time and Five-year prevalence of homelessness in the states*. New York: Division of Epidemiology, School of Public Health, Columbia University.

Slagg, N., Lyons, J., Cook, J., Wasmer, D., & Ruth, A. (1994). Profile of clients served by a mobile outreach program for homeless mentally ill persons. *Hospital and Community Psychiatry, 45* (11),1139–1140.

Torrey, F. (1988). *Nowhere to go*. New York: Harper & Row.

Ugarriza, D., & Fallon, T. (1994). Nurses' attitudes toward homeless women: A barrier to change. *Nursing Outlook, 42*(1),26–28.

Williams, L. (1991). *Mourning in America: Health problems, mortality, and homelessness*. Washington, DC: National Coalition for the Homeless.

Wright J., & Weber, E. (1987). *Homelessness and health*. Washington, DC: McGraw Hill's Healthcare Information Center.

Wright J. (1990). Poor people, poor health: The health status of the homeless. *Journal of Social Issues, 46* (4).

CHAPTER 23

Incarceration

Brenda V. Smith
Cynthia Dailard

Introduction

Until recently, the critical health care needs of women prisoners have been virtually ignored by correctional officials, the medical and public health communities, and society at large. This long-standing neglect stems not only from the lack of resources directed toward prisoners, but also from the low value society places on providing health care to low-income women.

Although the health care needs of incarcerated women still largely go unmet, advocates, policymakers, and health care providers are beginning to direct attention toward this medically vulnerable population. This attention is due in part to the dramatic increase in the women's prison population over the past 15 years. It also stems from the recognition that low-income women with serious health problems and high-risk behaviors, such as drug use and prostitution, increasingly find themselves in prison. As a result, correctional systems across the nation have been forced to assume the responsibility for providing treatment to large populations of women with significant health care needs. Moreover, the intersections of the recent health care debate—with its heightened attention to women's health—and the national debate on crime and justice, has placed a spotlight both on conditions of confinement and on the increasing costs of providing health care to growing populations of prisoners.

Prisons, much like homeless shelters, can provide an important focal point for efforts to address some of the more persistent public health problems, including acquired immunodeficiency syndrome (AIDS), tuberculosis (TB), and addictions. Because women at risk for incarceration are often disconnected from health care, treatment services, and public health messages in the community, they enter prison with a host of health problems and limited preventive information. For many women prisoners, the prison medical system is the first health care system with which they have direct, sustained contact. As a result, prisons are becoming a common place for women who are socially or economically marginalized to receive health care. However, correctional functions of security and control often operate at cross purposes with established principles for disease prevention and treatment. At the same time, prison health facilities are rarely equipped to treat and prevent a full range of health problems, especially those particular to women. With increasing numbers of women in the criminal justice system, it is crucial not only to have a more complete picture of the health status of women prisoners, but also to have a better understanding of the roles that prisons can play in either ameliorating or exacerbating the health problems of low-income women.

Profile of Incarcerated Women

At the end of 1993, 55,365 women were incarcerated in federal and state prisons (Gilliard & Beck, 1994, p. 4). Women accounted for 5.8% of the total prison population and 9.3% of the jail population (individuals generally incarcerated for less than a year) nationwide (Gilliard & Beck, 1994, p. 4; Jankowski, 1992). Between 1980 and 1993, the growth rate for the female prison population increased approximately 313% compared to 182% for men (Gilliard & Beck, 1994, p. 4; Greenfeld & Minor-Harper, 1991). The primary reason for the marked increase in the number of incarcerated women has been the nation's "war on drugs," along with the advent of mandatory minimum sentences for many drug offenses. The emphasis on interdiction, along with more stringent sentences, has had a substantial impact on women. In 1991, 64% of women in federal prisons and 32% of women in state prisons were serving sentences for a drug-related offense (Kline, 1992, p. 34; Snell & Morton, 1994, p. 3). This represents a substantial increase over 1980, when only 11% of women in state prisons were serving sentences for drug offenses (Greenfeld & Minor-Harper, 1991, p. 4).

Women prisoners are overwhelmingly low-income women of color struggling with poverty and addiction. Although women of color comprise 21% of all women, they account for 58% of the women's prison population. Forty-six percent of women in prison are African American, 14% are Hispanic, and 3.6% are categorized as "other" (Snell & Morton, 1994, p. 2). The vast majority of women prisoners are young—between the ages of 21 and 34—in their childbearing years (Snell & Morton, 1994, p. 2). Many of these women are single mothers raising families with little family or social support. Fifty-three percent of women in prison and 74% of women in jail were unemployed before their incarceration (Snell, 1992; Snell & Morton, 1994, p. 2). High rates of poverty and unemployment explain why women are overwhelmingly convicted of nonviolent crimes with economic motives—income-generating crimes such as drug sales, theft, forgery, and prostitution. A 1991 study of the federal prison population by the Federal Bureau of Prisons found that drug offenses and property crimes such as larceny, theft, bribery, and fraud accounted for 76% of the crimes that led to women's incarceration compared to 65% for men (Kline, 1992).

The majority of women prisoners have drug and alcohol dependency problems. Conservative estimates suggest that 70% to 80% of all women prisoners are addicted to alcohol or other drugs. The correlation between drug use and crime is inescapable. For example, Bureau of Justice statistics reveal that in 1991, 36% of women in state prisons reported that they were under the influence of a drug at the time they committed the offense for which they were incarcerated (Snell & Morton, 1994, p. 7). Women were more likely than men to be under the influence of a major drug at the time of their offense; one in four women prisoners reported they had committed their offense to obtain money to purchase drugs compared to one in six male prisoners (Snell & Morton, 1994, p. 7). The increasing number of incarcerated women with addictions and related high-risk behaviors has severe implications for already overburdened prison health care systems that have long neglected the medical treatment and health education needs of female inmates. Nonetheless, prisons provide a valuable opportunity for delivering services and resources to high-risk women—services necessary to break cycles of crime and drug use while encouraging healthy behaviors.

Health Status of Incarcerated Women

Before their incarceration, women prisoners are largely disconnected from medical institutions in their community. Low-income women often do not have the transportation, child care, job flexibility, or income necessary to gain access to systems of care. Additionally, primary health care and health education may simply not be a priority for women who devote much of their energy to making ends meet, providing for children, avoiding homelessness, or grappling with trauma caused by physical or sexual violence. Moreover, often the systems of care constructed to serve low-income people are inefficient and demeaning, requiring women to wait for many hours with no guarantee of seeing a health care provider. Women often fear the consequences of obtaining services and may avoid seeking care purposefully rather than out of ignorance. For many, accusations of drug abuse or a diagnosis of AIDS could mean the loss of custody of their children or the loss of public benefits such as housing or financial assistance. Feelings of shame related to sexual encounters or drug addiction may inhibit others from seeking treatment for sexually transmitted diseases (STDs) or other health problems.

Ultimately, low-income women's estrangement from the public health care system only becomes exacerbated when they enter the prison setting, which can be inhospitable—if not hostile—to the health care and health education needs of women prisoners. Although medical care for all prisoners is poor, the situation is far worse for women prisoners. Because prison health care systems were created for men, routine gynecologic care, such as Pap smears, breast examinations, and mammograms, is extremely rare. As a result, women fail to receive preventive services necessary to maintain their gynecologic health and frequently receive treatment only when their condition has deteriorated to the point that they require emergency care.

The structure of prison health care systems is also not conducive to either long-term treatment or health maintenance. Prison health services generally operate according to a "sick-call" model of health care, designed to respond to discrete and immediate health problems such as the flu or an injury. This system requires prisoners to follow a specific protocol whenever they need to see a physician or seek medication. In some facilities, prisoners must report to the medical unit for sick call. In others, prisoners "sign up" for sick call and a member of the medical staff screens the patient on the housing unit, referring those who require treatment to a physician. Treatment for these patients often depends on the availability of transportation or guards to escort them to the medical facility, which may impede their access to care. The influx of medical staff onto the housing unit also affords little confidentiality to prisoners and may deter prisoners who do not want to appear vulnerable from seeking necessary treatment. The sick call protocol also often lacks the flexibility needed for individuals with acute or chronic health problems that require regular monitoring or quick intervention. Because inmates are not entrusted with the responsibility of controlling their own medication, prisoners who require medication on a regular basis must follow this procedure several times a day. As a result, prisoners often miss doses of medication whenever they are too sick to reach necessary services, or when staff is inadequate to transport them to the pharmacy or bring their medications.

The health of women prisoners is also adversely affected by the severe staffing shortages and inadequately trained staff found in many prison health facilities. Because economic resources are generally directed toward maintaining security, rather than providing medical care to inmates, prison health care facilities routinely lack sufficient numbers of physicians or nurses, as well as the medical technology, necessary to provide appropriate care (General Accounting Office [GAO], 1994, p. 2). The lack of staffing commonly means that physicians do not have enough time to supervise physician assistants who provide the bulk of primary care to inmates (GAO, 1994, p. 2). Furthermore, many physician assistants do not meet the training and certification requirements of the general medical community (eg, Inmates of Three Lorton Facilities v. District of Columbia, 1994). The inability of prison health care facilities to recruit and retain qualified medical staff commonly translates to significant delays in scheduling tests, obtaining test results, and receiving treatment, and may result in deficient, and potentially inappropriate, care. For example, because of staffing shortages, half of 56 women with abnormal mammograms at the Lexington Medical Referral Center, which specializes in providing medical care to women in the Federal Bureau of Prisons, left the facility without being notified of their test results (GAO, 1994, p. 17). It also means that few resources are available for coordinating the treatment of women with chronic health problems after their release. Consequently, many women with significant health problems such as human immunodeficiency virus (HIV) infection are released to the community without linkages to necessary medical services.

Moreover, the correctional mandates of security and control are often antagonistic to public health messages that encourage individuals to take an active role in maintaining their health and seeking primary care. Security protocols emphasizing custody, rather than care, may impede women's access to treatment. For example, correctional institutions may not be equipped to provide reliable transportation to appointments at medical facilities outside the correctional institution (Geballe & Stone, 1988, p. 4; Women Prisoners v. District of Columbia, 1994). As a result, women prisoners may miss a series of scheduled appointments or be transported to a clinic after it has closed. Others may be forced to wait for several hours with their hands and feet shackled without ever receiving treatment because their medical records were not transported to the medical provider. Prison guards may deny prisoners access to medication and health services as a form of punishment or as a means of social control (Burris, 1992, p. 300). These experiences, and the feelings of frustration and disempowerment they engender, reinforce the distrust of health care providers that women developed in the community and deter many women prisoners from seeking necessary treatment for their medical problems.

Chronic Conditions

Typically, women enter prisons and jails with a host of medical problems, including disorders associated with poor nutrition and poverty, such as obesity, diabetes, anemia, and hypertension, and other chronic conditions such as asthma, seizures, and ulcers. Patients with chronic conditions often require frequent observation and monitoring. This is particularly true for prisoners because conditions of confinement exacerbate many of these disorders (Wilson & Leasure, 1991, p. 34). However, prison systems rarely have the facilities or resources available to implement appropriate protocols for monitoring patients with chronic conditions. Instead, prisoners with chronic conditions must appear at sick call or schedule a clinic appointment themselves when they require care. The sick call model of health care renders health monitoring and continuity of care virtually impossible (GAO, 1994, p. 10).[1] However, continuity of care is critical to women with chronic health problems.

Moreover, according to the GAO, relying on inmates with chronic problems to schedule their own appointments or appear at sick call is inefficient insofar as some chronically ill prisoners may not recognize that their symptoms warrant medical attention until the condition becomes serious (GAO, 1994, p. 9). Because low-income women have not been the targets of public health education efforts in their community, many women prisoners are not trained to identify the early signs of illness or problems requiring early medical intervention. At the same time, public health advocates have failed to make these public health messages accessible to women while they are incarcerated.

Addiction

The vast majority—between 70% and 80%—of incarcerated women are addicted to alcohol or other drugs. Fifty-four percent of women inmates, compared to 50% of male inmates, said they had used a drug in the months before their offense, and over 41% said they had used drugs on a daily basis (Beck et al., 1993, p. 22). In the month before their offense, 19% of women, compared with 10% of men, had used crack, and an additional 17% of women, compared with 15% of men, had used cocaine. Approximately 20% of women in state prisons reported daily alcohol use during the year preceding their incarceration (Snell & Morton, 1994, p. 10). Not only do women have higher rates of drug use than men, but they are more likely to have

---

1. The Lexington Medical Referral Center closed its chronic care unit in 1990 because it did not have a sufficient number of nurses to staff the unit. Consequently, most inmates with chronic conditions were housed in units that did not have frequent monitoring by nurses. The GAO review of the facility indicated that women with chronic conditions were not receiving the health care they needed, and thus, incarcerated women die needlessly because of the absence of proper monitoring (GAO, 1994, p. 10).

used more serious drugs such as crack cocaine and to be injection drug users: a third of female inmates in state prisons reportedly used a needle to inject drugs, compared to a quarter of male inmates (Snell & Morton, 1994, p. 7). An estimated 18% of the women and 12% of the men also said that they had shared a needle at least once in the past (Snell & Morton, 1994, p. 7).

Drug treatment, however, is still largely unavailable to low-income women in the community, especially pregnant women. Notwithstanding the large populations of women who require drug treatment while they are incarcerated, many prison systems have failed to provide the services necessary to meet their needs. As a result, women prisoners commonly must withdraw from alcohol and other drug addictions outside the medical unit, without direct medical supervision (Geballe & Stone, 1988, p. 4). Pregnant women addicted to heroin or methadone may detoxify without proper supervision during crucial stages of their pregnancy, despite risks to themselves and their fetus (Geballe & Stone, 1988, p. 4). Approximately half the women in state prisons in 1991 reported that they had never participated in a drug treatment or drug education program (Snell & Morton, 1994, p. 8). After their admission to prison, 38% of incarcerated women had participated in a drug treatment program (Snell & Morton, 1994, p. 9). These figures signify a promising improvement over statistics for 1990, which indicated that only 8% of federal prisoners and 11% of state prisoners were enrolled in drug treatment programs (Stephan, 1992). However, even the 1992 figures may be misleading because the quantity and quality of drug treatment services provided by correctional institutions vary dramatically. Consequently, many women with alcohol and other drug addictions routinely leave prison without the resources necessary to break cycles of drug use and incarceration or to curb behaviors related to drug use that place them at high risk for disease.

Sexually Transmitted Diseases

Drug addiction is also linked to high rates of STDs, including HIV disease, among women in prison. Drug addiction forces many women to trade sex for drugs, or for money to buy drugs, often with multiple partners. Although many women find it difficult to practice safe sex because of the power imbalance in their relationships, these difficulties become amplified while they are under the influence of alcohol or drugs (Schilling et al., 1994, p. 540). Many women fear that proposing condom use to their partner will jeopardize either their relationships or their means to support their drug habit. The nature of these sexual encounters, compounded by histories of sexual victimization and physical abuse, create situations in which women feel powerless to insist on barrier protection.

Consequently, women prisoners experience high rates of STDs such as gonorrhea, syphilis, herpes, human papillomavirus (HPV), and chlamydia. In one study of 114 female detainees at a large New York City jail, 8% had abnormal Pap smears, 35% had HPV, 7% had gonorrhea, and 22% had syphilis (Bickell et al., 1991). In another study of 101 women at Rikers Island, 27% tested positive for chlamydia (Holmes et al., 1993). The detection and treatment of STDs among this high-risk population is critical given that many untreated STDs lead to irreversible complications such as infections and infertility or birth defects in newborns. Moreover, HPV is recognized as a premalignant condition, leading to cervical cancer in a significant percentage of women who contract the disease.

Public health experts have indicated that Pap smears and pelvic examinations should not only be a routine intake procedure for incarcerated women, but should be provided on an annual basis thereafter (and more frequently for women with HIV or histories of abnormal test results). This is particularly imperative given that early signs of HIV disease in women are frequently gynecologic problems such as chronic yeast infections, pelvic inflammatory disease, and cervical dysplasia. However, many prison systems have failed to implement these protocols.[2] In some prison systems, women may wait months to receive their test results, or may never be notified of abnormal test results. As a result, women are at risk of having undetected or untreated gynecologic disorders and cancers progressing toward a serious condition before they receive attention.

HIV and AIDS

Perhaps the greatest challenge for prison health facilities, however, is treating the increasing number of HIV-positive women prisoners. High rates of HIV infection among this population can be explained by the congruence in risk factors for both HIV and incarceration in women—race, poverty, and drug use (Smith & Dailard, 1994). Women currently account for only 13% of persons with AIDS (U.S. Department of Health, 1994a). As of June 1994, women comprised 51,235 of the 396,015 adult and adolescent AIDS cases in the United States (U.S. Department of Health, 1994a, pp. 8, 10). Yet, they represent the fastest growing rate of HIV infection of any identifiable group in the country. Statistics show that AIDS is the fourth leading cause of death nationwide for women between the ages of 25 and 44 and is now the leading cause of death among women in 15 of the 135 largest cities (Altman, 1995).

Women with AIDS are poorer than the general population, and 74% of them are African American or Latina (compared to 45% of men with AIDS) (U.S. Department of Health, 1994a). Women of color accounted for 75% of new AIDS cases in 1994 (*Time Magazine*, 1995). The primary route of infection for women is through injection drug use and related heterosexual transmission. Forty-eight percent of women with AIDS in June 1994 were current or former injection drug users, and 19.5% were infected as the result of heterosexual contact with male partners who contracted the HIV virus through intravenous drug use (U.S. Department of Health, 1994a).

The congruence in risk factors for both HIV infection and incarceration in women has resulted in distressingly high rates of HIV infection among women prisoners. Contrary to patterns in the community, the prevalence of HIV infection

2. Although the Federal Bureau of Prisons requires that female prisoners receive pelvic examinations and Pap smears on intake and annually thereafter, the GAO reported that at the Lexington Medical Referral Center, Pap smears "were not done in a timely manner and in some cases may not have been doen at all. In fact, these tests were often only performed when the patient had a problem that brought her to sick call." Due to medical staff shortages, the center was about 6 months behind in performing pelvic examinations and Pap tests (GAO, 1994, p. 4).

among incarcerated women exceeds that for male prisoners. As early as 1988, a study conducted by the Centers for Disease Control and Prevention, Johns Hopkins University, and the National Institute of Justice of 11,000 entrants to 10 prison and jail systems throughout the country found rates of HIV infection ranging from 2.1% to 7.6% in men and from 2.5% to 14.7% in women. Seropositive rates were higher for women than for men in 9 of the 10 jurisdictions, and the rate of infection for women under 25 years of age more than doubled the rate for males in the same age group (5.2% compared to 2.5%) (Vlahov et al., 1991).

Another 1988 study of entrants to New York State prisons found that 18.8% of the women compared to 17.4% of the men were HIV positive (Smith et al., 1991). Furthermore, a recent Bureau of Justice Special Report indicates that 3.3% of women prisoners who reported test results in 1991 were HIV positive compared to 2.1% of men (Harlow, 1993). This represents the self-reported incidence of HIV infection in U.S. state and federal prisons, including the nation's 503 largest jails. Reportedly, 6.8% of Hispanic women and 3.5% of African American women were HIV positive compared to 1.9% of Caucasian women (Harlow, 1993). These figures probably greatly underestimate the incidence of HIV because test results were self-reported and because prison testing policies vary greatly across jurisdictions. Prison systems with mandatory testing policies (the minority) are likely to have much more accurate estimates of HIV infection that those with voluntary policies (Hammett, Harrold, Gross, & Epstein, 1994, p. 26). Correctional facilities housing women prisoners from urban areas have the highest rates of HIV infection, with experts now estimating that 27% of women in New York's Rikers Island—the largest U.S. jail—are HIV positive (Rosenthal, 1994).

The AIDS epidemic has magnified the significant deficiencies in prison health care systems, highlighting the incompatibility between existing principles for security and health maintenance. The National Commission on AIDS (1991) stated that the disproportionate concentration of persons with HIV in correctional facilities has placed an "intolerable stress on marginal prison health care capabilities." This has devastating implications for HIV-positive women, whose health care needs have traditionally been ignored by correctional institutions. Although the presence of HIV disease in correctional facilities has been a great concern for prison administrators since the mid-1980s, few correctional facilities have developed comprehensive strategies for treating and supporting infected prisoners, or for preventing or reducing the transmission of HIV infection among prisoners during and after their incarceration. The lack of medical resources directed at incarcerated women means that prisons are especially unprepared to shape these programs to meet the needs of women prisoners.

Few correctional systems have developed or implemented adequate protocols for treating HIV-infected women. For example, the Federal Bureau of Prisons requires that patients with AIDS be seen on a monthly basis. However, staffing shortages at the Lexington Medical Referral Center, which specializes in providing medical care to women in the Federal Bureau of Prisons, were so severe that women with AIDS were scheduled to be seen by physicians every 6 months (GAO, 1994, p. 10). Moreover, the isolation of prison physicians and nurses from the rest of their profession means that prisoners often do not receive state-of-the-art care (Dixon et al.,

1993), such as access to innovative new drugs therapies. In addition, the problems that women commonly face gaining access to treatment in prison are compounded by the general lack of knowledge concerning both the progression of HIV disease in women and gender-appropriate treatments. Although health care providers are generally not trained to identify the particular manifestations of HIV in women, the absence of routine and consistent gynecologic care means that prison health care providers are unlikely to detect the early signs of HIV disease in women. Moreover, the high incidence of STDs, gynecologic complications, and other health problems in this population may confound the identification of HIV. Physicians who care for women prisoners may only treat the STDs or other health problems associated with HIV infection, while the underlying HIV goes undiagnosed until it has progressed to full-blown AIDS. Consequently, women prisoners infected with HIV lose out on the significant benefits of early intervention and treatment.

Education for women prisoners is desperately needed to reduce the transmission of AIDS both during and after their incarceration. This includes exploring topics related to drug use, violence, sexuality, and safer sex practices. These programs must also focus on empowering women to take a proactive role in obtaining health care. Unfortunately, issues of institutional control have historically frustrated AIDS education efforts in prison. Although experts believe that the most effective means of controlling the spread of AIDS is through grass roots mobilization and community empowerment (Hammett et al., 1994, p. 41), opportunities for self-empowerment are extremely limited due to the intrusion of prison authority on all aspects of life. In a few systems, women prisoners have successfully organized themselves to educate, support, and counsel their peers. However, prison administrators generally disfavor prisoner initiatives, viewing them as a threat to prison security. As a result, prison officials may work to undermine efforts of women prisoners to organize themselves in an effort to combat the spread of AIDS and the discrimination facing HIV-positive women (Clark & Boudin, 1990, p. 91; Mason, 1994, p. 150).

Tuberculosis

The prison setting also increases women's risk for contracting TB, hepatitis, and other airborne communicable diseases that thrive in prisons and jails. TB, in particular, is a major problem in prisons, occurring three times more often in correctional facilities than in the community (GAO, 1994, p. 3). Because incarcerated women frequently enter prisons from other high-risk settings, such as homeless shelters, public hospitals, and crowded urban environments, they may be exposed to TB. The rapid movement of women prisoners back and forth from the correctional system to other high-risk environments provides the population turnover that fuels high rates of TB in prison.

Although TB is not a new problem in prisons, the rapid growth of overcrowded prison populations living in unsanitary and poorly ventilated facilities, the lack of access to health care in the community, and the increasing number of prisoners with HIV have resulted in a resurgence of the epidemic. Prisoners who have a positive TB test result and do not complete their course of medication risk developing active TB disease—which can be spread to other inmates, correctional staff, and individuals in the community—or an often fatal, drug-resistent form of the disease. Women with compromised immune systems caused by HIV or diabetes are particularly vulnerable to TB and are more likely to progress to active TB.

Although many correctional systems have taken the initial steps necessary to counter the threat of widespread TB, many have failed to implement programs that effectively contain the epidemic and treat affected prisoners (Hammett & Harrold, 1994). For example, in 1992 the Bureau of Prisons facility in Lexington, Kentucky hired two Public Health Service pharmacy students to review patient records and to ensure that inmates who tested positive for TB were complying with treatment. They found that among those women who tested positive for TB, 27% were not following their prescribed treatment regimen (GAO, 1994, p. 10). On learning these results, the medical staff immediately instituted a counseling program to ensure compliance, which successfully achieved a compliance rate of close to 100% 3 months later (GAO, 1994, p. 10). However, most correctional systems do not have the staff necessary to ensure compliance with treatment regimens or the resources available to promote prisoner education. Because women prisoners typically serve short sentences, this inability to effectively treat prisoners exposed to TB fosters thriving rates of the disease both in prisons and in the community.

Pregnancy

In addition to the general health problems of women prisoners, many women must address pregnancy-related health concerns while they are incarcerated. Although statistics from a recent Bureau of Justice study indicate that 6% of women incarcerated in state prisons are pregnant on intake (Snell & Morton, 1994, p. 10), this study may significantly underestimate the number of pregnant prisoners, insofar as protocols for pregnancy testing at intake vary widely across jurisdictions. This figure also does not account for the number of prisoners who become pregnant by guards, other prisoners, and visitors while incarcerated (Smith & Dailard, 1994, p. 81; Women Prisoners v. District of Columbia, 1994). Moreover, an additional 15% of women prisoners are estimated to be postpartum (Greenfeld & Minor-Harper, 1991). Low-income women generally experience high rates of complications during pregnancy because of chronic health conditions, problems caused by drugs, alcohol, smoking, poor nutrition, and the lack of prenatal care in the community. Researchers are beginning to study incarceration as a risk factor for adverse birth outcomes. One study (Fogel, 1993) of 89 prisoners found the following incidence of health problems in pregnant prisoners:

- anemia (38%)
- diabetes (9%)
- hypertension (9%)
- STDs (18%)
- urinary tract infections (33%)

Another study of 69 pregnant prisoners found that 36% of the women reported drug use, primarily cocaine, during pregnancy, and 68% smoked cigarettes (Egley,

Miller, Granados, & Fogel, 1992).[3] Prison medical facilities are also encountering increasing numbers of pregnant prisoners who are HIV positive.

Despite the significant population of women in prison who are at increased risk for pregnancy complications, neither adequate prenatal care nor abortion services are routinely provided to incarcerated women. Correctional systems typically do not have the prenatal protocols, staffing, and equipment necessary to provide pregnant women—especially those at risk for complications—with the timely and regular examinations or the careful monitoring they require (Barry, 1989, p. 190). In some prisons, pregnant women never see an obstetrician during the entire course of their pregnancy because of the absence of resident obstetricians or gynecologists. Women prisoners commonly do not have access to exercise, proper diets, and the nutrition supplements necessary for healthy pregnancies. The absence of regular prenatal care for women prisoners and the attendant neglect of high-risk pregnancies significantly jeopardize the health of pregnant prisoners and their infants.

The lack of prenatal care also means that pregnant women who are HIV positive may not receive antiviral drugs necessary to prevent the transmission of HIV to their newborns. One recent study found that the drug Zidovudine (AZT) dramatically reduced the transmission of HIV from infected mothers to their infants, without increasing the risk of birth defects; of newborns whose mothers received a placebo during pregnancy 26% were born HIV positive compared to 8% of the newborns whose mothers received AZT (U.S. Department of Health, 1994b). Because transmission from mother to infant is not guaranteed, pregnant women face many issues, including whether to terminate the pregnancy or whether to carry it to term. For many women, this decision may be based on their access to AZT. Virtually all prisons claim to make AZT available to prisoners (Hammett et al., 1994, p. 69), but the absence of prenatal care means that female prisoners may not receive appropriate AZT therapies during crucial stages of their pregnancies. Also, obstetricians are often not trained specifically in protocols for working with HIV-infected pregnant women and may not even be aware that these women should receive AZT.

Mental Health Problems

Women prisoners constitute a population of women at high risk for mental health problems. In a recent study funded by the National Institute of Mental Health, Teplin, Abram, and McClelland (1994) found substantial psychiatric morbidity among a sample of almost 1300 female jail detainees. More than 80% of the women studied had experienced one or more lifetime psychiatric disorders, and 70% were symptomatic within the 6 months before the interview. The 6-month prevalence study revealed that almost 15% of the women had experienced severe psychiatric illness, including a major depressive episode (13.7%), a manic episode (2.2%), or schizophrenia (1.8%). Moreover, a significant percentage experienced antisocial personality disorder (13.5%) or dysthymia (6.5%). Lifetime prevalence rates for specific conditions were as follows:

3. The prevalence of drug use may have been underestimated because the study relied on self-reporting.

- major depressive episode (16.9%)
- manic episode (2.6%)
- schizophrenia (2.5%)
- dysthymia (9.6%)
- substance abuse/dependence (70.2%)
- posttraumatic stress syndrome (33.5%)
- antisocial personality disorder (13.8%)

Many of these prevalence rates are significantly higher than rates for the general population, including major depression (which is three times higher) and dysthymia (which is twice as high). The researchers note that the high prevalence rates of these two disorders are particular problems in correctional facilities because suicide is one of the leading causes of death among prisoners.

Although the high rates of mental illness among women prisoners may result from chronic poverty and harsh living conditions such as homelessness, the stress of incarceration may cause a relapse in women with a history of mental illness. Moreover, histories of sexual or physical abuse may lead to depression or other psychological problems including posttraumatic stress syndrome. Teplin, Abram, and McClelland (1994) found that one-third of the female jail inmates studied had experienced posttraumatic stress syndrome during their life and 22.3% within the previous 6 months. Most of these women were victims of rape or other sexual assault. This corresponds to Bureau of Justice statistics, which indicate that 43% of women in state prisons and 44% of women in jail had either been physically or sexually abused at some point during their lifetime before their incarceration (Beck et al., 1994, p. 9). Thirty-one percent of women in state prisons had been abused before the age of 18 and 24% after age 18 (Beck et al., 1994, p. 9). Moreover, prolonged separations from their children cause incarcerated women to experience depression, nervousness, and extreme anxiety. The majority of women prisoners require psychological and other support services that target women and address the root issues triggering drug and alcohol abuse and crime. These issues include adult and childhood physical and sexual victimization, along with the poor self-esteem, pain, and disconnectedness that follows from such experiences.

Despite the tremendous need for psychological counseling and other mental health care, these services are largely unavailable to incarcerated women. In 1991, approximately 23% of women in state prisons received mental health care such as group or individual counseling after their admission (Snell & Morton, 1994, p. 10). However, these statistics are misleading because mental health care in prison is rarely consistent and does not meet optimal standards. For example, the GAO reports that many female psychiatric patients at the Lexington Medical Referral Center were not receiving regularly scheduled individual and group therapy necessary to improve their psychological condition (1994, p. 5).[4] Experts indicate that many women prisoners are overmedicated or medicated inappropriately, noting that it is "a common practice in correctional institutions to give medication without psy-

4. The Chief of Psychiatry at Lexington has stated that he could not provide the type of psychiatric care that each female patient needed and "he was lucky if he could 'eyeball' each patient daily" (GAO, 1994, p. 5).

chotherapy and to medicate inmates for minor psychosomatic complaints or as a 'cure' for behavioral problems" (Wilson & Leasure, 1991, p. 36).[5] Although women prisoners are less violent than their male counterparts, women are more likely to receive psychotropic medications than are men (Wilson & Leasure, 1991, p. 36).[6] Nearly one in six women in 1991 received medication prescribed by a psychiatrist or other doctor for an emotional or mental problem since their admission to prison (Snell & Morton, 1994, p. 10). Moreover, prison facilities rarely have the facilities or the staff necessary to provide appropriate psychiatric care to patients with more acute mental health problems. These staffing shortages place inmates at risk of receiving poor or untimely psychiatric assessments and inadequate monitoring of their mental conditions.[6] Women with mental health problems who do not receive appropriate psychiatric treatment or counseling while incarcerated are at high risk for homelessness, violence, and repeated involvement in the criminal justice system once they are released to the community.

Conclusion

When women enter prisons, they bring with them the major health problems of low-income communities. Unfortunately, prisons have become incubators for the most serious and life-threatening diseases in our communities. Because women typically serve relatively short sentences, women who do not receive treatment services while they are incarcerated reenter society, potentially carrying with them contagious diseases that place their families and communities at risk. The startling lack of health education in prison also means that on their release women do not have the information necessary to use preventive services in the community such as mammograms, Pap smears, or timely prenatal care, or the resources available to curb behaviors that place them at high risk for HIV and STDs, addiction, TB, unplanned pregnancies, and reproductive cancers.

Prisons, however, provide public health advocates and health educators with a valuable point of contact with high-risk women who are not receiving public health messages in the community. Prisoner and health advocates must assist correctional officials to realize the potential preventive and rehabilitative roles that prisons can play in educating prisoners about high-risk behaviors and in reducing morbidity among women both during and after women's incarceration. Correctional facilities, community health care providers, and other organizations serving low-income women must work together to empower incarcerated women to gain access to systems of care and to curtail high-risk behaviors to break cycles of infection.

---

5. Overmedicating women with psychotropic drugs is not unique to the prison setting. In the United States, women receive two-thirds of all prescriptions for psychotropic drugs (Cafferata & Meyers, 1990). The overmedication of women in the prison context, however, takes on a unique coercive dimension.
6. The Federal Bureau of Prisons maintains that a single psychiatrist for every 20 to 25 inmates is an ideal staffing pattern. According to this standard, the Lexington Medical Referral Center for women prisoners should have nine psychiatrists serving its 237 acute and chronic care mental health patients. However, in 1992, the Center was only authorized to have three psychiatrists on staff, and only had two serving the entire inmate population (GAO, 1994, pp. 5-6).

Ultimately, comprehensive public health initiatives targeting incarcerated women must become a major component of public health strategies both in prison and in the community to improve the health of low-income communities.

References

Altman, L. K. (1995, January 31). *The New York Times.*

Barry, E. (1989). Pregnant prisoners. *Harvard Women's Law Journal, 12,* 189-205.

Beck, A., Gilliard D., Greenfeld, L., Harlow, C., Hester, T., Jankowski, L., Snell, T., Stephan, J., & Morton, D. (1993, March). *Survey of state prison inmates, 1991* (Bureau of Justice Statistics). Washington, DC: U.S. Department of Justice.

Bickell, N. A., et al. (1991). Human papillomavirus, gonorrhea, syphilis, and cervical dysplasia in jailed women. *American Journal of Public Health, 81,* 1318-1320.

Burris, S. (1992). Prisons, law and public health: The case for a coordinated response to epidemic disease behind bars. *University of Miami Law Review, 47,* 291-335.

Cafferata, G. L., & Meyers, S. M. (1990). Pathways to psychotropic drugs. *Medical Care, 28,* 285.

Clark, J., & Boudin, K. (1990). Community of women organize themselves to cope with the AIDS crisis: A case study from Bedford Hills Correctional Facility. *Social Justice, 17,* 90-109.

Dixon, P., Flanigan, T., DeBusno, B., Laurie, J., DeCiantis, M., Hoy, J., Stein, M., Scott, H., & Carpenter, C. (1993). Infection with the human immunodeficiency virus in prisoners: Meeting the health care challenge. *American Journal of Medicine, 95,* 629-635.

Egley, C., Miller, D., Granados, J., & Fogel, C. (1992). Outcome of pregnancy during imprisonment. *Journal of Reproductive Medicine, 37,* 131-134.

Fogel, C. I. (1993). Pregnant inmates: Risk factors and pregnancy outcomes. *Journal of Obstetric, Gynecologic, and Neonatal Nursing, 22,* 33-39.

Geballe, S., & Stone, M. (1988). The new focus on medical care issues in women's prison cases. *National Prison Project Journal, 15,* 1-4.

General Accounting Office. (1994). *Bureau of Prisons health care: Inmates' access to heath care is limited by lack of clinical staff* (GAO/HEHS-94-36). Washington, DC: Author.

Gilliard, D. K., & Beck, A. J. (1994, June). *Prisoners in 1993* (Bureau of Justice Statistics, p. 4). Washington, DC: U.S. Department of Justice.

Greenfeld, L. A., & Minor-Harper, S. (1991). *Women in prison* (Bureau of Justice Statistics Special Report, p. 7). Washington, DC: U.S. Department of Justice.

Hammett, T. M., Harrold, L., Gross, M., & Epstein, J. (1994, January). *1992 Update: HIV/AIDS in correctional facilities, issues and options* (National Institute of Justice). Washington, DC: U.S. Department of Justice.

Hammett, T. M., & Harrold, L. (1994, January). *Tuberculosis in correctional facilities, issues and practices* (National Institute of Justice). Washington, DC: U.S. Department of Justice.

Harlow, C. (1993, September). *HIV in US prisons and jails* (Bureau of Justice Statistics Special Report, p. 5). Washington, DC: U.S. Department of Justice.

Holmes, M. Safyer, S., Bickell, N., Vermund, S., Hanff, P., & Phillips, R. (1993). Chlamydial cervical infection in jailed women. *American Journal of Public Health, 83,* 551-555.

Inmates of Three Lorton Facilities v. District of Columbia, Civil Action No. 92-1208 (D.D.C. 1994).

Jankowski, L. W. (1992, June). *Jail inmates* (Bureau of Justice Statistics, p. 1). Washington, DC: U.S. Department of Justice.

Kline, S. (1992). A profile of female offenders in the Federal Bureau of Prisons. *Federal Prisons Journal, 47,* 33-35.

Mason, C. (1994). HIV-positive women in prison, women with HIV: Breaking the silence. *Berkeley Women's Law Journal, 9,* 149-152.

National Commission on AIDS. (1991, March). *HIV disease in correctional facilities,* p. 9.

Rosenthal, E. (1994, January 1). Doctors behind bars balance safety and care. *The New York Times,* p. A1.

Schilling, R., El-Bassel, N., Ivanoff, A., Gilbert, L., Su, K., Safyer, S., Vermund, S., Holmes, M., Safyer, & Burk, R. (1994). Sexual risk behavior of incarcerated, drug-using women, 1992. *Public Health Reports, 109,* 539.

Smith, B. V., & Dailard, C. (1994). Female prisoners and AIDS: On the margins of public health and social justice. *AIDS & Public Policy Journal, 9,* 78-85.

Smith, P., Mikl, J., Truman, B., Lessner, L., Stevens, R., Lord, E., Broaddus, R., & Morse, D. (1991). HIV infection among women entering the New York State correctional system. *American Journal of Public Health, 81,* 35-40.

Snell, T. L. (1992, March). *Women in jail, 1989* (Bureau of Justice Statistics Special Report, p. 3). Washington, DC: U.S. Department of Justice.

Snell, T. L., & Morton, D. C. (1994, March). *Women in prison: Survey of state prison inmates, 1991* (Bureau of Justice Statistics Special Report). Washington, DC: U.S. Department of Justice.

Stephan, J. (1992, May). *Census of state and federal correctional facilities, 1992* (Bureau of Justice, p. 12). Washington, DC: U.S. Department of Justice.

Teplin, L., Abram, K., & McClelland, G. (1994, October 20). *The prevalence of psychiatric disorder among incarcerated women: Pretrial jail detainees.* Delivered at the 25th annual meeting of the American Academy of Psychiatry and the Law, Miami, FL.

Time Magazine. (1995, February 20). p. 16.

U.S. Department of Health. (1994a). U.S. HIV and AIDS cases reported through June 1994. *HIV/AIDS Surveillance Report, 6* (1) 9-10.

U.S. Department of Health. (1994b). Recommendations of the U.S. Public Health Service Task Force on the Use of Zidovudine to Reduce Perinatal Transmission of Human Immunodeficiency Virus. *Morbidity and Mortality Weekly Report, 43* (RR-11), 3.

Vlahov, D., Brewer, T., Castro, K., Narkunas, J., Salive, M., Ullrich, J., & Munroz, A. (1991). Prevalence of antibody to HIV-1 among entrants to U.S. correctional facilities. *Journal of the American Medical Association, 265,* 1129-1132.

Wilson, J. S., & Leasure, R. (1991). Cruel and unusual punishment: The health care of women in prison. *Nurse Practitioner, 16,* 32-39.

Women Prisoners of the District of Columbia Department of Corrections v. District of Columbia, No. 93-2052, slip.op. at 25 (D.D.C. Dec. 13, 1994).

CHAPTER 24

Poverty

Linda Burnes Bolton

"Our women are falling from the skies," exclaims an ancient African chieftain. He was describing the escalating number of women dying in Western Africa in the late 1800s. Women, the heart and soul of every community, are sick more often and have their human and economic potential limited more often than their male counterparts. This is especially true of women living in poverty. At any point in time over the last century, adult women have been twice as likely as men to live in poverty. This phenomenon correlates with the diminished value of women expressed in the lack of access to resources to sustain human development–nutrition, housing, safety, health, and education. Seventy-five years after women won the right to vote, 25 years after they won the right to control their reproductive lives, and 30 years after purportedly breaking the glass ceiling, many women remain trapped within the ranks of poverty. Regrettably, the social condition of poverty with its deleterious effect on women and families is accepted and tolerated by our society.

Gender, education, and income are part of the multidimensional construct of social class that too often is correlated with human potential. The status of women in society is measured by income derived from employment out of the home, which changes over time (Grella, 1990). Throughout their lives women must struggle against the mutually reinforcing social pressures of gender and poverty (Andes, 1992). The experience of being poor, undereducated, and female is life shattering and robs women of dignity, respect, self-esteem, and potential.

This chapter explores the effects of poverty on the health status and life experiences of women. A description of the scope and dimensions of poverty is presented. Data on the health of impoverished women are included to illustrate fully the deleterious effects of poverty. The chapter concludes with a review of programs that seek to improve the living environments of women and their families, and with a call for social action to reduce the level and scope of poverty among women.

The Concept of Poverty

Poverty is commonly defined in the United States by a federally designated index, derived from family size and the dollars needed to purchase food and housing (O'Hare, 1985). In 1987, poverty was defined as an annual income of $15,000 for a family of four (U.S. Bureau of the Census, 1992). The federal designation does not consider other human needs such as access to education, health care, transportation, and supportive services. Poverty is a relative, not an absolute experience. Poverty has been described by others as a social condition (Lillie-Blanton, 1993). Poverty interacts with other dimensions of socioeconomic status to adversely affect the lives of women and increase their vulnerability.

The equitable distribution of life resources remains a challenge for women and their children (Mahowald, 1993). Without equitable access to financial resources, women are vulnerable and subject to many forms of oppression, such as discrimination in education, employment, housing, and transportation systems (Mahowold, 1993). Poverty adversely affects women—their liberty, freedom, and pursuit of well-being.

The condition of social inequality, caused in part by economic inequality, cannot be rectified without working to achieve economic opportunity for women. Women, especially non-Caucasian women, are more likely to be single heads of families. As such, they represent the largest population of impoverished people in the United States (Pearce, 1978). One-third of all women and 75% of all African American women live in poverty (U.S. Bureau of Census, 1992). This "feminization of poverty" is also characterized by the low earning capacity of single women, the lack of child support from noncustodial fathers, and the economic marginal benefits received from governmental assistance programs (McLanahan et al., 1989).

Poverty and its related stresses adversely affect women's ability to parent (Larner, Halpern, & Harkavy, 1992). Limited social and financial resources can negatively affect women and their children. For example, children who live in households headed by a single woman are less likely to graduate from high school, more likely to be victims and perpetrators of violence, and less likely to receive adequate health care (National Center for Health Statistics [NCHS], 1995a). Women without economic resources and social support underutilize preventive health services (Bolton, 1988).

Pearce (1978) described the compelling effect of gender inequality and poverty on human potential and predicted an exponential growth in the absolute number and percentage of impoverished women. She predicted that nearly two of three poor people in the 1990s would be women. The faces and voices of poverty may look different but they all sing the same sad song—loneliness, despair, and lack of choices. Poverty is experienced by women as lack of opportunity, lack of access to education, a struggle to exist and survive.

The following excerpts illustrate women's experiences and the effect poverty has on their lives. The comments were drawn from various sources including interviews conducted over a 3-year period of women enrolled in an community program, entitled Great Beginnings for Black Babies.

VOICES OF POVERTY

I'm Jacqueline. I had my first child at age 14. My mother kicked me out. I went to live with my boyfriend. He left me when the baby was 6 months old. I went on welfare. I have three kids now. I can't work. I don't know how.

My name is Liza. I'm 19. When I graduated from high school I thought the world would open up for me. I had a diploma! I make less today than I did 3 years ago in the Twenty Twenty Program. I worked half the week and went to school the other half.

My name is Mary Jo. Everyday I work. I'm so tired of working for nothing! I have two jobs so I can pay rent and feed my kids. I don't have time to talk to my kids. They're growing up without me. I pray God will keep them safe.

My two daughters and sons have lived with me with all their lives, except when they were in jail. Two of them just got out. They don't work and I'm afraid for them and myself. My blood pressure is so high the doctor told me I should quit working and go on disability. I can't do that. Disability won't pay for my kids.

When my husband died my life ended. He did everything. I didn't know about the money. I had no idea what it costs to live. I don't live anymore. I exist. I'm 76 years old. I wish I had died instead of Morrie. (Senior enrolled in community program).

I'm tired of working. The girls on the job talk about making it. They're different. They got somebody to listen to them, to encourage them, to help them. I got myself. Careers are what White women have; jobs are what Black women do (Boyd, 1993).

Voices of despair and disillusion are often associated with poverty. It does not discriminate. Caucasian, African American, Jew, Gentile, old and young, poverty affects them all. And perhaps its most ravaging effect is on the health and well-being of women.

Adverse Effects of Poverty on the Health of Women

In the book *Women and Children Last,* Sidel (1986) observes that a person who is poor is more likely to be sick, less likely to receive adequate medical care, and more likely to die at an early age. Poverty takes away the future of so many women and young people.

Poverty has previously been described in this chapter as a social condition with multiple effects. Its effect on the health status of women and children is most notable. Women living in poverty have shorter life spans, limited access to health care services, higher incidence and prevalence of disease and illness, and are less likely to use preventive health services. Impoverished women are stricken by the same diseases and conditions that are killing most Americans, but their survival rates are lower. Children living in poverty experience higher rates of disability, are much more likely to have higher elevated blood lead levels, and show a higher incidence of acute asthmatic episodes (NCHS, 1994). The following review of the effect of poverty on health illustrates the many conditions that limit impoverished women.

Cardiovascular Disease

Forty-nine percent of poor women die within a year of experiencing a myocardial infarction as compared to 31% of their male counterparts (NCHS, 1995a). One in nine women between the ages of 45 and 54 has cardiovascular disease and one in three women over the age of 65 experiences severe cardiovascular disease resulting in massive myocardial infarction and stroke. The paucity of research on the effects of gender, age, and poverty on women has limited sustained interventions to address this critical health problem. What is known is that women living in poverty die at two times the rate of all women experiencing cardiovascular disease. In the United States, 15 million women have hypertension and 11 million have heart disease (NCHS, 1995b). Impoverished women with limited access to prescription drugs, clinical research trials, and comprehensive services die from undetected and untreated malignant hypertension and other disorders of the cardiovascular system. The Office of Research on Women's Health has launched a major women's health initiative to enroll women in longitudinal studies regarding the health of women. However, without support and aggressive outreach most poor women will not participate.

Cancer

Lung cancer, not breast or cervical cancer, remains the leading cause of death from cancer among women (NCHS, 1995a). The 400% exponential growth in the death rate from lung cancer since 1985 has largely occurred among poor women with substandard living conditions. The American Cancer Society data suggest that controlling for poor socioeconomic status affects the incidence, prevalence, and mortality disparities observed between racially and culturally diverse groups so that the gap between groups is diminished (American Cancer Society, 1991). Disparities also exist in cancer screening and detection that are associated with income. Only 40% of women 35 years of age and older with annual incomes of less than $10,000 have ever had a mammogram compared to 60% of women in the same age group with gross annual incomes of $20,000 or more (NCHS, 1995). Poverty and socioeconomic status are the most significant factors associated with decreased breast cancer survival rates (McCoy et al., 1994). Yet, programs exist that can improve survival if cancers can be detected early. Unfortunately, poor women underutilize preventive health services such as screening and detection programs (NCHS, 1995b).

AIDS and Sexually Transmitted Diseases

Women comprise the fastest growing group of persons with human immunodeficiency virus (HIV) and acquired immunodeficiency syndrome (AIDS). Seventy-five percent of all women with AIDS are African American or Hispanic with the majority at or below the poverty level (NCHS, 1995b). Poor women seek care later, have their diseases detected at later stages, and die earlier. Syphilis, gonorrhea, and chlamydia infections have increased dramatically in the past decade among all women. However, the epidemic has claimed the lives of poor women more often (NCHS, 1995a).

Reproductive Health

Twenty-seven percent of children born to women below the poverty line are unplanned at conception (NCHS, 1995b). Women with incomes above the poverty line are more likely to have planned pregnancies, prenatal care, and insurance to cover the costs of care. In the last decade, births to unmarried adolescents increased 30%, and at higher rates among poor, ethnically and culturally diverse populations. The infant mortality rate for women without adequate prenatal care and support has increased dramatically (NCHS, 1995b).

Although the maternal mortality rate remains low, it is an important issue for impoverished women who die from the lack of ability to obtain care (NCHS, 1995b). Women classified as poor are more likely to forgo care (Himmelstein & Woolhandler, 1995). The lack of access to primary health care services for poor women and children remains one of the critical public health issues. In the United States, 80% of all deaths are preventable, particularly in the areas of women's health, through the combined forces of preventive health behaviors and early detection and screening of disease.

Violence

Homicide is the second leading cause of death among poor and vulnerable women and specifically among women of color (NCHS, 1995a). This phenomenon is associated with a plethora of interweaving social factors such as the lack of basic resources, dependence, stress, poor living conditions, and increased risk-taking behaviors such as substance abuse. One-third to one-half of the 10 million people who abuse drugs and alcohol are women. Drug abusers are vulnerable to becoming victims. Every 60 seconds 60% of the poor women in this country are physically, emotionally, sexually, or psychologically abused (Bolton, 1995). These frightening statistics are part of the everyday lives of women without hope and economic well-being. There are countless untold stories of women and children who suffer from the effects of poverty. The media sensationalizes violence by reports of a 5-year-old child thrown from a window or of husbands who beat their wives. However, the daily insults of poverty and abuse experienced by poor women receive little attention from the media, policymakers, or the community at large.

Health Insurance

Women are three times more likely to suffer from chronic conditions than men (NCHS, 1995a). Yet, Medicare, the number one insurance coverage for women, provides more acute than chronic care coverage. Fifteen million women of childbearing age are without insurance coverage and an additional 5 million have minimal coverage (Abel, 1994). Women pay higher premiums for coverage than men and receive less. Feminists have termed this as "gender-based insurance" (Abel, 1994). These policies have adversely affected the ability of women to care for themselves and their children. Women, the caregivers of the world, are also more likely to lose insurance at higher rates than men. This phenomenon occurs most often from disruptions in employment caused by pregnancy or serious illness. Women experience greater difficulty reentering the job market and finding insurance coverage. Data from multivariate analyses indicate that women experience increased rates of illness and disability days and mortality associated with acute and chronic illnesses all related to income and their living environments (Montgomery & Carter-Pokras, 1993). Working poor women are less likely to have access to basic health care services and their children are more likely have poor health status (Weitzman & Barry, 1992). These women and their families have limited access to health and social services compared to women receiving governmental assistance.

Health Policy

Women account for more than 70% of all Medicaid beneficiaries and 60% of all Medicare beneficiaries. One-third of all births in the United States are paid for by Medicaid. Seventy-one percent of female Medicare beneficiaries have disabilities (Employee Benefit Research Institute, 1995). What would happen if Medicare and Medicaid were reduced in the United States? How would such a health policy affect poor women? According to the Kaiser Commission on the Future of Medicaid (1995), a 15% cut in funding would result in the following:

- 350,000 women would not receive breast and cervical cancer screening.
- 200,000 women would not receive prenatal care.
- 400,000 women would not receive primary care.
- 600,000 women would not receive family planning services.
- 180,000 women would not receive AIDS/HIV testing and counseling.
- 2 million women would not receive disability services (Davis, 1995; Kaiser Commission, 1995).

The potential consequences of cuts in programs and services for poor women could be higher incidences of infant mortality, delays in disease detection and treatment, and more deaths from preventable causes. We are one of two nations in the world (the other is South Africa) without a national family policy that protects women and children. We must actively work together to reshape health and human services policies if poor women and children are to be adequately served.

Programs

In the 1960s the Great American Antipoverty campaign was launched to counter the devastating effects of poverty on women, children, and families. The war on poverty had lofty goals and no substantial impact, except for Head Start. It relied on the federal government for design, implementation, and, most importantly, funding. When President Lyndon B. Johnson called on the American people to help each other, he chided them to be charitable and help their fellow humans because it was the right thing to do. The images in the mass media of Appalachian poor families, homeless children, and sick and frail elderly men and women launched a public policy initiative and led to most of today's social entitlement programs. The problem was thought to be simple—provide a little help for the most needy, give them a hand. Unfortunately, the war on poverty failed. Today, millions of women and children remain in poverty—25% of all families in the United States with children and 50% of all African American families, mostly female, single heads of household, exist in poverty (NCHS, 1995).

How shall we prevent our women and children from "falling from the sky"? Relying on federal or state entitlement programs to be the social safety net is not the answer. We must take steps to improve the living environments that perpetuate inequity and limit human potential. As Dr. Bernice Johnson Reagan, a community activist and cultural anthropologist of the Smithsonian Institute, states, "we must develop a bond between those who are of the community." We must believe and be guided by the beliefs of what allows humans to flourish. It will take individuals, organizations, corporations, neighborhoods, and communities standing up together to address this issue—one family at a time. We must engage in the public policy debate about what does and does not work.

Some programs have worked. The successful ones have the following core themes:

1. Focus on families and communities.
2. Avoid focusing solely on individuals with special risks.
3. Provide intensive and sustained social supportive services.
4. Use family members, community workers, and supportive networks to provide primary services.
5. Integrate assistance with education, information, and support.
6. Set and maintain time commitments for financial support.

Fair Start Story

The seven demonstration projects funded by the Ford Foundation grants program entitled, "Child Survival/A Fair Start for Children" are excellent examples of antipoverty programs that work (Larner et al., 1992). The collective results from this effort have improved the chances for development of children from low-income families. The interventions were performed by parents and extended family or community networks. The researchers and caregivers helped women and their families to shed the bonds of poverty by providing them with education, social support, and opportunities to build their self-efficacy. The faces of poverty within these projects included women from immigrant families, working poor women, teen-age mothers, women living in rural areas, and abused and hopeless women. What worked for the seven projects that took place throughout the United States from 1982 and 1989 was winning the active participation of families and communities in addressing the social and health issues, investing funds in terms of employment of community workers, and encouraging women to develop themselves. The unique interventions were education, social support, practical assistance, and building trust relationships.

Opportunity International

Opportunity International provides small to modest loans and training to impoverished women and families (Calonius, 1995). Over the last 25 years, this successful program has slowly made entrepreneurs out of poor people in developing countries. The founder, Alfred Whittaker, believed that people with an idea, willingness to work, and support could live and thrive if they had two basic resources—capital and training. Opportunity International does not give money to any individual or community. Rather it forms a local board of directors made up of the community to lend money to local entrepreneurs. The loans can be as small as $25 to buy a plastic cooler to sell frozen fruit pops or $1700 to purchase a tricycle-taxi service. Most of the businesses have survived and prospered. The women have been excellent investments. The loan repayment rate is 98%. The 24,468 loans given out in 1994 generated 64,302 jobs. Opportunity International has successfully improved the living conditions of communities by helping them move from existence and dependency to interdependence and living.

Unfortunately, the program has only recently been tried in the United States in one city, Boston. The rationale for not implementing the program in the United States was the belief that the poor in the United States do not have the drive and support to become independent. Women in the United States have the drive; they need the collective support of families, professionals, social scientists, policymakers, and communities. If we remove the barriers to human potential—poverty, poor education, violence, limited choices, and dependency—women can be successful.

Last Call

The Fourth World Conference on Women was held in Beijing in September 1995. It was envisioned as the culmination of 20 years of success on the women's agenda of equality, development, and peace. The conference proceedings have not been released. However, the media reports on international cable networks indicated the need for additional work to achieve the conference's identified goals. The goal to achieve more equal, peaceful, and people-centered development for women's families, cities, and nations cannot be achieved without recognition of the impact on women of sexual and racial discrimination, illiteracy, violence, hunger, joblessness, poor health, and limited life choices.

As long as women are reared and live in environments that diminish their value, we will not achieve equality, development, or world peace. We must demonstrate how to improve living environments and involve poor women in our efforts to improve their living environments. It is essential that individuals, organizations, communities, and governments join forces to reshape policies and practices targeted to improve the quality of life of women and their families. We must speak out against economic systems that marginalize entire groups. We must empower women with education and confidence. If you educate a woman, you educate a nation. We must foster among ourselves the strength and the will to take full responsibility for our community of women while supporting poor women through the transition from poverty and isolation to communal interdependence and fulfillment. We must heed the words of an ancient Chinese proverb in our efforts to promote the well-being of women. "Tell me, I forget. Show me, I remember. Involve me, I understand."

We must all become better "servant leaders "if we are to create the living environments in which women will flourish. Servant leaders are guided by the desire to be in service to humanity (Bower, 1994). In assuming this role, we acknowledge that being human and being of service means more than charity and handouts. We must work harder at keeping women from the ledge so that they don't fall into the abyss of poverty rather than perpetuate the reinvention of the "safety net" of programs to catch them.

America, according to the Committee for Economic Development (1987), is subject to becoming a nation of limited human potential. When one-third of our entire nation is limited by poverty, we run the risk of limiting our entire nation's potential. We must examine and replicate public policies and programs that mitigate the effects of discrimination and poverty. We must envision our communities as better places for women and work to bring that vision to reality. Women can and will help themselves and their families. We must answer the last call to action by providing nonstigmatizing, community-based, non-authoritative, family-focused, and supportive programs to keep women and families from falling into the vicious cycle of poverty and dependence. In the near future, we must within our own living environments take steps to remove the barriers to human potential by advocating for equitable and just public health, education, and social policies.

References

Abel, E., & Sofaer S. (1990). Older women's health and financial vulnerability: Implications for the Medicare benefit structure. *Women's Health, 16,* 47-67.

American Cancer Society. (1986). *Cancer in the economically disadvantaged: A special report.* New York: Author.

Andes, N. (1992). Social class and gender: An empirical evaluation of occupational stratification. *Gender and Society, 6* (2), 231-251.

Bolton, L. B. (1988). Analysis of prenatal care utilization patterns. Doctoral dissertation, University of California, Los Angeles.

Bolton, L. B. (1995, Summer). The protection of women and children: A call to action. The HCQA Quality Forum. Washington, DC.

Boyd, J. (1993). *In the company of my sisters.* New York: Dutton.

Bower, F. (1994). Servant leadership. *Reflections, 20* (4), 4-5.

Callahan, J., & Smith, P. (1994). Liberalism, communitarianism and feminism. In Reynolds, N., Murphy, C., & Moffat, R. (Eds.), *Liberalism and community.* New York: Leviston.

Calonius, E. (1995). *Creating a world of opportunity: An interview with Alfred Whittaker* (pp. 21-24). Greensboro, NC: Hemispheres, Pace Communications.

Committee on Economic Development. (1987). *Current population survey.* New York: Author.

Davis, K. (1995). The federal budget and women's health. *American Journal of Public Health, 85,* 1051-1053.

Employee Benefit Research Institute. (1995). *Picture of health of middle and older women.* Washington, DC: Author.

Grella, C. E. (1990). Irreconcilable differences: Women defining class after divorce and downward mobility. *Gender and Society, 4* (1), 41-55.

Himmelstein, D., & Woolhandler, S. (1995). Care denied: US residents who are unable to obtain needed medical services. *American Journal of Public Health, 85,* 341-344.

Kaiser Commission. (1995). *Medicaid and Medicare Facts.* Washington, DC: Author.

Kreiger, N. (1991). Women and social class. *Journal of Epidemiology and Community Health, 45,* 35-42.

Larner, M., Halpern. R., & Harkavy, O. (1992). *Fair start for children.* New Haven, CT: Yale University Press. New Haven.

Mahowald, M. (1993). *Women and children in health care* (pp. 3-17, 217-227, 255-273). New York: Oxford University Press.

McCoy, C. B., Smith, S. A., Metsch, L. R., Anwyl, R. S., Correa, R., Bankston, L., & Zavertnik, J. J. (1994). Breast cancer screening of the medically underserved results and implications. *Cancer Practice, 2* (4), 267-274.

Montgomery, L., & Carter-Pokras, O. (1993). Health status by social class and/or minority status. *Toxicology and Industrial Health, 9* (5), 729-773.

National Center for Health Statistics. (1994). *National health and nutritional examination survey II.* Hyattsville, MD: U.S. Department of Health and Human Services.

National Center for Health Statistics. (1995a). *Measuring the health of women in America. National health interview survey.* Hyattsville, MD: U.S. Department of Health and Human Services.

National Center for Health Statistics. (1995b). *Measuring the health of women in America. National survey on family growth.* Hyattsville, MD: U.S. Department of Health and Human Services.

O'Hare, W. P. (1985). "Poverty in America trends and new patterns. *Population Bulletin, 40* (33).

Pearce, D. (1978). The feminization of poverty: Women, work and welfare. *Urban and Social Change Review, 11,* 28-36.

Royce, J. (1885). *The religious aspect of philosophy.* Boston: Mifflin.

Sidel, R. (1986). *Women and children last* (pp. 122-156). New York: Penguin Books.

U.S. Bureau of the Census. (1992). *Poverty in the United States: Current population reports, population characteristics.* Washington, DC: U.S. Department of Commerce.

Weitzman, B., & Berry, C. (1992). Health status and health care utilization. *Women and Health, 19* (2/3), 87-105.

Bibliography

Agency for Health Care Policy and Research. (1994). America's women's health care: A patchwork quilt with gaps. Bethesda, MD: U.S. Department of Health and Human Services.

Blanton-Lillie, M., Martinez, R., Lidd-Taylor, A., & Garman Robinson, B. (1994). Latina and African American women: Continuing disparities in health. *International Journal of Health Services, 23* (3) 555-584.

Farley, R., & Allen, W. (1987). *The color line and the quality of life in America.* New York: Russell Sage Foundation.

Frisancho, A. R., & Ryan, A. S. (1991). Decreased statures associated with moderate blood lead concentrations in Mexican-American children. *American Journal of Clinical Nutrition, 54,* 516-519.

Lin-Fu, J. S. (1992). Modern history of lead poisoning. In Needleman, H. L. (Ed.), *Human lead exposure* (pp. 23-43). Boca Raton, FL: CRC Press.

McLanahan, S., Sorenson, A., & Watson, D. (1989). Sex differences in poverty. *Signs: Journal of Women in Culture and Society, 15* (11), 107-110.

Montgomery, L. E. (1992, November 9). Increased effects of poverty on the health of children and young people since 1976. Presented at the American Public Health Association annual meeting. Washington, DC. November 9.

O'Hare, W. P., Mann, T., Porter, K., & Greenstein, R. (1990). *Real life poverty in America: Where the American public would set the poverty line.* Washington, DC: USA Foundation, Center on Budget and Policy Priorities and Families.

CHAPTER 25

Women's Health in the Workplace

Naomi G. Swanson
Ami B. Becker

Magnitude of the Problem

In the last 100 years, the participation of women in the work force has increased dramatically. In 1890, approximately one in seven women worked outside of the home (ie, 18% of the work force). Today, nearly two of every three women work outside of the home, and women constitute 47% of the work force (Fullerton, 1993). More than half of the 30 occupations projected to grow most rapidly through the year 2005 are occupations traditionally dominated by women. These include occupations such as home health aides, human services workers, paralegals, child care workers, manicurists, and flight attendants (Silvestri, 1993).

Although women represent nearly half of the work force today, research on workplace hazards in which women are the study population is not present to the same extent as research on working men. Working women encounter a wide range of physical and psychological workplace hazards, and some evidence indicates that their working experiences are quite different from those of men in some important aspects. However, thus far, researchers have concentrated to the greatest degree on areas that deal with the reproductive and maternal status of working women (eg, reproductive hazards, multiple roles), and far less attention has been given to other areas of occupational safety and health that may pose different injury and illness risks for working women than men.

Contributing Factors

Although women have made strides with regard to breaking down job barriers, there continues to be a dichotomy in underlying attitudes toward the health and well-being of women in the workplace. In some instances, gender differences are minimized when, in fact, certain differences may carry important health and safety implications. In other instances, gender differences, which have little to do with performance or health and safety considerations, are emphasized. These conflicting attitudes are discussed in greater detail below.

Minimization of Gender Differences

With respect to many physical hazards, women are regarded as small men who differ only with respect to their reproductive systems. This attitude is apparent, for example, when one finds that concessions to women in safety products originally developed for men (eg, personal protective equipment), generally involve offerings in smaller sizes only. The products are not redesigned to fit the different anthropometry of women, a practice that can seriously compromise the safety (and performance) of women using these products in the workplace.

This attitude also ignores some physiologic differences that may affect the health of working men and women. For example, women have a higher body fat content than men, and their storage volume for fat-soluble substances is greater. Thus, there is a potential for fat-soluble carcinogens to cause differential rates of cancer in men and women. Female hormones tend to inhibit anabolism, whereas male hormones are anabolic. Thus, where a difference in toxicity exists between oxidized and nonoxidized forms of a workplace chemical, its toxicity may vary for men and women (Poitrast, 1988).

Emphasis of Gender Differences

Discounting the physical differences between female and male workers can have a negative impact on women's health and safety in the workplace. Yet gender differences, which tend to have little impact on safety and health, or performance aspects of a job, are sometimes cited to dissuade women from pursuing certain jobs. An example is the frequently cited gender difference in strength (ie, in general, women possess only 65% of the lifting strength of men; Hayne, 1981). However, this attitude exaggerates gender differences that in today's workplace generally do not have an impact on safety and health or performance capabilities. Most jobs today are largely sedentary or do not require the extreme energy expenditures and strength capabilities that would render the job impossible for the average woman to perform.

Myths About Women Workers

In addition to the presumption that gender is an important determinant of performance quality on the job, other myths regarding women's capabilities, seriousness about their careers, and spheres within which they should be operating continue to color women's experiences in the workplace. These myths and their consequences are examined further in the sections dealing with discrimination and harassment. Other sections focus on various workplace hazards as they affect the health of women workers: stress, various physical and ergonomic hazards, and workplace violence. A review such as this is necessarily limited by space constraints. Interested readers can find additional information listed in the bibliography, where recommended readings are grouped by subject.

Health-Related Concerns

Job Stress

Psychological Benefits of Work

Work has the potential for both a positive and a negative impact on psychological health. The psychological benefits of work have been acknowledged for some time. Early stress theorists (Gardell, 1971; Herzberg, 1966; McGregor, 1960) wrote of increased motivation and esteem and self-actualization through work. Indeed, a recent study suggests that work has a strong, beneficial effect on women's health apart from the "healthy worker" effect (Jennings, Mazaik, & McKinlay, 1984). For women, some of the positive aspects of working outside the home can include increased social support, higher self-esteem and confidence, increased independence, and improved financial status (Cox, Cox, & Steventon, 1984; Sorenson & Verbrugge, 1987). Conversely, being unemployed may be harmful to health. Studies of the unemployed show increased levels of depression, anxiety, somatic disorders, and health care usage (Linn, Sandifer, & Stein, 1985).

Job Stressors

Although work has many psychological benefits, work may also negatively affect psychological health. Certain job and organizational characteristics can have deleterious effects on worker psychological and physical health. These characteristics fall generally under the rubric of job stress. Stressors for which the greatest amount of evidence exists include high workload demands coupled with little control over work, role ambiguity and conflict, lack of job security, poor relationships with coworkers and supervisors, and work consisting of repetitive, narrow tasks (Sauter, Murphy, & Hurrell, 1990). Unfortunately, these sorts of stressful attributes define many of the jobs that are traditionally available to women (eg, data entry, caregiving). These jobs often are monotonous and repetitive, have high workload demands and heavy responsibilities for the well-being of others, and allow little control over work tasks and work pace. It has been suggested that stress from such repetitive work can give rise to low job satisfaction, poor job performance, and impaired well-being (Cox, 1980; Cox, Cox, Thirlaway, MacKay, 1982; Sauter et al., 1990).

Health Consequences of Job Stress

Long-term exposure to job stress may have serious health consequences. Early work by the National Institute for Occupational Safety and Health (NIOSH) identified a number of women's occupations (eg, health technicians, practical nurses, nurses' aides, waitresses, and secretaries) that had much higher than average rates of admission to mental health centers (Colligan, Smith, & Hurrell, 1977). More recently, Eaton, Anthony, Mandel, and Garrison (1990) identified many of these same occupations as having elevated rates of major depressive disorder (eg, data entry operators, computer equipment operators, health and nurses' aides, and waitresses).

Women's Multiple Roles

A potentially serious stressor for many working women is that of juggling responsibility for work and families. Evidence certainly exists for the stressful effects of the multiple roles many women assume (worker, wife, mother). Most women who work still have primary responsibility for family care and housework, and these latter responsibilities can add up to 40 or more additional hours to their weekly workload (Quinn & Woskie, 1988). The lack of day-care facilities and family leave policies in many companies can compound these stresses (Friedman & Galinsky, 1992). However, recent studies have pointed to the fallacy of the assumption that multiple roles are always associated with stress and morbidity among working women. These studies suggest that multiple roles can enhance health and well-being because they expand resources and rewards and provide multiple sources of self-esteem and satisfaction. When problems arise in one role (eg, work), other roles are buffers or offer sources of support for dealing with these problems (Barnett & Baruch, 1985; 1987).

Ergonomics

Ergonomics refers to the study of human behavior in relation to work, particularly with regard to the adaptation and design of tasks, tools, equipment, and work environments to fit human capabilities and characteristics (Grandjean, 1986). The end goal of ergonomics is the improved health and well-being of workers (eg, redesigning a tool so that its use no longer results in injury to the musculoskeletal system).

Design Considerations

A primary problem that women have faced in moving into the workplace is that tools, equipment, workstations, and personal protective equipment have been designed and built for men. For example, workstation surfaces are too high, promoting poor work postures; reaches are too great; chair seats cannot be adjusted low enough; and protective clothing is too large and baggy, making it prone to being caught in equipment. These ergonomic deficiencies can result in increased risk of injury for women.

Upper Extremity Musculoskeletal Disorders

Many predominantly female occupations carry the risk of exposure to repetitive motions and awkward postures that can result in injury to the musculoskeletal system (Quinn & Woskie, 1988). Neck, shoulder, and upper limb disorders have been identified in various assembly jobs (Maeda, 1977), teleoperator jobs (NIOSH, 1992), and cash register jobs (Grant, Habes, & Baron, 1994). Musculoskeletal discomforts and disorders suffered by keyboard operators have been described in numerous articles (Grandjean, 1987; Sauter, Gottlieb, Jones, Dodson, & rohrer, 1983; Sauter & Swanson, 1991; World Health Organization, 1987) and have been linked with poor design of workstations, work environments, and jobs. Additionally, the stresses associated with these types of jobs may interact with the physical demands of the work to create or exacerbate musculoskeletal problems (Sauter & Swanson, 1996). For example, Brisson, Vezina, and Vinet (1992) found increased risk for severe musculoskeletal disability, anxiety, and depression among female garment workers working under a piecework system. Time pressures (ie, a job stressor) were greater among these workers because the rapidity with which they performed their work affected their pay. The time pressures may have increased the repetitiveness of the tasks, changed the temporal distribution of work and rest, or increased general muscle tonus.

Lifting

A number of industrial jobs, as well as traditionally female jobs (eg, nursing, child care), involve frequent or heavy lifting, increasing the risk for low back pain and injury. Magora (1970) found that substantially more women (ie, up to seven times as many) in jobs requiring heavy lifting reported low back pain as compared to women whose work did not require heavy lifting.

Pregnancy may make lifting more dangerous (Quinn & Woskie, 1988). Increases in body size make it difficult to keep the object being lifted close to the body, and the body's center of gravity shifts as the pregnancy progresses, altering the capacity to lift. The ligaments and muscles of the stomach and back are stretched, and joints become more flexible and mobile during pregnancy, potentially increasing the risk of injury with heavy lifting. Some evidence suggests an increased risk of low back injury for women who do heavy lifting (Quinn & Woskie, 1988), and heavy or strenuous industrial work (including lifting) has been associated with an increased risk of spontaneous abortion and premature birth (Saurel-Cubizolles & Kaminski, 1987).

Strength differentials between the sexes are often cited to show that women are unsuitable for some jobs requiring heavy lifting. On average, women are only two-thirds as strong as men for tasks involving upper body strength (Hayne, 1981). However, despite this difference, there is a substantial overlap in strength distributions of men and women. This overlap is as much as 50% or more for certain muscle groups (Quinn & Woskie, 1988). In industry, strength testing is often used to select individuals for lifting jobs under the premise that greater strength is associated with a lower risk for injury. However, there is no strong evidence that strength testing predicts an individual's risk for injury, and there is a danger that strength testing may unnecessarily exclude individuals who would not suffer injury. These tests do not measure factors that may be protective against the stress of heavy lifting, such as endurance or flexibility. Also, there is no epidemiologic evidence that women suffer more musculoskeletal injuries than men when performing the same task (Quinn & Woskie, 1988).

Other Physical Hazards

Industrial Hazards

Women are exposed to a wide variety of physical, biologic, and chemical hazards in the workplace. Although many women work in office environments, which are comparatively free of dangerous chemical and biologic toxins, many other women work in environments where such exposures are a real hazard. For example, many women work in food processing, health care, clothing/textile, laundry/dry cleaning, and janitorial occupations. Others work in nontraditional jobs (eg, construction, machining), manufacturing, and agriculture. Many of these jobs contain the potential for exposure to suspected carcinogens, allergens, or asthmatogens, and increased rates of certain occupational illnesses and diseases have been documented for some of these industries. Following is a sample of some of the occupational exposures that have been linked with morbidity among women.

Meat Industry. Women working in the meat industry are exposed to a number of chemical and biologic hazards. More than 90% of the workers who wrap and label meat are women. Heat is used to cut and seal the plastic used in the meat wrapping process and also to adhere the labels to the plastic wrapping. Workers are heavily exposed to fumes emitted from the thermal decomposition of the plastic, which can result in an acute respiratory disorder called "meatwrapper's asthma" (Vandervort & Brooks, 1977). Long-term exposure to these fumes, which often contain the suspected carcinogen benzene, may be linked with an increase in myeloid leukemia, non-Hodgkin's lymphomas, and lung cancer (Johnson, Fischman, Matanoski, & Diamond, 1986). Women working in slaughterhouses and meatpacking plants are at increased risk of animal-borne infections, such as leptospirosis, brucellosis, Q fever, and psittacosis (Copplestone & Kaplan, 1972),. Those involved in meat curing or smoking can be exposed to smoke, nitrosamines, or antioxidants, which have been associated with tumor production in animals.

Laundry/Dry Cleaning Industry. Women working in the laundry/dry cleaning industry are exposed to a number of solvents, such as chlorinated hydrocarbons and tetrachloroethylene. Mortality and cohort studies of laundry/dry cleaning workers have found an excess of kidney, cervical, bladder, and skin cancer, as well as an excess risk for primary liver cancer among women (Lynge & Thygesen, 1990). Laundry workers are also at risk for exposure to dangerous workplace substances from the clothes that they wash (eg, pneumoconiosis from exposure to silica-contaminated clothing).

Textile Industry. Textile workers are susceptible to a variety of lung diseases. Workers in cotton mills, exposed to raw cotton dust, may develop byssinosis. Beckett, Pope, Xu, and Christiani (1994) found a relationship between levels of dust in the workplace and chronic respiratory symptoms (cough, phlegm, shortness of breath, and wheezing) among women textile workers in China. Workers in mills that produce synthetic fibers or process wool, flax, and other natural fibers may develop pulmonary hypersensitivity that can lead to the onset of chronic lung disease (Stellman & Stellman, 1983).

Metal Working Industry. Increased risk for lung cancer has been found among women metal workers (ie, metal surfacers, foundry workers, and welders). These workers may be exposed to coke oven emissions and dust, fumes, and smoke containing a number of carcinogens, such as inorganic arsenic, polycyclic aromatic hydrocarbons, organic vapors, and metallic aerosols (Wu-Williams et al., 1993). Women metal workers have also been found to have an elevated risk of bladder cancer (Silverman, Levin, & Hoover, 1990). An increased risk for bladder cancer has also been found among women rubber processing workers (ie, exposure to fumes and dust such as talc and carbon black), chemical processing workers, pharmacists, structural painters, printers, and gardeners (Silverman, McLaughlin, Malker, Weiner, & Ericsson, 1989; Silverman et al., 1990).

Agriculture. Some evidence points to an increased risk of cancer among women agricultural workers. Zahm et al. (1993) found an increased risk for non-Hodgkin's lymphoma among women in rural Nebraska who had directly mixed and applied pesticides (chlorinated hydrocarbon and organophosphate insecticides) to livestock, farm buildings, or lots. Fingerland (1982) found an increased risk for lung cancer among women cooperative farm workers in the former Czechoslovakia. The workers were exposed to a number of potential carcinogens: aflatoxins from rotten hay and dust from grains, mercury compounds in grain pesticides, formaldehyde used in fumigation, and herbicides.

Ceramics Industry. A little recognized occupational hazard is pneumoconiosis/silicosis among ceramics workers and among those involved in the manufacture of scouring powders. Gerhardsson and Ahlmark (1985) found that women potters in Sweden showed greater susceptibility to silicosis than men and that the progression of the disease was more rapid and more severe among women potters. The more rapid progression of the disease may have been due to the type of work being performed. Women potters were primarily finishers of fired wares (ie, involving exposure to large amounts of dust), whereas men worked primarily with moist materials.

Health Care. Health care workers are exposed to a number of toxic and allergenic substances. For example, formaldehyde is heavily used in pathology, renal hemodialysis, and histology, and can compromise pulmonary function (Kilburn, Warshaw, & Thornton, 1989). Hospital wet work (eg, cleaning of patient units, kitchen work) is commonly associated with dermatoses. Different studies have found that 15% to 44% of women engaged in hospital wet work suffered from hand eczemas and dermatitis (Hansen, 1983; Nilsson & Back, 1986). Disinfectants are a major cause of allergic contact dermatitis because many contain allergens (eg, formaldehyde) and have an irritant effect on skin. Rubber and nickel allergies are also common causes of dermatitis. Soaps and detergents may contain irritants (eg, alkaline agents), but more typically they magnify the effect of other cleaning substances (eg, disinfectants). Soaps and detergents increase the permeability of the epidermis, consequently increasing the risk to the skin of irritants and allergens (Hansen, 1983).

Health care workers are also exposed to radiation, anesthetic gases, infectious diseases, chemicals, and other toxic substances. A review of the hazards faced by health care workers, along with guidelines for preventing these hazards, is provided by the National Institute for Occupational Safety and Health (NIOSH, 1988).

Reproductive Hazards

Recent legislation prohibiting the exclusion of women of childbearing age from working with substances that may cause fetal damage (Brushwood, 1991) underscores the volatility of the issue of women's right to work in jobs of their choice versus prohibiting women from performing certain work suspected of adversely affecting their reproductive capabilities.

Given the excellent reviews on the reproductive health of working women that currently exist, only a few examples of occupational links to adverse reproductive outcomes will be given. For example, many potentially genotoxic and fetotoxic chemicals (eg, solvents) are used in semiconductor manufacture and assembly, and increased frequencies of spontaneous abortions, low birth weight infants, and birth defects have been observed among workers in this industry (Eskenazi, Guendelman, & Elkin, 1993; Huel, Mergler, & Bowler, 1990; Lipscomb, Fenster, Wrensch, Shusterman, & Swan, 1991). Cadmium exposure among metallurgic workers may be linked with lower infant birth weight (Huel, Everson, & Menger, 1984). Intense physical activity, increased standing, heavy lifting, and exposure to temperature extremes have been associated with various adverse pregnancy outcomes (Evanoff & Rosenstock, 1986). Health care workers and veterinarians are exposed to a number of physical and chemical hazards that can adversely affect reproduction, such as radiation, infectious diseases, surgical instrument sterilants (eg, ethylene oxide), anesthetic gases, and antineoplastic drugs (Hunt & Smith, 1982; Moore, Davis, & Kaczmarek, 1993; NIOSH, 1988).

Sex Discrimination

Definition

Workplace sex discrimination is loosely defined as a pattern of conditions, attitudes, and behaviors that reflects a gender-based bias in the relative treatment of female and male employees. Although sex discrimination against men is not unheard of, it is directed disproportionately against working women. Discrimination may manifest itself in an organization's hiring practices, distribution of monetary rewards and promotions, and attitude toward "family-friendly" leave policies. Although sex discrimination is prohibited under Title VII of the 1964 Civil Rights Act, it continues to pervade many work environments in both obvious and subtle forms.

Salary Differential

One of the more obvious forms of sex discrimination is the pay discrepancy that exists between equally qualified men and women working at the same jobs. For example, Jagacinski, LeBold, and Linden (1987) found that equally qualified female engineers were not being as well compensated as their male counterparts. Similarly, Reskin and Ross (1992) found that female managers earned an average of $10,487 less per year than male managers although the sexes were matched for education, experience, and managerial level. A salary gap also exists between female and male blue collar workers (Schroedel, 1990).

Career Advancement

Employment practices that effectively keep working women out of top rank-ing positions are often referred to collectively as the "glass ceiling." In their study of male and female managers, Reskin and Ross (1992) found female man-agers predominantly at the bottom of the chain of command. Women were un-derrepresented in middle management and were virtually absent in the top ranks. Their data also revealed that managers were typically assigned to super-vise employees of their own gender and that female managers were less likely than males to have decision-making authority within their departments or divi-sions. Perhaps their most disturbing finding was that female managers are often given influential sounding titles, yet the work they do actually remains low level. Such a tactic allows employers to avoid discrimination and affirmative ac-tion litigation.

In another study of the work life of female and male managers (Metcalfe, 1987), female managers reported a variety of obstacles that threatened their career advancement. The women indicated that, as compared to their male colleagues, their accomplishments were not recognized, their potential was undervalued and underutilized, and their access to important people and information was restricted. They also reported being targets for male resentment. In turn, the female respon-dents expressed resentment at having constantly to prove themselves and having to reflect the male success stereotype by engaging in aggressive, competitive be-havior. Galinsky, Bond, and Friedman (1993) and Jagacinski et al. (1987) also re-ported problems in career advancement for female managers and engineers, respectively.

Professional women are not the sole victims of employment discrimination. In a study of blue collar women, Schroedel (1990) discovered similar impedi-ments to career advancement. For example, the women in that study reported that job assignments were not given in an impartial manner. Sometimes women were consistently given the more difficult job assignments, presumably to pro-mote failure. At other times, women were invariably given low-level, repetitious tasks to perform, compromising their skill development, value to the company, and marketability.

Sex Discrimination and Culture

Societal support in the United States for women's career aspirations remains less than optimal. Of 75 industrialized countries, only the United States has no govern-ment-sponsored, paid pro-family policy, such as paid family leave, paid maternity benefits, or subsidized child care (Silverstein, 1991). The absence of such a policy differentially affects men and women. It ignores the fact that two-thirds of working women *must* work to support their families (Bursten, 1986) and that women who work outside the home continue to be primarily responsible for housework, chil-dren, and child care arrangements (Friedman & Galinsky, 1992; Nakamura, McCarthy, Rothstein-Fisch, & Winges, 1981). Thus, it is not surprising that working women experience a great deal of stress when it comes to making decisions about career, marriage, and motherhood. In their study of male and female engineers,

Jagacinski et al. (1987) found that the women were more likely than the men to be divorced or separated and were also more likely to remain unmarried or childless because of the stress engendered by the conflicting responsibilities of family and career. Similar findings regarding the stress of role conflict in the lives of working women have been reported by Beckman (1978), LaCroix and Haynes (1987), and Metcalfe (1987).

The Weaker Sex

A number of misconceptions regarding women's abilities can influence their treatment at work and often underlie sex discrimination (Warren, 1982). One is that women are unsuited to work because they are physically the weaker sex. Thus, women have been encouraged to seek sedentary activities and not to develop their physical strength. However, as Warren (1982) points out, this particular belief is not grounded in reality for many of the world's women. The International Labor Organization has estimated that, worldwide, the "weaker sex" works 80 hours for every 50 hours that men work (Wysocki & Ossler, 1983). Additionally, in the United States, the physical demands of work today are enormously reduced, and the need for strength is not a factor in most cases.

Demise of the Family

Another attitude underlying sex discrimination pertains to the view that women's influx into the workplace violates social norms (Chester & Grossman, 1990) and undermines the strengths and traditional values of the nuclear family. Working mothers have sometimes been accused of materialism and selfishness, as well as indifference toward their children's emotional and moral development. At the extreme end, working mothers have been blamed for a variety of social ills, ranging from the divorce rate to teenage crime.

Problems associated with maternal employment (eg, maternal stress and fatigue, latchkey children) appear to be mediated by the lack of societal and governmental support systems for working women, noted earlier. Many organizations have continued to maintain outdated leave policies and have resisted efforts to introduce more flexible work schedules and inhouse child care facilities (Friedman & Galinsky, 1992).

Sex Role Stereotypes

Stereotypes about women and women's behavior may also foster workplace sex discrimination, in particular misconceptions regarding women's emotional lability and intellectual capabilities. In a cross-cultural study of male and female business students, Schein and Mueller (1992) found that male students from the United States, Great Britain, and Germany strongly sex typed successful managerial characteristics as male. The same was true of the German women. Female management students from Great Britain also sex typed the position as male, but less so than the German women. Only the American women indicated that a successful manager was equally likely to have male and female qualities. The authors concluded that the American women had benefited from this country's sex discrimination laws, in that many more women have achieved management status in the United States as compared to Great Britain and Germany. The great paucity of women in management positions in Germany explains the German women's acceptance of the masculine model of success, as well as their low expectations for their own success.

Schein and Mueller's (1992) results are somewhat unusual in that the American women did not sex type the successful managerial candidate as a man. Other studies (Crowley, Levitin, & Quinn 1981; Kouach, 1981; Lott, 1985) have shown that in laboratory, academic, and business settings, women as well as men tend to express a bias against hypothetical and actual female job candidates who have the same credentials as male candidates. However, a more encouraging finding shows that when a real, *known* woman is evaluated on the job, she tends not to be devalued, suggesting that with increasing experience, gender becomes a less salient cue, and stereotyped responses to the individual are diminished (Lott, 1985). In a similar vein, the results of a large, national study demonstrated that female and male employees gave same sex and opposite sex supervisors equally high ratings for management style, effectiveness, and overall supportiveness (Galinsky et al., 1993).

Job Performance and Health Implications

Sex discrimination can have adverse effects on health and performance. Workers who believe they have been discriminated against, or who feel that they have limited opportunities for advancement because of their gender, express less loyalty toward their employers, are more likely to feel burned out by their jobs, are less satisfied with their jobs, and are less committed to performing their jobs well or helping their employers succeed (Galinsky et al., 1993). Additionally, perceived lack of opportunities for a career and financial advancement have been linked to psychological distress (ie, anxiety symptoms), musculoskeletal complaints, and more frequent visits to physicians (Piotrokowski & Love, 1987).

Sexual Harassment

Acts of Harassment

In cases of sex discrimination, the issue is unfair or inequitable treatment based on gender, without any overtly sexual overtones (Bursten, 1986). However, when unsolicited sexual behavior becomes an issue in work relationships, this is considered sexual harassment. Sexual harassment includes a variety of unwanted, threatening, demeaning sexual behaviors and overtures, which can be either verbal or physical in nature. Verbal behaviors may range from sexual remarks and jokes to explicit sexual threats and coercion. Physical behaviors may range from "accidental" touching to outright physical assault, including rape (Schroedel, 1990). Indeed, some have taken the view that sexual harassment is, by definition, a form of workplace violence, whether the harassing acts are physical or verbal and whether threats of violence or retribution are explicit or implied (Fitzgerald, 1993).

Another view of sexual harassment, though, is that it is a *tool* of sex discrimination (McKinney, 1994), or a *type* of sex discrimination (Bernstein, 1994). In the former case, sexual harassment may be used as a technique to keep workers out of top-ranking positions or out of the workplace entirely. In the latter case, sexual harassment is viewed as a type of wrongful discrimination or unequal treatment, in which the victim suffers an injustice akin to unequal pay (Bernstein, 1994). Sexual harassment as a manifestation of unequal treatment is currently the prevailing view, and is subsumed under Title VII of the Civil Rights Act of 1964.

Legal Definitions

Two broad varieties of sexual harassment are recognized by U.S. courts. "Quid pro quo harassment" refers generally to a one-on-one situation in which an employee makes sexual threats or unwelcome verbal or physical advances to a coworker. In a textbook case, a male superior threatens a female subordinate with demotion or job loss should she refuse to grant him sexual favors. Although men may be victims of sexual harassment, quid pro quo harassment is typically found in male-supervised, traditionally female, occupations.

Although the goal of quid pro quo harassment is sexual contact, the objective of the "hostile working environment" is the marginalization of a gender as a collective (Goldsmith Kasinsky, 1992). In extreme cases, the hostile working environment is characterized by threatening behavior, sexual taunts and jeers, demeaning graffiti, posters, and calendars, and so forth. *Individuals* are not necessarily sought out for sexual favors, and typically the power structure of the organization is such that the offenders themselves do not have the authority to level job-related sanctions against a noncompliant employee. Rather, the focus of the hostile environment is on making all members of one gender uncomfortable to the point that they will feel compelled to seek employment elsewhere. Hostile working environments are usually found in traditionally male occupations, where women are not yet fully established. Such occupations may be blue collar (eg, construction) or white collar (eg, corporate management).

Models of Sexual Harassment

Several models have been devised as explanatory mechanisms for sexually harassing behavior. These are reviewed in greater detail in Saal, Johnson, and Weber (1989) and McKinney (1994). The *biologic model* emphasizes the natural sexual attraction between women and men and suggests that the man's harassing behavior is a result of his stronger sex drive. This model does not account for female to male or homosexual harassment, but it does allow for the fact that in some cases there is no *intent* to do harm on the part of the offender (eg, asking for a date or complimenting a coworker's appearance).

The *organizational model* of sexual harassment suggests that the power structure of a company or business determines the level and incidence of harassing behaviors. An organization that sexually discriminates in terms of hiring, pay, and promotion provides fertile ground for sexual harassment. In addition, the absence of a formal policy against sexual harassment and appropriate grievance procedures increases the probability that female employees will be harassed on the job.

The *sociocultural model* provides an illustration of sexual harassment based on the traditional sex roles of, and power relationships between, women and men. In this view, sexual harassment derives from the greater power and status that men have historically held in this society. The influx of women into the work force has challenged this power structure. Thus, according to this model, sexual harassment is used by men to reclaim their lost authority and benefits.

Other models of sexual harassment ascribe the behavior to sex-role spillover, in which the individual's gender biases and expectations "spill over" into the workplace (Gutek, 1985); individual characteristics, such as the offender's age; and interpersonal factors, such as miscommunication between the sexes (McKinney, 1994). Few tests of these models have been conducted although it seems reasonable that all of the influences mentioned above can have a role in the harassment of working women.

Prevalence

Sexual intimidation has been a feature of working life since women first began working outside of their homes (Bernstein, 1994; Fitzgerald, 1993). It is estimated that 50% of working women will be harassed at some point during their academic or professional lives (Fitzgerald, 1993). In traditionally male occupations (eg, academia, truck driving), the percentage of women in those occupations who encounter sexual harassment can rise to as much as 80% (Bursten, 1986; Fitzgerald, 1993). According to Goldsmith Kasinsky (1992), sexual harassment may be one of the most prevalent health hazards for working women. No woman is immune because of race, ethnicity, social status, or age.

Economic Consequences

Women who are sexually harassed at work can be at economic risk. The fear and humiliation engendered by the harassment may compel the victim to avoid the offender and the workplace. At the very least, a woman encountering sexual harassment is distracted from her work. Such a state of affairs may culminate in diminished performance, negative evaluations, wasted career opportunities, and eventual job loss. Other work-related consequences of sexual harassment include diminished job satisfaction and morale, as well as loss of confidence and self-esteem (Fitzgerald, 1993; McKinney, 1994).

It is not only the victim of sexual harassment who is faced with economic losses. Companies and organizations, both private and public, waste resources when employee absenteeism and turnover rates are high, and productivity is low. For example, it has been estimated that during the 2-year period, 1985 to 1987, sexual harassment cost the federal government $267 million. This is a conservative estimate. The figure is even higher when other factors, such as health care costs, are considered (Bernstein, 1994; Goldsmith Kasinsky, 1992).

Psychological Consequences

Psychological and emotional effects of sexual harassment have been documented, including anxiety, depression, fearfulness, rage, insomnia, weight change, and feelings of guilt and shame (Fitzgerald, 1993; Goldsmith Kasinsky, 1992; McKinney, 1994). Sexual dysfunction and marital conflict may also ensue (Bursten, 1986). Finally, the Institute for Research on Women's Mental Health (1988) has identified sexual harassment as a severe stressor that has the potential to activate or aggravate psychological disorders.

Physical and Physiologic Consequences

Goldsmith Kasinsky (1992) has suggested that the distraction and emotional stress resulting from sexual harassment may contribute to the hazards of occupations requiring a high level of control and alertness (eg, police work, firefighting, and nuclear power plant operations). In terms of the physiologic sequelae of harassment, symptoms include headache, nausea, gastrointestinal disorders, fatigue, psychogenic pain, fainting, muscle spasms, and hypertension (Bursten, 1986; Fitzgerald, 1993). These symptoms may be severe and may persist for extended periods of time, even after the actual harassment has ceased.

Workplace Violence

Fatal and Nonfatal Violence

Violence in the workplace is a leading cause of injury and death for women workers. Currently, the leading cause of fatal injury in the workplace for women is homicide. Although far more men than women are victims of workplace homicide, homicide accounts for a disproportionate amount (40%) of fatal workplace injuries for women (Bell, 1991; Bureau of Labor Statistics, 1994; NIOSH, 1993). There are some indications that women are primary victims of some types of nonfatal workplace violence as well (eg, rape, hitting, kicking, beating, biting, squeezing, pinching, scratching). The Bureau of Labor Statistics (1994) has released figures on the frequency of various types of nonfatal workplace violence, which resulted in days away from work. Overall, women workers were victims of 56% of the incidences of violence and constituted up to 84% of some categories of victimization. Many of the victims of nonfatal violence were female health care workers who were injured by patients. There are also questions of the extent to which domestic violence may spill over into the workplace for women. Although recent Department of Justice data (Bachman, 1994) do not address this issue directly, it is interesting that women are most likely to be attacked by someone they know rather than by a stranger, whereas the opposite is true for men.

Characteristics and Risk Factors

There appear to be some important differences between fatal and nonfatal workplace violence in terms of perpetrators, motives, and victims. With respect to workplace homicides, evidence indicates that robbery is the primary motive and that the majority of perpetrators are strangers. Certain working conditions appear to increase the risk of homicide in the workplace. NIOSH (1993) has listed the following as possible risk factors:

- exchanging money with the public
- working alone or in small numbers
- working late night or early morning hours
- working in high-crime areas
- guarding valuable property or possessions

Workplaces and occupations with these risk factors tend to have higher rates of homicide in the workplace. Those with the highest rates of occupational homicide include taxicab establishments, liquor and convenience stores, gas stations, detective and protective services, grocery and jewelry stores, hotels and motels, and eating and drinking establishments.

Less is known about nonfatal workplace violence, but recent data point to the following. In general, physical attacks and threats appear more likely to be directed at men and perpetrated by customers and strangers (Northwestern National Life, 1993). Indeed, men are much more likely than women to experience the most violent attacks (eg, stabbing, shooting) in the workplace (Bureau of Labor Statistics, 1994; Bachman, 1994). In some settings (eg, health care) women appear more likely to be the victims of less violent types of assaults, such as pinching, scratching, kicking, and so forth, where the primary perpetrator is the client or patient (Bureau of Labor Statistics, 1994). In general, various kinds of harassment appear most likely to be directed at women and perpetrated by others at work (Northwestern National Life, 1993). In contrast to workplace homicides, where almost all of the perpetrators appear to be strangers, a sizable proportion of nonfatal workplace violence may be perpetrated by coworkers (ie, Northwestern National Life data indicated that 27% of attackers, 37% of those making threats, and 86% of harassers were fellow workers).

Strategies for Intervening

Controlling Job Stress

The preferred strategy for preventing work-related stress involves *eliminating* the stressor (primary prevention) rather than focusing exclusively on individual stress-reduction techniques (secondary prevention), or the treatment of individual illness or pathology (tertiary prevention). Ideally, however, employees would have access to elements of all three prevention techniques. That is, their workplace would have a program combining organizational and job redesign initiatives (where needed) with stress management training and psychological counseling (Sauter et al., 1990). Job redesign can control or remove job stressors, such as work overload, lack of control over one's work, work role ambiguity, and lack of skill utilization. For further information on job stress and various stress intervention strategies, see the bibliography.

Ergonomic Solutions

There are a wide range of ergonomic solutions to the poor design of work tasks, tools, workstations, and work environments that reduce visual, musculoskeletal, physical, and mental loads. For example, design solutions for differences in size or anthropometry include making the work equipment and workstations adjustable for a range of sizes, designing for the smallest or largest individual in circumstances where a facility must "fit" everyone (eg, designing doors to fit the taller end of the height continuum and stairs to fit the shorter end), and providing protective clothing or equipment that is designed specifically for women (Matzdorf, 1987; Redgrove, 1979). Design solutions for repetitive tasks can include job rotation to other tasks that do not stress the same musculoskeletal structures (Grandjean, 1987), or designing rest schedules that allow for the relief of musculoskeletal fatigue and discomfort (Sauter & Swanson, 1991; Swanson & Sauter, 1993; Swanson, Sauter, & Chapman, 1989). Many other design solutions must necessarily be workplace or situation specific (see bibliography).

Reducing Physical and Reproductive Risks

Control measures and methods have been developed for limiting or preventing exposures to physical, biologic, and chemical hazards in the workplace. These methods vary, depending on the type of work being performed and the exposure. They can include installation of local and general ventilation systems, use of shower and change rooms, personal monitoring for exposure (eg, to radiation), use of personal protective equipment, and changes in work practices (Quinn & Woskie, 1988). All chemicals used in the workplace should be carefully labeled, and documentation regarding the nature of these chemicals should be readily available to the workers. Physicians should obtain an occupational history of women who are pregnant, or who are contemplating pregnancy, to ensure that exposure to reproductive hazards that may compromise the pregnancy is not occurring. Relevant clinical information and occupational history questionnaires are presented by Hunt and Smith (1982). For further information, see the bibliography.

Sex Discrimination and Sexual Harassment

Litigation has often been used by victims of sex discrimination and sexual harassment to seek redress for their injuries. However, primary prevention strategies should be emphasized in ensuring the fair and equal treatment of all members of the work force. Such strategies focus on organizational changes in practices and policies toward female employees. For example, organizations need formal policies against sex discrimination and sexual harassment that are clearly articulated, easily accessible to employees, and reliably enforced. A formal set of grievance procedures must also be developed. In addition, education and training of employees and managers, and, in the case of sexual harassment, appointment of a sexual harassment information officer, may help to deter discriminatory behavior (eg, Bernstein, 1994; Fitzgerald, 1993; Goldsmith Kasinsky, 1992; McKinney, 1994). Organizational strategies to prevent sex discrimination can also include affirmative action programs, pro-family policies, and subsidized child care for needy working families (Fitzgerald, 1993). (For several examples of organizational programs benefiting working families, see Friedman and Galinsky [1992].)

Bernstein (1994) has argued that American organizations can learn a valuable lesson about combating sexual harassment from the experience of their European counterparts. In European countries, sexual harassment is conceptualized not as an actionable civil rights violation, but as an occupational health issue. The goal of redressing sexual harassment under such a system is cessation of the offending behavior, rather than litigation. Thus, inhouse, informal resolution strategies involving confrontation of the offender are popular and encouraged. Typically, the victim of harassment confronts the offender directly, in the presence of a third party, or the offender is confronted indirectly via an intermediary.

Bernstein (1994) urges organizations to begin treating sexual harassment as a workplace hazard and take proactive steps to safeguard employee health, rather than waiting for harm to be inflicted to address the problem. Clearly, an organization that protects its employees also protects itself. A business that seeks to eradicate sexual harassment preserves valuable resources and avoids the costly damages and loss of reputation associated with litigation.

Preventing Workplace Violence

Recommendations for preventing workplace homicides center around changing the physical work environment, work practices, or personnel policies. These include improving the visibility of the work area to the outside, installing external lighting, keeping limited amounts of cash on hand, installing silent alarms and surveillance cameras, providing bullet-proof barriers or enclosures, increasing number of staff on duty, and training in conflict resolution and nonviolent response (NIOSH, 1993).

The motives for nonfatal workplace violence have not been clearly established, and preventive practices and policies have not been empirically tested. There are hints that organizational factors and workplace stressors may exacerbate nonfatal workplace violence. Work by Chen and Spector (1992) indicates a linkage between workplace stressors (eg, role conflict, interpersonal conflict) and aggression and sabotage at work. Chen and Spector (1992) postulated that frustration resulting from factors (ie, stressors) that interfere with the accomplishment of work goals is the mediating variable between job stress and workplace aggression. Northwestern National Life (1993) data indicated that workplaces with greater work group harmony, higher levels of employee control and autonomy, and more coworker and supervisor support had lower rates of workplace violence. Further inferential analyses of these data have indicated that both structural and environmental variables (eg, money handling, working at night) and workplace climate and stress variables (eg, work group harmony, coworker and supervisor support) were linked with threats, harassment, and fear of becoming a victim of violence. Most interesting, however, is that the work climate and stress factors tended to be more predictive of violence than the structural variables (Cole, Grubb, Sauter, Swanson, & Lawless, 1995).

Much more work needs to be done to determine the causes and characteristics of nonfatal workplace violence and the best preventive measures. General, although untested, prevention recommendations from Northwestern National Life (1993) include the following:

- fostering a supportive, harmonious work environment
- providing training in conflict resolution
- developing effective harassment, grievance, and security programs
- providing counseling services for employees
- setting up a crisis plan for dealing with violent incidents

Recommendations for promoting safety in health care settings involve the identification of security hazards and engineering administrative and work practice controls for these hazards. The California Department of Industrial Relations (1994) recently published a set of guidelines for preventing violence among health care workers, and similar recommendations were published by the British Health and Safety Executive in 1987 (Health Services Advisory Committee, 1987). With respect to dealing with the aftermath of a violent episode in the workplace (ie, violence-induced trauma), guidelines for assessing the scope of the problem and determining appropriate responses have been published by White and Hatcher (1988).

Conclusions

The continued influx of women into the work force and the unique job hazards faced by women point to the increasing importance of women's occupational health issues. Unfortunately, research to date on women's occupational safety and health has largely focused on a narrow aspect of this issue (ie, reproductive and maternal health concerns). With regard to other areas of occupational safety and health the male experience at work has often been considered to be representative of the female work experience. Although in many cases this assumption is valid, in other cases it can be inaccurate and may lead to workplace designs and practices that compromise the working woman's health and safety. Additionally, few men experience two work hazards that a large number of working women face, namely, gender discrimination and sexual harassment. Future research should be aimed at exploring the female experience at work. Such attention can significantly improve working conditions for women.

References

Bachman, R. (1994). Violence and theft in the workplace. *Crime data brief*. Washington, DC: U.S. Department of Justice.

Barnett, R. C., & Baruch, G. K. (1987). Social roles, gender, and psychological distress. In R. Barnett, L. Biener, & G. Baruch (Eds.), *Gender and stress*. New York: Free Press.

Barnett, R. C., & Baruch, G. K. (1985). Women's involvement in multiple roles and psychological distress. *Journal of Personality and Social Psychology, 49,* 135-145.

Beckett, W. S., Pope, C. A., Xu, X. P., & Christiani, D. C. (1994). Women's respiratory health in the cotton textile industry: An analysis of respiratory symptoms in 973 non-smoking female workers. *Occupational and Environmental Medicine, 51,* 14-18.

Beckman, L. J. (1978). The relative rewards and costs of parenthood and employment for employed women. *Psychology of Women Quarterly, 2,* 215-234.

Bell, C. A. (1991). Female homicides in United States workplaces, 1980–1985. *American Journal of Public Health, 81,* 729-732.

Bernstein, A. (1994). Law, culture, and harassment. *University of Pennsylvania Law Review, 142* (4), 1227-1311.

Brisson, C., Vezina, M., & Vinet, A. (1992). Health problems of women employed in jobs involving psychological and ergonomic stressors: The case of garment workers in Quebec. *Women and Health, 18,* 49-65.

Brushwood, D. B. (1991). Women of childbearing capacity may not be excluded from working with hazardous substances because of their gender. *American Journal of Hospital Pharmacy, 48,* 1281-1283.

Bureau of Labor Statistics. (1994). Violence in the workplace comes under closer scrutiny. *Issues in labor statistics* (Summary 94-10). Washington, DC: Author.

Bursten, B. (1986). Psychiatric injury in women's workplaces. *Bulletin of the American Academy of Psychiatry and Law, 14,* 245-251.

California Department of Industrial Relations. (1994). *Guidelines for security and safety of health care and community service workers.* Los Angeles: Department of Industrial Relations, Division of Occupational Safety and Health, Medical Unit.

Chen, P. Y., & Spector, P. E. (1992). Relationships of work stressors with aggression, withdrawal, theft and substance use: An exploratory study. *Journal of Occupational and Organizational Psychology, 65,* 177-184.

Chester, N. L., & Grossman, H. Y. (1990). Introduction: Learning about women and their work through their own accounts. In H. Y. Grossman & N. L. Chester (Eds.), *The experience and meaning of work in women's lives* (pp. 1-9). Hillsdale, NJ: Erlbaum.

Cole, L. L., Grubb, P. L., Sauter, S. L., Swanson, N. G., & Lawless, P. (1995, September 13-16). Predictors of non-fatal workplace violence. Paper presented at *Work, Stress and Health '95: Creating Healthier Workplaces*, Washington, DC.

Colligan, M. J., Smith, M. J., & Hurrell, J. J., Jr. (1977). Occupational incidence rates of mental health disorders. *Journal of Human Stress, 3,* 34-39.

Copplestone, J. F., & Kaplan, J. (1972). *Encyclopedia of occupational health and safety.* Geneva, Switzerland: International Labour Office.

Cox, S., Cox, T., & Steventon, J. (1984). Women at work: Summary and overview. *Ergonomics, 27,* 597-605.

Cox, S., Cox, T., Thirlaway, M., & MacKay, C. (1982). Effects of simulated repetitive work on urinary catecholamine excretion. *Ergonomics, 25,* 1129-1141.

Cox, T. (1980). Repetitive work. In C. L. Cooper & R. Payne (Eds.), *Current concerns in occupational stress.* Chichester: Wiley.

Crowley, J. E., Levitin, T. E., & Quinn, R. P. (1981). Seven deadly half-truths about women. In J. O'Toole, J. L. Scheiber, & L. C. Wood (Eds.), *Working changes and choices.* New York: Human Sciences Press.

Eaton, W. W., Anthony, J. C., Mandel, W., & Garrison, R. (1990). Occupations and the prevalence of major depressive disorder. *Journal of Occupational Medicine, 32,* 1079-1087.

Eskenazi, B., Guendelman, S., & Elkin, E. P. (1993). A preliminary study of reproductive outcomes of female maquiladora workers in Tijuana, Mexico. *American Journal of Industrial Medicine, 24,* 667-676.

Evanoff, B. A., & Rosenstock, L. (1986). Reproductive hazards in the workplace: A case study of women firefighters. *American Journal of Industrial Medicine, 9,* 503-515.

Fingerland, A. (1982). Lung cancer in women and its relation to occupation. *Studia Pneumologica Et Phtiseologica Cechoslovaca, 42,* 462-467.

Fitzgerald, L. F. (1993). Sexual harassment: Violence against women in the workplace. *American Psychologist, 48,* 1070-1076.

Friedman, D. E., & Galinsky, E. (1992). Work and family issues: A legitimate business concern. In S. Zedeck (Ed.), *Work, families, and organizations* (pp. 168-207). San Francisco: Jossey-Bass.

Fullerton, H. N., Jr. (1993, November). Another look at the labor force. *Monthly Labor Review*, 31-39.

Galinsky, E., Bond, J. T., & Friedman, D. E. (1993). *The changing workforce: Highlights of the national study.* New York: Families and Work Institute.

Gardell, B. (1971). Alienation and mental health in the modern industrial environment. In L. Levi (Ed.), *Society, stress and disease: Vol. 1. The psychosocial environment and psychosomatic diseases*. London: Oxford University Press.

Gerhardsson, I., & Ahlmark, A. (1985). Silicosis in women. *Journal of Occupational Medicine, 27,* 347-350.

Goldsmith Kasinsky, R. (1992). Sexual harassment: A health hazard for women workers. *New Solutions*, 74-83.

Grandjean, E. (1987). *Ergonomics in computerized offices*. New York: Taylor & Francis.

Grandjean, E. (1986). *Fitting the task to the man*. London: Taylor & Francis.

Grant, K. A., Habes, D. J., & Baron, S. L. (1994). An ergonomics evaluation of cashier work activities at checker-unload workstations. *Applied Ergonomics, 25,* 310-318.

Gutek, B. (1985). *Sex and the workplace*. San Francisco: Jossey-Bass.

Hansen, K. S. (1983). Occupational dermatoses in hospital cleaning women. *Contact Dermatitis, 9,* 343-351.

Hayne, C. R. (1981). Manual transport of loads by women. *Physiotherapy, 67,* 226-231.

Health Services Advisory Committee. (1987). *Violence to staff in the health services*. London: Health and Safety Executive.

Herzberg, F. (1966). *Work and the nature of man*. Cleveland, OH: World.

Huel, G., Mergler, D., & Bowler, R. (1990). Evidence for adverse reproductive outcomes among women microelectronic assembly workers. *British Journal of Industrial Medicine, 47,* 400-404.

Huel, G., Everson, R. B., & Menger, I. (1984). Increased hair cadmium in newborns of women occupationally exposed to heavy metals. *Environmental Research, 35,* 115-121.

Hunt, V. R., & Smith, D. M. (1982). The health of working women. In M. H. Alderman & M. J. Hanley (Eds.), *Clinical medicine for the occupational physician*. New York: Marcel Dekker.

Jagacinski, C. M., LeBold, W. K., & Linden, K. W. (1987). The relative career advancement of men and women engineers in the United States. *Work and Stress, 1,* 235-247.

Jennings, S., Mazaik, C., & McKinlay, S. (1984). Women and work: An investigation of the association between health and employment status in middle-aged women. *Social Science and Medicine, 19,* 423-431.

Johnson, E. S., Fischman, H. R., Matanoski, G. M., & Diamond, E. (1986). Occurrence of cancer in women in the meat industry. *British Journal of Industrial Medicine, 43,* 597-604.

Kilburn, K. H., Warshaw, R., & Thornton, J. C. (1989). Pulmonary function in histology technicians compared with women from Michigan: Effects of chronic low dose formaldehyde on a national sample of women. *British Journal of Industrial Medicine, 46,* 468-472.

Kouach, K. A. (1981). Implicit stereotyping in personnel decisions. *Personnel Journal, 60,* 716-722.

LaCroix, A. Z., & Haynes, S. G. (1987). Gender differences in the health effects of workplace roles. In R. C. Barnett, L. Biener, & G. K. Baruch (Eds.), *Gender and stress* (pp. 96-121). New York: Free Press.

Linn, M. W., Sandifer, R., & Stein, S. (1985). Effects of unemployment on mental and physical health. *American Journal of Public Health, 75,* 502-506.

Lipscomb, J. A., Fenster, L., Wrensch, M., Shusterman, D., & Swan, S. (1991). Pregnancy outcomes in women potentially exposed to occupational solvents and women working in the electronics industry. *Journal of Occupational Medicine, 33,* 597-604.

Lott, B. (1985). The devaluation of women's competence. *Journal of Social Issues, 41,* 43-60.

Lynge, E., & Thygesen, L. (1990). Primary liver cancer among women in laundry and dry-cleaning in Denmark. *Scandinavian Journal of Work, Environment and Health, 16,* 108-112.

Maeda, K. (1977). Occupational cervicobrachial disorder and its causative factors. *Journal of Human Ergology, 6,* 193-202.

Magora, A. (1970). Investigation of the relation between low back pain and occupation. *Industrial Medicine, 39,* 465-471.

Matzdorff, I. (1987). Women at work in workplaces designed for men: Anthropometry and ergonomics. *Work and Stress, 1,* 293-297.

McGregor, D. (1960). *The human side of enterprise*. New York: McGraw-Hill.

McKinney, K. (1994). Sexual harassment and college faculty members. *Deviant Behavior: An Interdisciplinary Journal, 15,* 171-191.

Metcalfe, B. A. (1987). Male and female managers: An analysis of biographical and self-concept data. *Work and Stress, 1,* 207-219.

Moore, R. M., Jr., Davis, Y. M., & Kaczmarek, R. G. (1993). An overview of occupational hazards among veterinarians, with particular reference to pregnant women. *American Industrial Hygiene Association Journal, 54,* 113-120.

Nakamura, C. Y., McCarthy, S. J., Rothstein-Fisch, C., & Winges, L. D. (1981). Interdependence of child-care resources and the progress of women in society. *Psychology of Women Quarterly, 6,* 26-40.

National Institute for Occupational Safety and Health. (1988). *Guidelines for protecting the safety and health of health care workers* (DHHS NIOSH Publication No. 88-119). Cincinnati, OH: Author.

National Institute for Occupational Safety and Health. (1992). *Health hazard evaluation report: US West Communications, Phoenix, Arizona, Minneapolis, Minnesota, Denver, Colorado* (NIOSH Report No. HETA 89-299-2230). Cincinnati, OH: Author.

National Institute for Occupational Safety and Health. (1993). *Preventing homicide in the workplace* (DHHS NIOSH Publication No. 93-109). Cincinnati, OH: Author.

Nilsson, E., & Back, O. (1986). The importance of anamnestic information of atopy, metal dermatitis and earlier hand eczema for the development of hand dermatitis in women in wet hospital work. *Acta Dermato-Venereologica, 66,* 45-50.

Northwestern National Life. (1993). *Fear and violence in the workplace.* Minneapolis: Author.

Piotrokowski, C. S., & Love, M. (1987). Quality of supervision and well-being of women workers. National Institute for Occupational Safety and Health Order No. 85-35692.

Poitrast, B. J. (1988). *Women in the workplace.* U.S. Air Force Occupational and Environmental Health Laboratory Report 88-130CO0111JCE.

Quinn, M. M., & Woskie, S. R. (1988). Women and work. In B. S. Levy & D. H. Wegman (Eds.), *Occupational health. Recognizing and preventing work-related disease* (2nd ed.). Boston: Little, Brown.

Redgrove, J. (1979). Fitting the job to the woman: A critical review. *Applied Ergonomics, 10,* 215-223.

Reskin, B. F., & Ross, C. E. (1992). Jobs, authority, and earnings among managers: The continuing significance of sex. *Work and Occupations, 19,* 342-365.

Saal, F. E., Johnson, C. B., & Weber, N. (1989). Friendly or sexy? It may depend on whom you ask. *Psychology of Women Quarterly, 13,* 263-276.

Saurel-Cubizolles, M. J., & Kaminski, M. (1987). Pregnant women's working conditions and their changes during pregnancy: A national study in France. *British Journal of Industrial Medicine, 44,* 236-243.

Sauter, S. L., Gottlieb, M. S., Jones, K. C., Dodson, V. N., & Rohrer, K. M. (1983). Job and health implications of VDT use: Initial results of the Wisconsin-NIOSH study. *Communications of the Association for Computing Machinery, 26,* 284-294.

Sauter, S. L., Murphy, L. R., & Hurrell, J. J., Jr. (1990). Prevention of work-related psychological disorders: A national strategy proposed by the National Institute for Occupational Safety and Health (NIOSH). *American Psychologist, 45,* 1146-1158.

Sauter, S. L., Schleifer, L. M., & Knutson, S. J. (1991). Work posture, workstation design, and musculoskeletal discomfort in a VDT data entry task. *Human Factors, 33,* 151-167.

Sauter, S. L., & Swanson, N. G. (1991, September 2-6). *Increased restbreaks yield increased productivity in repetitive VDT work.* Paper presented at the 35th annual meeting of the Human Factors Society, San Francisco.

Sauter, S. L., & Swanson, N. G. (1996). An ecological model of musculoskeletal disorders in office work. In S. Moon & S. L. Sauter (Eds.), *Beyond Biomechanics: Psychosocial factors and musculoskeletal disorders in office work.* New York: Taylor and Francis.

Schein, V. E., & Mueller, R. (1992). Sex role stereotyping and requisite management characteristics: A cross cultural look. *Journal of Organizational Behavior, 13,* 439-447.

Schroedel, J. R. (1990). Blue-collar women: Paying the price at home and on the job. In H. Y. Grossman & N. L. Chester (Eds.), *The experience and meaning of work in women's lives* (pp. 241-260). Hillsdale, NJ: Erlbaum.

Silverman, D. T., Levin, L. I., & Hoover, R. N. (1990). Occupational risks of bladder cancer among white women in the United States. *American Journal of Epidemiology, 132,* 453-461.

Silverman, D. T., McLaughlin, J. K., Malker, H. S. R., Weiner, J. A., & Ericsson, J. L. E. (1989). Bladder cancer and occupation among Swedish women. *American Journal of Industrial Medicine, 16,* 239-240.

Silverstein, L. B. (1991). Transforming the debate about child care and maternal employment. *American Psychologist, 46,* 1025-1032.

Silvestri, G. T. (1993, November). Occupational employment: Wide variation in growth. *Monthly Labor Review,* 58-86.

Sorenson, G., & Verbrugge, L. M. (1987). Women, work and health. *Annual Review of Public Health, 8,* 235-251.

Stellman, J. M., & Stellman, S. D. (1983, November). Occupational lung disease and cancer risk in women. *Occupational Health Nursing,* 40-46.

Swanson, N. G., & Sauter, S. L. (1993). The effects of exercise on the health and performance of data entry operators. In H. Luczak, A. Cakir, & G. Cakir (Eds.), *Work with display units 92.* Amsterdam: Elsevier.

Swanson, N. G., Sauter, S. L., & Chapman, L. J. (1989). The design of restbreaks for video display terminal work: A review of the relevant literature. In A. Mital (Ed.), *Advances in industrial ergonomics and safety I.* London: Taylor & Francis.

Vandervort, R., & Brooks, S. M. (1977). Polyvinyl chloride film thermal decomposition products as an occupational illness. *Journal of Occupational Medicine, 19,* 188-191.

Warren, B. (1982). *Hazards to women in the workplace.* National Technical Information Service Report No. HRP-0906079.

Wu-Williams, A. H., Blot, W. J., Dai, X. D., Louie, R., Xiao, H. P., Stone, B. J., Sun, X. W., Yu, S. F., Feng, Y. P., Fraumeni, J. F., Jr., & Henderson, B. E. (1993). Occupation and lung cancer risk among women in Northern China. *American Journal of Industrial Medicine, 24,* 67-79.

White, S. G., & Hatcher, C. (1988). Violence and trauma response. *Occupational Medicine: State of the Art Reviews, 3,* 677-694.

World Health Organization. (1987). *Visual display terminals and worker's health.* Geneva, Switzerland: Author.

Wysocki, L. M., & Ossler, C. (1983). Women, work and health: Issues of importance to the occupational health nurse. *Occupational Health Nursing, 31,* 18-23.

Zahm, S. H., Weisenburger, D. D., Saal, R. C., Vaught, J. B., Babbitt, P. A., & Blair, A. (1993). The role of agricultural pesticide use in the development of non-Hodgkin's lymphoma in women. *Archives of Environmental Health, 48,* 353-358.

Bibliography

Stress

Hurrell, J. J., Jr., Murphy, L. R., Sauter, S. L., & Cooper, C. L. (1988). *Occupational stress: Issues and developments in research.* New York: Taylor & Francis.

National Institute for Occupational Safety and Health. (1987). An overview of organizational stress and health. In L. R. Murphy & T. F. Schoenborn (Eds.), *Stress management in work settings* (DHHS NIOSH Publication No. 87-111). Cincinnati, OH: Author.

(1988). *Controlling work stress: Effective human resource and management strategies.* San Francisco: Jossey-Bass.

Ergonomics

Ayoub, M. M., & Mital, A. (1989). *Manual materials handling.* London: Taylor & Francis.

Eastman Kodak Company. (1986). *Ergonomic design for people at work* (Vols. 1-2). New York: Van Nostrand Reinhold.

Sauter, S., Dainoff, M., & Smith, M. (1990). *Promoting health and productivity in the computerized office: Models of successful ergonomic interventions.* New York: Taylor & Francis.

Waters, T. R., Putz-Anderson, V., & Garg, A. (1994) *Applications manual for the revised NIOSH lifting equation.* Cincinnati, OH: National Institute for Occupational Safety and Health.

Physical and Reproductive Hazards

Council on Scientific Affairs. (1985). Effects of toxic chemicals on the reproductive system. *Journal of the American Medical Association, 253,* 3431-3437.

Himminki, K. (1980). Occupational chemicals tested for teratogenicity. *International Archives of Occupational and Environmental Health, 47,* 191-207.

Jaffery, F. N., & Viswanathan, P. N. (1986). Women workers as specific high risk group in occupational and environmental toxicology. *Journal of Scientific and Industrial Research, 45,* 109-118.

Lidstrom, I. (1990). Pregnant women in the workplace. *Seminars in Perinatology, 14,* 329-333.

Office of Technology Assessment. (1985). *Reproductive hazards in the workplace.* Washington, DC: Author.

Women's Bureau. (1993). *1993 handbook on women workers: Trends & issues.* Washington, DC: U.S. Department of Labor.

INDEX

NOTE: A *t* following a page number indicates a table; an *f* following a page number indicates a figure; and a *d* following a page number indicates a display. Drugs are listed under their generic names. When a drug trade name is listed, the reader is referred to the generic name.